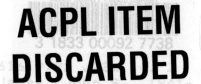

# AIDS TREATMENT NEWS

## VOLUME 2

Issues 76 through 125

April 1989 through April 1991

_____

JOHN S. JAMES

_____

with

Denny Smith, Michelle Roland, and Laura Thomas

Introduction by Paul Reed

## CELESTIALARTS

_Berkeley, California_

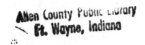
*The publisher assumes no liability for any injuries sustained in conjunction with use of any therapy, substance, protocol, or treatment described in this book. Individuals are cautioned that this material appears for informational use only, and the publisher advises that individuals seek professional medical counsel regarding any therapy described in this book.*

*Cover design by Nancy Austin*
*Text design by Nancy Austin and Jeff Brandenburg*
*Composition by ImageComp, San Francisco*
*Index by Ed Serdziak*
*Production by Mary Ann Anderson*

FIRST PRINTING 1991

Library of Congress Cataloging-in-Publication Data

James, John S., 1941–
    AIDS treatment news.

    Includes bibliographies references and indexes.
    Contents: v. 1. Issues 1 through 75, April 1986 through March 1989 — v. 2. Issues 76 through 125, April 1989 through April 1991.
    1. AIDS (Disease)—Treatment.   2. AIDS (Disease)—Alternative treatment.   I. Title.
RC607.A26J35   1989      616.97'9206      89-7399
ISBN 0-89087-553-7 (v. 1)
ISBN 0-89087-614-2 (v. 2)

1      2      3      4      5      /      95      94      93      92      91

# CONTENTS

# INTRODUCTION

Hope for AIDS treatment has always lain in experimental therapies, for no existing conventional or alternative therapies have consistently arrested the progression of the human immunodeficienty virus (HIV). Since 1986, John S. James has reported on the expanding field of AIDS treatment research, consistently bringing to public attention therapies that are promising and often neglected or controversial. Patients, scientists, doctors, medical personnel, and journalists have learned to rely on AIDS Treatment News for groundbreaking coverage of new treatments.

This twice-monthly newsletter grew out of the grassroots response to the AIDS epidemic. When institutional responses were painfully lagging, James dug in the trenches and started the work that needed to be done — finding out what was out there that could help save people's lives, and commenting on the public policy issues that needed to change in order to deliver life-saving therapies to people with AIDS, ARC, and HIV disease.

His work was an historical step in the community response to AIDS. The politics of AIDS, coupled with the immense sluggishness of scientific and medical institutions, often leave the HIV patient in the uncomfortable situation of having nowhere to turn for help. For this reason, the AIDS community has done the work itself, from the early days of New York's Gay Men's Health Crisis and San Francisco's Kaposi's Sarcoma Foundation through the magnificently empowering strategies of Project Inform and the dazzling power of AIDS activist organizations, most notably the AIDS Coalition to Unleash Power (ACT UP).

And the community continues to do the work itself. For more than a decade, the unfortunate reality of AIDS has remained the same: We must save our own lives. Some progress has been made in forcing our medical and governmental institutions to do their job — to save lives and to safeguard the public health — yet therapies and medications — many potentially close to a cure — remain untested, sitting on shelves in pharmaceutical research units, backlogged and clogged up by bureaucratic red tape, commercial disincentives, legislative lethargy, and the near-criminal lack of national leadership.

Now, more than five years after the first issue of AIDS Treatment News appeared, the need is greater than ever. The World Health Organization has estimated that by the end of this century, twenty-five million to thirty-million people will have been infected with the AIDS virus. While significant progress has been made in treating the many opportunistic infections associated with HIV disease, the immune dysregulation wreaked by HIV infection has yet to be effectively treated.

Again: We must save our own lives. To do that, we must educate ourselves about the disease, about its treatment, about its potential cure, and about the roadblocks that prevent rapid progress in the field. We must take what knowledge we gain and convert it to practical use, taking our health care into our own hands, seeing that our doctors adequately monitor us, insisting on treatments that may save our lives despite their unpopularity, neglect, or controversy.

And we must inform each other. That HIV patients go without treatment and prophylaxis, still developing such largely preventable infections as pneumocystis pneumonia, is testimony to the public education effort yet required. AIDS Treatment News is one such organ of education, allowing patients and doctors alike to know, as soon as possible, about advances in the treatment of AIDS.

This volume represents the most definitive resource on the comprehensive treatment of HIV disease and its ramifications. It is not to be read from start to finish, as though it were a novel (though such a reading illuminates the devastation of the epidemic in a startling way). Rather, it is best used as a reference text — using the index to locate symptoms, infections, medications, or other topics of interest to the reader.

Please bear in mind that no treatment should be undertaken in the absence of reliable care by a health care practitioner. AIDS Treatment News contains information on many promising and experimental treatments, but these should only be undertaken in conjunction with sound health care.

By remaining active, by seeking aggressive treatment against AIDS and its infections, by pressuring our institutions to be responsible to their duties, and by keeping ourselves informed, we can extend good health, improve quality of life, and save lives. The work is urgent.

—PAUL REED
*October 1991*
*San Francisco*

# Issue Number 76
# March 24, 1989

## HPMPC: POSSIBLE CMV (CYTOMEGALOVIRUS) TREATMENT

A major struggle continues over access to ganciclovir (DHPG) and foscarnet, the only accepted treatments for CMV retinitis, which can cause blindness in persons with AIDS—or with serious immune deficiencies from other causes, such as medications given to organ-transplant recipients. (For more information, see *AIDS Treatment News* # 71). CMV can also infect many other organs. Some experts believe it is the most common cause of death in persons with AIDS (Snoeck and others, 1989).

Both ganciclovir and foscarnet, however, have important drawbacks. Therefore the AIDS community should also know about HPMPC (also called "(S)-HPMPC"), a chemical developed by Belgian researchers, which appears in test-tube studies to be much more active then either ganciclovir or foscarnet against CMV. While HPMPC has not yet been given to humans and therefore is not an immediate treatment option, community awareness, investigation, and involvement may be necessary to make sure that it is not lost by lack of followup before clinical trials, or in the usual five-year to eight-year "drugjam" of new treatments going through clinical trials for U. S. approval.

HPMPC is also effective against some other viruses, including herpes simplex. It may be part of a new class of broad spectrum antivirals.

A major article on HPMPC was published last December in *Antimicrobial Agents and Chemotherapy* (Snoeck and others, 1988). These are the major points from that article:

• The scientists measured an "inhibitory index," the ratio of the drug concentration which inhibited cell growth by 50 percent to the concentration which inhibited the virus by 50 percent. This ratio provides an early indication of the possible usefulness of the drug. A large value suggests that there may be a wide margin between effective and toxic doses, increasing safety and also allowing physicians to increase doses when necessary without unacceptable toxicity.

In tests against CMV, the ratios for foscarnet, ganciclovir, HPMPA (a relative of HPMPC), and HPMPC were 14, 150, 200, and 1,500, respectively. (Using another strain of CMV, the ratios were 20, 200, 100, and 1,000.) These results suggest that HPMPC might have about ten times the range between effective and toxic doses as ganciclovir—and even more when compared to foscarnet.

• HPMPC completely suppressed the growth of CMV at concentrations of 0.1 microgram per milliliter, about ten times lower than required for ganciclovir.

• Like ganciclovir, HPMPC suppressed CMV plaque formation when added two, 24, or 48 hours after infection. Both failed to do so when added after 72 hours. But the two differed in that HPMPC protected cells even after it had been removed from the culture, while ganciclovir did not.

• For those who are interested, the full chemical name of HPMPC is (S)-1-(3-Hydroxy-2-Phosphonylmethoxypropyl)Cytosine.

It is not known exactly how it works. In one experiment, several natural nucleosides were tested to see if they could inhibit the antiviral effect of HPMPC. None of them did.

• Based on their results, the researchers suggested testing HPMPC in animals as a CMV treatment. They pointed out that appropriate "animal models" for CMV infection are available — for example, the mouse or guinea pig.

• All funding for the above research was from institutions in Belgium. The researchers synthesized their own HPMPC, by a procedure outlined in the article. We do not know of any pharmaceutical company involved in this work, although Bristol-Myers researchers have also published a paper on synthesis of HPMPC (Webb and others, 1988).

## Comment

We suggest that the AIDS community follow HPMPC, and become familiar with its current status and future prospects. Are there any financial or other obstacles to further research, which community awareness could help to overcome? It would be inexcusable for this drug to take the usual five to eight years or more to become available in the United States.

Except for red tape, enough preliminary testing could be completed in a few weeks or months. Volunteers for whom nothing else works would be willing to try the drug, after brief tests in animals. Only cultural inertia stands in the way—in particular, the unwillingness to respond to AIDS as an emergency, instead of business as usual.

## REFERENCES

De Clercq E., Holy, A., Rosenberg I., Sakuma T., Balzarini J., and Maudgal P. C. A novel selective broad-spectrum anti-DNA virus agent. *Nature* volume 323 number 2, pages 464-467, October 1986.

De Clercq E., Sakuma T., Baha M., Pauwels R., Balzarini J., Rosenberg I., and Holy, A. Antiviral activity of phosphonylmethoxyalkyl derivitives of purine and pyrimidines. *Antiviral Research* number 8, pages 261-272, 1987.

Snoeck R., Sakuma T., De Clercq E., Rosenberg I., and Holy, A. (S)-1-(3-Hydroxy-2-Phosphonylmethoxypropyl)Cytosine, a Potent and Selective Inhibitor of Human Cytomegalovirus Replication. *Antimicrobial Agents and Chemotherapy* volume 32 number 12, pages 1839-1844, December 1988.

Webb R. R. II, Wos J. A., Bronson J. J., and Martin J. C. Synthesis of S-N-1-3 Hydroxyl-2-Phosphonylmethoxypropylcytosine S-HPMPC. *Tetrahedron Lett.* 29 (43) pages 5475-5478, 1988.

# DEXTRAN SULFATE: CONFUSION CONTINUES

During the past year dextran sulfate has become one of the most widely used "underground" HIV treatments—based on laboratory tests showing that the drug stopped HIV in the test tube, plus the fact that oral dextran sulfate has been used for other purposes for 20 years in Japan, where it is available without a prescription. (For background, see *AIDS Treatment News* #50.)

But despite the widespread use in Japan, there have long been questions of whether dextran sulfate is absorbed from the intestines into the bloodstream well enough to be effective.

Recently, new data has increased these doubts about the "bioavailability" of the drug. The new information has been widely reported in the press, beginning with a story in the February 19 *Los Angeles Times*. But experts disagree on how certain or conclusive the new data is.

At least until recently it has not been possible to measure dextran sulfate levels in the bloodstream. So at first an indirect test was used. Six people took 1800 mg each of the drug, and then were given before and after measures of a blood clotting parameter known to be affected by dextran sulfate. Later, a direct chemical test was devised. Both studies concluded that less than one percent of dextran sulfate taken orally was absorbed into the bloodstream.

All seem to agree that these findings cast doubt on dextran sulfate. But questions remain. Was a single dose of 1800 mg enough for the test? Could even a small amount absorbed be of some benefit—especially if combined with AZT or other drugs? Is the new blood-level test accurate? Could the Japanese have been taking a useless drug for 20 years and not noticed? How do we explain the apparent benefit seen in some of the data collected by physicians whose patients are using dextran sulfate? And even if the drug is not absorbed into the bloodstream, might it still benefit some people by treating HIV infection in the intestinal lining itself, by direct contact?

At this time, the case for oral dextran sulfate seems weak. But confusion remains because solid answers are not yet available. We hope that the clinical trials now in progress will be completed so that physicians can answer the bottom-line question: Does the drug help patients?

There has been some controversy about the early release of preliminary information on dextran sulfate absorption, before formal publication. We think it was right to tell people early. Final analysis and publication of the results may take months—and meanwhile thousands of people are making vital decisions about their health care. They need the best information available. We hope that this controversy does not deter other scientists and officials from releasing unpublished results when there is an urgent need to do so.

For more information, see: the *Los Angeles Times*, February 19, 1989 (home edition), page 1; statement by Martin Delaney of Project Inform, to be published in *PI Perspectives* this month (415/558-9051 to be added to Project Inform's mailing list); and an investigative article by Tim Kingston to be published in *Coming Up!* newspaper in San Francisco, April 1989.

## PHYSICIANS: FDA SEEKS GANCICLOVIR INFORMATION (DEADLINE APRIL 21)

On May 2, the FDA's Anti-Infective Drugs Advisory Committee will review the status of ganciclovir—a review which could lead to approval of the drug. Health-care providers with summaries of data or other clinical information about ganciclovir should contact the Committee preferably by April 10; however information will be accepted as late at April 21.

If you have any information which might be useful, please contact Tom Nightingale, the executive secretary of the Anti-Infective Drugs Advisory Committee, at 301/443-5455. Send summaries as soon as possible to him at the Center for Drug Evaluation and Research (HFD-9), Food and Drug Administration, 5600 Fisher Lane, Rockville, MD 20857. Ophthalmologists are encouraged to address the Committee; anyone who wants to present data must call ahead of time. The meeting is open to the public, but seating is limited so attendees must preregister to assure access.

## SAN FRANCISCO: WEIGHT LOSS/MEGACE STUDY

The San Francisco County Community Consortium is currently recruiting patients for a phase III study of megestrol acetate (Megace), a drug which may be useful in reversing HIV-related wasting syndrome (cachexia). Marked weight loss is a serious problem for some people with HIV disease. It can further impair an immune system already damaged by the virus, resulting in an increased susceptibility to opportunistic infections.

The rationale for this study is based on observations from another study conducted at the University of Maryland which found that 28 of 30 patients being treated for breast cancer with Megace experienced increased appetite and weight gain. Although this side effect was beneficial for the patients, it was also unexpected, so that important nutritional data was not collected.

The trial, conducted by Consortium physicians through their private practices, is one of the first community-based trials in the greater Bay Area. The trial seeks to determine if the weight gain associated with Megace is comprised of protein or fat, or merely water retention, and what relationship there is between immune status and general or specific nutritional status. This is a placebo-controlled study, but it is also a "cross-over" study, which means that halfway through (after eight weeks), the treatment/placebo arms will be switched, so that by the end of the study everyone will have received active drug.

Note that Megace is a prescription drug; if someone is now seriously anorectic, they could discuss the immediate use of Megace with their physician. Last December, *AIDS Treatment News* #71 reported on the good results with Megace for AIDS-related cachexia published in the November 15, 1988 issue of *Annals of Internal Medicine.*

We were assured that participants will be closely monitored by physicians, nurses and nutritionists to watch for any weight loss severe enough to warrant withdrawal from the study. Megace and all laboratory tests required by the study are provided free of charge. In addition, all patients will receive monthly feedback on their nutritional status by a registered dietitian.

Eligibility criteria for the study include either asymptomatic HIV infection or ARC and a documented loss of at least 5% of usual body weight. Persons with AIDS-defining diagnoses are excluded.

## OPINION SURVEY ON U. S. DRUG-APPROVAL PROCESS: STUDY SEEKS VOLUNTEERS

Persons with AIDS or ARC or who are HIV-positive can participate in a survey of attitudes and opinions toward the FDA and the new-drug approval process in the United States.

This study began as an undergraduate project by Kenneth James and Ira Nydick at Worcester Polytechnic Institute, Worcester, MA, but it has gone well beyond the usual student project. Assistance is being provided by the AIDS Center at the University of California Los Angeles, where most of the research will be conducted. AIDS organizations which assist in the study will receive a copy of the results.

# Issue Number 77
# April 21, 1989

## ABOUT THIS ISSUE

*AIDS Treatment News* skipped its scheduled April 7 publication; the last published issue was #76, dated March 24.

We never cancel an issue because of lack of news to report. At this time there is more news than ever, more than we can keep up with. We skipped the last issue because of the unusual difficulty of integrating and making sense of what is going on at the present time.

Today we have the best news ever on treatment developments. But the human and organizational failures in both the medical-research establishment and the AIDS community itself are so profound that it is hard to see how the potential advances now in view will get to the persons who need them, except through grassroots or underground movements.

These human and organizational failures are not new; they have been pervasive since the beginning of the epidemic. But today's improved prospects for treatment development are greatly increasing the cost in human life of squandered opportunities and institutional bankruptcy.

In "The Drug-Trials Debacle" (below) we provide a simple mathematical model supporting a conservative estimate of fifty thousand *unnecessary* deaths over the next several years—barring policy changes or lucky developments, such as a much better treatment becoming available underground. We show that behind the flimsiest fig leaf, provided as a service for those who prefer denial, the research establishment has written off people with AIDS. Besides the remarkable lack of urgency, we propose that the crux of the problem is a scientific and medical issue, in which the research establishment is correct in its own terms, but wrong in its choice of terms. We show that the refusal to accept the fact that patients and physicians must and do make decisions under uncertainty—and the narrow insistence that all drug-treatment research be geared to developing statistical proof of safety and efficacy—has inadvertently turned the commendable effort to develop a more proven, scientifically-based medicine into a gruesome public disservice.

We will suggest practical ways, through coalition building and through community-based research, for bringing the real issues of AIDS research into the light of day where they can be discussed and decided on their merits.

The interview with friends of Terry Sutton, a San Francisco treatment activist who died this month, brings a human and spiritual perspective to the issues of drug access and clinical trials, and of the AIDS community's slowness to face these issues and insist that deficiencies be corrected.

# COMPOUND Q (GLQ223)

In the last few weeks a potential AIDS treatment, so far tested only in the laboratory, has generated enormous public and scientific interest. We have followed compound Q (also called GLQ223) and do agree that it is important (we listed it as one of eight treatments to watch in 1989, in our January 13 issue). But we are not yet ready with an in-depth report. Instead, this note will refer readers to authoritative, accessible published information—and also include cautions about use of a similar drug from China, should it become available.

The reason for the interest is that laboratory studies suggest that compound Q *might* kill infected macrophages, and eliminate this major reservoir of HIV from the body. No other treatment has been found to do so.

Two good, readily-available articles summarizing information on compound Q were published in *The New York Times*, April 18, 1989, Medical Sciences section, and *Business Week*, April 24, 1989, page 29.

For technical background, see the article by Michael S. McGrath and others, "GLQ223: An Inhibitor of Human Immunodeficiency Virus Replication in Acutely and Chronically Infected Cells of Lymphocyte and Mononuclear Phagocyte Lineage," *Proceedings of the National Academy of Sciences, USA*, April 15, 1989. Also see the United States Patent, number 4,795,739, date of patent January 3, 1989.

The active ingredient in compound Q is a protein called trichosanthin, which is extracted from the root of a Chinese cucumber, *Trichosanthes kirilowii*. It must be given by injection. This protein is also used in China to induce abortions, and to treat ectopic pregnancy, hydatidiform moles, and one particular kind of cancer, choriocarcinoma. (For an overview of the Chinese medicinal use of trichosanthin, see Yu Wang and others, "Scientific Evaluation of Tian Hua Fen (THF)—History, Chemistry, and Application," *Pure and Applied Chemistry*, volume 58, number 5, pages 789-798, 1986. "Tian Hua Fen" is the name of the herbal preparation from which trichosanthin, the active ingredient, can be extracted.)

**Injecting impure preparations of the protein could cause fatal side effects.** In China there are three different grades of trichosanthin prepared for injection: crude extract, purified extract, and crystallized, which is the highest purity. Only the crystallized form can be used safely; the others cause severe side effects. (Animal tests cited by Wang and others, reference above, showed a lethal dose to be only three times higher than the effective dose for the least pure grade, only six times for the intermediate, so-called "pure" grade, but over 75 times higher than the effective dose for the purest, crystallized grade.) Fortunately it is fairly easy to test for impurities, using a standard chemical technique called gel chromatography, so it should be straightforward to test that a drug claimed to be the "crystallized" grade really is.

We have heard that side effects (of the Chinese "crystallized" grade) can include fever, muscle weakness, and possible electrolyte imbalance, lasting 12 to 18 hours. These problems may not start for about 12 hours. Because of the possibility of electrolyte imbalance, the patient must be monitored by a physician, so that treatment can be given if necessary. Wang and others (reference above) mention 1,042 cases of human use of the crystallized grade, by intra-amniotic or intramuscular injection, in their paper published in 1986. They said there were no significant side effects; a low fever of 37.5 degrees occurred in 79 percent of the cases. (Since there are no side effects of compound Q in animals unless the dose is extremely high, the side effects of the Chinese crystallized version may result from some remaining impurities, or from the intended killing of target cells, which presumably would not occur in animal toxicity tests.)

There may be additional precautions. For example, repeated use could conceivably cause anaphylaxis, although no such problem has been seen in animal tests. We do not know if there is any Chinese experience with repeated use.

This drug may be dangerous, and must not be used without knowledgeable professional supervision.

A story widely reported in the press claims that six people in Florida used a Chinese version of compound Q, and had to be hospitalized due to side effects. We have heard serious doubts about the truth of this rumor, and have not been able to confirm it.

We plan to publish further reports on compound Q in future issues.

# HYPERICIN UPDATE

*AIDS Treatment News* reported about hypericin, a chemical in the St. John's wort plant which has shown antiretroviral activity in laboratory and animal tests, in issues number 75, 74, and 63. In the last two months, a number of people have started using commercially-available St. John's wort extracts which have been tested and found to contain significant amounts of hypericin. It is too early to be confident that the treatment is valuable, but the results continue to look good:

• Of the handful of people who were P24 antigen positive before starting hypericin, and had another P24 test after using it and reported the results to us, every one either became P24 negative, or had a greatly reduced antigen level. Some were using AZT in addition to hypericin, others were not using AZT. (Note: as we went to press we heard of two cases in which P24 antigen failed to improve after use of hypericin. We do not know how long it was used, or what dose.)

P24 antigen, a measure of HIV activity, only occasionally becomes negative without treatment. AZT is known to reduce its level.

• Almost everybody whose results have been reported to us has had at least one dramatic, unexpected improvement in symptoms within six weeks after starting hypericin (except of course for those who were asymptomatic, who had nothing to improve). However, many of them have also had other symptoms which failed to improve. These observations are based on fewer than 25 people and are far from conclusive

Our current impression from the few cases reported so far is that improvements might be *most* likely to be seen in increased energy level and reduced fatigue, neuropathy, certain cases of diarrhea but not other cases, weight loss, and (as already discussed) P24 antigen levels. T-cell counts seem to improve, very slowly if they start from very low values, more rapidly otherwise.

Dr. David Payne in Mesa, Arizona, who has the most experience with hypericin with 70 patients now using it, believes that improvements are *least* likely in symptoms which may be autoimmune, such as low platelet levels or certain skin rashes. We have also heard of other symptoms failing to improve (for example, one case of KS, and one case of diarrhea), but there are too few reports so far for a pattern to have developed.

• We have not heard of any case of a person believed to have been harmed by St. John's wort extracts. We have received one report of slightly increased sensitivity to sunlight, and several of drowsiness, especially with large doses.

*AIDS Treatment News* #75 reported one case of a patient taken off of hypericin extracts by his physician because his liver enzymes were found to be too high. Since then we have heard of another case of elevated liver enzymes; this patient was using many drugs, in addition to hypericin. There is no way to be sure whether or not the hypericin (St. John's wort extract) was responsible. However, Dr. Payne has found no evidence of any such problem in his 70 patients using hypericin, even though he has been looking for it.

As a precaution, we continue to urge that anyone using hypericin be monitored by a physician, with the monitoring including a blood-chemistry panel.

## Doses

There is still much uncertainty about the best dose and schedule for using hypericin.

Dr. Payne has increased his dose slightly, from 120 drops a day of the Hyperforat tincture to 160. (Some of his patients are using a different brand, Yerba Prima St. John's wort tablets, which is less expensive and easier to obtain in the United States.)

Because animal studies suggest that less frequent or intermittent doses might work better, some of Dr. Payne's patients are trying an intermittent schedule. They are taking two of the tablets every four hours on Monday and Tuesday only, and no hypericin during the rest of the week. (The four-hour schedule does *not* include the middle of the night, so the total dose comes to ten tablets each day, 20 total for the week. Hypericin is believed to be eliminated slowly from the body, so some will remain for several days or weeks.)

As more information about hypericin becomes available, we will report it.

## MEGACE CAUTION

Issue #76 of *AIDS Treatment News* announced recruitment for a study of Megace (megestrol acetate) through the San Francisco County Community Consortium. The goal of the trial is to determine whether Megace, a prescription drug used to treat breast cancer, also has the potential to enhance appetite and weight gain in people with ARC who are experiencing cachexia, or wasting syndrome.

James Kahn, M.D., the principal investigator of this study was notified earlier this month by the manufacturer, Bristol-Myers, that one participant in another Megace study had developed a severe rash covering most of his body after eight days of Megace, 1200 mg each day. The rash was later diagnosed as Stevens-Johnson Syndrome. It was treated with benadryl and steroids and resolved slowly. Because the participant had a diagnosis of AIDS and had been receiving other medications, there is not a conclusive link between the rash and Megace. Nevertheless, Dr. Kahn felt that we should caution people on Megace to be aware of any allergic reactions (which must be seen immediately by a physician).

## THE DRUG-TRIALS DEBACLE—AND WHAT TO DO ABOUT IT (PART I)

by John S. James

Today the news is better than ever on AIDS treatment developments. But even the good news cannot dispel a widespread despair that no matter what comes out of the laboratory, the treatments will not be tested rapidly, and will not become available to physicians and patients in time to prevent massive, unnecessary deaths.

One long-term survivor and treatment expert noted recently that almost nothing was being done to save lives. And a leading AIDS physician commented off the record that the research community had convinced itself it would take ten years to cure this disease, and that "they want to milk the grants and appropriations."

*AIDS Treatment News* has long criticized the treatment-research establishment for having written off those now ill with AIDS or HIV, and for the remarkable lack of urgency about saving lives. Recently we have had more contact than previously with this establishment, and we have found the situation even worse than we had realized. So entrenched and near-universal is the commitment to unworkable viewpoints, approaches, and programs, that in meetings and conversations we must temporarily suspend our own view of what is happening, and operate from the prevailing mindset in order to allow any communication to take place. **The real issues of how to save lives in this epidemic are so far removed from the conventional wisdom of the research and regulatory professionals, that if these issues are put forward in meetings, no dialog is possible.** Many professionals as individuals would want to challenge the prevailing ideas; but they have lacked a conceptual infrastructure that is developed enough to hold its own against the conventional views—views which *started with* the inevitable deaths of those now ill, accepted *a priori* without looking at facts or doing any analysis.

Here we will outline the real issues as we see them, and suggest analytical tools for bringing these issues out of their current limbo and into the light of day, where they can be considered openly and decided on their own merits.

In particular, this article will:

• Show that, barring a miracle, fifty thousand unnecessary deaths over the next several years is a conservative estimate of the cost of continuing with current policies and directions.

- Provide a simple mathematical model which anyone can use to calculate the number of unnecessary deaths caused by any given treatment research and access delays. We will also show how to use this model to analyze proposals for regulatory reform, how to do the arithmetic to determine whether or not a given proposal could possibly help to prevent these deaths, even if it worked perfectly.

- Show that even if an AIDS "penicillin" is developed—a dramatically successful new treatment—all bureaucratic incentives would be not to release it, but rather to conceal it for as long as possible. We will show that such concealment of dramatic breakthroughs may have happened already.

- Explain the crucial scientific dispute which underlies these problems. We will show that the research establishment is *right*, of course, in its own terms—but wrong in its choice of these terms, and in its uses of them. We will show that the fundamental dispute is not a scientific but a human one—rooted in the failure of academic researchers to acknowledge that at least for now and for some time to come, patients and physicians must and do make decisions under uncertainty—and that trials de-signed to statistically prove isolated drugs safe and effective after several years may serve the interests of drug companies, the regulatory system, and research profession-als, but that there are much better research strategies for supporting the actual decisions which must be made now in the course of medical practice.

- Suggest examples of the kinds of research which need to be done. We will show that much of it is legally possible in the United States today, and can be done very economically, without the financial support of the research establishment, with money raised directly from the community. We will also show that some of the research needed cannot be done in the United States under the current regulatory climate—and that the AIDS community must let the world know that other nations cannot rely on the United States to do anything in these areas, but must do their own work independently.

- Show where to start in building a coalition to bring the real issues in AIDS research into the open, to force an open choice: a research effort oriented to saving lives vs. writing people off *a priori*.

## Estimating Unnecessary Deaths:
## A Mathematical Model

How many deaths are caused by each month or year that red tape, malice, or unworkable policies or systems delay AIDS treatment development? A simple math-ematical model provides rational estimates. We propose this model as an intellectual tool to help in analyzing the costs and benefits of public policies (or lack of policies).

AIDS deaths have increased approximately at a geometric progression—meaning that they tend to double, and then double again, and so on, during the same fixed amount of time. (Fortunately the doubling time for AIDS deaths had increased somewhat over time, meaning that the death rate is not exactly a geometric progres-sion; this variation does not greatly affect our model, however.) We have not looked up the latest epidemiological figures, but an estimate of national (or world) AIDS deaths doubling every 18 months is close enough for the purpose of illustrating this model.

In any geometric progression (or any other sequence which doubles repeatedly), it turns out that the *last* doubling accounts for at least half of the cumulative total—no matter how long the sequence has gone. To illustrate with simple arithmetic, if we take the geometric progression 1, 2, 4, 8, 16, 32, 64, 128, 256, the last value, 256, is very close to half of the total of all the numbers, which is 511. No matter where we stop the sequence, the last doubling will account for half of the grand total of all the numbers.

How does this model apply to AIDS deaths? Someday there will be a cure or effective treatment. What the model shows is that no matter when the cure is found, the *last* doubling before that time (about 18 months) will account for half of the cumulative total of AIDS deaths throughout the entire epidemic.

Therefore, a delay of 18 months anywhere in the treatment research and development process will account for half of the total deaths of the epidemic. An unnecessary delay of 18 months, anywhere in the political mobilization, funding, coordination of research, conducting of the trials themselves, analysis of the data, or regulatory approval, means that half of the total deaths which will ever be due to AIDS will be unnecessary. A delay as long as 36 months (3 years) in treatment development will cause three quarters of all the deaths of the epidemic—deaths which would otherwise not have occurred.

If there is no single cure, but instead a gradual, incremental improvement of treatments which brings the deaths to an end, then the calculations become more difficult, but the bottom-line result of the model does not change.

There have been fifty thousand AIDS deaths in the United States so far. No major drugs are likely to come out of the regulatory pipeline for at least another 18 months—during which time an additional fifty thousand deaths will occur. Therefore, the cost of any unnecessary 18-month delay, in research or in patient access to whatever treatment turns out to be effective, can be estimated at fifty thousand lives.

But what delays are unnecessary? The research establishment tells the public that there are none—that we are going as fast as we can, that the only issue is whether to compromise the standards of Good Science, due to public impatience, and replace it with Bad Science. Researchers who break with this party line will jeopardize their future projects and future careers, so few will speak out. Journalists, politicians, and others involved with public education and public policy naturally tend to follow the consensus of recognized scientists on scientific questions—especially since one could otherwise be accused of wanting to weaken the standards of science. Good Science, like God, patriotism, and the flag, are rhetorical devices designed to be impossible to argue against—devices often used in the absence of a good case on the merits.

Later in this article we will show how the most important drugs in the pipeline could be tested and made available in weeks or months, not the years which will be required under present procedures. First, however, we must provide some additional background necessary for the defense of this statement, which understandably may seem preposterous to the reader. How, one might ask, could drugs be tested properly in weeks, when the scientific establishment has said that such testing takes years?

# What Will Happen When a Cure Is Found?

Researchers have told us that if an AIDS "penicillin" is discovered—a drug which works dramatically well—it will be made available to patients very quickly. However, it is hard for us to understand how all existing procedures will suddenly be suspended, in favor of a new set of procedures which so far as we know have never been written down or even thought through, let alone implemented as public policy. Governments, corporations, and professional bodies seldom work that way.

In fact, all bureaucratic incentives would be *not* to release such a drug, but rather to conceal it. To release it would mean that some person or institution would have to take responsibility for a momentous decision, with little preparation or lead time—something bureaucracies seldom do. It would be very difficult to develop a consensus to abandon all existing procedures and move into uncharted territory.

But another consensus would be easy to reach. Almost by definition, the research and political establishments agree that underground, unauthorized use of a treatment is undesirable. And unless the treatment could be tightly controlled, a large grassroots use of it would be inevitable if the public knew that the drug clearly worked. There would also be extensive political activity, which would be troublesome to the establishment.

**This means that the incentives built into the system would be to conceal an effective drug from the public, not to release it.**

Large-scale clinical trials cannot be hidden, because too many patients are involved. Successful concealment is only possible at the early stages of a treatment's development, before anyone knows for sure that it works. Phase I trials could either be postponed, or drawn out. We are not suggesting that anyone would do this deliberately to have people killed. But institutional pressures lead inexorably toward this kind of institutional denial, motivated by the normal bureaucratic fear of making major decisions and being forced unprepared into uncharted territory.

Long-term concealment of major advances in AIDS treatment may have happened already. One example is Compound Q. On April 18 *The New York Times* reported that "The researchers were so afraid of raising false hopes in people with AIDS that they did not disclose their findings for two years, until they were ready to test the drug in people." One of the researchers explained, "If I told you that we had found a drug that selectively kills HIV-infected cells in a single dose but then told you that it won't be available for two years, you'd go nuts." However, a version of the drug was already available and in routine use in China; it could easily have been tested in people two years ago, as soon as it was found to work in the test tube. But in fact, the secrecy around the Compound Q research largely ended on the day the patent for it was issued—suggesting that the wait for patent approval may have been what really held up not only release of the laboratory results, but also the testing in people with HIV (which could not have been kept secret) for as long as two years. (FDA rules would have accounted for some portion of this time even if the patent were not an issue.)

Companies normally keep their work secret until they receive a patent. Otherwise, rivals could learn what they were doing and file their own patent application. While the original party would normally be protected because it filed first, its application might be found to be defective and thrown out, losing its priority and perhaps losing the patent to the rival. The time taken to receive a patent is variable, because there may be negotiation with the patent office over specific claims.

During the approximately two years of quiet development of compound Q, laboratory and animal research did proceed. But in view of the prior human experience in China, where the same active ingredient is given by injection in comparable doses, laboratory work has little practical relevance to the safety and usefulness of the drug as an AIDS treatment. Only tests in patients can show how well it can work. Such tests will start now, with tiny, useless doses of the proprietary drug, much as they could have been done two years ago with active doses of the Chinese version.

If Compound Q does work as well as some people think that it might, this delay in its development could by itself account for half of the total deaths to date (see the mathematical model above). We should not blame the developers, who seldom have control over the key decisions. The fault is with the lack of national will to treat the epidemic as an emergency and make the system work.

And if, as expected, it takes yet another two years to get compound Q through clinical trials before it becomes widely available, then we can add another 50,000 unnecessary deaths, from this second delay alone. For if the drug does have dramatic effects, it would take only weeks at most to discover that fact. And long-term toxicity is little danger in a drug already widely used in humans elsewhere without any such problems. Certainly it is less of a danger than untreated AIDS.

Of course, compound Q may turn out not to work at all. But eventually, whatever drug finally does work will face the same kinds of delays. The public policies in effect today make the massive unnecessary deaths which we have predicted inevitable, regardless of whether compound Q or some other substance turns out to be the particular occasion where the delays cause the deaths.

Another example of a major advance in AIDS treatment concealed from the public and from many physicians is fluconazole (an antifungal for opportunistic infections, not a treatment for HIV or AIDS itself). When *AIDS Treatment News* first reported about fluconazole over 18 months ago (September 25, 1987), it was so little known in the United States that few physicians had heard of it. Yet even at that time two thousand persons in Europe had used the drug. Today fluconazole is approved in England; yet in the United States many physicians have never heard of it, and few know how to get it for their patients if they need it.

A third example of deadly concealment of treatment information is pneumocystis prophylaxis. This treatment, using aerosol pentamidine, bactrim, or other drugs, is now becoming the standard of care for persons with AIDS. But what few people realize is that pneumocystis prophylaxis (with bactrim) was already the required standard of care for persons at risk for pneumocystis for any reason *except* AIDS—ever since the 1970s, before AIDS was known. A few physicians have used this treatment all through the epidemic, and their patients are among the long-term AIDS survivors today. Most patients, however, were never told about this option.

The point of these examples is that major AIDS treatment advances can be and are concealed from the public, and sometimes from the medical and scientific communities, at major cost in loss of human lives.

Many people believe that the commercial pressures of capitalism are driving drug research and development as fast as it can safely go. In fact, even today the AIDS market is considered too small to be very profitable. Companies are better off waiting for this market to expand. They know that nothing will beat them to the market, because they can see for months or years ahead what is coming (or not coming) through the clinical-trials pipeline. This long pipeline delay, required by FDA rules, rationalizes and protects the investments of the entire pharmaceutical industry. This is why the clinical-trials pipeline is not being seriously shortened, although empty "reforms" (those which in practice could not save lives in the foreseeable future, even if everything went right and the reforms worked exactly as they were designed to) may be provided as public-relations diversions.

AZT, the only AIDS drug ever allowed to move rapidly through the clinical-trials pipeline, was unique in that there was no competitive product ahead of it to be threatened. However, there will never be such a slot again.

(Note: Part II of this article will appear later.)

# TERRY SUTTON, 1955–1989

Terry Sutton, 33, who died of AIDS on April 11, 1989, had quickly become one of the most important AIDS treatment activists, helping to make foscarnet and other treatments more available in San Francisco. He is also the one who suggested blocking the Golden Gate Bridge, which took place in the early morning of January 31.

We spoke with two of Terry's close friends, Marty Blecman and Michelle Roland, asking them to speak about whatever came to mind. The following is part of that 90-minute interview:

Marty: Terry took on the fight of drug access, and went up against what many seem to feel are overwhelming odds, an overwhelming bureaucracy. Terry saw it clearly, cleanly, and simply: Unless I get drug access, the treatments I need, my life will be shorter and I won't be here for the cure.

People need to understand that there isn't an army of activists fighting for this access, and that people can be powerful as individuals. Terry Sutton was not Gandhi, he was just an average guy who used to teach school, who came down with HIV and got his power—and spiritually wouldn't let a government that did not care about him, wouldn't let even a community that did not seem to care about him, stop him from going after what he wanted for himself, and ultimately for everyone.

Foscarnet could treat CMV, and allow him to go back to AZT, which could keep him alive longer. Terry was determined to stay alive until there was a cure. But he was realistic, that probably he didn't have enough time to do that.

Finally he went into the hospital. CMV was on the ravage, and he was told that he would lose sight in his right eye. So they went to full-dose DHPG—what he had to do to save his sight.

The result of DHPG was that his white blood cells kept dropping. They went so low that he eventually became septic, had an infection throughout his system. The day came when the doctor said, this is it, the antibiotics aren't working.

Terry died a fighter. He was not giving into death and being metaphysical about it and letting go. He was comatose throughout most of this, but the last day he came back to consciousness, and he was having seizures, and was alert enough to know what was going on in the room, and he was definitely terrified and panicked. He was biting his tongue and grinding his teeth in seizures, and it was horrible; he died a horrible, frightening death.

The irony is that he didn't have a lot of choices. When Terry wanted foscarnet, he couldn't get it.

This has to change. We're in the middle of an epidemic. People don't have seven years [the usual time for new-drug approval—*ed*], some don't have two years, some don't have two months. The system has to recognize this and turn it around—not take five years to turn it around, but do so now.

Unfortunately it's human nature not to feel the urgency to turn it around. Those who really feel the urgency for drug access are those who are going blind, or looking at death's door, and knowing that the only thing that's going to keep them from dying is this drug.

Denial plays into it, thinking it's never going to be my issue. To fight for drug access while you're healthy is saying to yourself that you might end up in a terminal position. This holds many people back from fighting.

Michelle: Terry turned around on the treatment access issue when he was diagnosed with CMV. He knew he could not survive on DHPG—he would ultimately fail that drug. He would either go blind and die of some other opportunistic infection, or die because DHPG wiped out his white blood cells, which is what happened.

When he was diagnosed with CMV, treatment issues were his reality. When the foscarnet issue came along, he said, "Maybe this will work. Maybe I can treat the HIV [with AZT, which can be combined with foscarnet but not with DHPG], and keep the CMV in check. I know that I can't do it with the DHPG, so why not try the foscarnet?"

Marty: Terry studied the Black Plague of Europe. In mass hysteria, people were bludgeoning themselves with clubs, to ward off or deal with the epidemic. In our time that doesn't make much sense. But maybe when history looks back on the epidemic, they'll say, "Everybody was caregivers."

Terry said that he could do without the support of organizations like PAWS, or Open Hand. "Take away everything, and just give me people who will fight for my life, and fight for drug treatments, to give me a drug to help me live longer. I'll take care of the rest of the support."

What's wrong now is that we're eight years into the epidemic, and the caregivers can't seem to take on the fight. Not only are they getting burned out, but they haven't got it through their heads that after they've watched so many people die, when will they say, "Enough is enough," and stand up and do something?

Terry Sutton stood up, and motivated people by his anger and desperation to get a drug, and brought a whole treatment-access issue into the forefront. He had discussions with Dr. Anthony Fauci (Director of the National Institute of Allergy and Infectious Diseases) which moved this man to go back to Washington and speak compassionately, saying he had met with people in San Francisco, and we must change the system. That foscarnet now has "salvage protocols" in San Francisco is directly related to Terry Sutton bringing the fight forward.

People have got to start telling the truth about what's going to stop the epidemic, and not what's going to support it.

Michelle: I saw Terry in Washington at the Quilt. I was very uncomfortable, watching the volunteers in the clean, white clothes running around shoving Kleenex at everybody who let a little tear run down the side of their face. I wondered how many of the people willing to volunteer for this quilt, and for Shanti, Open Hand, and other support organizations, were going to show up at the FDA that Monday?

Terry wouldn't walk on the Quilt. I looked at him and said, "Are you feeling it too?" We sat down and just raged on the side of the Quilt. We saw that we as a community have made this epidemic OK. We take care of ourselves—not only physically, we've even learned how to take care of our grief. But we're not doing anything to stop the epidemic. It's so infuriating that everybody is patting themselves on the back about how good they are, taking care of each other, and just creating this whole system where it's OK to watch people die and die and die. People had a hard time hearing that. And I told Terry, "If I ever make a panel for you, it's going to say, 'Terry Sutton hated this fucking Quilt'."

That's when he started thinking of San Francisco as not a model community—it's a myth. First, we don't really take care of everybody in the community, as we say we do. And second, taking care of people is not stopping this epidemic; in fact, by itself, it's enabling the epidemic to continue. And nobody from the outside has to deal with it, because we're taking care of it and making it OK.

Marty: I could swallow the Quilt more easily if at least they acknowledged that in the face of genocide, we must have a Quilt, to enlighten people. And in the face of genocide, we have Shanti. And in the face of genocide, we have PAWS, and in the face of genocide, we have the AIDS Emergency Fund, because society has looked at us and said, "It's not our problem," because society thinks we're faggots and drug users and blacks and Hispanics, and it's not our problem—that we're not going to get infected because we're good, straight, clean people. When society takes a segment of the population and turns its back on them, it's genocide.

Many gay men don't want to acknowledge that they're hated, despised enough to be let go by the wayside—because that goes to the root of their coming out, and acknowledging that they're OK. The layers of denial around the epidemic—people must start telling the truth.

If Terry stood for anything, it's the truth. He told the truth about himself most of the time, the good and the bad. He told the truth about his doctors, and the treatments, and the issues, and the straight society and the gay society. He kept telling the truth, and he shut a lot of people down.

But he moved a lot of people, moved them into action. He moved me into action. Everybody he touched he moved. Because he told the truth. And they didn't want to hear it, and then they went home and cried because they knew it was right.

Michelle: The sad thing is that when he was screaming and shouting, "Help save my life, now, do it now, I need the foscarnet and I can't do it by myself, you guys have to help me," it didn't happen. I'm glad that now people are mobilized around Terry's death, but it's sad that it had to take Terry's death to mobilize people to make the sense of urgency real.

Terry made the salvage protocol happen, but that salvage protocol didn't work for Terry Sutton, and it isn't working for the vast majority of people who want to try foscarnet. They have to get sick enough that the drug probably cannot be effective anyway. Terry knew he had to fail DHPG in order to get access to foscarnet. I watched him day after day in the hospital trace the fall of his white cells, until he said to me, "I'm eligible for foscarnet now."

Marty: "But I'm almost dead."

Michelle: When he told me his doctor was going to get him foscarnet, I wanted to support him, to say that's great, but what happened inside, I felt that if that doctor walks in with that drug I'm going to strangle him—"How dare you offer him foscarnet now when he has 700 white cells, when he's been saying for six months that he wanted a chance to try this drug."

Marty: Terry heard through one of his Deep Throats that foscarnet wasn't working for people. And the assumption was that they were so sick when they got on the foscarnet that it wasn't working.

Michelle: The other issue was that you have to pay for your hospitalization to administer the drug, about a thousand dollars a day. You have to be in the hospital for the first 14 days of foscarnet.

Marty: We need an information network among physicians. I spoke to an ophthalmologist in Los Angeles. He has a patient failing DHPG, going blind; he's trying to get DHPG to use for direct injection into the eye. The drug company said, "No, you can't have the drug."

The doctor didn't know there were salvage protocols going on in Houston or San Francisco. And he's an ophthalmologist in Los Angeles.

What this comes down to is that if there are five thousand caregivers in San Francisco, there's probably at most five hundred who would actually go to a demonstration, and maybe only 100 people who are politically activated, who are really fighting the epidemic in San Francisco. The proportion who are fighting to stop the epidemic, it's screwed up. People have got to get it, or this thing is going to go on and on.

Michelle: One of the things Terry was able to do was to fight it from many perspectives. He really moved doctors; when he first met them they were willing to do placebo trials with CMV patients. And after Terry had known them for a while, they were willing to fight for ethical protocols.

He motivated me to be able to move from being a caregiver 100 percent, to being able to decide to spend part of my time caretaking and part doing political work, and find more time to do it. He moved many people. There were friends in his life for years who had never done anything political, who were on the roof of Burroughs Wellcome getting arrested, who were at the FDA getting arrested, who were on the Golden Gate Bridge getting arrested.

Marty: Terry said to his mother, "If you're not willing to fight for my life now, while I'm alive, don't you dare come to my death scene."

We talked a lot about what's going on in the community. To be able to fight, you have to have a will to live. I think somewhere deep down, people have lost touch with their will to live. They question what do they have to live for, and do they deserve to live. People have to look at these issues to get in touch with their power. If a government is denying you access, and a protocol is denying you access, and a doctor is denying you access, and they're killing you because you're being denied access, how can you go to healing circles, how can you go to support groups, and how can you learn to live powerfully with AIDS, and live this metaphysically OK life, and go to your grave without fighting? The natural human spirit would be to fight back, to fight the death squads. If people were marching through the streets and gunning us down, we would still need support groups to deal with the grief and the anger around the death squads, but the support groups would be telling the truth about the death squads, and mobilizing people to fight them.

Something has gone wrong—a mass psychological hysteria . . . something is wrong with the picture. I don't know how to straighten it out, or who's going to straighten it out.

What people do catch onto are squeaky wheels. Fortunately, squeaky wheels get oiled. It's that simple; if people get diagnosed with HIV and they lay down with it, and they don't stand up for their rights, and they don't stand up for their spirit, and they don't stand up for the right to live, because they deserve it as a human being and a citizen of the United States and as a citizen of the planet, if they don't stand up for their rights, then they will get walked over.

People just have to squeak, and I don't know what's holding them back—fear, being overwhelmed.

Michelle: Terry ran himself ragged. There were many breakfasts he just didn't have time to eat because he was off to a meeting, trying to straighten this mess out.

And it wasn't just for him. He was very much aware of trying to save his own life. But when some brave soul in the medical community was going to pull strings, and pull illegal strings, to get Terry foscarnet, and he wouldn't do it. If not for everyone, then it's not right.

People have got to start telling the truth. And then the answer to the epidemic is clear, it's give us treatments and keep us alive.

The fund-raisers that go on are great—but God forbid that anyone would do a fund-raiser and give a million dollars to ACT UP. It's unthinkable.

They all want to do the same thing, direct service. It's natural to want to help the people who are sick. People should. But they must realize that they'll be helping the people who are sick from now till eternity unless they start helping to find a cure, or treatments.

I'd gladly take pills the rest of my life; if I could play my life out to a basically normal old ripe age, and get all the grey hair I deserve, I'll take drugs for the rest of my life. But I won't sit here and live powerfully with AIDS, and go off to healing circles and enrich my life and smell the roses and go to my death without screaming about it.

Michelle: It's such a complex situation. Where do you fight? We fought the drug companies, and we went to the FDA and fought there, and we meet with Congresswoman Pelosi about drawing up legislation. Terry took the time, and spent the emotional and mental energy, to try to figure out where the appropriate targets were. He had file cabinets full of files, and phone numbers of contacts in every file. He spent hours and weeks and months, sorting that out and educating people. I feel scared about what's going to happen without Terry. We are trying to pick up where Terry left, and not let this work fizzle out, but it's a full-time job.

Terry had the ability to mobilize people, as very few have. People would meet him, and you either fell in love with Terry or you didn't. If you didn't, fine, but if you did, you listened and you were moved. Who's going to be able to do that—be able to move the doctors, the officials like Fauci, and all the people who came into his life?

Who will take up the fight? It doesn't take very many people. People say, "They'll take care of it, there's ACT UP, they'll fight for me, there's Terry Sutton and he'll fight for me, there's Mobilization Against AIDS and they'll fight for me." People go on with their lives because it's hard enough just getting through the day, let alone taking on the

FDA, or taking on a drug company, or taking on a major issue. But one of Terry's favorite quotes was, "If not now, when? And if not me, who?" There aren't a lot of people out there doing it.

The philosophy of Terry hopefully will live on, and the people he inspired will continue to inspire other people, and the fifty thousand people who have gone before Terry will not be forgotten.

Terry didn't have a lot of patience for PWAs who weren't fighting. He would get angry with them. "How can you sit there and get infused every day, and throw up your guts on the floor, and not be willing to come to San Francisco General and sit down on the floor and get arrested? What have you got to lose?"

What do people have to lose—except their denial, maybe, and their fears? And what they have to gain is everything. You gain victories, you gain power, and you gain personal insight and knowledge, you gain control over your life, you gain hope, you gain all kinds of things from action. Plus you gain just getting yourself out of bed to do something.

How many people died of pneumocystis while aerosol pentamidine was hanging out there for two years?

Michelle: He was forced into wanting that diagnosis. He didn't really have the option of going to work, but as we know, people with ARC are not acknowledged as disabled most of the time. There's no way Terry could have worked 40 hours a week.

Marty: He was wasting away. Work was going to start in September, and he was freaked out. He was also freaked out when he got his diagnosis, but there was also a sigh of relief, "Now I can fight, and get paid for it"—barely.

Michelle: Then he had to ask how he could live on $600 a month.

Marty: When I asked him to be my roommate, he cried.

Michelle: Terry was involved in the formation of AIDS Action Pledge, and Burroughs Wellcome was a kick-off.

Marty: Terry was one of the first Shanti volunteers, back around 1982 or 1983, before he knew he had HIV. He was one of the first volunteers at Kaiser who supported the AIDS ward.

Michelle: He did the Kaiser work up through his diagnosis. And he would come home after going to Kaiser, and he had to talk about what he had just seen and experienced. One of the problems that Terry had, and one of the problems in the AIDS activist movement, is that he couldn't talk about his emotional experience with activists. AIDS activists are very separate from the actual experience of living with AIDS. Terry was one of the rare people who could do both of those things, but had a hard time finding people who could support him and listen to the terror and the anger and the fear and the sadness that came in that work, helping people die.

Marty: He did a workshop by Sally Fisher called the AIDS Mastery. A friend said that after the mastery, he got in touch with his power. Before the mastery he was very shy, and quiet. The mastery lit his fire.

When the "Midnight Caller" episode came up, Terry was the first one to light everybody's fire; he found out about the script, and plugged everybody into it, and became a negotiator.

After "Midnight Caller," he took on foscarnet, which led to the sit-in at San Francisco General—which of course brings up the [blockade of the Golden Gate] Bridge.

Michelle: I remember Terry saying that we had to do something, something really radical to shake people up; that we have to increase the militancy in the AIDS activist movement, we can't just sit in front of empty buildings or even full buildings, that's not doing it.

Terry's phrase around the Bridge was, "Bridge the treatment gap." Because there were many people from different organizations represented in the Bridge, people wanted it to include more issues, so it became "AIDS equals genocide."

On the day of the Bridge itself Terry was really sick. He went out there and sat in the fog, and got arrested. And after the Bridge, when everybody was celebrating and feeling really good about ourselves, Terry came home and went to bed.

In my mind, the Bridge was Terry Sutton. That there were people in the community who hadn't been involved in AIDS activism before, who were willing to take the risk of shutting down the Golden Gate Bridge, infused him with a lot more hope, more belief in the possibility that people would come around and start doing this work.

And partly the Bridge came off out of respect for Terry. People knew how important it was to Terry.

Marty: The Bridge was a tremendous success. The media hoopla that swelled around it was pretty much expected. It was expected that many in our community would snub their noses at it at first, and say that these stupid people were going to turn everybody off. And it was also expected that they would turn around and get it, after they had thought about it for a while. It's like, "What have we got to lose—and if not now, when?" And as for those poor commuters who were inconvenienced for an hour and a half, well, excuse me, my life's been put on hold.

Michelle: The power that it had in the AIDS community was more important than in the general community. It shook people up in the service community, and in the Democratic clubs, and even in the AIDS activist community. It's a challenge. It said that we have to do things that are more militant, and we have to be more committed.

Marty: More people have died of AIDS in this country than died in the Vietnam War, but with Vietnam it was easier to connect, to find the enemy.

In the AIDS fight, there might be a problem because the people who feel the epidemic the most are in a constant state of mourning. They're depressed, and may be shutting down. If you lose a friend in February, and lose one the next month, and again the next week, and you can't even get through the grief and the mourning process of the last friend, emotionally you start to shut down. Maybe that's what's going on.

Michelle: The other difference is that it's easier to fight for other people. When the Vietnamese are the victims, we can get out and say that our government is wrong. But when we're the victim, saying that our government is wrong is acknowledging that our government doesn't give a shit about us. People can't do that. People are so totally invested in believing that the government and the research community are doing everything that they possibly can to end this epidemic, and you guys just have to be patient, and it's a virus and we don't know that much about viruses, and on and on.

It makes perfect sense why we're so invested in that. It's terribly painful to think, "My country, my government, and my society are willing to watch me die."

Terry pushed us to confront AIDS as genocide. Even some activists felt, "Intellectually I can get it, but emotionally it's so horrifying, that I want to figure out all the rationalizations why it's not true." Terry's the one who said, "You've got to tell the truth, this is what it's about."

Marty: People shut down. I can talk about how Terry died, how gruesome it was, and people still keep open and listening. And I can talk about emotional things, and people still listen. But when I talk about politics, and about genocide, and about maybe getting up off their ass and doing something to stop the epidemic and facing the reality that maybe we're disliked, then they shut down. I see them drifting off into space, and looking the other way, and feeling uncomfortable, and wanting to get out and away from me. That's when I lose it. What scares me more than having HIV is watching people shut down to the truth.

(We asked about the scattering of Terry's ashes at sea.)

Michelle: We had balloons with "Silence Equals Death" written on them, and we let them go symbolically, to let go of Terry a little bit, of the grief.

From the time we pulled out of the dock and headed toward the bridge, it was the first time since he started dying that it felt really real. I guess that's why we do these services and go through these rituals, because we need ways to accept what's happening, and to deal with the reality of it. I was very upset and I cried almost the whole way to the bridge. And then when they shut off the motor under the bridge, to be underneath the Golden Gate Bridge to say good-bye to Terry was such a powerful and sad and exciting experience. I felt it from everyone; the grief on that boat, and the pride, to be underneath the Bridge doing this for Terry.

Marty: We did an "Act Up, Fight Back, Fight AIDS" chant under the bridge, and another chant for Terry.

Marty: Terry was a teacher and emotional support person, and he urged people continuously to get their powers of attorney signed, and their wills taken care of. And because Terry constantly joked about having just a mild case of AIDS and not having to get this together yet, he never did get together his power of attorney or his will. The havoc that caused throughout his hospital stay when he went unconscious was horrible—practical and emotional. It was very hard on his friends and caregivers, and on his family, and on his doctors, trying to make decisions and not knowing exactly what he wanted.

Don't stay in denial about getting your powers of attorney and wills done, because "If not now, when?"

Michelle: Terry asked three of his friends to do the power of attorney. And I believed and he believed that he would get out of the hospital and we'd do that. Guess what, less than one week later he was unconscious, and it didn't happen. Thank God we'd had the conversations, he had them with the three of us, so we knew what he wanted. We were able to work with the doctors and the family.

Marty: The obit we wrote, it was not, "Terry died peacefully in the arms of his friends and his lovers and went peacefully to the light beyond." It was basically, "He died a gruelling, uncomfortable, drawn-out, horrible death."

Michelle: That truth has to be told, too. We all live in this illusion that there's this peaceful passing. There was nothing peaceful, nothing OK or reassuring, about Terry's death.

Marty: If more people were scared—it's like, "Don't make me not scared of death, please. Don't make me not afraid to get sick, and to watch my body fall apart. Don't make me not scared to not be supported, and to be financially broke." We're putting bandaids over these natural reactions to the holocaust. Maybe we've put too many bandaids on people. I'm plugged into the AIDS Mastery, and I've seen hundreds of

PWAs come through and learn to live powerfully, and get their lives back, and get out of that state. But to get beyond that, and to fight, is a different story.

And that's the only way we see out of the epidemic. Unless a miracle happens.

Michelle: And even with a miracle, it will take seven years to get that miracle out.

Marty: And if compound Q is the answer, God forbid you are on DHPG or foscarnet or whatever. Who are they going to exclude from the protocol right off the bat, and when will they make it acceptable and accessible to everybody? When do the HIV babies get it?

We're talking about people shutting down and not wanting to stand up and fight for foscarnet, when too many gay men in this town won't even get tested. How are they ever going to stand up and fight? How do you move these people from not knowing what their status is, to fighting to save their lives?

People are not telling the truth, all the time, all the truth. They're putting it in candy wrappers.

And when you know the truth, and you don't get the support of people around you, you start to think you're crazy. And Terry Sutton would listen to people say, "You're crazy," and then look at it and say, "No, no I'm not. This is the truth."

If people want to make donations in Terry's name, they should donate to ACT UP. That's probably the closest thing to him.

Marty: His experience in teaching emotionally disturbed children got him his power. All of us to some degree are emotionally disturbed around AIDS. He got us to understand. To get an emotionally disturbed child to calm down and listen to something—he got me calm enough to accept the fact of genocide, he affected people as a teacher.

Michelle: And he could play, and he could be crazy, and silly, and have fun, and really act out. That helped us emotionally, too, because there was all this heavy shit going on, and then we could just crack up, with Terry.

Marty: He was happy, actually. He was a pretty happy guy.

Michelle: He had a lot of friends.

# Issue Number 78
# May 5, 1989

## COMPOUND Q WARNING, AND UPDATE

Compound Q, an experimental AIDS treatment extracted from the root tuber of a Chinese cucumber, has received wide publicity in the last month. On May 5 we heard the first report of a severe adverse reaction to a bogus "compound Q," apparently homemade from the root which was obtained from a health-food store, and injected. According to Martin Delaney of Project Inform, who is now warning buyers' clubs, the person almost died as a result, and was in intensive care for three days. This case occurred in Kansas City.

We have also heard that some health-food stores are exploiting the situation and promoting a dried root or extract by suggesting that it contains compound Q. People should know (1) that the root also contains lectins, which are poisonous when injected because they cause blood cells to clump together, which can cause heart attacks or strokes, and (2) that compound Q (which is a protein called trichosanthin) is almost certainly destroyed by drying, so the dried root used as an herbal medicine for other purposes does not contain the active ingredient.

It is generally believed that a good-quality equivalent of compound Q does exist in China, and has been used there for other purposes for several years (see *AIDS Treatment News* #77). However, this drug is tightly controlled and very difficult to obtain. We have heard from knowledgeable persons (but have not yet been able to confirm independently) that only half a million doses a year are manufactured, all by one factory in or near Shanghai, and that some of it did reach a few persons with AIDS in the U.S. While extracting the active ingredient (trichosanthin) from the Chinese cucumber root is not too difficult for a protein chemist, there are practical problems, especially the need to obtain large quantities of the fresh or frozen root, as well as the usual difficulties of setting up effective manufacturing and quality control for pharmaceuticals.

Any credible, good-quality data which may develop from use of the Chinese compound-Q equivalent would be very important in speeding the authorized clinical trials. At this time, the only clinical trial planned anywhere in the world is a "phase I" study to take place at San Francisco General Hospital. This trial may be slowed by the current budget crisis of the City and County of San Francisco, since hospitalization is required for the study but there is not enough funding to staff the nursing support for the hospital beds.

The San Francisco trial will also be slow because it is designed primarily to test for toxicity and determine the maximum tolerated dose, not to determine whether the drug can help patients. A tiny dose which no one believes could be effective will be tried first, followed by a wait to look for side effects. This process will be repeated several times, with a wait each time. This dose-escalation study could take as little as three to six months, or as long as a year. By contrast, "underground" users of the Chinese drug will test reasonable doses right away—the same which have already been used in China—so they can get results far ahead of the official trials. If such use should happen to produce credible evidence that the drug is useful in treating AIDS, then far more pressure would develop to speed the research and regulatory system and make compound Q available through authorized channels. We will continue to report on compound Q as we learn more about it.

# DDI INFORMATION PUBLISHED

At a recent Washington, DC meeting of the American Federation for Clinical Research, Dr. Robert Yarchoan summarized results so far of the longest-running clinical trial of ddI (dideoxyinosine), being conducted by himself and others at the National Cancer Institute. DDI is a relative of AZT, but it may be considerably less toxic.

No written paper accompanied the talk, and the researchers are not giving interviews until their presentation at the V International Conference on AIDS in Montreal in early June. But the *Los Angeles Times* covered the Washington meeting in a page-one story published May 1; other newspapers reprinted parts of the *Los Angeles Times* report. That article may have the latest news available on DDI until June. (For background information, see *AIDS Treatment News* #72).

The National Cancer Institute study, conducted in Bethesda, Maryland, should not be confused with a separate phase I trial conducted at New York University and the University of Rochester by the National Institute of Allergy and Infectious Diseases and Bristol-Meyers, which obtained an exclusive license to ddI from the National Institutes of Health.

According to the *Los Angeles Times*, Dr. Yarchoan reported that most of the patients improved, with "minimal toxicity"—at least for the six months observed so far, even for those who cannot tolerate AZT. Two patients had seizures, which might or might not have been caused by the drug; two had low white counts; and some reported minor side effects such as headaches or insomnia. These problems, which can occur without drug treatment in persons with HIV, were fewer than would be expected in such a study.

ddI can be taken by mouth, if used with antacid, and it does cross the blood-brain barrier.

ddI has not been released for compassionate use, even for those who cannot tolerate AZT. We have heard that the phase I trials have been delayed by failure to find toxicity, since rules require that such trials continue until a maximum tolerated dose is found—meaning that the safer the drug is, the longer the trial will take. Caution is understandable, as other drugs of the same class (AZT and ddC) have had serious toxicities which did not show up immediately. But the risk of some hypothetical side effect which appears only after months must be balanced against the risk of untreated AIDS for persons who cannot tolerate AZT and have no alternative. Persons with AIDS and their physicians should have some role in making this decision. Today they are shut out.

On March 30 of this year, the news service Reuters reported that the Japanese company Ajinomoto had set up mass production facilities to produce ddI from uridine, under contract with Bristol-Meyers for use as an AIDS treatment.

## AEROSOL PENTAMIDINE, GANCICLOVIR RECOMMENDED FOR APPROVAL

On May 1 an advisory committee of outside experts set up by the Food and Drug Administration recommended full new-drug approval for aerosol pentamidine, used for prevention of pneumocystis. The next day, the committee recommended similar approval for ganciclovir (DHPG) for treating CMV retinitis. Official approvals are expected within several weeks or months.

What will be the practical effect of these approvals of drugs which have already been available under a variety of arrangements?

For aerosol pentamidine, full approval will help with insurance reimbursement. Until now, some insurance companies and government agencies have refused to pay for the treatment, claiming that it was "experimental". Others have paid, since the cost of preventing pneumocystis with aerosol pentamidine is far less than the cost of treating it in a hospital. It is widely suspected that companies which refused to pay have calculated that they could save money in the long run by having their clients die.

For ganciclovir, approval will allow the manufacturer to charge for the drug, currently provided free under a treatment IND. We do not know what the price will be. Insurance presumably will pay since the drug will be approved, but many do not have insurance, or do not have policies which cover prescription drugs.

One advantage of the approval is that physicians will be allowed to use ganciclovir to treat CMV infection in the intestines or elsewhere besides the retina, even though the FDA approval will not specifically cover such use. Physicians may be reluctant to prescribe for such "unlabeled" uses, however, and insurance companies may refuse to pay.

Another advantage of the approval of ganciclovir is that it will now become possible to conduct a trial to compare this drug directly with foscarnet for treating CMV retinitis, a trial specifically recommended by the advisory committee. Until now such a trial has been blocked by the prohibition against using more than one "experimental" drug in the same study.

# OBTAINING TREATMENTS FROM ABROAD

Buyers' clubs in New York and San Francisco recently began helping people import drugs with promise for AIDS/HIV and opportunistic infections, from countries where these drugs are approved. This is possible because a physician can legally prescribe any drug for her or his patient if it is approved for human use in the country of origin; the FDA recently said it would not obstruct shipments ordered only for personal use, at least for drugs that the agency deems safe.

The PWA Health Group in New York is able to obtain fluconazole, roxithromycin (see *AIDS Treatment News* #75), dextran sulfate, isoprinosine, ribavirin, and hypericin herbal extracts (which are also available in the U.S.). It will consider requests for other drugs if approved for prescription use in other countries. The PWA Health Group can be reached at 212/532-0280. A long tape message will answer first with a comprehensive explanation of available products and prices, so have a pen and paper on hand.

The Healing Alternatives Foundation in San Francisco can order dextran sulfate, fluconazole, hypericin herbal extracts, and possibly roxithromycin. Healing Alternatives may be able to ship orders to customers. Their number is 415/626-2316.

This development is a vital step in the direction of people gaining urgent access to potentially life-saving drugs—drugs like fluconazole which could languish out of reach for years if we have to wait for FDA approval or NIH or drug-company funding. If other buyers' clubs are able to follow suit, we would like to hear from them, especially regarding treatments not mentioned above.

# AMFAR FUNDS COMMUNITY-BASED RESEARCH IN 15 CITIES

On April 27, the American Foundation for AIDS Research awarded $1.4 million in development grants for community-based research—efforts to organize community physicians and patients to test treatments under the supervision of research professionals, but outside the major medical centers where such trials would usually be run.

Organizations receiving the awards are located in Atlanta, GA, Austin, TX, Boston, MA, Brooklyn, NY, Dallas, TX, Houston, TX, Los Angeles, CA, New Haven, CT, New York, NY, Portland, OR, Redwood City, CA, San Francisco, CA, Santa Fe, NM, Springfield, VA, and Westwood, NJ.

In San Francisco, the Community Research Alliance (see *AIDS Treatment News* #70, December 1, 1988) received $30,000 under this program for organization development. The County Community Consortium received two grants, one for development and another for its AZT and HIV alternative-treatment databases.

# THE DRUG-TRIALS DEBACLE, PART II:
# WHAT TO DO NOW

*by John S. James*

*"If you ask researchers the question, as I have several of them, 'If you did not need to deal with the FDA regulations, if you did not need to face all the questions of marketing and licensing, etc., and just get an answer, could you determine within six months whether a drug is going to be useful in the fight against AIDS?' If you just ask the question in that simple way, all of them I've asked say, 'Well, of course we could.'*

*"That being the case, let's get some of this baggage out of the way, and get these answers more quickly, and act like this really is the emergency that everyone says it is."*

> Martin Delaney, co-founder and director of
> Project Inform, on KQED public radio
> "Forum" program, May 3, 1989.

Part I of this article (*AIDS Treatment News* #77), presented a simple mathematical model which anyone can use to calculate the loss of human life caused by delays in AIDS research and treatment access. We showed that because of the geometric progression of the epidemic, a delay of 18 months to three years[1] would cause half of the total of all the deaths due to AIDS—deaths of people whose lives can be saved if the delay can be avoided. This model brings home the cost of the widespread unspoken attitude that everyone infected with HIV is going to die anyway, and therefore we can write them off and ignore research and access delays, in favor of other things such as services for the dying short of saving their lives, or grief support. If we assume that the epidemic will someday be controlled, then it is certain that we can save many thousands of lives by eliminating some of the unnecessary delays now built into the research and treatment access and delivery systems.

In Part I, we also showed that if a cure were found, there would be no mechanism to release it to people quickly—that in fact the bureaucratic incentives are to avoid risks and therefore to conceal treatment advances rather than release them. We pointed out that delays in the new-drug research and regulatory "pipeline," delays long enough to cause tens of thousands of deaths, serve the interests of major corporations by rationalizing and protecting their drug-development investments—and that perhaps as a result, the "reforms" allowed to take effect have been only those which could not change the outcome, even if they worked perfectly as intended.

Part I showed what is wrong. Here we suggest what we believe can and should be done toward correcting the problems. We will show what kinds of studies could quickly and inexpensively produce information that would assist the treatment decisions physicians and patients must make now—and why the research establishment largely rejects such studies. We will show that the mainstream research tradition in the United States has become skewed toward producing the kinds of information which corporations and regulators need to make their decisions—not the information which patients and physicians need to make theirs.

We will show that much of the needed research could be done legally in the United States today, using community funding to bypass the financial control and ineffectual bureaucracy of the research establishment—and that some of the studies which could not be conducted in the United States could be done elsewhere.

Politically, we will suggest that a key, doable first step is to develop clearer statements of consensus within the coalition of individuals and groups already committed to saving lives, then use this consensus to get our friends on board.

## The Mainstream View Of Research

One school of thought has come to dominate government funding and permissions, and therefore research careers, in the United States. This establishment approach is not, of course, all bad. The problem is that it has achieved such dominance that it can insist on applying its own ways of doing things to all situations, no matter how inappropriate the result.

Mainstream treatment research is based on the following mindset:

• The first goal of clinical research is to prove, to a statistically stated degree of confidence, that a drug does work better than nothing, or better than some existing treatment.

• There must be a control group, as otherwise there would be no way to justify the statement that the drug to be tested is better than something else.

• Above all, clinical trials must guard against the danger that a drug which is useless and perhaps harmful could become accepted and generally used in medicine, as has happened many times in the past.

• Since most drugs being tested will show only a small benefit, trials must be designed to distinguish a small benefit from none at all.

• If patients use other treatments during a trial, their effects could interfere with the results. Therefore subjects must refrain from other treatments—even if the drug being tested will in fact be used with other treatments after it is approved.

• The fact that a trial imposes an unrealistic environment which may never occur in practical use of the new drug does not matter. What is important is to learn about a drug in isolation, not a therapy in practical use.

• If for whatever reason (such as lack of national political will) it is impossible to arrange a trial which meets these and all other standards of pure research, then it is better to do nothing until such future time as trials may be done, instead of doing any other kind of a study, which could lead to error.

• There is no need to design trials in such a way that it is feasible for any particular patients to volunteer, or for physicians to recommend their patients. If the trial fails to recruit subjects, that is not the fault of the researcher, whose job concerns pure science, not practical medicine.

• It is ethical to deny access to treatments until the trials are complete or at least well along—either to force patients into trials, or to maintain a stockpile of untreated patients available for future studies which may occur when someone gets around to paying for them.

• If the necessary trials do not get done, no one is responsible, since no one has the job of expediting trials, or untangling the snafus which block them.

• No one is responsible for the tens of thousands of unnecessary deaths which will result from this approach. All involved can make the case that they have done their jobs. The final outcome is no one's responsibility.

This system developed to serve the needs of the powerful players: drug companies and Federal agencies. The companies want above all to get their "NDA" (new drug approval), allowing them to market a drug which they have exclusive rights to and have chosen to push. The Food and Drug Administration, supported by consumer protectionists in Congress and elsewhere, wants above all to protect the public from unsafe or unproven drugs. The National Institutes of Health wants to pursue studies which are scientifically interesting. No one has the mission of making sure that trials which are critically important for saving lives get done quickly, or making sure that patients have access to treatments which are clearly beneficial but which for any of a multitude of reasons have not gone through all the steps necessary for full marketing approval.

## Prospective Monitoring Studies: Another Kind of Trial

The main problem with controlled, randomized trials, the kind the U.S. research establishment has insisted on, is that they are very difficult to get going. They are difficult because the procedures which take place in these trials are so different from those in the normal practice of medicine. There are major ethical and practical difficulties in giving patients a placebo—or in asking them to submit to any random- ized study, in which they do not know which of two or more medicines they will receive. Only large, well-financed institutions can manage such trials, and the red tape involved usually creates months or years of delay.

It may seem that these trials, however cumbersome, are the only way to get credible information. After all, researchers can show with statistics that using fewer patients, or deviating from their rules for running trials, may cause wrong answers to be found. It is well known that many inadvertent biases in the design or conduct of clinical trials can cause a drug to appear appear effective when really it is not, or vice versa.

But these arguments assume that the goal of the trial is to prove (or fail to prove) that a drug is effective. This is the information which drug companies and regulators need for their decisions, and of course this information is useful to patients and physicians too. However, there are other kinds of studies which do not even try to prove whether or not a drug is effective, which can produce information useful to patients and physicians (but much less useful to corporations and regulators).

One of the problems we face today is that if the large, cumbersome trials have not been done, then the only alternative has been anecdotal information, which is notori- ously unreliable, and often under the control of self-interested parties—true believers or promoters with a product to sell. The obvious problems of such reports have discredited any information not confirmed by big-money, big-bureaucracy trials.

If you are considering a new treatment now, you have several alternatives, all of them unsatisfactory:

• Wait several years or more until official trials have been done and the drug is approved.

• Try to get into a trial—but it may not start for a year, the nearest site may be hundreds of miles away, you may not qualify, you may have to stop other drugs (or have never used them), and then you may get a placebo.

• Ask around. Maybe a friend knows two people who used the treatment and whose T-cells went up. Maybe they forgot to say that the before and after tests were at different labs, that they began other treatments at the same time, and that other blood values deteriorated.

• Read articles about the treatment. Unfortunately, the writers may have an interest in promoting it. And even if not, they will usually have had to base their articles on anecdotal reports, since good information is not available.

There is another alternative, however—very well managed collection, handling, and presentation of data about a particular treatment, in the environment and context in which that treatment is actually used. Community-based research organizations can take treatment information out of the hands of the true believers and promoters, and have it controlled instead by professionally guided research teams which serve no interests except those of the patient community.

Besides waiting for years for randomized trials, or using anecdotal reports to make treatment decisions, there should be another choice. Prospective monitoring studies could provide another source of treatment information. Here is how they can work:

When persons with AIDS or HIV start using a new treatment (for example, hypericin), a research organization could offer to monitor perhaps 20 to 50 persons, paying for blood work and physical examinations. The study would be designed in advance (that is why it is called "prospective") and approved by a scientific advisory committee, so all the important data would be collected for every patient, in a uniform way; for example, all blood work would be done by the same lab, to avoid inter-lab variations. All physical exams and medical histories would be conducted uniformly. Identical patient diaries can be used. All patients would be accounted for. Data handling would be audited and would meet the same standards as in any other clinical trial.

A purely monitoring study cannot ask patients to change what they were doing for the sake of the research. Therefore patients can use whatever other treatments they want during the study, as long as they tell the researchers what they are doing.

As the study proceeds, data is statistically summarized and given to one or more leading HIV physicians for their interpretation. Is anything happening which is dramatically different, either better or worse, from what would have been expected without the treatment being tested? Or is it unclear whether or not the treatment has helped—meaning that the benefits, if any, are less than dramatic? These evaluations by the physicians, along with the statistical summaries, would be published as the report of the study. Because there is no control group and no randomization, this study is not designed to "prove" the drug safe or effective. The treatment group is in effect being compared with the expectations of the expert physicians chosen to evaluate the data obtained—a method not as statistically precise as using a placebo control, but certainly able to pick out a decisively effective treatment, which is what these studies will be looking for.

Instead of asking for statistical proof, the important question for judging a monitoring study is whether it provides information useful for making treatment decisions.

Primary-care physicians will make this determination, when they decide what studies are credible. Our own expectation, after reporting on AIDS treatments for three years, is that for many unapproved therapies, a single such study, scientifically designed and professionally managed by an unbiased research organization and collecting complete data from several dozen patients, could produce better information on the use of the treatment for HIV than all of the world's anecdotes and rumors put together, even for substances which had already been widely used for months or years.

Perhaps most importantly, such monitoring studies could be used as a quick screening for the most promising treatments now entering human trials (such as compound Q, ddI, or D4T). The goal would be to look for very dramatic benefits, in order to bypass years of ineffectual bureaucracy for any treatment found to work so well that there could be no dispute about its value.

Monitoring studies have several advantages of flexibility and ease of use:

• No FDA permission is required, because the study does not give any drug to people—it only collects data. Major delays are therefore avoided.

• The cost is low. Less than a thousand dollars per patient will pay for physical examinations and for six to eight months of blood work more complete than that of many official "phase II" studies. Therefore this research can be supported directly by contributions from the public, bypassing government agencies which often take more than a year to award money—a year **after** completion of the ponderous applications, which can run to hundreds of pages. Since there is no major overhead cost, monitoring studies can start with whatever funding is available and add more patients later as additional money comes in, or let patients pay for their own blood work until funding can be found.

• Reports can be compiled and published at any time, not just after the study is done, as is usually the case with randomized trials. Mainstream medical journals may reject these papers because there is no control group. But the results can be distributed immediately by community organizations to patients and physicians, without being restricted for months by pre-publication secrecy.

• The fact that patients can use other treatments during the study will make the results more difficult for the physician(s) engaged for that purpose to interpret. But in return there are two advantages of not restricting other therapies. First, the treatment is studied in the actual context of its use, not in an artificial context of a single drug tested in isolation. And second, in the traditional trials which kick people out for using additional treatments not in the protocol, patients whose lives are at stake often use other drugs anyway, and conceal what they are doing. The difference is not whether other drugs are used, but whether the researchers know about it.

• Since these studies do not require any medical sacrifice of the patient—they simply offer free blood work—recruitment can be much easier. Randomized trials are often delayed for months and sometimes cancelled entirely because they cannot recruit patients.

• Since no big institution is needed to run monitoring studies, this research can be more responsive to community needs than the official, randomized drug trials.

• Monitoring studies can legally be done in the United States, provided that patients can obtain and use the drug without the help of the researchers. If patients cannot obtain a drug here, the study might be conducted abroad.

Monitoring studies are already occurring—for example, an antabuse project of the Community Research Initiative in New York, and monitoring of AZT, and of alternative therapies in general, by the County Community Consortium in San Francisco. Although the idea of community-based research is to conduct trials through physicians' offices, monitoring studies might work better if the blood tests, physicals, and patient interviews were handled at central locations when possible, so that staff can be trained to do these consistently. The research organization must coordinate with primary-care physicians, of course, and give them copies of laboratory reports and other information. But most primary-care physicians are too busy to go out of their way to collect data in a specified, uniform manner. This job can be done by medical staff trained by the project and following written guidelines.

## Treatment Politics: Challenging the Death Consensus

The fast, inexpensive kind of study suggested above is only one example of how AIDS treatment research could be improved. The political task is more basic: how to overcome the widespread fatalism which makes even friends of the AIDS community unwilling to deal with treatment issues, as they have already given up on saving the lives of persons now ill or infected, and written them off as dead. How do we respond to the widespread, often silent assumption in professional and institutional circles that saving the lives of those now infected or ill is either impossible or not worth doing?

Congress, for example, is today largely a wasteland on the issues addressed here. The usual attitude toward those who bring the subject up has been described by one treatment advocate as, "You are the doomed or advocates for the doomed, and the doomed always want more drugs." End of conversation—and of any effort or interest in dealing with the issue.

To change this attitude, which today forms a consensus even among many friends of persons with AIDS in Congress, we need to start in our own community.

Recently a leading gay rights lobbyist, describing his commitment to AIDS work, was quoted in a major newspaper as saying, "I feel compelled to use my professional skills to make it easier for those who will die, and to prevent others from getting sick." Too many organizations have written off much of their constituency as dead and left out any involvement in saving the lives of the tens of thousands who will die unnecessarily as a result of current policies. No wonder Congress and the research community have failed to examine their own fatalism, their unwillingness to lift a finger to change policies which make thousands of unnecessary deaths inevitable, since even the AIDS community's organizations and advocates have not done so. How can we expect others to speak for us when we will not speak for ourselves?

Why have most AIDS organizations been so reluctant to work on treatment issues? There seem to be many reasons. One is that they fear differing with their political allies, usually liberals, who for years have been fighting for consumer protection. Consumer protectionists want to see the strongest possible FDA, strong regulations, and the most exhaustive testing of new drugs before they are released. They are afraid that AIDS will allow the pharmaceutical industry to weaken the regulatory system they have worked so hard to build, and that flexibility in treatment access will facilitate quackery and unscrupulous exploitation of persons who are desperate. (We too support consumer protection—but not at the cost of human lives. AIDS must be treated as an emergency, as it would have been if it had not first been perceived as a gay disease. It is not enough to simply apply old battle lines in utter disregard of the existence of this emergency, and of the effects of its eight years of its malign neglect under the Reagan White House.)

A second reason is that AIDS service organizations are usually publicly funded, sometimes with Federal funds, so they may be fearful of questioning Federal agencies.

A third reason is the emotional issue of HIV testing. Of hundreds of AIDS organizations in the country, only a handful, mostly in San Francisco, are now willing to recommend that persons at risk of AIDS seek voluntary, anonymous testing. The others may be deterred from becoming involved in treatment issues, because if they did, they would face the contradiction that people cannot obtain early treatment (such as aerosol pentamidine before a first attack of pneumocystis) unless they seek testing to find out whether they need it. Organizations must re-evaluate strongly held positions in light of the fact that early, voluntary testing has now become a medical issue, as there are many patients who clearly should receive preventive treatment even though they feel fine and have no outward sign of illness.

The AIDS community needs to tell its advocates what kind of representation it wants. Are we satisfied to accept projections of tens or hundreds of thousands of deaths, without making any effort to change a system which keeps new treatments in the drug development and regulatory "pipeline" for years longer than necessary? Are we willing to accept a consensus which keeps designing trials which are so unworkable and inhumane that it is widely believed that patients must be denied access to treatments outside of trials, or else nobody would volunteer and the trials could not be conducted?

The death consensus is so entrenched that it is hard to know where to begin to change it. One Washington, DC-based PWA organizer made what seems to be an excellent suggestion. The way to start, he suggested, is to develop a coalition of those who already agree, then use that coalition to force other friends of the AIDS community to face the issue. He only saw three groups already mobilized for saving the lives of those now infected or ill: persons with AIDS or HIV, "treatment physicians," and some AIDS activists.

While today the picture is bleak, there are great pressures for change. Treatment will inevitably become a central issue in AIDS, as more and more people see that it affects them. Meanwhile, the first steps are clear. We need to develop explicit consensus among those already committed to saving the lives of persons with AIDS or HIV, and then talk with those among our friends who have so far refused to become involved.

## Footnote:

[1] The 18-month figure for the doubling time of the AIDS death rate, used in part I of this article, is approximately consistent with the projection of the U.S. Public Health

Service of 179,000 deaths at the end of 1991. In San Francisco, however, the projections fortunately indicate a longer doubling time, between two to three years. There are many possible reasons for this difference, among them different statistical methods used, the later stage of the epidemic in San Francisco, and much earlier safer-sex education in San Francisco than nationally.

# Issue Number 79
# May 19, 1989

## PERSANTINE: ANTI-CLOTTING DRUG MAY ENHANCE AZT, DDC

*by John S. James*

An inexpensive prescription drug used orally to prevent blood clots in persons with certain heart conditions has been found to substantially increase the effectiveness of AZT in laboratory tests, without increasing its toxicity to bone marrow or other human cells. This finding, by a team of researchers at the U.S. National Cancer Institute, was published this week in the *Proceedings of the National Academy of Sciences, USA* (volume 86, pages 3842-3846, May 15, 1989). The drug has not yet been tested in patients in combination with AZT, so its safety and effectiveness for anti-HIV use are not known.

The drug, dipyridamole (abbreviated DPM—the brand name is Persantine) had little or no antiviral effect by itself. But in laboratory tests, it allowed AZT concentrations to be reduced by a factor of five to ten times and still have the same anti-HIV activity as the larger amount of AZT without the DPM. The concentration of DPM needed to achieve this effect was greater than or equal to two micromoles; usual oral doses of 100 to 400 mg per day produce blood levels of two to six micromoles, suggesting that such doses would likely be effective.

These tests were done in human macrophages, which are believed to be the major reservoir of HIV. DPM also enhanced the anti-HIV effect of ddC, an experimental antiviral in the same class as AZT, in macrophages.

The researchers discovered this effect of DPM by chance. They do not know why it occurred, but suspect that the mechanism may be one which would apply only to nucleoside analogs (such as AZT, ddC, or ddI), not to other kinds of antivirals.

DPM is an old, well-known drug and generally considered safe. We checked medical reference books and found no indication of serious toxicities when the drug is taken by mouth (toxicity from larger intravenous doses has been reported). According to the *Physician's Desk Reference*, there are no known contraindications; only a few precautions are listed. Adverse reactions "are usually minimal and transient"; side effects generally disappear with long-term use. However, as far as we know the drug has never been tested with persons with HIV, and there may be need for special precautions. For example, since DPM works as an anticoagulant by inhibiting the action of platelets, it could be dangerous for persons with low platelet counts; a hematologist we spoke to was very concerned about this risk. Physicians will need to weigh potential risks and benefits.

According to a May 15 report in the *San Francisco Chronicle*, DPM has already been reviewed by a committee at the U.S. National Institute of Allergy and Infectious Diseases (NIAID), and plans are being developed for a clinical trial combining DPM and AZT, although no date for the trial has yet been set. Trials are necessary because the laboratory results do not prove that the drug will be useful against AIDS, or even safe when combined with AZT.

DPM should not be confused with heparin or dextran sulfate, which are also anticoagulants. DPM is different in that it is not an antiviral by itself.

## Comment

We see these laboratory findings as especially important because of the ease with which this potential treatment can be tested, and if found to be useful, made widely available. Physicians can legally prescribe DPM for any use, although understandably they may be reluctant to do so, since as of this date the drug may never have been tried in patients for the purpose of enhancing AZT. DPM costs little—about 50 cents a day or less in its generic versions—so cost will seldom be an obstacle to availability.

We are concerned that trials will take too long, either because of bureaucracy before they even start, or because of inherently slow designs, such as having to wait for opportunistic infections or deaths (in an AZT-plus-placebo group) to gain irrefutable statistical proof of efficacy. Much faster trials are possible, for example looking for clear benefit from giving DPM to persons who are already taking AZT but not getting enough results from it.

Since many people cannot wait for trials to be completed, it seems inevitable that some patients and physicians will try DPM in combination with AZT; if they get good results, more will follow. Community-based or other research organizations could perform an important service by monitoring and documenting the results of any such use.

The example of DPM illustrates one of the major although largely unrecognized public policy problems in the management of research on AIDS and other diseases—the lack of any institutional advocacy for the interests of patients in getting treatment sooner. The FDA and the NIH do not do this job; neither do drug companies, medical associations, most physicians, universities, foundations, or AIDS service organizations. It is tragic that in a major emergency we have had to take the time to develop new organizations (such as ACT UP) from scratch, because existing institutions have refused to become involved.

# HYPERICIN CAUTION

While we are continuing to hear many good reports on hypericin, an antiviral available in St. John's wort extracts (see *AIDS Treatment News* issues # 77, 75, 74, and 63), we have also heard of two more patients taken off the treatment by their physicians because of abnormally high values on liver-function tests.

Both patients had been using tablets containing St. John's wort extracts for four or five weeks (we do not know what kind of tablets, or what doses), when transaminase levels were found to be about five times normal. In both cases the levels returned to normal after the patients stopped using the tablets. Neither was using any other treatment likely to cause the high levels. Both were asymptomatic, and neither had baseline tests run before they started using the herbal extracts.

We talked to Dr. David Payne in Mesa, Arizona, who has several dozen patients who are using hypericin extracts (many from St. John's wort tablets), and he has not seen any problem of abnormal liver-function tests. He has seen many HIV-positive patients with elevated liver-function values without any treatment. In those using hypericin, the values often go down.

At this point we do not know whether St. John's wort extracts are causing abnormal liver-function tests in some people, or whether those patients would have had high values anyway. The tests have returned to normal after the treatment was stopped, and there is no evidence of any lasting harm. But it would be dangerous to ignore a potential problem by not getting the tests (which are usually given as part of a blood-chemistry panel). Anyone using St. John's wort should tell their physician, and should have a blood-chemistry panel including liver functions probably within the first few weeks of starting, if they plan to continue using the herb, so that the treatment can be discontinued if necessary.

# NEW NIH HOTLINE FOR CLINICAL TRIALS INFORMATION

The National Institutes of Health (NIH) has set up a new toll-free hotline to provide information about all NIH clinical trials of experimental AIDS treatments. Persons considering volunteering for a trial can call 800/TRIALS-A between 9:00 AM and 7:00 PM Eastern time, Monday through Friday. Three health workers (including one who speaks Spanish) will provide the information from a computer database which is updated weekly.

At this time the hotline has information about NIH trials—about a third of all AIDS trials in the United States. Within the next few months, the system plans to expand to include the other trials also, by incorporating a database of non-NIH trials currently being developed by the FDA. There are also plans to make this information directly accessible to the public by personal computer, through database services already provided by the National Library of Medicine.

NIH trials are currently being conducted at over 100 hospitals and medical centers throughout the United States, and at the NIH Clinical Center in Bethesda, MD. There are trials for adults and for children, and for persons at all stages of HIV infection, including those who are asymptomatic.

The hotline is sponsored by the National Institute of Allergy and Infectious Diseases (NIAID), in cooperation with the Centers for Disease Control (CDC).

## Comment

It has long been difficult for those who want to volunteer for trials to find out what trials are available. At the same time, many trials have been greatly delayed because they cannot find volunteers. The new NIH hotline service should help with these problems. We need to see how well it works in practice, and would appreciate hearing from our readers about their experiences in using it.

Persons considering volunteering for trials should also obtain *A Practical Guide to Clinical Research*, published by the American Foundation for AIDS Research (AmFAR), with support from NIAID. It was published as a special issue of AmFAR's *AIDS/HIV Experimental Treatment Directory*, February, 1989. It can be obtained for $10 (free for persons with HIV who cannot afford it) from AmFAR, 212/719-0033; or by mail, send a check to AmFAR, 1515 Broadway, Suite 3601, New York, NY 10036.

## BETA INTERFERON TRIAL SEEKS PATIENTS WHO HAD TO REDUCE AZT DOSE

A clinical trial of beta interferon and low-dose AZT is recruiting patients who could not tolerate full-dose AZT and had to reduce the dose. Beta interferon is an antiviral which may work like alpha interferon but have fewer side effects.

In the laboratory, beta interferon reduced the amount of AZT needed to stop HIV replication by up to two-hundredfold, according to a physicians' fact sheet prepared by the developer. Patients using the drug have had a much lower than expected incidence of opportunistic infections, although it is still too early to be sure that this effect was not due to chance.

The trial is taking place at 20 sites in 12 cities in the U.S.: Baltimore, Boston, Chicago, Cleveland, Galveston/Houston, Irvine (CA), Los Angeles, New York City, Philadelphia, San Francisco, Tampa Bay Area, and Washington, DC. One third of the patients will receive high-dose beta interferon (45 million units), one third low dose (9 million units), and one third placebo; all patients will also be using AZT. The interferon is self-administered once per day by subcutaneous injection.

There is no charge for participating in the trial; however, the study will not pay for the AZT. If beta interferon proves effective, patients who complete the study or are dropped through no fault of their own will be able to receive the interferon free indefinitely.

To qualify for the study, patients must have AIDS or T-cell counts under 200, must not currently have poorly controlled opportunistic infections, extensive KS, or HIV wasting syndrome, and must have hematologic toxicity which required AZT dose reduction but allows 500-600 mg per day to be used. There are several other requirements in addition, such as acceptable liver and kidney function. Full information on eligibility requirements can be obtained from the number below.

The trial is sponsored by Triton Biosciences (a subsidiary of Shell Oil Company), of Alameda, CA. For more information, patients or physicians can call 800/432-2828.

## SAN FRANCISCO: HIV TREATMENT AWARENESS WEEK, JUNE 22–25, 1989

A series of events sponsored by several San Francisco AIDS and health agencies will discuss treatment-related issues including medical strategies for AIDS/HIV treatment, immune system monitoring for asymptomatics, access to insurance, HIV discrimination and the law, and political action for access to treatment. Sponsoring organizations are Project Inform, AIDS Service Providers Association of the Bay Area, Bayview Hunter's Point Foundation, Latino AIDS Project of Instituto Familiar de La Raza, Mobilization Against AIDS, San Francisco AIDS Foundation, and the San Francisco Department of Public Health.

A public-policy symposium on Thursday, June 22, from 9 AM to 5 PM, will focus on economic issues and access to treatment, especially for the disadvantaged. Rev. Jesse Jackson will give the closing address.

A medical symposium on the following day, Friday June 23, includes an opening address by Anthony Fauci, M.D., Director, National Institute of Allergies and Infectious Diseases, and concurrent sessions on psychosocial/medical issues, clinical roundtable on case management, and adjunctive therapies, including nutrition and Eastern medicine.

On Saturday, June 24, there will be an all-day health fair, with roundtables and exhibits. The program will close with a tea dance fundraiser party, Sunday June 25, 4:00 PM to 9:00 PM at The Arena, Civic Auditorium

## NEEDED: COMPULSORY LICENSING OF PHARMACEUTICALS?

*by John S. James*

Compulsory licensing, a concept used in the copyright law in the United States and many other countries, is also applied to patented pharmaceuticals in Canada. Under this part of Canadian patent law, a company can in certain circumstances market a drug patented by another company. It pays a royalty to the patent holder; the royalty percentage is set by a government agency. This system is called **compulsory** licensing because the patent holder cannot stop the other company from using its drug (and paying it a royalty for doing so).

In the United States, it would probably be impossible to pass such a law over the opposition of the pharmaceutical industry; too many lawmakers are more influenced by campaign contributions than by the public interest. We suggest the concept because a limited kind of compulsory licensing might be in the interest of pharmaceutical companies (and therefore politically possible), as well as in the interest of persons with serious or life-threatening illnesses. Compulsory licensing could overcome the liability problems which otherwise block the treatment use of new drugs even when government agencies ask for their release. It could place responsibility for emergency access to drugs clearly in the hands of the government, which has public accountability, as private companies do not. It would not open the door to quackery, because compulsory licensing would only be used for drugs requested by government bodies for emergency treatment use. And it might be acceptable to the industry, because whenever it was used it would turn an unmarketable drug which was only a loss to the company which held the patent into a risk-free, trouble-free source of profit instead.

In Canada, compulsory licensing of pharmaceutical patents has been the law since 1923. Its main purpose is to keep drug prices low by encouraging generic pharmaceuticals. Compulsory licensing was not used very often until 1969, however, because until that year the generic drug had to be manufactured in Canada in order to qualify for such a license. In 1969, an amendment allowed imported drugs to qualify also, and compulsory licensing became more widely used.

According to a 1985 Canadian report (by the Commission of Inquiry on the Pharmaceutical Industry), the law had succeeded in greatly reducing drug prices, at no cost to the overall profitability of the Canadian pharmaceutical industry. However, that industry has bitterly opposed compulsory licensing, and after great controversy significant restrictions were adapted in 1987.

As far as we know, Canada is the only country with compulsory licensing of pharmaceuticals. In the United States, a bill proposing such a system was introduced in the House of Representatives in 1981.

In the United States today, compulsory licensing could be most important when patent holders have refused to allow the use of irreplaceable drugs for treating AIDS or other serious diseases (through compassionate use or through the "treatment IND"), even when the FDA has pleaded with them to do so. Under current law, there is no public recourse for access to such drugs. And companies have no incentive to make the drugs available, since it is expensive to do so and the manufacturers are seldom allowed to charge anything, even to reimburse their costs. In addition, they could face product liability lawsuits in the future, another reason to deny use of the drug, for which they are usually the only legal source. All existing incentives are for companies to deny access to potentially lifesaving drugs, before completion of the years-long process of obtaining full marketing approval. In the United States today, allowing physicians to use any experimental drug is all cost and no benefit to the company which holds the patent rights.

Under compulsory licensing, a government body (probably a commission set up within in the Public Health Service) could designate drugs urgently needed for treatment use (not for general marketing), and issue a license to any qualified company which contracted to supply the drug. The price would be set in the contract. The commission would also set a fair royalty (probably a percentage of the contract price), which would be paid to the patent holder. The patent holder would therefore receive a royalty without any trouble or expense—or any risk of liability, since it had done nothing to provide the drug. It would also benefit from data which could speed full marketing approval, and also from the favorable publicity of having its drug selected by an independent body as beneficial and indeed essential.

The cost for this system would be minimal, for several reasons. The price for the drug would presumably be low, near the generic price; this emergency access system would not have to pay for the cost of development of the drug, since compulsory licensing places no additional cost on the licensor, but only provides pure profit. If the government paid for the drug, the total cost would also be kept low by the fact that few drugs would be distributed this way, as this system would be used only when urgently necessary. The cost of deciding which drugs to release would also be low, since only a few obvious candidates would ever be considered. (By contrast, the FDA must consider thousands of drug applications, and apply much more thorough criteria to approve for general marketing than would be appropriate to approve for treatment use in an emergency.)

In the United States, the concept of compulsory licensing of patented pharmaceuticals has been absent from public discussion. We suggest that the idea be investigated and considered, so that legislation to provide this access to essential treatments can be proposed if necessary.

## REFERENCES

Chromecek, M. The amended Canadian patent act: general amendments and pharmaceutical patents compulsory licensing provisions. *Fordham International Law Journal*, volume 11 number 3, pages 504-548, Spring 1988.

Hayhurst, WL. Food for thought: compulsory licensing of patents. *Intellectual Property Journal*, volume 1 number 1, pages 73-76, July 1984.

Shulman, SR, and Richard, BW. The 1987 Canadian patent law amendments: revised pharmaceutical compulsory licensing provisions. *Food Drug Cosmetic Law Journal*, volume 43 number 5, pages 745-757, September 1988.

U.S. House of Representatives. HR 915, compulsory licensing of prescription drug patents (12 cosponsors). *House Proceedings*, 97-046, page H1049, March 23, 1981.

# PML, TOXOPLASMOSIS AND MAI: SURVEYING THE OPTIONS

*by Denny Smith*

The early years of the epidemic made clear that people who are immunocompromised are susceptible to infections from various bacteria, fungi, viruses and protozoa which would ordinarily be harmless. Since these microorganisms take advantage of a disarmed immune system, they are described as "opportunistic" infections (OIs).

The most familiar of these is a pneumonia caused by the organism *Pneumocystis carinii* (PCP). *P. carinii* is found everywhere in the environment and exposure to it is impossible to avoid. But PCP has become one of the most treatable of OIs, if diagnosed early enough. And the FDA recently acknowledged what thousands of people with HIV and their physicians already knew: that a decline in T-helper cells to 200 or less warrants the use of a prophylaxis (preventive measure) such as dapsone, sulfa trimethoprim or aerosol pentamidine to ward off even a first bout with PCP.

Other opportunistic infections have generally been handled less successfully than PCP, particularly MAI, toxoplasmosis and PML. But new experimental approaches to all three of these are receiving attention, and it is possible that the risk for developing the first two can be lessened by avoiding routine exposure to the responsible pathogens. This article suggests some precautions, and surveys the drugs now being tried or considered to control active infections. Many of the drugs mentioned are FDA approved, and a doctor can prescribe them as she or he determines appropriate for any condition. If they are only investigational in the U.S. we will indicate so, although new guidelines allow the importation of drugs approved in other countries if prescribed by a physician for personal use. As any treatments, approved or unapproved, gain a strong consensus as effective (or ineffective) therapies, we will report on them in depth. Until then we want to name the possibilities we are aware of in order to maximize the choices of people with these diagnoses and their physicians.

## PML

Progressive multifocal leukoencephalopathy (PML) is an uncommon but devastating brain infection with an historically bleak outlook, and many physicians have opted not to initiate treatment, or simply rely hopefully on AZT for its antiviral and CNS access capacity. The results of intervention in the progress of PML have increased the possible options, however, enough to justify an aggressive attempt to treat.

This OI probably results from reactivation of a latent papovavirus to which most people gain immunity after childhood exposure. Some symptoms of PML, such as headaches, confusion, visual impairment in one or both eyes, aphasia (difficulty with verbal comprehension or expression) or loss of muscle coordination on one side of the body, can resemble toxoplasmosis, herpes encephalitis or meningitis. Each of those infections, as well as PML, can be imminently life-threatening and should be seen immediately by an AIDS-knowledgeable physician, who may consult a neurologist. Someone experiencing these symptoms may become too disoriented to respond quickly to the situation, so the observant help of friends or family could make a difference. The time from appearance of symptoms to diagnosis to treatment is crucial for PML or other AIDS-related neurological infections.

*AIDS Treatment News* recommends to interested readers a very comprehensive, well-researched report on experimental treatments for PML compiled by two concerned AIDS activists in Los Angeles, Lisa A. Muller and Peter L. Brosnan, with an introduction by Ronald Webeck, a long-term survivor of PML. The treatments discussed in this report were drawn from current medical literature and include beta interferon, vidarabine (adenine arabinoside, or ARA-A), cytarabine (cytosine arabinoside, or ARA-C), alpha-2 interferon, acyclovir, clonazepam, trimethoprim with sulfamethoxazole, and dexamethasone combined first with sulfadiazine and then with pyrimethamine. The first three in the list appeared to be more effective when administered intrathecally (injected into the spinal fluid) instead of intravenously. The others were tried only intravenously. (Clonazepam is probably useful to control convulsions which may accompany PML, but not as a primary treatment.)

Some of these drugs have side effects which people with HIV and their doctors would usually weigh carefully, but the gravity of an untreated PML infection may override these concerns, and AIDS-experienced physicians often make similar compromises in treating other OIs. None of these drugs have been proven to work repeatedly, but accumulated attempts to treat PML **have** resulted in better survival rates than nontreatment. The articles referenced from the literature are included in entirety in the report's appendix, making it self-contained and practical for outpatient clinics and AIDS-care health professionals

❏

## Toxoplasmosis

AIDS-related toxoplasmosis is a serious infection of the central nervous system caused by the protozoan *Toxoplasma gondii*. The symptoms of toxoplasmic encephalitis can be difficult to diagnose with certainty, but as mentioned above call for urgent attention.

Various mammals and birds can be infected with *T. gondii*, but only cats appear to harbor the reproductive forms of the organism. Resting forms called oocysts are shed by cats in their feces, where they can survive in the soil for more than a year. Here they are a ready source of infection for other animals and humans. In humans the oocysts themselves are not damaging, but when the multiplicative forms, or active parasites, break out of the cysts they are capable of causing disease in infants and immunosuppressed adults. Active parasite forms of *T. gondii* can also be transmitted to people in undercooked meat.

The standard treatment for toxoplasmosis is pyrimethamine with sulfadiazine. These drugs are effective against the parasite, but they do not destroy oocysts, so a continuous maintenance dose is necessary to squelch emerging parasites. Some people reach toxic intolerance of these drugs, and folinic acid (Leucovorin) is then used to diminish this toxicity. Pyrimethamine is also being studied in combinations with dapsone, trimetrexate, clindamycin and spiramycin (investigational), instead of sulfadiazine. Clindamycin is probably substituted most often.

Issue #75 of *AIDS Treatment News* reported on two other promising options for toxoplasmosis: roxithromycin, approved in France, and azithromycin, approved in Yugoslavia. They may be as effective as pyrimethamine/sulfadiazine but more easily tolerated. However, we do not know results of human use for toxoplasmosis at this time. Roxithromycin might be obtainable through buyers' clubs (see paragraph above).

The abstracts of the 1988 Interscience Conference on Antimicrobial Agents and Chemotherapy (ICAAC) presented results of varying combinations of pyrimethamine, sulfadiazine and arprinocid (investigational) against *T. gondii* in mice. Arprinocid was found to work poorly when combined with pyrimethamine, and pyrimethamine alone was somewhat more effective that either sulfadiazine or arprinocid alone. But arprinocid and sulfadiazine together worked synergistically, the best combination tried. Additionally, a metabolite of arprinocid called arprinocid-N-oxide was more effective alone in smaller doses than arprinocid (Luft and Frankel, abstract number 1420). Unfortunately, another study found that AZT made pyrimethamine much less effective in animal tests (Israelski, Tom, and Remington, abstract number 349).

In January 1988 in *The Journal of Infectious Diseases*, Drs. Benjamin L. Luft and Jack S. Remington authored a comprehensive discussion of diagnostic procedures and potential therapies for toxoplasmosis. In addition to many of the drugs mentioned above they proposed the investigational agents gamma interferon and interleukin-2 as candidates against *T. gondii*.

Lastly, researchers at the Robert Koch Institute in Berlin found that monophosphoryl lipid A, or MPL (not FDA approved), enhanced resistance in mice when administered before or at the same time they were injected with *T. gondii* (Masihi and others, 1988). This raises the possibility of prophylaxis or chronic suppressive therapy for toxoplasmosis. Also, we have heard anecdotally that people who are taking Septra for PCP show a reduced incidence of toxoplasmosis. Hopefully some trends will be identified for practical use.

Most physicians we spoke with feel that AIDS-related toxoplasmosis is a reactivated infection from early, common exposure to *T. gondii*; and indeed a large portion of the world's population is chronically but asymptomatically infected. Of people with AIDS who have the antibodies which verify this latent infection, at least 30% develop toxoplasmic encephalitis. This incidence may reflect the comparative virulence of different parasite strains operating within a context of immunodeficiency. But another consideration factor for the progression from latent to symptomatic infection is inoculum threshold—the amount or concentration necessary to cause illness in someone. "Superinfection", or repeated exposure, could be a mode of reaching this threshold. It seems reasonably possible, especially for an immunocompromised person, that some infections might be avoided or suppressed by minimizing exposure to the organism.

Obviously, cat litter boxes could be kept away from food preparation and eating areas, and the litter disposed of by someone who is not at risk for toxoplasmosis. Cats should not be fed raw meat, and anyone who handles a cat or changes the litter should wash their hands thoroughly afterward. In this regard, toxoplasmosis is a "zoonotic" disease, one that can be transmitted from animals to humans.(1) Since birds, cats, fish, reptiles and rodents can all carry various zoonotic diseases, people with pets should **observe careful handwashing** after handling pets and before meals or food preparation.

# MAI

MAI (*Mycobacterium avium intracellulare*) is one of a group of mycobacteria, others of which can cause tuberculosis and Hansen's disease (leprosy). MAI is found widely in soil, dust, untreated water and bird droppings. Formerly a lung infection occurring primarily in people who have chronic lung disease or are on steroids, MAI infection (or *M. avium* Complex—MAC) in PWAs is usually disseminated throughout the body and can cause fatigue, fever, sweats, anemia, diarrhea and serious weight loss. There are quite a few drugs being tried for MAI, although it appears to respond very slowly.

The March 30, 1989 edition of Treatment Issues, published by the Gay Men's Health Crisis, reports on the following drugs for consideration in the treatment of MAI: isoniazid (INH), rifampin (Rifadin), rifabutin (Ansamycin), ethambutol (Myambutol), amikacin (Amikin), imipenem (Primaxin), ethionamide (Trecator), clofazimine (Lamprene), ciprofloxacin (Cipro), ofloxacin, cycloserine (Seromycin), erythromycin (Robimycin) and azithromycin. Usually several of these are tried in combination. The article includes diagnostic information about MAI, as well as MTB *(Mycobacterium tuberculosis)*, for which PWAs are also at risk. To obtain this article, write to GMHC, Department of Medical Information, 129 West 20th Street, New York, NY 10011. Be sure to specify volume 3, number 2 on mycobacterial infections. We spoke with Shelley M. Gordon, M.D. who is an infectious disease specialist with Pacific-Presbyterian Medical Center in San Francisco. She has observed the best response so far in MAC from a combination of rifampin, ethambutol and clofazimine, with amikacin included as warranted.

Researchers at Shimane Medical University in Japan have strengthened the rifampin activity against *M. avium*-infected macrophages in mice by encapsulating rifampin in liposomes. Liposomal vescicles are already widely used to enhance the delivery of other antimicrobial drugs, and the researchers suggest that this technique is particularly suited to treat persistent infections like MAI. Of related interest, three separate studies presented at last year's International Conference on AIDS in Stockholm suggested that rifabutin in v*itro* demonstrated anti-HIV activity, especially when combined with heparin. This could provide an option for many people with MAI who cannot take AZT, although some physicians, including Dr. Gordon, feel it is neither convincingly active against HIV nor noticeably better than rifampin for treating MAI. Despite its investigational status, rifabutin was widely available to physicians who wished to prescribe it; recently the manufacturer cut off compassionate access for new patients.

Amikacin, azithromycin and roxithromycin have been examined in various combinations with tumor necrosis factor (TNF), a natural product of the immune system which is synthesized and being tested for other diagnoses, particularly Kaposi's sarcoma. *M. avium*-infected human macrophages were more susceptible *in vitro* to each antibiotic when tried with TNF than compared to any antibiotic alone. The mycobactericidal action was strongest when TNF was combined with both amikacin and roxithromycin. The researchers of that study suggest that the pairing of immunomodulators with antimicrobial agents could be a useful treatment for MAI. In addition to some of the drugs mentioned above three more possibilities were presented at the 1988 ICAAC conference: fusidic acid (Fusidin), which may also have anti-HIV activity and which is approved in Canada and the U.K. but not in the U.S., temafloxacin, and sulfisoxazole (Gantrisin).

As a prophylactic measure to keep a latent MAI infection inactive, San Francisco physicians working with the County Community Consortium are studying the effect of low-dose clofazimine (50 mg daily). People taking clofazimine, however, should be aware that in rare cases it can accumulate as crystals in various parts of the body, including the liver, spleen and intestinal membranes. One friend of ours who was taking clofazimine experienced a mildly enlarged liver and elevated liver enzymes which eluded diagnosis. He looked up the warnings for the drug in the *Physicians Desk*

*Reference* and brought this to his doctor's attention. The clofazimine was discontinued but it is too early to draw a clear connection. We hope physicians prescribing MAI treatments carefully explain any side effects to watch for (such as anemia, dizziness, allergic rashes, kidney impairment, emotional depression, skin discoloration, etc), especially since some drug side effects can be confused with symptoms of AIDS-related infections.

As with toxoplasmosis, active symptoms of *M. avium* are often assumed to originate from an old exposure which remained unnoticed as a latent, immune-controlled infection. Although MAI is widely present in water and soil, it may be feasible and advantageous to decrease exposure to it. Keith Barton, M.D., of Berkeley recommends to all his patients with AIDS that they not eat raw foods, especially salad and root vegetables, or unpasteurized milk or cheese, and that the water they drink be boiled. The bacteria are killed at around 80 degrees centigrade, which means any conventional cooking (oven, stove, steamer) is sufficient to neutralize MAI in vegetables and meat. An alternative to cooking vegetables or fresh fruit is to peel and rinse any surface which could have been exposed to soil or irrigation water. Of Dr. Barton's patients who follow this advice, only three have developed an active MAI infection, a much lower incidence than he would have expected otherwise. This suggests that while it is not possible to avoid exposure to MAI completely, it may be worth taking precautions to minimize the risk.

We want to acknowledge that many physicians and people with HIV discount the practicality of avoiding microorganisms which are pervasive in the environment. While the measures suggested above may not completely eliminate exposure to pathogens like *M. avium* or *T. gondii*, they might keep the quantity and frequency of exposure below a disease-causing threshold. More importantly, the search for the optimum treatments of these infections should be intensified before they surpass the toll wrought by PCP early in the epidemic.

For example, we have heard from some readers that their doctors do not attempt to treat an MAI infection on the lethargic assumption that there is no treatment proven conclusively to control MAI. When we called the offices of the National Institute of Allergy and Infectious Diseases (NIAID) to clarify the status of some promising drugs, the person we spoke with was very helpful but repeated the same idea with nearly the same words: NIAID does not recommend a treatment for MAI because none has been shown to be so effective that it could win FDA approval as an MAI treatment, even though most of them are approved for other infections and have been available to physicians for the entire epidemic. While waiting for the perfect treatment, disregarding some that only might be useful, how many people with MAI (or Kaposi's sarcoma, or plummeting T-helper cells) discovered the consequences of waiting?

Current medical literature sometimes asks a more laissez-faire question: "Did this patient die **with** MAI or **from** MAI?" The question would be unnecessary if new potential treatments were pursued aggressively and intelligently until a potent choice or combination of choices surfaced. MAI, like HIV, is damaging partly for its tendency to invade the disease-fighting cells called macrophages. An unchallenged MAI infection could tip the scales on a depleted immune system, clearing the path for other opportunistic infections and providing another reason for treating MAI. The approach to toxoplasmosis has a similarly pessimistic history but for different reasons. The drugs of choice have been clearer than for those for MAI, but they are seriously limited by toxicity. Now the possibilities for treating toxoplasmosis are growing, those for MAI are being refined, and some for PML are getting initial recognition. The pessimistic prognosis surrounding these OIs appears to be changing, and the rate of change could use a push by recognizing these infections early and intervening with as many treatment options necessary.

# REFERENCES

Hawkins, CC and others. *Mycobacterium avium* Complex infections in Patients with the Acquired Immunodeficiency Syndrome. *Annals of Internal Medicine*, volume 105, pages 184-188, August 1986.

Bermudez, LEM and Young, LS. Activities of Amikacin, Roxithromycin, and Azithromycin Alone or in Combination with Tumor Necrosis Factor against *Mycobacterium avium* Complex. *Antimicrobial Agents and Chemotherapy*, volume 32, number 8, pages 1149-1153, August 1988.

Henry-Toulme, N and others. Immunomodulating properties of the N-(1-deoxy-D-fructos-lyl) derivative of amphotericin B in mice. *Immunology Letters,* volume 20, pages 63-67, 1989.

Masihi, K. Noel and others. Effects of Nontoxic Lipid A and Endotoxin on Resistance of Mice to *Toxoplasma gondii. Journal of Biological Response Modifiers,* volume 7, number 6, pages 535-539, 1988.

Suzuki, Y and others. Differences in Virulence and Development of Encephalitis During Chronic Infection with the Strain of *Toxoplasma gondii. The Journal of Infectious Diseases*, volume 159, number 4, pages 790-794, April 1989.

Hajime,S and Haruaki, T. Therapeutic Efficacy of Liposome-Entrapped Rifampin against *Mycobacterium avium* Complex Infection Induced in Mice. *Antimicrobial Agents and Chemotherapy*, volume 3, number 4, pages 429-433, April 1989.

(1) People often derive therapeutic companionship from pets and do not need to choose between staying healthy and having a pet. A San Francisco organization, Pets Are Wonderful Support (PAWS), acknowledges the value of a pet while encouraging people to observe precautions which minimize the risk of contracting infections from an animal. To receive their *Safe Pet Guidelines*, write to PAWS, P.O. Box 460489, San Francisco, CA 94146.

# Issue Number 80
# June 2, 1989

## CRYPTOSPORIDIOSIS: IMPORTANT TREATMENT ADVANCE?

*AIDS Treatment News* has heard credible rumors that a new drug used to kill parasites in animals might be effective for treating cryptosporidiosis, a serious opportunistic infection which causes severe diarrhea in persons with AIDS.

The drug, diclazuril (trade name Clinacox), kills parasites and their cysts in chickens, when added to their feed in as little as one part per million, or when given as a single dose of 5 mg/kg. We have heard that a few people have used diclazuril in Africa and in the United States, and that a dose of 200 mg per day or slightly more may completely eliminate cryptosporidiosis in many cases, killing both the organism and the cysts in a few days. However, the drug is not approved anywhere for human use, and we have **not yet confirmed** that the 200 mg dose is safe or effective. And no one is sure how long the treatment may need to be continued.

We do not know in which countries diclazuril is currently marketed for agricultural use.

We decided to publish this short article, despite the fragmentary information, so that others can help us investigate and learn more. If you have any information about diclazuril, please contact John James at *AIDS Treatment News*, 415/255-0588, or by mail.

## REFERENCES

No human research has been published. We obtained the following references by computer searches and have not yet seen the articles.

*Animal Pharm World Animal Health News* : Number 139, page 18, October 9, 1987; Number 140, pages 8-9, October 23, 1987; Number 166, page 14, November 4, 1988; Review issue, page 14, January 6, 1989.

Jensen, JF. Comparison of the new coccidiostat diclazuril and an approved coccidiostat in research with broilers (English translation of Danish title). *Statens Husdyrbrugsforsoeg*, number 724, October 6, 1988.

Kutzner, E and others. Diclazuril—a new anticoccidial agent for broilers (English translation of German title). *Wiener Tierarztliche Monatsschrift*, volume 75 number 11, pages 415-419, 1988.

Maes, L and others. In vivo action of the anticoccidial diclazuril (Clinacox) on the developmental stages of Eimeria tenella: a histological study. *Journal of Parasitology* volume 74 number 6, pages 931-938, December 1988

Mathis, GF and others. Anticoccidial efficacy of diclazuril in chickens. *77th Annual Meeting of the Poultry Science Association, Inc. Poult Sci* 67 (supplement 1), 115, 1988.

Verheyen, A and others. In vivo action of the anticoccidial diclazuril (Clinacox) on the developmental stages of Eimeria tenella: an ultrastructural evaluation. *J Parasitol*, volume 74 number 6, pages 939-949, December 1988.

# ITRACONAZOLE: AFFORDABLE FLUCONAZOLE SUBSTITUTE?

Fluconazole is a very good antifungal which is taken by mouth; it is effective for cryptococcal meningitis and many other fungal infections. It is approved in England, but not in the United States, apparently because of bureaucratic snafus. Some people have obtained personal supplies from England, but the drug is very expensive; maintenance doses for cryptococcal meningitis can cost almost as much as AZT, and insurance will not pay for fluconazole because it is not approved.

Another drug, itraconazole (brand name Sporanox) may be almost as good as fluconazole but much less expensive. Itraconazole is used to treat many different fungal diseases. It may be less effective than fluconazole for cryptococcal meningitis, however, although it is sometimes used for that condition (see references, below). Itraconazole is available in Mexico, and it either is or is soon expected to be available in the UK. We do not have exact price information, but have heard that treatment with itraconazole (obtained from Mexico) costs about $1.50 to $3.00 per day, depending on the dose.

Anyone considering using fluconazole or itraconazole should also consider the more conventional options. Amphotericin B (AMB), which is readily available, is probably at least as effective as fluconazole. Its drawbacks are that it must be given intravenously, it can cause unpleasant side effects, and some patients cannot tolerate it at all.

If AMB cannot be used, a patient may be able to qualify for a trial of fluconazole, or for compassionate use—in which case the drug will probably be free. **Physicians only** who want to find out how to enroll their patients should call the developer, Pfiser Inc., at 203/441-4112.

If these options do not work, then for more information about obtaining fluconazole or itraconazole from abroad, patients can call the PWA Health Group, 212/532-0280.

## REFERENCES

De Gans, J and others. Itraconazole as maintenance treatment for cryptococcal meningitis in the acquired immune deficiency syndrome. *British Medical Journal* 296/6618 (339), 1988.

Dismukes, WE. Azole antifungal drugs: old and new. *Annals of Internal Medicine* volume 109 number 3, pages 177-179, August 1, 1988.

Dupont, B. Attack and maintenance cure of cryptococcal meningitis in AIDS patients. (English translation of French title.) *Med. Mal. Infect.*, volume 18, special issue 215, pages 737-741.

Saag, MS and Dismukes, WE. Azole antifungal agents: emphasis on new triazoles. *Antimicrobial Agents and Chemotherapy* volume 32 number 1, pages 1-8, January 1988.

Tucker, RM and others. Treatment of mycoses with itraconazole. *Annals of the New York Academy of Sciences* number 544, pages 451-470, 1988.

Wishart, JM. The influence of food on the pharmacokinetics of itraconazole in patients with superficial fungal infection. *Journal of the American Academy of Dermatology* volume 17 number 2 part 1, pages 220-223, August 1987.

# SAN FRANCISCO: HYPERICIN, OZONE MONITORING PROJECTS BEGIN

*by John S. James*

San Francisco area community groups have begun two small, prospective monitoring studies to collect reliable information about potential AIDS/HIV treatments which have come into use by patients but are not being studied in formal clinical trials.

"Monitoring" studies do not give treatment to anyone; they only collect data. Therefore they are much easier to set up and administer than the large-scale, randomized trials favored by large institutions. "Prospective" means that these monitoring studies are designed in advance, allowing clean, uniform data gathering: the same blood tests for every patient, on the same schedule and at the same lab; uniform physical examinations, medical history interviews, and patient diary forms; and an overall study design approved in advance by a scientific committee. If successful, these studies can serve as precedents for rapid, community-controlled research projects to get reliable data for patients and physicians, as soon as new treatments come into use.

## The Hypericin Study

We have previously reported on hypericin, an antiretroviral found in St. John's wort, a plant long used in herbal medicine (see *AIDS Treatment News* #63, 74, 75, 77, and 78). While mainstream researchers are synthesizing the chemical, running animal studies, and negotiating for FDA permission to begin "phase I" human trials this year or next, probably hundreds of people are already using herbal extracts. We are hearing anecdotal reports of benefits, but this information is inherently limited because of unknown self-selection biases, and because different blood tests and different labs were used.

The new monitoring study, formally approved May 22 by San Francisco's Community Research Alliance (CRA; for background on this community-based research organization, see *AIDS Treatment News* issue # 70), is for people who have not used hypericin in the last six months, but plan to start using a standardized herbal extract. (Standardized extracts are those which have been chemically tested during their manufacture and adjusted to contain a uniform strength of an active ingredient in every batch. Examples of St. John's wort extracts standardized for hypericin content are Yerba Prima tablets, Psychotonin tincture, and Hyperforat tincture.)

The study will last four months. "Baseline" testing (before treatment begins) includes P24 antigen, T-cell subsets, CMI, Beta 2 microglobulin, CBC, ESR, and SMA 25, as well as a physical examination and medical history. Blood tests are given monthly; the last visit includes a second physical exam. A total of five monthly visits is required.

All tests are paid for by the CRA. At this time, the CRA has enough money to enroll 30 patients. More will be enrolled if the money can be raised.

Note: Ten patients per month will be enrolled in this observational study. If you are interested in volunteering, call the Community Research Alliance at 415/626-2145. If more than ten qualify for the study, ten will be chosen by a lottery; those not chosen the first month will be considered again at later months. The first ten may be able to start by late June. However, no starting date can be guaranteed, and there will probably be more volunteers than can be accepted.

It is very important that people who enter this study have not used hypericin in the previous six months. Otherwise, benefits may have already occurred before the first physical exam and blood test, and therefore the study would miss them and misleadingly underestimate the value of the treatment.

All other treatments (AZT, etc.) are OK, however, either before or during the study. One of the rules of a monitoring study is that it does not ask people to change the treatments they would be using anyway. These must be reported to the researchers, of course.

The Community Research Alliance is also looking for volunteers for office work, etc. If you can help, call the number above.

## Ozone Study

Ozone is being studied as an AIDS/HIV treatment in Germany, but aside from a small trial for AIDS-related diarrhea at the Veterans Administration Hospital in San Francisco, there are no government or corporate clinical trials in the United States. Recently, however, a group of ten persons with AIDS or HIV jointly purchased an ozone machine for their own use, and before beginning the treatment they organized their own monitoring study, with the help of research nurse Leland Traiman. Mr. Traiman runs mainstream AIDS clinical trials professionally, and he volunteered to help coordinate the patients' ozone trial.

This eight-month study includes the same blood tests as the hypericin protocol described above. (These tests are becoming a core subset of uniform blood work and data collection forms, to be used in many prospective monitoring studies.) Laboratory work, medical history, and physical exams were given before treatment started, to obtain baseline values; eight additional appointments were scheduled over the next eight months. The baseline and two other blood drawings have already occurred; the fourth blood draw is scheduled for the end of May.

At this time, the ozone trial is not officially sponsored by any organization; it belongs entirely to the people in the study. When they obtained the ozone machine, the Community Research Alliance was newly organized and not ready to approve and administer a study. But the patients were ready to start, and of course they did not want to wait for a study. So the Healing Alternatives Foundation (the San Francisco buyers' club) donated $2500. for initial blood work; without that support at a critical time, the baseline values could not have been obtained and the study would have been lost. The entire trial will cost about $10,000, almost all of it for lab work, as Mr. Traiman's time is volunteer. Money from an anonymous benefactor, from *AIDS Treatment News*, and from Mr. Traiman himself has kept the study going so far.

Recently the Berkeley Gay Men's Health Collective offered to assist, by housing the ozone monitoring project in the Berkeley Free Clinic building.

After seven weeks of ozone treatment, no dramatic changes have been found. At three weeks, lymphocyte counts had improved substantially for many of the patients; other blood work showed no meaningful change. By the seventh week, however, these counts had returned to close to their baseline values. At this time there is no evidence of any benefit, or of any harm, from the ozone treatment.

The lack of early results does not discourage Mr. Traiman. "There are no conclusive results so far; it's too early to tell... I don't believe or disbelieve that ozone is an effective therapy. I've heard some strong positive anecdotal reports, and I want to learn if there is any scientific basis behind them."

## A New Model for Community Response?

One of the most successful responses to the AIDS epidemic so far has been the "San Francisco model"—close cooperation between public agencies and private, mostly volunteer organizations, in providing prevention education and services to those who are ill. However, this model has traditionally not included any involvement with research.

The ozone and hypericin studies suggest a new, additional model for the years ahead. Small but well-conducted research studies are within the capabilities of grassroots organizations. The key test of the success of these projects is whether they produce information which is credible to front-line AIDS physicians, and useful to patients and physicians alike in making treatment decisions. Community groups responsive first and foremost to patients' interests can move much faster than Federal or corporate bureaucracies ever will; if they can generate solid treatment information, they will make a major contribution to saving lives and improving quality of life.

These small studies which combine the work of professionals, activists, and other volunteers are also relevant to public policy in a time of scarce resources. Monitoring studies cost very little to run. If they produce useful treatment information, they should pay for themselves many times over—by reducing the need for hospitalization and other treatment, by keeping people productively employed instead of ill, and by developing very low cost treatment options (such as hypericin herbal extracts) which other U.S. research institutions seldom or never do.

## HOW TO USE HYPERICIN

*by John S. James*

*AIDS Treatment News* has published several articles and updates on hypericin, an antiviral available in extracts of the St. John's wort plant (see *AIDS Treatment News* numbers 79, 77, 75, 74, and 63). Almost all the reports we are hearing from users are good—a fact not always reflected in our articles, as we have felt obligated to publish reports of side effects or possible dangers immediately, but have not hurried into print with the reports of benefits. Few people who have told us about their use of hypericin have failed to report benefit—usually objective improvements in symptoms, blood-test results, or both, often entirely unexpected. However, we have only received about 25 reports overall, and it is possible that we have seen a biased picture because persons who did not see any effects may not have bothered to contact us. We hope that the survey elsewhere in this issue will help to correct such bias. And the upcoming prospective monitoring study by San Francisco's Community Research Alliance (also described in this issue) should obtain better information than any survey could.

There has also been confusion about how to use hypericin. We have reported several different dosage regimens, and different brands. *AIDS Treatment News* has a policy against making its own treatment recommendations; but we have closely followed the use of hypericin herbal extracts, and since little information is available, we decided to summarize the picture as we see it.

The following three standardized extracts contain significant amounts of hypericin: Yerba Prima St. John's wort tablets, Psychotonin tincture, or Hyperforat tincture. "Standardized" means that the concentration should be uniform from batch to batch.

Of the three, the Yerba Prima tablets are much less expensive than the other two, which must be imported from Germany. As far as we know, the tablets are just as good.

*AIDS Treatment News* had a chemist test several brands, as we previously reported. Two other products, St. John's wort tinctures from Herb Pharm and from Jarrow Formulas, were found to contain comparable amounts of hypericin. These products are not standardized for hypericin content, however, so the concentration may vary.

**Not** acceptable are products which have not been independently tested. As there are no standards for herbal products in the United States, a product can be labeled "St. John's wort" no matter how little St. John's wort or hypericin it contains. Even some European extracts may have ten times less hypericin as the products we named above. We could not test everything, however, and other products we do not know about may also be good.

Also **not** acceptable are teas made from dried St. John's wort, which is sold in health-food stores. As previously reported, we have heard of little or no benefits from these teas, and one report of possible harm.

Hypericin may be especially effective for persons who are also using AZT.

What about the dose? For the Yerba Prima tablets, with which we are most familiar, the usual dose is two or three of the 250 mg, 0.14 percent hypericin tablets per day. Some people are using as many as six tablets every day. (The dose recommended on the bottle is two.) There are also intermittent schedules being tried, in which the tablets are not used every day.

Absorption and blood-level studies are now being done, with hypericin being administered intravenously, intramuscularly, and orally. Dose recommendations may change in the future. *AIDS Treatment News* will report information as it develops.

The most important safety precaution, in our view, is to have liver function tests (often included in a blood-chemistry panel) within several weeks of starting hypericin. In a handful of cases, persons using hypericin have been found to have elevated transaminase values, and their physicians had them stop all treatments which might have been responsible. While no one is sure that St. John's wort caused the problem, it would be unsafe to take risks until more is known.

Another precaution is to avoid exposure to sunlight or ultraviolet light. Photosensitivity (abnormal sensitivity to sunlight) due to St. John's wort extracts has been so rare in humans that there is debate about whether it happens at all. But again it seems better to err on the side of safety.

Drowsiness has been reported when people have used large doses of hypericin-containing extracts.

One conservative strategy for using hypericin would be to continue it only if there are clear benefits. In most of the reports we have heard, unmistakable improvements in symptoms and/or blood work were seen within a few weeks. One approach to risk reduction would be to accept the probably small risks of the treatment provided that there is clear benefits to balance the risk, but to discontinue use if there was no evidence that it was helping.


# CIMETIDINE (TAGAMET) AS IMMUNOMODULATOR, ANTITUMOR TREATMENT?

*by Denny Smith*

Cimetidine (Tagamet), commonly used to treat stomach ulcers and one of the most widely prescribed drugs in the U.S., has shown immune enhancing and antitumor activity in recent studies. In its original use, cimetidine worked by blocking the receptors on stomach cells which control digestive acid secretions, and it has also been shown to be useful for controlling herpes simplex and herpes zoster outbreaks, as well as chronic Epstein-Barr infection. (Cimetidine can slow the metabolism of other drugs, leading to increased concentrations of them in the bloodstream. This is important for drug interactions/half-life considerations.)

The results of the current studies demonstrated variously that cimetidine appeared to increase *in vitro* the proliferation and potency of lymphocytes, probably by stimulating interleukin-2 production; increased the median survival time of patients with gastric cancer and possibly lung cancer as well; enhanced natural killer activity in patients with leukemia; and reduced T8-suppressor cell activity in patients with hypogammaglobulinemia. The most interesting research relating to HIV was done at the University of Essen in West Germany. 1200 mg of cimetidine was given daily to 33 patients with ARC for five months. All of the participants showed improvement of symptoms, such as decreased fevers, diarrhea and lymph node size, and increased body weight and sensitivity to skin antigen tests. Significant increases in several immune functions were noticed, including elevated T-helper cell counts. These effects were reversible when cimetidine was stopped, and reproducible when resumed.

We spoke with S. Jeanne Bramhall, M.D. who conducted her own informal cimetidine monitoring project with five patients in Seattle. All five patients experienced relief from a number of AIDS or ARC symptoms, apparently after several weeks of Tagamet, 300 mg three times daily. Here is a brief summary of the results:

*Patient 1:* After three weeks on Tagamet and imipramine, her fatigue, night sweats and lymphadenopathy disappeared completely. These symptoms returned when the patient stopped the Tagamet, and disappeared again when she resumed. Her T-cell ratio returned to normal and the symptoms did not recur when she discontinued the Tagamet after a second three- month trial. This patient has since been lost to follow-up.

*Patient 2:* Experienced relief of disseminated herpes lesions and thrush after two weeks of Tagamet, and after three months a diagnosed Kaposi's sarcoma lesion in his mouth vanished. His T-cell ratio was improving after eight months, and he had added amitriptyline, acyclovir and ketoconazole to his medications. He also wanted to start AZT, but was apprehensive about the potential for cimetidine to increase the toxicity of certain drugs. To avoid this he replaced Tagamet with ranitidine (Zantac), a related drug which studies found somewhat as active as an immunomodulator but less likely to potentiate the toxicity of other drugs. After switching he suffered several bouts with a persistent staph infection and two episodes of PCP. He was also lost to follow-up.

*Patient 3:* Started Tagamet after hospitalization for pneumocystis. He noticed increased energy levels and diminished oral thrush and enrolled in a local AZT study. After three months the AZT had caused anemia severe enough to warrant a transfusion (bone marrow toxicity is not unusual with AZT but perhaps the potential for toxicity was enhanced with Tagamet). He elected to discontinue both medications and after a month the anemia was corrected. He now takes no medication other than Chinese herbs, but seven months after the Tagamet he has seen four KS lesions subside and has gained 25 pounds.

*Patient 4:* After a month on Tagamet, his persistent leukoplakia, intermittent fevers and diarrhea all subsided. After five months, he discontinued the Tagamet and megavitamins, thinking that they were causing a recurrence of diarrhea. At the time he was lost to follow-up, he was not on any medication and had remained symptom-free.

*Patient 5:* Fatigue decreased dramatically after one week on Tagamet, but oral thrush persisted until he increased the dose to 400 mg three times a day for a week. He discontinued Tagamet and continues to be in good health.

Dr. Bramhall is not a researcher and did not have access to substantial funds or resources. But her anecdotal results should be a springboard for more and larger studies. She points out that cimetidine is relatively a very safe drug and is available now to people with HIV and their physicians. Our thanks to Dr. Bramhall for her work and to Jonathan Lax and Jim Tavitian for helpful information. We hope to find more information on this potential treatment at the V International AIDS Conference in Montreal.

## REFERENCES

Brockmeyer, NH and others. Immunomodulatory properties of cimetidine in ARC patients. *Clinical Immunology and Immunopathology*, number 48, pages 50-60, 1988.

Tonnesen, H and others. Effect of cimetidine on survival after gastric cancer. *The Lancet*, October 29, pages 990-991, 1988.

Gifford, RRM and Tilberg, AF. Histamine type-2 antagonist immune modulation II. Cimetidine and ranitidine increase interleukin-2 production. *Surgery*, volume 102, number 2, pages 242-247, August, 1987.

Allen, JI and others. Cimetidine modulates natural killer cell function of patients with chronic lymphocytic leukemia. *Journal of Laboratory Clinical Medicine*, volume 109, number 4, pages 396-401, April 1987.

White, WB and Ballow, M. Modulation of suppressor-cell activity by cimetidine in patients with common variable hypogammaglobulinemia. *The New England Journal of Medicine*, volume 312, number 4, pages 198-202, January 24, 1985.

Armitage, JO and Sidner, RD. Antitumour effect of cimetidine? *The Lancet*, pages 882-883, April 21, 1979.

# BOOK REVIEW: EPIDEMIC POLITICS UNDER MICROSCOPE
*by Denny Smith*

*AIDS: Cultural Analysis/Cultural Activism*, edited by Douglas Crimp, is an excellent anthology published by MIT Press last year and available in its second printing this year. Fourteen essays examine the culture of contempt and disinformation which has shaped the character of AIDS in America. Four essays recommended in particular are: "AIDS, Homophobia, and Biomedical Discourse: An Epidemic of Signification," by Paula A. Treichler; "AIDS and Syphilis: The Iconography of Disease," by Sander L. Gilman; "Is the Rectum a Grave?," by Leo Bersani; and "How to Have Promiscuity in an Epidemic," by the editor.

Treichler writes: "The 'free-floating' iconography of disease attaches itself to various illnesses (real or imagined) in different societies and at different moments in history. Disease is thus restricted to a specific set of images, thereby forming a visual boundary, a limit to the idea (or fear) of disease. . . the 'taming' of syphilis and other STDs with the introduction of antibiotics in the 1940s left our culture with a series of images of mortally infected and infecting people suffering a morally repugnant disease—without a sufficiently powerful disease to function as the referent of these images. . . AIDS appeared then as the perfect referent."

In the following passage Douglas Crimp quotes Senator Jesse Helms in the right-wing lawmaker's effort to foment support for an amendment to deny Federal funds for gay safe sex education.

" . . . about 10 days ago I went down to the White House and I visited with the President. I said, 'Mr. President, I don't want to ruin your day, but I feel obliged to hand you this and let you look at what is being distributed under the pretense of AIDS educational material . . .'

"The President opened the book, looked at a couple of pages and shook his head, and hit his desk with his fist."

The book in question was "precisely the sort of safe sex education material that has been proven to work, developed by the organization (Gay Men's Health Crisis) that has produced the greatest amount of safe sex education material of any in the country, including of course, the Federal government . . . when we see how compromised any efforts at responding to AIDS will be when conducted by the state, we are forced to recognize that all productive practices concerning AIDS will remain at the grass-roots level."

# Issue Number 81
# June 16, 1989

## NEWS FLASH 6/28: UNOFFICIAL "COMPOUND Q" STUDY

*by John S. James*

A so-called "secret study" of trichosanthin, the experimental AIDS treatment also called Compound Q, became a focus of national controversy after one of the patients died. All indications so far are that the drug **did not** contribute to the cause of death. But the controversy has furthered a much-needed national discussion over the design and implementation of clinical trials during a public-health emergency.

The project, a treatment program organized by Project Inform of San Francisco, included very thorough monitoring of laboratory test results and the clinical condition of over 30 patients in four U.S. cities, treated by their physicians with trichosanthin. The drug was obtained from China, where it has been widely used for almost two decades. All patients received the lowest dose used for any purpose in China; this dose was repeated three times at weekly intervals. The patients selected were very ill and had failed all other treatments. No one was charged anything to participate; all labor and expenses were donated by the physicians, or by Project Inform or others.

While early indications are promising, Project Inform emphasizes that it is too early to tell if trichosanthin will be useful as an AIDS treatment; the organization hopes to make a full report available in one to two months. Also, the drug is similar to chemotherapy and can cause severe side effects in some patients; it must not be used without proper medical supervision. A major reason for organizing this monitoring project was that people were already using the drug as an AIDS treatment, with unknown and potentially serious risks.

We will cover the trichosanthin monitoring study (and the debate around it) in depth in future issues. Meanwhile, readers can learn the basic facts from newspapers such as the *San Francisco Chronicle*, *San Francisco Examiner*, *The New York Times*, and the *Los Angeles Times*.

## Comment

This monitoring study is as thorough, professional, and careful as any trial we have seen, and it promises to be a turning point in efforts to control the AIDS epidemic. It shows that clinical trials can develop useful information very quickly when they are organized to do so, and when patients are well informed of the unavoidable risks and willing to accept them.

If trichosanthin turns out to be valuable as an AIDS treatment, then this project could save thousands of lives. Everyone involved deserves our gratitude and support.

# MONTREAL CONFERENCE: OVERVIEW AND COMMENT

*by John S. James*

The "V International Conference on AIDS", June 4-9 in Montreal, was the major AIDS conference of 1989. We have found it difficult to cover this meeting.

Why the difficulty? With over 5,000 papers on AIDS presented, we could easily have filled several issues with interesting facts and stories, each one safely documented. But these would have been isolated stories with no particular use or relevance. We want to present this information within a meaningful framework.

The widespread myth of objectivity, a myth cultivated to support the status quo, has obscured the fact that viewpoints, interpretations, or relationships can be essential tools for effective communication, not just extraneous opinion. The lack of coherent, well-formed viewpoints explains the seeming paradox of having simultaneously too little AIDS information, and too much. Persons seeking information are flooded with unconnected facts but unable to find what they need.

It is hard to cover the Montreal conference because viewpoints must be constructed for this purpose. No single theme emerged.

As many as fifteen official meetings ran simultaneously, together with hundreds of poster presentations, as well as press conferences and private or miscellaneous meetings. We had to choose certain areas, and leave important subjects to others. We did not focus on AZT, for example, because we knew that many physicians would be paying close attention to this treatment, and therefore important developments would probably not be lost. Instead, we sought information which could be overlooked by the mainstream, but which the AIDS community might use to save lives.

Several different themes emerged as most important:

(1) Lack of progress on getting new drugs ready to use;

(2) Promising drugs in the research/approval pipeline;

(3) More information (mostly negative) on certain "alternative" treatments;

(4) New treatment ideas; and

(5) Access issues, including early treatment and developing countries.

## Lack of Progress

The central impression from the conference is disappointment at the lack of productivity of the clinical-trial system during the last several years. Dozens of promising drugs are in the research/regulatory pipeline; the problem is getting them **out** of the pipeline.

Two years ago, when the same conference was held in Washington, D.C., some of the AIDS physicians said, "Next year, in Stockholm." A year ago, after the Stockholm conference, it was, "Maybe next year, in Montreal." This time we did not hear the same expectations for the 1990 conference in San Francisco. The experimental drugs are more promising than ever. But people are learning that the research designs now in use could not possibly release important antivirals for years—even when we already have every reason to believe that the drugs are safe and probably will make an important contribution to therapy.

The world according to press releases designed by public-relations professionals is a world where everybody involved shares a sense of urgency, and is proceeding as fast as good science will allow, but no faster. In this world, new treatments could appear almost any time, as if by magic. But a look behind the press releases at the actual design and operation of clinical trials shows clearly that there will be no decisive advances in AIDS treatments by the 1990 San Francisco conference, or the 1991 Florence conference either, if the design and management of trials continues as it is going today.

Fortunately, the impediments to productivity are becoming more clear. Our article below ("Why No Antivirals: A Case History of Failed Trial Design") analyzes as a case history an upcoming trial of the major antiviral which is furthest ahead in the clinical-trials pipeline. We show why it would be almost impossible for this drug (or any other major antiviral) to be ready within two years, even though there are dozens of candidate drugs which appear promising in laboratory, animal, and even human studies—unless a widespread professional consensus about how to design trials of AIDS drugs can be changed. We show why the trial was designed the way it was (making rapid results impossible), what assumptions motivated this design, where those assumptions are wrong, and what can be done instead (or in addition).

The central problem is not with any one agency, company, or other institution, but with a professional consensus which crosses organizational boundaries and if not changed, will stop any decisive treatment advance from being available for years. Instead of waiting until the 1991 Florence conference, for example, to ask once again why there are no new antivirals to replace or supplement AZT, we can raise the issue now. Some of the failures of upcoming trials are so predictable that we can analyze them before the trials even begin—when some of the problems might be bypassed or avoided—instead of waiting years to only recount the same failures after they have happened.

The professional consensus which guarantees lack of results has been allowed to persist because of national and international lack of leadership on treatment development, lack of commitment to saving lives. In the United States, for example, 97 percent of the 5,100 largest foundations have not given one penny to AIDS (December 1988 report of the Foundation Center, cited in May 17 talk by Dr. Timothy Wolfred, outgoing executive director of the San Francisco AIDS Foundation); of the three percent which have contributed at all, it is well known that most will not touch research or research advocacy. This lack of commitment, so clearly seen in the above tabulation, operates less openly behind the technical complexities of human trials, the legitimate need for caution and control in human research, the cleverly concocted press releases, and the widespread lazy assumption that the experts know best and therefore no further thinking or action by anyone else is necessary.

It is understandable that people and institutions are reluctant to look closely at clinical trials, a complex, technical area where human life is at stake. But in the resulting vacuum, the failure of national leadership and commitment has combined with pre-existing problems in the medical and research systems to lead to a "conventional wisdom" which includes assumptions which guarantee that the clinical-research system will fail to respond to the AIDS public-health emergency.

Something can be done. When the AIDS community is well informed, it can bring key issues into the open and force them to be addressed. Our "Why No Antivirals" article, below, shows the precise errors and design flaws which guarantee that an upcoming clinical trial will fail to meet the needs of the AIDS emergency, no matter what happens in the trial. Since this study is one of the better ones, and since the drug itself is ahead of all the important antivirals in the regulatory pipeline, the flawed assumptions and design illustrated in this trial almost guarantee that no decisive advance in AIDS treatment will be available for years—even though the drugs which will be available then are in many cases already well known today.

This issue has not been widely understood; until the Montreal conference, we ourselves did not see it clearly. By detailed understanding and by persistence, the AIDS community can force key weaknesses in trial design and administration to be addressed, force the spokespersons for the conventional wisdom to state the case for their positions before other medical and research professionals. When their case is weak, the professional consensus which controls clinical research will shift, and much faster shepherding of drugs through the research and regulatory system can quickly become possible.

## Outline on Promising Treatments

Many attenders at the Montreal conference (including this writer) agreed that ddI may be the most important single drug in the AIDS research pipeline now. Most of the information presented was not new, but confirmed previous informal accounts (see "ddI Information Published," *AIDS Treatment News* # 78). We are still analyzing the conference information, and will follow ddI closely in the future.

Compound Q was not discussed at the conference, although one abstract was published (abstract number C.596).

Soluble CD4 received much favorable attention in talks by Robert Gallo, M.D., and other researchers. So far, however, the efficacy results have been disappointing. While we are not listing this treatment as one of the most promising, some of the scientists who have worked with it remain enthusiastic about this line of research, especially later generations of the drug.

Two posters were presented and three other abstracts were published on hypericin, which continues to look good, although it received little attention at the conference. No human results were included,  since no human research has yet been completed.

There were many posters on treatment of opportunistic infections. Except for pneumocystis prophylaxis, the most important single drug was probably fluconazole, a broad-spectrum antifungal used in Europe but still not marketed in the United States.

We will report further on promising treatments in future issues.

## New Information On Non-Approved Treatments

Treatment possibilities which look **less** attractive now than they did before the Montreal conference include ribavirin, isoprinosine, dextran sulfate, AL 721, and roxithromycin. Often the new information is ambiguous, so we want to study it further before writing a report. We cover roxithromycin, which failed in treating advanced toxoplasmosis, below.

## New Treatment Ideas

A number of new ideas were presented, especially in some of the poster presentations.

For example, scientists at the University of Pittsburgh tested an organic arsenic compound which had been used to treat syphilis before penicillin was available (abstract number M.C.P.133). The compound, oxophenarsine, was found to be extremely effective against HIV in the test tube, in concentrations as low as 0.035 micrograms/ml. According to one of the presenters whom we met at the poster, it is the only drug known to be able to block the virus in chronically-infected H9 cells. In a similar test, AZT showed no antiviral effect.

We asked about toxicity, as some of the early syphilis treatments were notorious. This one was apparently not as bad as some of the others.

One advantage of this drug, which was once FDA approved, is that much information about human use is already available, published in old medical journals.

Unfortunately no pharmaceutical company anywhere still manufactures this drug, which was used by injection. The Pittsburgh scientists are trying to get the original manufacturer to produce enough for a test. Since the original patent rights have long since expired, other companies could legally do so; the drug is easy to make. (The University of Pittsburgh has applied for a use patent for HIV treatment, in order to make the project attractive to investors and obtain financial support.)

Oxophenarsine could be tested quickly and inexpensively to see if it might be helpful as an AIDS antiviral. Unfortunately it is more likely to be overlooked and ignored, regardless of merit. Few people have both the capability and incentive to make anything happen toward getting this potential treatment tested. We hope that this article will bring the drug and the project for its development to wider attention.

## ROXITHROMYCIN FAILS IN ADVANCED TOXOPLASMOSIS

On March 10, *AIDS Treatment News* reported that roxithromycin had been found effective in treating toxoplasmosis in mice, and had also been found to reach extremely high concentration in brain tissue when the drug was given to humans scheduled to undergo neurosurgery (so that the brain concentration could be measured). This preliminary work suggested that roxithromycin should be tried as a treatment for toxoplasmosis. We could only find one human case where the treatment had been tried, however, and the result was inconclusive. No trials were planned in the United States, where 20,000 to 40,000 cases of toxoplasmosis have been predicted by 1991 (Luft and

Remington, "Toxoplasmic Encephalitis", *The Journal of Infectious Diseases*, January 1988). We mentioned that we had heard a report that a small trial would soon begin in France.

At the Montreal conference, physicians from a hospital in Paris reported that they gave three times the usual dose of roxithromycin to eight patients who could no longer tolerate pyrimethamine/sulfadiazine (P/S), the conventional treatment for toxoplasmosis (poster # W.B.P.29 in the conference abstracts). However, symptoms of toxoplasmosis reappeared after 28 to 45 days of treatment. In four of these eight patients, P/S treatment could be started again, and it was successful. The conclusion was that the roxithromycin was not effective.

In addition, on June 6 a French physician wrote to us that roxithromycin had been found ineffective, at least when used after cerebral abscesses had already formed, although he noted that it might prove useful earlier.

## IN MEMORIAM: BARRY GINGELL

Dr. Barry Gingell, who died last month at age 34, was a New York activist, physician and PWA who inaugurated the invaluable publication *Treatment Issues* for the Gay Men's Health Crisis. He embodied the idea of empowerment for people with HIV and AIDS, working to make drugs like ribavirin and isoprinosine accessible as early as 1985. His leadership in advocating aggressive and intelligent treatment choices will be very much missed.

## WHY NO ANTIVIRALS: A CASE HISTORY OF FAILED TRIAL DESIGN

*by John S. James*

AZT provides limited benefits to persons with AIDS or HIV, and many people cannot use it at all. Many promising new antivirals have long been in the research and regulatory pipeline: for example, ddI, AZDU (CS-87), D4T, ddC, hypericin, and trichosanthin (compound Q). None has become available since AZT was released almost three years ago. And at the Montreal AIDS conference earlier this month, we learned why none will become available for years—unless certain current practices in the design of clinical trials can be changed. This article will illustrate some of the problems, and suggest solutions.

The basic problem lies not in any single agency, company, or other institution, but instead in a conventional wisdom which cuts across institutional boundaries. A professional consensus guides the design and conduct of clinical trials, and the shepherding of experimental drugs through the testing system. This consensus today includes certain assumptions which make it impossible for the existing system of clinical trials and drug approval to respond successfully to AIDS as a public-health emergency.

**Note and disclaimer:** Readers may notice that this issue of *AIDS Treatment News* has a call for volunteers (above) for the same trial analyzed below as an illustration of a failure of the clinical-trial system. This is not an oversight or contradiction.

This trial is no worse than other AIDS studies. It seems to be ethical in its treatment of volunteers. The problem is that it will not produce results for years. But for now it is the trial we have, so we must support it.

For the same reason, this article is not intended as a criticism of persons conducting this trial, nor of it's sponsor. They have done well within the system of shared assumptions which controls all mainstream AIDS research. It is this system which needs reform.

## A Case History: New DDC Trial

ddC (dideoxycytidine), an antiviral like AZT but with different toxicities, is not the most important new drug. But it is farthest ahead in the drug-approval pipeline among major antivirals. Because it is ahead of the others, and plans for a major new study have been revealed, it provides an excellent case study of the problems which will impede the approval of all important new antivirals, not only ddC but also more interesting drugs such as ddI.

## DDC Background

ddC, like most of the new AIDS antivirals, was discovered to have anti-HIV activity by U.S. Government scientists. The United States then asserted exclusive worldwide rights, and assigned these rights to a pharmaceutical company (in this case, Hoffmann-La Roche, Inc. of Nutley, New Jersey).

Several trials have already been conducted. In early studies, some patients developed severe peripheral neuropathy, causing numbness or pain in the feet. Later human studies found that lower doses could reduce P24 antigen levels, a sign of antiviral activity, with manageable toxicity.

On June 5, 1989, Hoffmann-La Roche announced new trials, designed in cooperation with the FDA (U.S. Food and Drug Administration). A major phase II trial, which could lead to marketing approval for the drug, will compare low-dose ddC head-to-head with AZT "in persons with AIDS or advanced ARC."

The problem with this trial is that because of the design chosen, it is unlikely to produce any conclusion for two and a half years.

And since ddC is ahead of all other major antivirals in the drug-approval pipeline, and the delays in this study design are generic to AIDS antivirals and not specific to ddC, it is likely that all major new AIDS drugs will face a similar delay. This fact alone strongly suggests that no major new treatment for AIDS will come out of the drug-approval pipeline for years, unless the assumptions currently guiding clinical trials can be changed.

An analysis of the design of the new ddC/AZT comparison trial, and the assumptions behind this design, will show exactly how this intolerable situation came about, and how it can be changed.

## DDC Rumor: A Treatment IND?

Rumors have circulated that ddC may become more available through a "treatment IND" before the end of 1989. We hope these rumors are true.

But we are skeptical. The FDA has interpreted the treatment IND very conservatively, using it only near the end of efficacy trials, when the drug is almost sure to get full marketing approval after the final paperwork is complete. If this procedure is followed for ddC, a treatment IND will probably be more than two years away, as we will show below.

The record is full of comforting but broken promises that things have changed and therefore AIDS research will move faster in the future. When the future arrives, the public has forgotten the promises.

## Why will the trial take so long?

This new phase II trial will compare ddC with AZT, using a randomized, double-blind design. No placebo will be used; every patient will get one of the drugs. The trial is scheduled to last two years; recruiting the subjects is expected to take about six months in addition.

In theory, the study could end earlier. A team of experts will periodically monitor the results, secretly breaking the code to see if there is statistical proof that patients getting ddC are doing much better or much worse than those getting AZT. In practice, however, for reasons explained below, it is almost impossible that this study will end this way. The researchers expect it to take the whole two years.

The reason that the study will take so long must be explained in several steps:

(1) The FDA will not approve a drug based only on "surrogate markers", meaning improvement in blood work such as reduction in P24 antigen, or T-cell rises. The FDA also wants statistical proof that the drug is helping people.

(2) After rejecting surrogate markers, the FDA has insisted on the slowest measure of clinical improvement—"clinical endpoints", meaning OIs (opportunistic infections) or deaths. This means that the drug being tested is not measured by improvements in the patients who receive it, but OIs or deaths in those who do not.

The ddC trial will compare that drug with AZT. Since AZT works fairly well for the first year, the number of deaths and OIs in the control (AZT) group will be low. Therefore, even if the drug being tested were perfect and everybody taking it were cured instantly, the clinical trial design would not recognize that fact **until enough deaths and OIs had accumulated in the control group** to provide statistical proof that ddC was no worse than AZT.

(3) This study, like some others, will use a team of experts (sometimes called a "data safety monitoring board") to meet periodically and secretly break the code and examine the results so far, to see if the study should be ended early. The public is told that such reviews can end studies as soon as statistical proof of effectiveness is obtained.

But in practice it is unlikely that this or any similar study will be ended early. The reason why not involves an esoteric problem in statistical interpretation. If researchers take an early look at their data to decide whether to stop the study early and call the drug a success, but then decide that the data does not justify stopping, meaning that the study will run to its normal conclusion, then the very fact that they looked early means that they must tighten their interpretation of the final results. A drug which otherwise could have been considered a success might now need to be counted a failure—just because the researchers looked at the data and **might** have acted on that information—even though in fact they did nothing different as a result of the look.

This seemingly preposterous conclusion is hard to explain even to scientists, let alone to readers with no statistical background. We will try to do so; those who are not interested in the details can skip the next four paragraphs.

[When researchers claim statistical proof that their drug works, they are usually claiming that the drug passed a test which only a small percentage of worthless drugs could have passed by chance; the smaller the percentage, the better. For example, if a journal article claims that a result is "statistically significant at the $p<0.01$ level," this means that the probability (p) that a worthless drug could have done as well or better by chance alone is less than one percent (0.01).

What happens, then, if you look at the data early? Suppose that the researchers did not know about the problem that we are describing here, and they decided to take an early look at their data, and end the trial immediately if the drug was good enough to have reached the $p<0.01$ level already. If not, they would continue the study and see if they achieved that level later.

Clearly then the chance of accepting a worthless drug at some time in their trial would now be greater than one percent. This is because there is a full one percent chance to accept such a drug at the early look—and if the worthless drug did not pass the test at that time, there is some additional chance that it could pass later. Since the overall probability of accepting a worthless drug is now greater than one percent, the researchers cannot correctly claim that their trial showed efficacy at the $p<0.01$ level. To honestly make that claim, the researcher must use a higher standard both for the early look, and also at the normal end of the study (if the early look did not result in the trial's termination).

This means that if researchers take an early look at their data but decide not to end the study as a result, they then must tighten their standard for judging a drug successful later. Drugs which would otherwise have been judged effective will therefore now be rejected. Clinical trial design can minimize this problem by making the early look be as conservative as possible.]

The practical effect of this statistical oddity is that researchers have a strong incentive to use an extremely conservative criterion for ending a study early. As a result, a "data safety monitoring board" provides less protection to the volunteers in a study than they may be led to believe. And the assurance to the public that experts are monitoring the trial and will end it as soon as the data justifies, thereby speeding final approval of the drug, is largely empty.

(Note: The AZT trial was stopped early in September, 1986, when there were 16 deaths in the placebo group, vs. only one death in the AZT group. No one knows why this extreme difference occurred, as later experience does not support a 16 to one difference in death rate with AZT. And despite this great difference in deaths, the decision to stop the study then has been controversial.)

During the Montreal conference, Hoffmann-La Roche conducted a press conference on ddC. The speakers were Thomas Merigan, M.D., principal investigator at the AIDS Clinical Trials Group at Stanford University, and Whaijen Soo, M.D., Ph.D., director of clinical virology at Roche. Few reporters came to this meeting, which was a mile away from the main conference. Our impression from the discussions at that press conference is that nobody expected the study to end before two years.

The important question is not whether to end studies early. It is whether the best way to prove a drug is to wait for deaths and OIs in those who do not receive it. This trial design makes studies inherently slow, whether they are ended early or not.

No one at the press conference raised the issue of whether a study design which will take more than two years to get results is an acceptable public health response to the epidemic. We are concerned that all the important AIDS antivirals are behind ddC in the pipeline. If they suffer the same delay as ddC, then we can almost guarantee that no major new AIDS antiviral will be generally available for at least two years.

## Recruiting Problems Likely?

One of the problems with many AIDS clinical trials is that entry criteria are designed purely for scientific reasons, without thought as to whether there will be patients available to fit them. As a result, many studies take much longer than intended, or even fail altogether, because of recruiting difficulties.

The ddC study may have this problem. Volunteers must have less than 200 T-helper cells, and also have had pneumocystis in the last four months or have certain ARC symptoms. And yet they must have never taken AZT. Most people will have already tried AZT before they have severe symptoms and under 200 T-helper cells.

Some may have never taken AZT because they chose not to. But they would be unlikely to volunteer for this study—because 50 percent of the people enrolled, chosen at random, will go into a control group and receive AZT instead of ddC.

It seems that the only volunteers left would be those who never took AZT because they could not afford it; in the study, the drug is free. But these people face another problem. The study also **requires** use of aerosol pentamidine, **but will not pay for it**. If persons could not obtain AZT in the past, how will they obtain aerosol pentamidine for the next two years into the future?

It would seem that these conditions, taken together, systematically exclude almost everybody from the trial. A few might get through, such as those whose first contact with the medical system is pneumocystis.

Notice how much of the problem with this study, including recruitment, stems from the decision to prove ddC by counting "clinical events" (deaths and OIs) in the control group. To get clinical events, the patients must be seriously ill—although never treated with AZT. But once on the study, for ethical reasons they must receive an antiviral and pneumocystis prophylaxis, reducing the clinical events and therefore requiring more volunteers (therefore a multicenter trial) and a two-year duration. All this to get enough deaths and OIs to allow the drugs to be compared.

An alternative would be randomized, double-blind trials designed to use patients' overall clinical condition as the outcome measure, not deaths and OIs. The problem seems to be that academic researchers do not trust physicians' evaluations in outcome measures in their experiments—even within a double-blind trial—because such evaluations involve some subjective element. A body-count outcome sounds more scientific.

## The Ideology and Public Relations of Clinical Trials

Having looked at the reality of the modern phase II clinical trial for AIDS antivirals, we will now look at the image. The image is important, because it is used to calm the public, justify the existing system, and impede calls for reform.

The ddC press packet from Hoffmann-La Roche provides a convenient look at this image. Any other public relations from a mainstream clinical trial would be similar, however, as government and other controls have imposed a research monoculture. Even the public front is uniform.

From a June 5 press release we learn that "Everyone collaborating on this project at Roche, the FDA and the National Institutes of Health is intensely aware of the urgency for developing safe and effective treatments for AIDS. Awareness of that urgency constantly compels us to work together as expeditiously as possible toward definitive results." We also learn that "Initial studies suggest that ddC may have an antiviral effect at the low doses that result in manageable toxicity. The studies now being planned are essential if we are to turn suggestions into medically useful conclusions."

An undated *Dideoxycytidine (DDC) Fact Sheet* includes a question and answer section on the availability of ddC. We quote it at length because it illustrates several aspects of the currently prevailing ideology of clinical trials.

"Q: When will ddC be available?

"A: That depends largely on the results of the new trials. When dealing with human life, the adverse effects profile and optimum dosage of a drug must be carefully studied no matter how urgent the need. As soon as the clinical data warrant, Roche will file a New Drug Application (NDA).

"Meanwhile, each of the new trials has entry criteria specific to its design, and some of the studies already have their full complement of volunteer patients. People who would like to participate in, or simply learn more about, the trials should call FDA [sic] at 800/874-2572 (800/TRIALS-A) or Roche (collect) at 201/235-2355.

"Q: Will Roche provide ddC on a compassionate plea basis?

"A: The urgent need for more effective weapons against HIV weighs heavily on everyone associated with this project at Roche, the FDA, and the NIH. However, at present, we are agreed that the clinical data now available are insufficient to justify distribution or use of ddC against AIDS outside of carefully controlled clinical trials. Only new data can change this situation. Consequently, we are working closely together to expedite the next round of therapeutic trials, from which the medically necessary data will flow.

"Q: When will Roche submit an NDA for ddC?

"A: Roche will submit an NDA as soon as the data from the pivotal studies allow. A special review board will continually evaluate data from all of the trials and make appropriate recommendations to FDA."

Some points to note about the world of AIDS treatment research according to press releases:

(1) Everyone involved feels urgency, and is working well with everyone else. (During the press conference, however, this reporter could find no shred of evidence of urgency.)

(2) More studies are, of course, essential. (300 people have already been given ddC in clinical trials.)

(3) The phrase "no matter how urgent the need," in the context of justifying withholding a drug until more studies collect still more information about "the adverse effects profile and optimum dosage," clearly illustrates the fact that no weighing of costs and benefits (of the extra studies and their associated delays) will be considered. Instead, persons with AIDS can simply get lost until the researchers are finished. In theory they might join the study, but in practice less than one percent of persons with AIDS or related conditions will be able to do so.

Incidentally, the dose has already been determined well enough to bet this entire phase II study on it, as only one dose will be used in this study.

(4) Unless they qualify for a trial, patients and their physicians have no role in the decision of whether or not to use a drug, until someone is ready to sell it to them. This decision is made for them, by agreement between government officials and potential vendors. For AIDS, the answer is almost always no. Other diseases have been treated more liberally.

(5) The public is not told that the reason the trial will take so long is that deaths and OIs must be accumulated. Instead, the public is told that the trial might not take two years but could end any time, because experts will watch over it and pull the plug as soon as medically possible, moving the drug to the next step in the approval pipeline. As we have seen, this study will almost certainly take more than two years.

(6) The *Dideoxycytidine (DDC )Fact Sheet* also said that the first comparison trial was expected to "begin" in July and last up to two years, "depending on results." Readers might assume that the maximum delay for this trial is therefore two years and one month. This assumption would be wrong.

The six months for recruiting subjects was an informal estimate mentioned by one of the researchers at the press conference. Past experience suggests that it is probably optimistic.

Note that a trial which "begins" in one month and lasts "up to" two years may take far longer than 25 months to be finished. This is because the trial "begins" with the recruitment of the first subject, but the two-year clock starts only with the recruitment of the last. In addition, multicenter trials often have recruitment quotas for different centers, meaning that the clock starts only when the slowest center is ready.

The difference recruitment can make is illustrated by a study of Imuthiol (DTC). Over two years ago, on April 10, 1987, *AIDS Treatment News* reported that this six-month study was underway. Most centers recruited patients promptly and completed their phase of the study. But because of stragglers, this six-month study was still running two years later, and the data from those subjects who completed the trial long ago has not been released.

The point is that press releases about clinical trials are designed to provide a comforting picture of reality. Since clinical research is a forbidding area—complex, esoteric, and involving risk to human life—few in the media or elsewhere have looked behind the image. It is much easier to trust the experts.

Because of lack of understanding of what is really going on, people are repeatedly surprised at the lack of new drugs for AIDS. Those who do look will realize that the current system of clinical trials could not possibly meet the needs of the AIDS emergency, and is very unlikely to release even a single important new AIDS drug for years—even though the drugs are there. The drugs which will provide the important treatment advances of 1992 and 1993 are already available and quite well known—we named some of them above. But ddC will take over two years for the upcoming trial alone, and all the other important antivirals are behind it in the pipeline, so they will take longer still.

## The Central Issue

The key reason no new antivirals are available is that clinical trials have waited for deaths and OIs, instead of looking directly at clinical benefit, which with some drugs is dramatic. Conservative trial designers have used deaths and OIs because the numbers seem more "scientific" than clinical ratings, which depend in part on judgments of physicians, and may not be identical from one researcher to the next; by contrast, everyone can agree precisely on the number of deaths in the treatment and control groups. However, "softer" kinds of data such as average ratings by panels of experts have been handled successfully in many fields of science. When we are looking for dramatic effects, as with ddI or Compound Q, these methods have more than enough precision to do the job.

The AIDS community must continue to raise the issue of whether counting deaths and OIs is truly the only legitimate way to tell whether an AIDS antiviral is working. Using "surrogate markers", such as T-helper cell count or P24 antigen level, is one approach to faster study design.

But we fear that surrogate markers alone are not enough—that to try to use blood work as the sole basis for approving new drugs would lead to a long and unproductive argument. A middle ground, which we believe will be most productive, is to use surrogate markers **and also** direct measurements of clinical benefit in persons taking the drug, such as numerical ratings based on examinations by physicians. The variability in the course of the disease, sometimes cited in arguing against this approach, can be controlled for by double-blind designs, and by well-known statistical methods. The purpose here is to find the dramatically effective drugs, the home runs, and to test them quickly; slower study designs are acceptable when researchers are looking for minor or marginal differences.

The issue of surrogate markers is already receiving serious professional attention. But the related issue of the reluctance of trial designers to use direct measures of clinical benefit as proof of efficacy of AIDS antivirals, instead of insisting on deaths and OIs in the control group as the only important measure, has been largely overlooked. The AIDS community must insist that this issue be considered on it merits, as this key reform will allow the most important new AIDS antivirals to be tested many times faster than by the methods now in use.

# Issue Number 82
# June 30, 1989

## COMPOUND Q UPDATE

*by John S. James*

Our previous issue included a last-minute report on a so-called "unofficial study" of Compound Q—actually a treatment program and data monitoring project—organized by San Francisco's Project Inform and including over 30 patients and nine physicians in four U.S. cities (San Francisco, Los Angeles, New York, and Miami/Ft. Lauderdale), using a version of the drug which is in common use in China. Probably no single story in the AIDS epidemic has generated as much coverage in San Francisco's major daily newspapers, the *San Francisco Chronicle* and *San Francisco Examiner*. Some of the information released by the San Francisco press is available nowhere else. Local press coverage has been even-handed and mostly sympathetic, despite vociferous opposition from some researchers in the official Compound Q study at San Francisco General Hospital. (A spokesperson for the California Medical Association took a middle position, describing the doctors involved as "respected physicians in the community working desperately to provide effective treatment and care," but expressing serious concern about phase I—dosage or safety—studies being conducted outside of a university medical center).

We believe that a loud debate "for" or "against" the unofficial study would be unproductive, the wrong issue for furthering the common fight against AIDS. The better question is what can we learn from this extraordinary response to an extraordinary situation. What can we learn about the drug, and also about how to improve the official system of authorized research, to get faster and better answers not only for AIDS but for other diseases as well?

Project Inform and others involved in this treatment program want to wait until it is finished, probably 30 to 60 days, to make a full report. This article is based on news already released but not widely available outside the San Francisco area.

## Background

*AIDS Treatment News* covered Compound Q in its issues of January 13, April 21, May 5, and June 16; the last issue went to press late and contained a news flash dated June 28. The active ingredient of Compound Q is a protein called trichosanthin, extracted from the root of a Chinese cucumber. The plant extract must be highly purified before injection; otherwise it is highly toxic and could be fatal. In the test tube, trichosanthin works by selectively killing macrophages infected with HIV. Infected macrophages are believed to be the major reservoir of the virus in the body.

In China, trichosanthin is used to induce abortion, because it selectively kills "trophoblast" cells, which line the uterus during pregnancy. It is also used to treat choriocarcinoma, a cancer of these cells, and may be better for this purpose than any treatment available in the U.S.

Dr. Hin-Wing Yeung, a scientist from Hong Kong, suggested trichosanthin as an AIDS treatment, based on earlier development of the drug by researchers in Shanghai. Michael McGrath, M.D., at San Francisco General Hospital, first thought that the drug might kill every macrophage in the body—a radical but possible treatment, as macrophages are normally replaced. In laboratory tests, he unexpectedly learned that it killed only those cells infected with HIV.

## The Unofficial Study

About three months ago, before Project Inform was involved with Compound Q, scattered groups of persons with AIDS, especially one group in Florida, had been able to obtain supplies of the drug from China. Because this drug is more dangerous than other non-approved AIDS treatments, the effort was made to obtain some answers quickly about its safety and efficacy through a highly professional treatment and data-monitoring program, before patients were harmed by self-medication or other improper use.

At a press conference on June 28, Martin Delaney of Project Inform explained the unofficial study, and the reason it was done. We edited his comments for length:

"This treatment use (of Compound Q) is no different from things like it that have been going on for the last five years. What is different is that the media has turned this into a high-profile event.

"Several points guided us and made us feel compelled to organize this treatment program. One was impending community use of this drug. Like other drugs before it— like ribavirin, AL 721, dextran sulfate—patients have ways to get these drugs into the country legally. When there is hope about new drugs, patients begin distributing and using them. Unfortunately, widespread distribution and use has often taken place before we had any sense of whether the drugs were safe, or whether they worked.

"For example, in 1985 when ribavirin started coming into the U. S. from Mexico, Project Inform was formed to ask the medical community to set up prospective data monitoring on patients using that drug. Nobody did so, and three years went by of use of that drug, and the government ultimately concluded that it was not useful, and might even be harmful in some patients. That's not an intelligent way to run an epidemic.

"Now Compound Q is perhaps the most hopeful drug, but also maybe a very toxic drug. Patients legitimately within their rights are preparing to use it. Once again we have the specter of hundreds if not thousands of people using a drug that we do not know is safe or effective. Once again, it will take years to get the answer by the standard methods.

"A hundred and fifty people a day are dying now because of bureaucratic delays, because of inability to access important drugs that are tied up in the pipeline. A good example is the drugs ddI and ddC; their promise has been known since 1986. The official researchers have now finished phase I testing on them, and now they are telling us it will be two to two and a half more years before efficacy tests are confirmed. AIDS patients don't have that long to live. That's beyond the life expectancy of most patients.

"We're already two and a half years into Compound Q, as scientists learned the basic facts about it two and a half years ago, and kept the information from us while there was a good equivalent drug in China, a drug that had been used there for nearly two decades.

"It is true that the ongoing official study of Compound Q might have been done in six or nine months—but it would not provide the answers we needed to guide community use. It will give limited answers about certain doses of the drug, one administration only, in certain patients. We have to answer to an entire community of people who are going to use the drug in any way they see fit, unless guidance is given.

"It is not OK, it is not acceptable morally, to just turn our backs and say, 'You guys shouldn't do it,' and feel that we've done our job. We have to give guidance, if people are going to have access to these drugs—and they do have that access, whether we want it or not.

"We also had experience going into this from people in Florida. We were not the first ones to use Compound Q in a clinical study. More than a dozen people in Florida had already used the (Chinese) drug for HIV, before we even began talking about doing what we are doing now. So we had considerable human experience before going in.

"What did we do? First we talked to people working on importation. We asked them this time, let's not distribute the drug, let's not sell it to people. Instead, let's try to channel it into controlled clinical use, rather than the old system which was pass it out and see what happens.

"We then collaborated to design a carefully controlled clinical process under which patients would be treated. This is not technically a study; it is a treatment program. People call it a study because of the extent of scientific processes being used to collect data from it. But the primary goal is treatment, not research.

"For the protocol design, we called upon a researcher who had run the research on another drug similar to trichosanthin, called ricin-A, which has been used in more than a thousand patients and is in the same family as trichosanthin. We used her help in putting this protocol together, along with the experience of the physicians involved. So the data gathering, the study part of what we are doing, was based on an existing FDA-approved study of the drug ricin-A; it is not something we made up.

"We also created an elaborate consent process to protect the patients and the physicians alike.

"We then shared the protocol with other interested physicians, pulled together a team of four groups in four cities, looking to treat about 60 patients.

[The next section of the statement, omitted here, concerned legal implications.]

"Baseline data was collected from all patients. Most of them already had more than a year of extensive laboratory work. After a complete workup, the patients were infused with a reasonable quantity of the drug—the smallest amount used for any purpose in China. It is a fraction of the dose used in China with cancer patients. It is a midpoint in the dose range proposed for the trials at San Francisco General Hospital; in another week they will have exceeded our dose. Our dose is the midpoint of expected therapeutic doses based on laboratory data—and the dose used by more than a dozen patients in Florida. It is a fifth of the dose that we've seen some patients use self-medicated.

"Basic safety precautions were followed. The criteria for entrance to this study were the criteria we lifted from San Francisco General's study. The same precautions were taken. Each patient was administered a test dose of the drug in a tiny quantity, to look for allergic reactions. They were followed for a 24 hour period of hospitalization, with vital signs taken constantly. They were in the physician's office nearly daily for the following week.

"Elaborate data gathering is going on, just as in a formal clinical study. 14 full physicals, 14 complete workups, blood chemistry, urinalysis, sedimentation rates, P24 antigen and antibodies, complete cellular immunity, all of what is being done in virtually every AIDS clinical study in the country.

"Additional safety precautions include use of standard adverse experience reporting forms that are approved by FDA, standard side-effect ratings from FDA-approved studies, and complete tracking of concomitant medications used. There is nothing missing here in what has been done.

"The outcome to date is that the vast majority of the more than 30 patients who have been treated in our treatment program have tolerated the drug very well.

"We seem to have made an interesting, perhaps major discovery about the effect of the drug on patients with HIV infection of the brain. Two patients experienced mental confusion, which cleared up in one to two weeks. And as you all know one patient entered a coma, a coma that lasted no more than 24 hours and was in the process of complete resolution when the incident occurred about a week later when the patient died.

"This patient vomited in his sleep and inhaled some of the vomit, and had to be resuscitated. The evidence at the scene suggested that the resuscitation process was quite successful, his vital signs had returned to normal. However, the patient had a living will, an agreement which called for no heroic measures, which the family interpreted this as being, and the family asked that the tube be pulled. It was the opinion of physicians on site that had that not been the case, the patient could well be alive today. We cannot say at this point if the problem was related to the drug or not.

"At this time we are not making statements about whether the drug is working. We have seen some interesting lab measures. But it would be irresponsible scientifically to say that therefore the drug is working. It will take time, to follow these patients for a longer period and see if these results hold up. It would give the wrong signal to our community to say we've concluded that the drug works. We need more information before people should start using this drug. The buyers' clubs and other groups that work with patients are completely cooperative with this; nobody is interested in endangering anyone.

"As to the future, there are questions we set out to answer here to protect our community; we intend to get the answers to those questions. The FDA has not shut us down; we do not know whether they will try to or not. We think where we should go is cooperation; we would like to collaborate, share our data with the people in San Francisco General Hospital and the Food and Drug Administration. That was the intention all along; and until the incident last week, they shared in that intention. We had discussed sharing data submissions, about the interaction of our data with theirs. It was only after this very unfortunate death that people headed for the hills.

"We intend to present our data to the Food and Drug Administration, the National Institutes of Health, and the medical journals. If the data suggests that the drug is useful, we will fight for early access to it on behalf of AIDS patients. And whatever the outcome, we will continue to press for faster action. It is unconscionable to accept five and a half years' typical time for the development of drugs for AIDS, when patients have an average lifespan of only two years. We have fought long and hard battles in Washington to improve this process, we think progress is being made, but it isn't being made fast enough."

## Neurological Side Effects: Bad News or Good?

As Delaney mentioned in the press conference above, a handful of patients with dementia or other evidence of HIV infection of the brain suffered neurological side effects—a period of mental confusion lasting one to two weeks for two patients, or a coma lasting less than 24 hours for one other.

Although no one knows for sure, it seems likely that the neurological effects may be evidence that the drug is doing its job—not a sign of toxicity.

What Delaney had heard from experts familiar with the study is that HIV does not infect neurons in the brain, but rather glial cells—supporting cells which the body can replace. The neurological effects seem to be a temporary result of killing a large number of infected cells at one time. If so, Compound Q might prove helpful for persons with HIV brain infection. It may need to be given in smaller doses at first, to control the side effects.

Further studies will be needed to answer this question. Meanwhile, because of the unknowns and risks involved, physicians are screening patients for evidence of HIV brain infection, because of the increased risk of treating them with Compound Q until more is known.

## The Future

The unofficial Compound Q study will end in 30 to 60 days. Until the results are reported, we will not know whether the drug is useful for treating AIDS or HIV, or not.

Readers should realize that there are other side effects, dangers, and precautions not touched on in this article. No one should use Compound Q without expert medical supervision.

What lessons have been learned? Medically, the unofficial study has taught re-searchers more in the last few weeks about Compound Q as a human treatment for HIV than had ever been learned before. And according to Delaney, the official study at San Francisco General Hospital has already used this information to skip some of its low test doses, which are now unnecessary. One result of the unofficial study, therefore, is that the official trials will produce results sooner—a major purpose of the unofficial treatment program all along.

Even more importantly, the unofficial Compound Q study is demonstrating that it is possible to get useful results quickly, if a research project is organized for that purpose. How is Project Inform's program getting useful results in only four or five months, while official trials take five years or longer to do the same?

A look at specifics of the trials will show part of the answer. The official Compound Q was kept secret for at least a year and a half, between May 29, 1987 when the patent application was filed for anti-HIV use of trichosanthin, and January 3, 1989 when the patent was granted. During this time a new method for extracting the drug from the Chinese cucumber root was developed. Then after the patent was granted, it took six months to get phase I tests going; and these tests are slow because phase I tests were designed for new chemicals never given to humans before. The Chinese experience was ignored.

In contrast, the unofficial study used the drug and medical information already existing in China. It proceeded immediately with a dose well known in human use and projected, based on laboratory data, to be therapeutic for HIV. By doing so, instead of developing a new patentable technology requiring new animal tests and phase I human trials, it avoided two years or more of delay. Note that this study could have been carried out two years ago, exactly as it is being done today, if the anti-HIV use of trichosanthin had not been kept secret during that time. As far we know, the intervening two years of official research added little or nothing to the unofficial study, which is based on pre-existing medical technology from China, not on the new technology created during the patent hiatus.

After the patent was granted on January 3 of this year, there was little media interest until April 15, 1989, when an article on Compound Q (also called GLQ 223) was published in the *Proceedings of the National Academy of Sciences.*

Another delay in the official research track is illustrative. After the patent was granted in January, it took some time for Genelabs, the developer of Compound Q, to get an IND (Investigational New Drug approval, meaning approval to test the drug in humans) from the FDA. We cannot know the full story of this delay, but we do know that at one point a San Francisco TV reporter called the FDA to ask why the IND had not been granted for this drug, and was told that the FDA had no application for the IND on file! Genelabs said that it had applied. Because of a misunderstanding, each party was waiting for the other. Apparently the FDA believed that what Genelabs had submitted was only a draft, not an official application—while Genelabs thought it had applied and was waiting for approval to begin the clinical trial at San Francisco General Hospital. We are all lucky that a chance call from a reporter straightened out this snafu, which had put the entire world's research program for one of the two most promising AIDS drugs on hold.

This kind of problem seems surprising only to the uninitiated. In our three years of covering AIDS treatment research, we have seen such mindless delays happen again and again. The difference is that usually there is no public interest in the details of the process, and nobody there to make the call or do what else may be needed to straighten the problem out.

For too long the public has accepted a stock answer that clinical research is going as fast as possible, that the delays are caused only by the requirements of good science. But analysis of what is actually happening shows that the system can be vastly improved.

In the field of industrial quality assurance, there are trained, professional specialists to solve just this kind of problem. If a company is taking too long to get its products developed, for example, it can hire experts to analyze what is happening and suggest solutions. Typically the problems are due to flaws in the system, not to faults of the individuals involved, as no one person alone may have the power and resources to produce results. Instead, the system must be improved, by identifying the problems and correcting them. Academic experts in quality assurance can and should be invited onto the team to examine how trials might be organized to get faster results, consistent with good science.

The unofficial study of Compound Q organized by Project Inform is now producing the most important results—practical information about whether, when, and how to use the drug—about ten times faster than the official research system has been able to do so, either for Compound Q or for other drugs.

Admittedly there are greater risks to the patients in an accelerated study. Some patients want a role in making this decision, however, in balancing the risks of using a new treatment against the risks of doing nothing. Some may also want to contribute to the benefit of others, realizing that tens of thousands of lives are likely to be saved if an accelerated study shows unequivocally that a drug is helpful, months or years ahead of the official trials.

The take-home lesson, we believe, is **not** to blame individuals, on either side. Nor do we believe that the official system, with its safeguards and protections for research subjects, should be abandoned. Instead, we should reform the official system of clinical trials to make it faster and more efficient. If this can be done, there should be no need for bypassing the system in the future.

The right approach to reform is a win-win approach. Nobody's interest needs to be sacrificed—and certainly the quality of scientific workmanship need not be reduced. Instead, careful, professional analysis and negotiation can find intelligent ways to make the system work better.

Who can implement this approach? Ultimately the only force which can do so is a professional consensus in the medical and research communities. Without that consensus, no one else—not the AIDS community, not the FDA, the NIH, the White House, or the pharmaceutical industry—can make it happen.

What if the consensus is not there? Physicians and scientists prize their independence; no one can tell them what to do. But we can appeal to their intelligence. The AIDS community can investigate and analyze exactly what is happening, and illuminate precisely what the problems are, what their consequences are, and what should be happening instead. Usually we cannot implement the reforms by ourselves. But we can make the problems and the opportunities for improvement so obvious that they cannot be ignored.

## FAUCI PROPOSES "PARALLEL TRACK" TREATMENT ACCESS

*by John S. James*

Anthony Fauci, M.D., the head of the largest AIDS clinical trials program at the U.S. National Institute of Allergy and Infectious Diseases, proposed a "parallel track" system whereby patients not able to enter clinical trials would be allowed to use some drugs which had passed safety tests but had not yet completed efficacy testing. The proposal, made public June 23 at a talk in San Francisco, was prominently reported in *The New York Times* and other newspapers the following Monday, June 26.

Although no new laws are required, Dr. Fauci stressed that this plan would work only if the FDA, the drug companies involved, and the scientists running the trials agreed. He cannot make it happen by his decision alone.

The way the plan could work is that when a clinical trial is being designed, the parties involved—the FDA, the drug company, and NIAID—would discuss whether a parallel track could be implemented. If all agreed, then the study protocol could specify that certain patients not eligible for the trial could be treated with the drug through the parallel track. Examples of those ineligible might be persons who had used AZT but had to stop because of the toxicity, if the particular trial excluded people who had ever used AZT. Others might be allowed in the parallel track because the study was full, or because there was no trial available in their area. Fauci emphasized that this parallel access must not interfere with the main trial needed to get scientific data about the drug—presumably meaning that those able to enter the trial would not be allowed to choose parallel-track access instead.

At a press conference after his San Francisco announcement, Fauci suggested that the parallel track would also be designed to collect data useful for evaluating the drug—and that community-based clinical trials might be ideal for conducting such studies.

Discussions on possibly implementing a parallel track are now going on with the FDA and with several drug companies.

## Comment

We commend Dr. Fauci for an excellent proposal, which could speed both access to drugs and final approval. However, there are important obstacles which might prevent the idea from being carried out.

For a parallel track to happen, three organizations must agree: Fauci's NIAID (if the trial is in the NIAID system), the FDA, and the pharmaceutical company which owns the rights to the drug. NIAID will be no problem, and the FDA seems willing to accept the idea, at least if the parallel track is able to generate scientifically sound data, as well as providing treatment access to the drug.

Most people familiar with the parallel-track concept think that the biggest problem will be with the drug companies. They will probably be expected to pay for the parallel track—since the government will not want to pay for it, and there would be problems in allowing patients to do so. The question, then, is what incentives the companies have to support this access to their drug?

What drug companies want above all is approval of their NDA (New Drug Application), meaning final permission to market the drug. If the parallel track will generate data likely to help them get the NDA sooner, then most companies will probably be willing or eager to have a parallel track when their drug is tested.

The key to the parallel track therefore depends on the FDA. If the FDA only halfheartedly permits it, then drug companies will know that paying for treatment access will do little or nothing for them in getting their drugs approved, and they will not agree. But if it is clear that the parallel track can collect data which the FDA is likely to accept as supporting the NDA, then the idea can work.

And even aside from the question of whether the parallel-track idea is ever implemented, the fact that Fauci proposed it has already furthered debate and consensus-building around the issue of earlier access to treatment for life-threatening conditions. For example, in private discussions of the idea before its public announcement, Fauci heard objections that drug companies would not accept the parallel track because they were afraid that what happened to Syntex with ganciclovir would happen to them. Syntex provided the drug free to thousands of patients on a compassionate basis, saving them from blindness, and it has been widely believed in the pharmaceutical industry that they were punished by the FDA for doing so. Fauci answered these objections by clarifying that Syntex got into trouble not for providing compassionate access to persons with AIDS, but for failing to conduct clinical trials early.

Fauci's suggestion is important in another way. As the U.S. government's leading AIDS researcher, he is the one most clearly qualified to challenge the unfortunate idea that providing wider access to treatment will make scientific trials difficult or impossible. By so doing he removes the issue from the realm of science, which most people consider themselves incompetent to think about, to the realm of cost and feasibility, where the public can address the issues on their merits.

## ACT UP/NEW YORK PROPOSES NATIONAL RESEARCH AGENDA

At the June 4-9 V International Conference on AIDS in Montreal, ACT UP / New York released A National *AIDS Treatment Research Agenda*, a 16-page document proposing public-policy changes in treatment research. The authors, in ACT UP's Treatment + Data Committee, are very well informed not only about new medical developments, but also about the procedures and politics of the Federal agencies and other organizations involved.

It is impossible to summarize this proposal adequately; but to give an idea of its scope, we will list the "12 Principles for a New AIDS Drug Testing System," which makes up one of the document's four sections. Note that the document contains explanatory material about each of these principles; it had to be omitted here because of limited space. The 12 principles:

1.   People with AIDS, HIV, and their advocates must participate in designing and executing drug trials.

2.   A comprehensive, coordinated, compassionate drug development strategy must ensure that all promising agents are evaluated thoroughly and, if found effective, distributed rapidly.

3.   Resources must be focused on drugs which treat or prevent opportunistic infections, not just on antiretroviral drugs.

4.   End the exclusion of women, poor people, people in rural areas, people of color, drug users, prisoners, hemophiliacs and children from experimental treatments. Expand staff and facilities in areas with high concentration of HIV-infected people so trials can take place there.

5.   End the exclusion of AZT intolerant individuals from trials for infections or other antivirals.

6.   Protocols should be flexible enough to accommodate new knowledge about HIV infection, allowing subjects to receive state-of-the-art care for opportunistic infections (OIs) as such standards evolve.

7.   Trials must be designed for the real world: prophylaxis permitted, placebos avoided, efficacy criteria and endpoints humane.

8.   Clinical costs associated with trials and not paid for by sponsors should be funded by third party payors to insure that personal income is not a *de facto* exclusion criterion.

9.   The Orphan Drug Act should be reformed so that products developed at public expense are priced fairly. In return for its multimillion-dollar investment in AIDS research, the government is entitled to demand low-cost drugs for AIDS. This will make treatments accessible to people who can't afford AIDS drugs in both the US and worldwide.

10.   The community-based clinical trials network, NIH, FDA and other drug development agencies require increased staff, funding and facilities to wage a successful effort against AIDS.

11.   Establish an accurate, up-to-date, accessible international directory of clinical trials and promising experimental treatments for HIV and for AIDS-related opportunistic infections.

12.   Promising new treatments for HIV and AIDS-related infections should be made accessible to anyone without regard to personal income.

Another section of the document, "AIDS Clinical Research Priorities," lists "5 Drugs We Need Now" (ddI, EPO [already approved—see below], fluconazole, foscarnet, and GM-CSF), and "7 Treatments We Want Tested Faster" (ansamycin, CD4-exotoxin, CD4-immunoadhesin, diclazuril, hypericin, passive immunotherapy, and peptide T). A short description is given for each drug.

Other sections of the proposal are "New Models for Clinical Trials," and "AIDS Drug Development Disasters."

# NEW DRUG APPROVALS: AEROSOL PENTAMIDINE, GANCICLOVIR, AND ERYTHROPOIETIN (EPO)

This month the FDA approved three drugs important in AIDS treatment.

## Aerosolized Pentamidine

On June 15 the FDA gave full approval to LyphoMed Inc. of Rosemont, IL for marketing aerosolized pentamidine to prevent pneumocystis— not only for patients who have already had pneumocystis, but also for anyone who has T-helper cell counts of 200 or less. The drug already had "treatment IND" status—official approval for early release of a treatment for a serious or life-threatening condition—but some insurance companies had used lack of final marketing approval as an excuse to deny reimbursement. The new approval announced this month should make it possible for many more patients to obtain the drug.

## Ganciclovir

On June 26, Syntex Corporation of Palo Alto, CA announced that the FDA had approved ganciclovir for treatment of CMV retinitis in persons with AIDS or other immune deficiencies. This approval resulted from negotiated compromises to end the very difficult situation of this drug (see *AIDS Treatment News* #71). This case, now hopefully behind us, made it much more difficult for persons with AIDS to receive compassionate use of other drugs.

The current approval will also allow physicians to prescribe ganciclovir for other CMV infections, such as colitis or pneumonia, although efficacy has not been officially established for these illnesses. Physicians may be reluctant to prescribe the drug for these "off label" uses, and insurance companies may refuse to pay.

The approval also removes an obstacle to research with other CMV treatments. Because it is unusual to get permission to use more than one experimental drug in the same trial, it would have been difficult to test other treatments such as foscarnet using ganciclovir as a control group. But since it was generally accepted that ganciclovir was effective, it was not ethical to use a placebo, either. Since no drug was approved for CMV, and yet one was generally known to work, it was not possible to have a control group for efficacy tests of any other potential treatments. The new approval should break this research deadlock.

## Erythropoietin (EPO)

Because this treatment for anemia has been involved in complex contract and pricing disputes, the drug has two separate approvals at this time. One will make it available to some persons with AIDS at no cost. The other makes it available to any patient who needs it, for AIDS or other conditions, but the official indication is only for kidney disease, so insurance companies will probably refuse to pay for other patients under that program.

The AIDS-related approval is a "treatment IND" obtained by Ortho Pharmaceutical Corporation, for its brand of EPO, Eprex. According to Ortho, the treatment IND was granted after earlier trials showed that the drug reduced anemia, and eliminated the need for transfusions in two thirds of the patients using it. EPO is used to treat anemia caused by AZT, or anemia caused directly by HIV.

At this time the AIDS patients eligible to receive EPO under the treatment IND must have a hematocrit less than 30 percent, and less than 500 mu/ml of EPO in their blood. (EPO is a hormone found naturally in the body.) They must also be patients of one of the 30 physicians who are already part of Ortho's EPO program. The company plans to enroll other physicians later.

Meanwhile, any physician can prescribe EPO for any patient who needs it, under an earlier (June 1, 1989) full marketing approval given to Amgen Inc (a competitor of Ortho Pharmaceutical) for Epogen, its brand of EPO. But since the official approval for this brand is only for kidney disease, the cost of this very expensive drug will probably not be reimbursed when it is used to treat anemia from other causes.

# Issue Number 83
# July 14, 1989

## DDI: COMPASSIONATE ACCESS ANNOUNCED

*by John S. James*

On July 13, Bristol-Myers Company announced that it would make the experimental anti-HIV drug ddI available to persons with AIDS who did not meet the criteria for clinical trials and had a "critical" need for the drug. This program, described by the company as "compassionate use," follows the "parallel track" ideas of NIAID director Dr. Anthony Fauci (see "Fauci Proposes 'Parallel Track' Treatment Access," *AIDS Treatment News* # 82). However, many important details are not yet available.

### DDI Overview and Importance

ddI emerged from the June Montreal AIDS conference with widespread professional consensus that it is the most important new AIDS antiviral at this time. The drug appears to be much less toxic than AZT, and the toxicities it does have are different—opening doors to more effective doses, as well as combination therapies.

Like AZT, ddI is not a cure, and will have to be used as a maintenance treatment. It can be taken less frequently than AZT, probably twice a day.

Although the drug is in the same general class as AZT, there does not appear to be cross resistance—meaning that strains of the virus which have become resistant to AZT are not automatically resistant to ddI. Therefore, ddI may be effective for people for whom AZT no longer works well. ddI may also be synergistic with AZT, meaning that the combination may work even better than would be expected by adding the efficacies of the two separate drugs together. But no one knows for sure, because as far as we know there have been no human tests of the combination.

Eventually AIDS virus strains will probably develop resistance to ddI, as with AZT. But the new drug should at least work for some time for people who cannot use AZT, or for whom AZT is no longer effective. And laboratory tests have suggested that when different drugs attack the virus in different ways (as suggested here by lack of cross resistance), it may take much longer for the virus to develop resistance to the combination than to any of the drugs separately.

Some scientists also suspect that bone-marrow toxicity from prolonged use of AZT might make it more difficult for the immune system to recover, even if the virus causing the immune deficiency can be stopped. ddI may provide evidence of whether or not this theory is true, by allowing AZT to be compared with an antiviral which has no bone-marrow toxicity. It will be important to see whether T-helper cells (for example) recover fastest with ddI alone, AZT alone, or a combination of the two.

In short, ddI will be most important for those who cannot use AZT. But also it may open doors to a whole range of new treatment possibilities, making possible creative research which can advance HIV management for the benefit of everyone.

These potential benefits, however, may be slowed or blocked by the ineffectual system of clinical research now in power. For example, no matter how clearly ddI works, the drug will have to go through a two-year ritual in which a statistically significant number of deaths and serious infections must accumulate in those in a control group **not** receiving the treatment. Trials to look directly at which patients do or do not improve while using the drug could be conducted much more rapidly, and would provide exactly the information patients and physicians want to know—but such trials would not be accepted for drug approval, because it is hard to measure patient improvement scientifically.

Since important antivirals will take years to go through the approval process, and patients cannot wait for reform of the current unproductive research system and the entrenched interests behind it, immediate discussion has focused on programs to make drugs available before full approval to those who need them most—after the drugs have passed safety tests and shown some evidence that they work. The basic fact shaping this discussion is the conflict between the interests of patients, who want to have more and better treatment options available, and the interest of institutions which, for differing reasons, want to restrict access.

Today there are increasing efforts to establish dialog among the different parties involved in treatment-access issues. Much of this dialog is focusing on the immediate and obvious point for negotiation—the specific rules on which groups of patients will or will not be allowed certain treatment options.

## DDI Negotiations

What made the recent Bristol-Myers announcement possible was the near-unanimous professional consensus coming from the Montreal conference that ddI looked good. (The only doubt we have heard so far was from a medical expert who questions whether HIV—which is inhibited by ddI—causes AIDS.) It would be hard for a company or for the FDA (U.S. Food and Drug Administration) to flatly deny access to a treatment when the medical profession is convinced that it could save lives. However, practical early access is not guaranteed, because there is still no consensus that the system should provide early access, even if the drugs clearly seem to work. And the all-important details of who will be able to get ddI have not been determined.

Bristol-Myers made its announcement after intensive negotiations involving the company, the FDA, Dr. Anthony Fauci of NIAID (the U.S. National Institute of

Allergy and Infectious Diseases), and the AIDS community, primarily represented by the Treatment + Data Committee of ACT UP/New York (the city where Bristol-Meyers is based). ACT UP's Treatment + Data Committee has done an outstanding job; without its work the current opening for ddI might not exist.

The Treatment + Data Committee defined four categories of patients who should have access to ddI:

• The AZT-intolerant, meaning those who cannot take AZT due to drug toxicity;

• The AZT-resistant, those for whom AZT is no longer working well, probably because the virus has developed resistance to it;

• The protocol-intolerant, including those too ill to qualify for the formal trials, those who need to stay on another medicine which disqualifies them, and those with symptomatic HIV infection but T-cells too high for the trial; and

• The protocol-inaccessible, including those living too far from a trial site, those who could not enroll because the trial was full, and those whose physicians were unable to enroll them and who could not change physicians (for example, those whose primary care was at a public-hospital emergency room where physicians could not take the time to get them enrolled in trials).

This list reflects the fact that those who most urgently need a new treatment are those who cannot effectively use any standard one. It also reflects the requirement of Fauci's "parallel track" access proposal, that use of experimental treatments must not be allowed to interfere with ongoing trials (see *AIDS Treatment News* # 82, cited above).

It is unclear at this time who will be allowed to use ddI. We have heard (but not confirmed) the following:

• At this time the only group fairly well assured of getting access is the AZT-intolerant—because the FDA is likely to insist that if a standard therapy is available it must be used in preference to an experimental one, unless, due to toxicity, the standard therapy cannot be administered.

• Informal discussions with FDA officials have raised some hope that four other groups might also be included: those too sick to qualify for the trials, those who must stay on another medicine which disqualifies them, those who live too far from a trial site, and those who cannot enter a trial because the trials are already full.

• The problem with the "AZT-resistant" group may be the difficulty of defining it. For example, one trial design being considered for AZT-resistant patients would accept anyone who has been on AZT for a year or more, since it is believed that the AIDS virus may develop resistance after that time. Even for a formal scientific study it is not feasible to do viral cultures for every potential subject to prove that viral resistance to AZT has in fact developed.

The potential difficulty in getting access to ddI for patients who can tolerate AZT but do not benefit from it recalls the example of trimetrexate, a pneumocystis treatment which at first was allowed only to those who could not tolerate the standard treatments, but not to those who could take them but did not respond and had no other alternative except death (see "Trimetrexate With Leucovorin: Decisions That Save Lives, Decisions That Kill, *AIDS Treatment News* #52). Following public outrage, these patients were also allowed access to trimetrexate. But what is not well known is that they were included through special procedures intended to avoid setting a precedent for the future. (We do not know why a special effort was made to preserve so clearly inhumane a procedure. One possible motive is that each early-access exception highlights a failure of the overall approval process, meaning that those who operate and support that process have reason to ration the exceptions as tightly as possible.)

## The Politics of Early Treatment Access

Ideally, persons facing a life-threatening illness should, with their physicians, be able to choose treatments based on medical merit, taking their whole medical situation into account. How can abstract, general rules make better decisions than those who know the specific, often unusual or even unique facts of a particular case? But the political reality is that institutions have more power to pursue their interests than patients do.

How do the different groups involved view the issue and perceive their interests? It would be difficult to answer this question fully. The insights and viewpoints below are some which have helped us in understanding what is happening. They refer to the general issue of access to treatments before full marketing approval, not specifically to DDI.

• Pharmaceutical companies. One clinical-trials expert described the position of pharmaceutical companies (toward the FDA) as, "Tell us what we must do, and that if we do it we will get the NDA." The NDA, or new-drug application approval, gives the company permission to market the drug—permission often worth hundreds of millions of dollars. Everything the companies do is seen in the light of whether it will help them get the NDA, or not.

Providing access to experimental drugs before the NDA (through "compassionate use," "treatment IND," or "parallel track,") is an expense and bother to companies. They must pay not only for the drug, but also for associated research and administrative expenses, and they can seldom be reimbursed, let alone profit from this activity. There may also be manufacturing, quality assurance, and liability concerns.

But the overriding issue is whether providing early access will help the company get the NDA. Early access primarily for treatment use could also provide data to help prove the drugs effective, and therefore support the NDA. But historically, the "compassionate use" system has provided poor data, probably because it relied on busy physicians to fill out forms which they would rather not deal with.

Starting almost two years ago, on October 26, 1987, compassionate-use access to drugs (at least for AIDS) became much more difficult to obtain. On that date an FDA advisory committee recommended against approval of ganciclovir (DHPG), and the pharmaceutical industry interpreted this rejection as punishment of Syntex for making its drug available to thousands of patients through compassionate use. Only recently, when NIAID's Dr. Anthony Fauci proposed his "parallel track" for access to certain treatments during trials, has the misinterpretation been corrected. When company officials said that they could not use the parallel track because they feared that what happened to Syntex would happen to them, Fauci pointed out that Syntex got in trouble not for making its drug available, but for failing to do scientific trials early.

A key difference between the old "compassionate use" system and the newer "treatment IND" or "parallel track" is that the newer systems provide access under a protocol, so that better data can be collected. Community-based research organizations may be able to monitor patients, collecting data according to the protocol and relieving primary-care physicians of unwanted paperwork.

(Why then did Bristol-Myers use the older term "compassionate use" in its announcement on ddI? Apparently the company did not want to be seen as taking sides in a fight between NIAID, with its "parallel track" proposal, and the FDA, which wants to revive its "treatment IND," which already exists but has not been used much because it has been interpreted so conservatively.)

For pharmaceutical companies, the bottom line is getting their NDA, which is granted by the FDA. Therefore, the most important factor determining whether or not these companies will be willing to provide their drug before marketing approval is the rules, often unwritten, set by the FDA. The public and the AIDS community have often failed to recognize this fact, in part because pharmaceutical companies and the FDA have an inner relationship between them which is hard for outsiders to penetrate. For example, which party takes the heat for an unpopular decision can be decided as part of a larger negotiated arrangement. For this reason, when treatments are not available, it is often hard to know whether the real problem is with the company which holds the exclusive rights to the drug, or with the FDA.

• The FDA. In discussions with FDA officials, the word "thalidomide" is likely to come up. Thalidomide was a drug disaster that led to the birth of thousands of deformed children in Europe in the early 1960s. No animal or other tests gave any advance warning of the problem. Fortunately, an FDA official noticed an obscure report suggesting other toxicity, and withheld U.S. approval long enough that the danger became known before the drug was distributed here.

After thalidomide, Congress amended Federal law to require proof of efficacy as well as safety before a drug could be marketed. This new law would not have stopped thalidomide, but in practice it has made new-drug approvals enormously more difficult. The current cost of drug development in this country is about $120 million for each new drug. And even aside from AIDS, analysts have questioned whether the current system saves as many lives as it destroys (see "FDA Reform: Major New Position Paper," *AIDS Treatment News* #58).

The FDA has taken its mission from thalidomide and the resulting Congressional mandate—to protect the public against dangerous or worthless drugs. Neither the FDA nor any other institution evaluates the risks or costs of not approving a drug which should be approved. People forget that thalidomide was a sleeping pill, and casually apply the standards appropriate for a new cold, cough, or baldness remedy for the development of life-saving treatments for diseases like cancer and AIDS. Thousands if not millions of people with diseases which are or should be treatable are sent away to die on their own, and there is no institutional responsibility. But if anyone is hurt by the other kind of mistake—approving a bad drug—then the FDA, the company, the researchers, and everyone else involved can expect to be blamed. The result is more than a distortion; it is a situation where half of the decision-making process does not take place at all.

The bottom line is not that we should weaken drug regulation, but rather strengthen it by balancing the costs of both kinds of errors. The rules of drug approval have immense and often hidden effects, not only on individual patients denied existing treatments, but also on the speed and creativity of the entire enterprise of medical research and development. Federal regulation largely controls the ability of medicine to respond quickly to new emergencies like AIDS, and to develop new treatments for old diseases like cancer.

• We do not have a clear picture of the other major institution in AIDS treatment development, namely NIAID (the National Institute of Allergy and Infectious Diseases), a branch of the National Institutes of Health. At this time the AIDS community is grateful that NIAID director Dr. Anthony Fauci proposed a "parallel track" system of allowing access to important new drugs while formal efficacy trials proceed. However, we are hearing of resistance to early access by some of the AIDS principal investigators working through NIAID contracts at sites around the country. Apparently these researchers fear that early access will deprive them of subjects for their trials, and as a result they are pressing to restrict such access. These reports have not yet been confirmed, but they have been greeted with anger in the AIDS community, which sees the NIAID research effort as unproductive in view of the time and money it has had, and which sees the notorious recruiting problems at academic research centers as being caused by poorly designed trials (that people cannot volunteer for even when they want to), not by the existence of other options for patients. This situation must be watched, because it could threaten access to lifesaving treatments.

## What Should Be Done?

Pharmaceutical companies and government agencies alike have been unenthusiastic if not hostile toward early treatment release. The old "compassionate use" system, for example, was supposed to apply to only a few patients. The "treatment IND" applied to groups, but the FDA has used this system after the full burden of proof has already been met, when only paperwork remains before approval of the NDA. And pharmaceutical companies have had little incentive to use either system.

What is needed instead is a flexible burden of proof that takes account of the uniqueness and potential value of a drug and the urgency of the need for it. For example, consider ddI:

• It will take probably two years or more to get statistical proof that ddI (or any antiviral) increases AIDS survival or reduces the frequency of major infections.

• During this time, 50,000 people will die in the United States alone, unless better treatment becomes available.

• Of the new treatment possibilities, ddI looks best at this time.

In this emergency the FDA should waive the requirement to prove reduced death or opportunistic infections. Instead, it could work with Bristol-Myers to design much faster trials using p24 antigen, T-helper count, and clinical measures such as weight gain to show drug efficacy, in a program of clinical trials involving perhaps several hundred patients, testing different doses and testing the drug in different patient populations. Placebos could ethically be used in some cases, because patients would not be on the trial for long—and after the trial would have the option of using the drug. If these rapid trials showed that the drug was useful, and the long-term experience available did not show serious problems, then the developer should get its NDA and be allowed to market the drug—provided that post-marketing studies continued. (The approval might be called an "emergency NDA," to alert physicians that the drug was approved with less testing than usual because of the urgent need, and therefore should be used cautiously.) No legislation would be needed to implement this approach; the FDA has the power to start tomorrow.

This system would be clean to administer, and would provide enough incentive to insure that pharmaceutical companies conducted their trials rapidly. Then the medical community could evaluate the evidence available and make recommendations to guide practicing physicians. Patients and physicians could then decide whether to use the drug or to choose other options instead.

Why hasn't such an approach been used already? The reason is that the outcome measures available—p24 antigen, T-helper cell count, and overall health of patients— all have flaws and therefore are not technically attractive in the academic world which sets the tone for these decisions. Fantastic scenarios can be concocted in which drugs could look good after the trials suggested above, but really not give any benefit to patients. But the small chance of mistakenly approving such a drug must be balanced against the certainty of tens of thousands of deaths caused by the built-in, two-year delay of the kinds of trials currently required.

## FOSCARNET INFORMATION NUMBERS

Many people with CMV retinitis are interested in the experimental treatment foscarnet, some because they did not obtain an effective response from the approved treatment, ganciclovir (DHPG), and others because they want to avoid the side effects of ganciclovir as well as make use of foscarnet's possible anti-HIV activity. In June, issue #80 of *AIDS Treatment News* printed the number of an ACT UP foscarnet organizing committee in San Francisco. The activists on this committee have done an excellent job of maintaining pressure on the Food and Drug Administration and the manufacturer of foscarnet, Astra, to develop wider access to the drug. The current alternatives for many people are to stay on ganciclovir but give up the option to use AZT because of the unacceptable combined bone marrow suppression, or to give up ganciclovir in order to stay on AZT. The first choice is life-threatening and the second one guarantees irreversible blindness. (For more background information, see *AIDS Treatment News* #71 and #77.)

Thanks to the efforts of activist Terry Sutton who died in April, more people who want to try foscarnet may be eligible for a "salvage" trial, and should call Astra's hotline number: 800/225-6333. This number may be useful for other questions regarding foscarnet as well. But the organizing committee still maintains a phone line to connect with people who are interested in challenging the basic restrictions on foscarnet: 415/431-6088.

## COMPUTER SYSTEM RECOMMENDATIONS FOR COMMUNITY-BASED RESEARCH ORGANIZATIONS

On July 7-9 a major conference on community-based research, sponsored by the Community Research Initiative of New York and the County Community Consortium of San Francisco and funded by the American Foundation for AIDS Research (AmFAR) and NIAID, brought together representatives of community-based research organizations, government agencies, and pharmaceutical companies. (For more information about this conference, see articles in *The New York Times*, July 9, 1989 and *The Washington Post*, same date.)

Plans were begun to set up electronic communication networks among organizations interested in community-based research, using conference calls, electronic mail, fax, and perhaps voicemail. A number of groups are buying computer equipment at this time, and it is important that a standard be suggested so that the groups will purchase compatible equipment and software to facilitate electronic mail and the sharing of text files and research data.

No official umbrella organization was formed at this time, so there was no body to decide on a standard. However, it is almost certain that the community-based trials organizations will follow the standard already set by NIAID's Community Programs for Clinical Research on AIDS. That is because many of the organizations involved have applied to that organization for funding, and those who receive contract awards will be required to purchase the specified computer equipment and software. (And from our own background in computers, we can tell that the recommended standard was clearly well selected and appropriate for the task.)

The following specifications are from instructions to community-based research organizations applying for NIAID grants:

> "Equipment will be required for computer-to-computer electronic mail communications, report generation, and data analysis. Specifically:
>
> * MS-DOS/PC-DOS microcomputer IBM compatible PC/AT or equivalent,
>
> * Monochrome display,
>
> * Minimum of 20 megabyte hard disk and 640 K memory; a 3.5" diskette drive is recommended,
>
> * A 2400 baud modem and cable (to be specified by AIDS Program),
>
> * 132-column printer and cable (Epson LQ-1500 or equivalent),
>
> * Communications software to be specified by AIDS Program,
>
> * WordPerfect word processing software (version 5.0 is preferred)."

The NIAID recommendations for communication software are not final, but they will probably include MCI Mail and Lotus Express. The modem specified will probably be any which is 2400 baud and Hayes compatible.

Any organization buying computer equipment for the purpose of community-based research should strongly consider following the recommendations outlined above. But if you already have a computer which is not compatible with these specifications, it might be OK for a time, so there is no need to rush to buy new equipment.

# AZT, ACYCLOVIR, AND THE CASE FOR EARLY TREATMENT

*by Denny Smith*

For several years the San Francisco-based organization Project Inform has developed a pioneering treatment strategy dealing with HIV infection. The key premise of this strategy asserts that HIV and AIDS are chronic, manageable conditions, not the death sentences bemoaned by the media/medicine/government complex. The prescription for action which grew from this premise is 1) early testing for the presence of HIV or immune dysfunction, and 2) flexible antiviral or immune-boosting treatment **before** the appearance of symptoms, possibly without waiting for the approval of a promising treatment by the Food and Drug Administration (FDA). Though much of the medical establishment still dismisses or ignores it, the message proposed by Project Inform is proving correct with the passage of time and with the accumulation of pointless deaths. Health officials from government and academia alike have been slow to advocate any plan of action, or "standard of care," to account for everyone with HIV, symptomatic or not.

Even within the limits of FDA-approved drugs there are treatment opportunities now available to seropositive asymptomatic people to optimize their chances of staying healthy. Two of them are AZT (Zidovudine) and acyclovir (Zovirax). Since its initial approval by the FDA, AZT has remained the most prominently discussed and intensively studied treatment for HIV and related infections. At the recent International Conference on AIDS in Montreal, for example, there were over 370 sessions which discussed some aspect of AZT. Despite pervasive and often unfounded mistrust of its efficacy, and despite its very real toxicity and the limits of its antiretroviral activity, AZT has proven to be of immune-preserving and life-prolonging usefulness for many people with HIV. In addition, its capacity to reach the central nervous system makes AZT useful for treating HIV neuropathy, and the neurologic impairment sometimes called AIDS dementia complex (ADC).

Side effects on the other hand, especially from the "high" dose of 1200 mg daily, completely prevent many people from using AZT. And for people who can tolerate the drug, long-term studies indicate that prolonged use of AZT on the originally approved dosing schedule often leads to unacceptable bone marrow suppression. Prolonged use may create AZT-resistant virus as well, although laboratory tests have shown that isolates of HIV which have become resistant to AZT are still susceptible to other anti-retrovirals such as ddI and ddC. AZT-induced anemia can be reversible if the drug is temporarily discontinued, or may be managed with periodic blood transfusions, or may possibly be prevented by also taking erythropoietin (EPO), a red cell growth factor recently approved by the FDA.

There are HIV and AIDS-related treatments which appear to enhance AZT. This has meant that the same anti-retroviral potency might be achieved by combining such an agent with lower, less toxic amounts of AZT. One possibility, reported in *AIDS Treatment News* #79, is the anti-clotting drug dipyridamole (Persantine). This is a prescription drug which extended the activity of AZT in the test tube. But there is no evidence yet that it will do the same, or do it safely, in people. The beneficial combination best studied is AZT and acyclovir (reported in *AIDS Treatment News* #47), although much more work has been published since then). Acyclovir is relatively nontoxic and two European studies presented at the Montreal conference (Walger, P and others, abstract W.B.P. 318, and Weber, R and others, abstract W.B.P. 321) suggested that AZT with acyclovir was superior to AZT alone. Acyclovir is also used to suppress latent infections of the herpes viruses, including herpes simplex, CMV, and herpes zoster, all of which have been discussed as factors that may facilitate the growth of HIV.

One small but illustrative AZT/acyclovir study, conducted by Harry Hollander and others at the University of California in San Francisco, began with 20 HIV+ asymptomatic participants almost two years ago. Ten of the participants were placed on 100 mg of AZT (half the dose originally recommended by the manufacturer, Burroughs-Wellcome) with 400 mg of acyclovir (twice the dose recommended for treating initial herpes infections) five times daily. The other ten participants received the same amount of AZT, with 800 mg of acyclovir.

Three participants withdrew from the study (two after 10 weeks and the other after 38 weeks) because of subjective toxicities (side effects that the patients told the physicians about, but were not measured by laboratory tests). Unfortunately, three other participants developed AIDS (at weeks 6, 8, and 62). These six participants had entered the study with a lower median T4-helper cell count than the other fourteen participants (210 versus 544), and the three who developed symptoms had each tested positive with the first p24 antigen results. The remaining participants continue to tolerate this drug combination without serious side effects and remain asymptomatic. Three have had at least one positive p24 titer, all below 25 pg/ml, and one participant who began the study with low titer antigenemia now tests negative. Helper cells have remained stable—from a baseline median of 503 to 588 at week 78.

The investigators concluded that the combination of AZT with acyclovir is generally well-tolerated, with no statistical consequences seen between the two acyclovir doses (although the three participants who withdrew for subjective toxicity were all on the higher dose). They added that larger trials are necessary to determine the efficacy of the combination.

Nevertheless, some implications may be useful for people now considering whether to treat an asymptomatic HIV infection, with or without AZT. The combination was apparently better tolerated by participants with a higher T4-helper cell count. Additionally, progression to illness was uniformly seen in those participants with the poorest laboratory predictors: depressed helper cells and elevated p24 antigen levels. A reasonable conclusion, one reflected by the Project Inform strategy, is that early intervention in HIV infection is easier to cope with, and more effective therapeutically, than applying an equivalent treatment **after** helper cells have been seriously depleted or AIDS-related symptoms have developed.

This was not a placebo-controlled study, fortunately, since there is ample epidemiological evidence that without any treatment intervention most people with HIV will eventually progress to illness. *AIDS Treatment News* has spoken to many people who are currently asymptomatic but watching their T4-helper cells fall or p24 antigen level rise (if they're lucky enough to get these tests). Many physicians would defend not treating these asymptomatic patients, with a rationale mentioned below. Other physicians are tending to treat earlier than the appearance of symptoms by following such progression markers as thrombocytopenia and elevated beta 2 microglobulin, in addition to helper cell counts and p24 antigen levels.

If most or all HIV infections eventually progress to illness, what is the basis for telling an asymptomatic seropositive person to "leave well enough alone" or "if it ain't broke, don't fix it"? And if the treatments now available for HIV are more effective the earlier they are initiated, what is the point of waiting until symptoms appear? There are objections which warn of "wasting" the AZT option by offering it early to asymptomatic people only to see them become anemic or reach resistance of the drug, leaving them without an antiviral if symptoms develop. This objection appears weak from two perspectives. For one, AZT or other early treatment options will not have been wasted if they forestall the progression to illness until another generation of anti-HIV drugs becomes available. Secondly, the option may be wasted precisely by waiting until symptoms appear, when drugs of all kinds are more difficult to tolerate and less potent against the immune deficiency.

If acyclovir or other agents can permit a decrease in the dosage of AZT, then many more people with HIV may have access to the only approved HIV treatment. And preliminary results of a large NIH study indicate that survival rates for patients on a full dose of AZT were no better than for those taking a low dose, without acyclovir as a factor. Whether AZT is absolutely more effective when combined with acyclovir or dipyridamole is not clear yet, but the originally recommended high dose of AZT appears to be unnecessary in any case. We have also spoken to many people who feel their physicians rely too heavily on AZT because they are unwilling to consider other potential antivirals such as dextran sulfate or hypericin which have not been approved for the treatment of HIV and AIDS. When AZT is routinely prescribed for someone who is not benefiting from it and who may benefit from another promising, but unapproved, treatment, then the letter of the law is obstructing the pursuit of the patient's health. Hopefully, accessibility to various treatments of promise will increase with growing public political pressure.

The indications which earned AZT an FDA approval were a T4-helper cell count below 200 or a diagnosis of AIDS. These could be exactly good predictors of a poor response to AZT, in light of the study described above and others. Many clinicians are prescribing AZT earlier than the FDA indications, but many insurance companies will only reimburse within the FDA parameters. Which means that without an FDA/NIH-backed "standard of care" which reflects the growing medical consensus, hundreds of thousands of U.S. citizens known to be HIV+ may not receive AZT or acyclovir or anything else, unless they can join an NIH drug trial or until they become ill (and are less able to manage AZT's toxicity). And for years, people who could not tolerate AZT were offered no other alternative by the NIH or FDA until the recent ddI announcement (see related article on ddI in this issue).

There were hundreds of drugs and drug combinations discussed at the Montreal conference, one or more of which may someday be a successful treatment for HIV. At present there is no NIH/FDA-approved treatment plan for everyone with HIV, which leaves thousands of doctors lacking authoritative leadership and a standard of care to apply to their HIV+ patients. Innovative physicians have been staying abreast of current treatment options without the guidance or permission of the national healthcare bureaucracy, and their patients are lucky for it: they tend to receive treatment, AZT or otherwise, before the appearance of opportunistic infections and they find out about other options if AZT ceases to be one. But people without innovative doctors will not fare as well, and for them the vacuum of leadership is unfair and perhaps deadly.

## For More Information

Project Inform's HIV treatment strategy can be requested by calling 800/822-7422 from outside of California, 800/334-7422 inside California, and 415/558-9051 from San Francisco or other countries. Fact sheets are also available which discuss potential treatments for HIV, both approved and unapproved. The following periodicals, like *AIDS Treatment News*, also report on new developments in the treatment of AIDS and HIV infection.

• *Treatment Issues* discusses new and now-standard therapies for HIV and related infections. Sent free of charge, but donation welcome. Write to GMHC, Dept. of Medical Information, 129 West 20th St., N.Y., NY 10011.

• *BETA*, (Bulletin of Experimental Treatments for AIDS) offers thorough coverage of anti-HIV drugs. Published by the San Francisco AIDS Foundation, three issues have appeared in the last year. Call 415/863-2437.

• *AIDS/HIV Experimental Treatment Directory*, published by the American Foundation for AIDS Research (AmFAR) lists and describes a wide spectrum of treatments currently in development or in clinical trials. Call 212/719-0033.

# Issue Number 84
# July 28, 1989

## OVERVIEW

The most important news now concerns the antiviral ddI, and the policies being developed about who will have access to it before full marketing approval, which is probably over two years away. This issue of *AIDS Treatment News* will show how you can have input into decisions being made this month about ddI, and about the "parallel track" or other systems for early access while formal trials continue.

The ddI situation is moving very rapidly, and there is much confusion. We will bring out some hidden ethical issues concerning treatment access. We will show what probably will happen, what should happen, and why it makes sense to work on both at this time.

ddI is not new, as many think. It has a history, with published references back at least to 1981. In a later issue, we will include a bibliography of published articles about ddI.

This issue of *AIDS Treatment News* also includes a historical overview of peptide T, by David Smyth of San Francisco. We first reported on peptide T over two and a half years ago (issue #22), after the drug had been given to four people in Sweden. Since that time peptide T has been the subject of unusually intense scientific controversy; the research in Sweden was stopped, for unknown reasons; and despite general agreement that the drug is safe, it is still in phase I (small dosage and toxicity studies) over two years later, with trials in Los Angeles and Boston. Although the evidence for peptide T appears weak at this time, the drug may have some usefulness. In any case its history illustrates a lack of practical judgment in the management of AIDS clinical research. When it was clear that the drug was safe, and that there were leading scientists on both sides of the efficacy debate, rapid efficacy testing should have been done. The scientific theories under dispute can serve only as guidelines as to what might work, and cannot substitute for experience.

The peptide T history is the first major article in 84 issues of *AIDS Treatment News* not written by a member of our staff. We first met the author about a year ago, and were impressed by his knowledge of peptide T, and his determination to research this treatment thoroughly and become an expert in the drug and its history.

# DDI AND PARALLEL TRACK: OVERVIEW AND EDITORIAL

*by John S. James*

Both the medicine and the public policy around ddI are developing rapidly. But the real progress should not obscure the fact that we still have a serious problem.

The bottom line is that unless major toxicity is found with ddI (which could still happen), the current plans, intentions, and directions will lead to an unprecedented situation of a clear medical consensus in favor of a treatment which is blocked by red tape. There will be adequate supplies of the drug, and it will not be especially expensive to produce. But treatment will be denied because of scientists' fears that they will not get subjects for trials of other drugs such as AZT or CD4 if patients have viable options, because of regulators' fears that precedents set with AIDS will damage their control over routine drugs in the future, and because even if the drug is inexpensive there is no way to charge for it, no one to pay for it, and reluctance to provide a free alternative to high-priced AZT. In other words, thousands of people will be denied lifesaving treatment because the lives of persons with AIDS are still not valuable enough to arouse the political will to treat this epidemic as an emergency.

Formal efficacy trials of ddI should start soon—hopefully within the next few weeks or months. There will probably be three different double-blind trials: ddI vs AZT for those who have never taken an antiviral before; low-dose ddI vs high-dose ddI for those intolerant to AZT; and AZT vs ddI for those who have already been on AZT for over a year. No one will get a placebo.

These trials appear to be ethical for those who can get into them. The problem is that they will take two years or more to get results—the time needed to wait for statistically significant numbers of deaths or serious infections to accumulate in the control groups. Meanwhile, for each person who can get into these trials, others who need ddI will be excluded, for various reasons.

It now seems clear that some form of early access—whether called "parallel track," "treatment IND," or "compassionate use"—will be provided for certain people who cannot get into the trials, during the two or more years it takes the trials to run, and the additional time for paperwork before ddI is approved for marketing. The issue then becomes what criteria are used to select those eligible for early access. There is much concern that the criteria will be narrow, in order to define away the parallel track as much as possible. Patients and their physicians benefit by early access, but other interests involved are likely to see it as an expense and bother, if not a threat.

An advisory committee including persons with AIDS or AIDS advocates is now being formed to advise Dr. James Mason, Assistant Secretary of Health, about the parallel track on or before August 21. You can write to Dr. Mason about the parallel track and access to ddI; for more information, see below. Telling Dr. Mason and the committee about your own situation, or that of your patients, could be especially helpful, as committees often produce inappropriate rules or criteria because they did not think of enough examples during their deliberations.

What will be done on ddI is haggling about the specific rules and boundaries of access—who will and who will not be allowed the option of using this treatment, with decisions being made primarily for institutional interests, not patients' interests. Consequently there will also be increasing activity around "underground" ddI. At this time it is hard to find, and costs about $600 per month or more; but several early samples have been tested and all were good quality. Further chemical testing will be essential, however, in order to prevent fraudulent and/or dangerously contaminated products.

What **should** be done is to move toward more control of treatment decisions by patients and their physicians. But clinical research will have to reform itself to work well in a more open environment (or in any environment, for that matter). Today it is argued that we must restrict patients' access to treatment options, in order to balance the interests of the "few" (those now ill with AIDS or HIV) against the interests of the "many" (those who will become ill in the future). The fear is that if patients have attractive treatment options, they will not volunteer for scientific trials, and therefore we will not get the answers needed. Even the more humane wing of the current professional debate, Fauci's "parallel track" proposal, is based on the idea that access must be denied those who could participate in trials, in order to force them to do so.

The cheap and easy way to get research subjects would seem to be to deny patients other treatment options. This approach not only is unethical, however, but also it has failed to produce subjects for trials even when there is no access to alternatives. The right way to get volunteers would be to reform what is currently wrong in clinical trial design. Too often trials are not designed for the real world. For example:

(1) If a trial asks a real, practical question, then it follows that all the treatment arms to which patients are randomized must be viable, medically sound therapeutic choices. Why ask patients to undergo a course of therapy which is known in advance to be unattractive and not a viable option? What useful knowledge is gained?

The answer is that commercial considerations often override scientific and medical ones. The drugs which get studied tend to be those with the most commercial and professional momentum behind them, whether they are the best scientific prospects or not. Or patients are forced to take single drugs only (when in practice those drugs will be used in combination with others), because each company wants its product to be approved by itself, not in combination with a rival's product.

When patients are asked to undergo bad medicine for the sake of "science," then naturally they will seek other options. But if trials were redesigned to compare good therapies with other good therapies, then few patients would object to the randomization and blinding which the researchers want, and the conflict would go away. An added bonus is that trials so designed would produce more useful information, because they would focus directly on obtaining the answers which physicians need.

It is finally being acknowledged that the information sought by the FDA for the drug-approval process, and the information sought by physicians for making treatment decisions, are not the same. How odd it is that they should be different! Imagine how much more efficient the system could be if clinical trials were designed to answer the same questions that good physicians will ask when they decide whether or not to use the drug. (One fundamental problem, however, is that the FDA is set up to approve products, not to approve treatments, and clinical trials are therefore designed accordingly.)

Some progress is being made. Trial design now is better than it was two or three years ago. But progress is inherently slow, because it means that academic researchers, who often look down on clinicians, need to learn new ways of thinking, and learn them well enough to be successful in using them.

(2) Another major problem in clinical trials is the discourtesy with which potential volunteers are often treated, the lack of concern for their interests and practical needs. For example, patients often must stop using other treatments which are important for their health in order to qualify for trials. Too often when they do so they are strung along, told that the trial is not ready for them at the expected date, and left to wait indefinitely without their standard medication, with no clear answers about when they can start the trial. (Notice that this problem is not considered in the ethical review of the trial, or the informed consent, because it occurs before the patient begins an official relationship with the study.)

Better administration is part of the answer, but not all of it. In addition, research on human beings must be recognized as a special calling. It differs profoundly from testing drugs on laboratory animals—and not only because stricter ethical guidelines are required. For human research to be successful, the whole approach to the problem must be different.

The practical effect that such reforms could have on recruitment is illustrated by community-based research organizations which have persons with AIDS or HIV on all their review boards and decision-making bodies. Organizations such as New York's Community Research Initiative have done far better than academic medical centers in recruiting volunteers for trials. The reason is that persons with AIDS and their physicians are well represented on the scientific and ethical review boards which approve these trials. Before studies begin, they are modified to take into account their medical and ethical impacts as felt by those most affected.

In contrast, the academic centers have done so poorly that a number of studies have gone through all the required steps of approval, at considerable trouble and expense, and then failed to recruit a single qualified volunteer. It is preposterous to blame the patients for this situation, or to blame access to "underground" treatment options, or sanctioned options such as the proposed parallel track—instead of analyzing the problem case by case to find out why patients do not volunteer, and how future trials could be improved so that they would.

# CONGRESSIONAL HEARING ON PARALLEL TRACK, JULY 20

*by John S. James*

On July 20, the U.S. House of Representatives Subcommittee on Health and the Environment, chaired by Henry A. Waxman (D-Los Angeles) held a public hearing on the "parallel track proposal for clinical drug development." The first panel was James Mason, Assistant Secretary for Health, testifying for the government, with FDA Commissioner Frank Young, NIAID director Anthony Fauci, and National Cancer Institute Director Samuel Broder available for questions. The second panel was Jim

Eigo of the Treatment and Data Committee of ACT UP/New York, and Martin Delaney of Project Inform, representing AIDS advocacy organizations. The third panel was John Petricciani, vice president of the Pharmaceutical Manufacturers' Association. We did not attend this hearing but have received copies of the prepared text submitted in advance by most of the speakers.

The opening statement by Congressman Waxman is an excellent neutral summary of the issues as they are conventionally viewed, so we reproduce it in full:

"Today's hearing is on the controversial and critical issue of release of experimental drugs. The hearing is specifically about recent proposals referred to as the parallel track for drug development.

"Food and Drug Administration law does not allow drugs to be *sold* until they are proven to be safe and effective. The same law prohibits distribution in any manner of drugs without permission of the FDA. This law was adopted to protect consumers from dangerous products and from snake-oil remedies. It was intended to establish a straightforward policy as to when manufacturers can profit from—and when consumers can take—drugs whose effectiveness is unknown.

"Exceptions have been carved out of the general rule. Drugs whose safety and effectiveness are unknown may be distributed for research purposes. Drugs whose safety is proven, but whose effectiveness is undemonstrated, may be distributed outside of strict medical trials under various labels—as Treatment Research or as Compassionate Use or as Open Protocols.

"But the law and its exceptions have run head on into the AIDS epidemic. Thousands of Americans find themselves without useful approved treatment and with steadily declining health. A handful can get into controlled trials, but most can just read about drugs they cannot get.

"During the course of the epidemic, this rationing has been scientifically and morally justified as necessary to the conduct of trials and appropriate for quickly meeting the needs of future Americans with AIDS. We have lived with a policy of limited distribution today so that we will have adequate information for tomorrow.

"But now, many people—patients, their families, and researchers—are questioning this policy. They argue that scientific trials do not require that everyone else be denied access to potential therapies; indeed, they say, the trials are better conducted with willing volunteers rather than desperate ones. And, they continue, it is, therefore, morally wrong to withhold promising drugs from patients with nothing else to turn to.

"From this questioning has grown the Parallel Track, a proposal that drugs be available for some distribution when they are known to be safe and when trials for effectiveness are fully enrolled. Doctors treating patients who receive such drugs would be asked to provide information back to researchers, thus forming a source of information that is parallel to the formal trials.

"This is an important proposal. It could change ground rules on research, clinical care, markets, and insurance. It could also provide access to drugs—the good ones and the worthless ones—long before data are available. If it works it could revolutionize drug development. If it fails it could cripple AIDS research for some time.

"Today's hearing is to form a record of the proposal, its reach and its limits as well as the questions that remain unanswered. I hope that with this hearing we can begin to form a consensus as to how AIDS drug development will proceed."

Congresswoman Nancy Pelosi (D-San Francisco) gave specific examples of problems with the current system:

"Each month, I hold an open meeting in my district for people with symptomatic HIV infection and their advocates. The group is very knowledgeable about HIV-related drugs and their potential uses. Their top priority is access to potentially lifesaving experimental drugs. Their stories are compelling.

"One young man participated in a NIH-sponsored phase I trial of ddC at Stanford. From his perspective, the drug worked well. He felt subjectively much better and his laboratory tests indicated a decline in p24 antigen level (a measure of viral activity) and limited increases in T-cell count (a measure of immune functioning). After 13 weeks, he received a phone call telling him that his participation in the study was no longer needed. Since then he has started AZT several times but has had difficulty tolerating even half of the standard dose. Although he has not yet received a formal AIDS diagnosis, as of last month his T-cell count dropped to 18. He is receiving no anti-retroviral therapy. He and his treating physician want him to try ddI or to go back on ddC. Given his history of prior use of AZT and ddC, he is a poor candidate for other clinical trials. Why can't this man and his physician be given access to either ddC or ddI?

"Another man from this group has been on AZT for just under two years. He did very well on this drug. However, in the last two months, his T-cell level has declined from over 300 to around 130. He is also beginning to experience symptoms which he has not had in the last two years, including disabling levels of fatigue. He and his physician believe it is time for him to switch to another anti-retroviral drug. Why can't this man and his physician be given access to ddI?"

We have not seen Dr. Mason's testimony. But Jim Eigo of ACT UP/New York's Treatment and Data Committee summarized the status of the parallel track after the hearings. According to his summary:

• Dr. Mason's testimony showed that the Public Health Service is committed to some form of parallel track—but that what parallel track means is so far undecided. The Public Health Service asked that an FDA advisory committee, to include AIDS advocates, report to Dr. Mason by August 21 and prepare recommendations on the parallel track.

• ddI will not be available under the "parallel track," at least not immediately, but it *will* be available under the "treatment IND" for people who are AZT-intolerant. However, FDA commissioner Frank Young admitted that Bristol-Myers has not yet applied for a treatment IND.

• The day after the hearing, Jim Eigo "argued with Dr. Ellen Cooper of FDA that ddI has to be made available under compassionate use to at least two other groups of people: those too sick to abide the rigors of the ddI clinical trials and those who can't go off medication that the ddI trials forbid. She said she believed that we could work that out."

• Parallel-track drugs will be open label (meaning that patients will know what they are getting, instead of being randomly assigned to two or more treatments and not told which).

• Parallel-track drugs will be judged individually—probably by an FDA advisory committee with AIDS-community representation. Drugs must show "some indication of efficacy." Persons receiving these drugs will sign informed-consent forms.

• There must be some way to prevent "secondary transfer" (i.e. an underground market) of drugs obtained under the parallel track.

On July 31 we spoke with Dr. Mason's office and learned:

• Dr. Mason wanted to emphasize that setting up the parallel track must not interfere with or delay access to ddI.

• The committee to advise Dr. Mason by August 21 has not yet been formed. However, it will probably consist of an FDA antiviral advisory committee which already exists, plus AIDS advocates brought in as consultants.

## COMMUNITY-BASED RESEARCH ORGANIZATIONS— AMFAR WILL COORDINATE

About 20 groups are organizing in cities around the country to do community-based research. Recently the American Foundation for AIDS Research (AmFAR) has hired a full-time coordinator to put together a communication network for community-based organizations doing clinical trials. The coordinator is Debbie Levine, who also organized the July 1989 New York conference on community-based trials.

AmFAR's community-based clinical trials program will set up a series of conference calls to address major topics:

• Putting together multicenter trials;

• Standardizing data collection and data management;

• Communication, by conference calls, electronic mail, fax, or voicemail;

• Examining the role of community-based organizations in the parallel-track system;

• Working on the relationship of community-based clinical trial organizations and NIAID's ACTG research centers;

• Fundraising for community-based research, including government and pharmaceutical-industry support;

• How to set up Institutional Review Boards;

• Recruiting, including equal access for poor or minority patients;

• How to work with the mass media;

• How to encourage community groups to have PWA representation on all decision-making bodies.

Immediate plans are for a conference call about once every three weeks, with one representative from each group on the call. There may also be a newsletter sent to each organization.

# PEPTIDE T
*by David Smyth*

Peptide T first gained notoriety in late 1986 and early 1987 when researchers at the Karolinska Institute in Stockholm reported in the *Lancet* improvements in lymphocyte counts, psoriasis and neuropsychiatric functions in four patients who had been given the drug on a compassionate basis (Wetterberg and others, 1987). Since that time the drug has undergone further tests in Sweden and the United States with scientists reporting some positive results.

Although there was considerable evidence from the earliest laboratory tests that peptide T is nontoxic, the drug has been bogged down for nearly two years in a small phase I toxicity trial in the U.S. Indeed, phase II efficacy studies have been delayed in part because of the drug's lack of toxicity. The questionable logic behind this policy dictates that phase II studies can not begin until a maximum tolerated dose is discovered in phase I. Researchers had ample warning this might be the case, because they could not find an LD50 dose (a dose potent enough to kill half the animals to which it is administered) in studies conducted before human trials began.

An application by the drug's sponsors for phase II studies of peptide T in the National Institutes of Health extensive testing system was denied in late July, 1989. And Bristol-Myers Co. in May, 1989 withdrew from a federal license to market and manufacture the drug.

Peptide T was discovered by Candace Pert, Ph.D., who was chief of the brain biochemistry section at the National Institute of Mental Health (NIMH). The mechanism of action of the drug is different from most antivirals in that it does not act directly on HIV or infected cells. Rather it is intended to block the virus from entering cells (Pert and others, 1986).

Eight amino acids which constitute part of the viral envelope called gp120 are thought by some scientists to be the key by which HIV gains entry through the CD4 receptor. Indeed, a common metaphor by which the drug's action is explained is the lock and key.

Pert theorized that if HIV could enter the CD4 receptor, it must mimic a chemical produced by the body that used the same receptor (Pert, 1987). She found a sequence of eight amino acids in a hormone called vasointestinal peptide (VIP) that duplicated a section of gp120 and designed peptide T as a way of plugging all the body's CD4 "locks" with artificial "keys," The drug's lack of toxicity is thought to derive from its similarity to a chemical produced by the body.

But the controversy swirling around the drug centers on its efficacy, not its toxicity. And the fact that the drug is plodding through a slow-moving toxicity study has done little to help resolve the issue in a timely fashion.

Six months after Pert and others asserted in *The Lancet* that peptide T helped Swedish AIDS patients, William Haseltine, Ph.D., of the Dana-Farber Cancer Institute in Boston reported that he and several other researchers found peptide T did not inhibit the virus in test tube experiments. Furthermore, the viral envelope was constantly changing, thus the sequence of amino acids in peptide T could not possibly duplicate a section of the viral envelope (Sodroski and others, 1987).

Two years later, Joseph Sodroski, M.D., one of the drug's critics, asserts, "There is no scientific basis for concluding that peptide T will perform the (blocking) function.

The first work that said the peptide T region is not the region on gp120 that interacts with the receptor was from our lab (Kowalski and others, 1987) and Larry Lasky's (Lasky and others, 1987) group at Genentech, which pointed more to the carboxyl terminus on gp120. Subsequently, Hans Wigsell (Nygren and others, 1988) at the Karolinska Institute has cleaved gp120 and they have a fragment that has cleaved off peptide T-related sequences completely and that still binds to CD4."

The drug's sponsors replied that Haseltine, Sodroski and others had used high concentrations of virus in their experiments (Ruff and others, 1987), and that no one knew what concentrations were actually present in the bodies of AIDS patients.

Frederick Goodwin, M.D., then director of NIMH, called a meeting where the opposing researchers could arrive at a consensus about the drug's mechanism of action. However, no agreement was reached (Barnes, 1987). Nevertheless the Food and Drug Administration, which had a representative at the meeting, granted permission to begin testing the drug in people, half a year after the application was filed.

At about this time, a researcher at Oncogen, a small Seattle-based company later acquired by Bristol-Myers Co., devised her own in vitro tests of peptide T and found the drug worked against low and moderate viral concentrations, but not against high concentrations (Barnes, 1987). This work helped influence the pharmaceutical giant's decision to seek a license for peptide T from NIMH, which has a patent pending on the compound.

Douglas Brenneman, M.D., of the Laboratory of Developmental Neurobiology at the National Institute of Child Health and Human Development has asserted in articles in *Nature* (Brenneman and others, 1988) and *Drug Development Research* (Brenneman and others, 1988) that gp120 is associated with neuronal cell death and that VIP and peptide T blocked the action of gp120 in the test tube.

In an interview, Dr. Sodroski said, "That work is of dubious significance. It's not clear what neuronal cell death in that system really means....The neuronal cells in that system are mouse cells. The problem is that gp120 does not bind to mouse CD4."

Although FDA allowed phase I testing to begin, the National Institutes of Health refused the sponsors' application for a phase I study of the drug in the agency's drug trials network. The agency wanted more documentation of the drug's mechanism of action as well as more studies in animals. NIMH (which is part of the Alcohol, Drug Abuse and Mental Health Administration, not the NIH) searched for months for a medical center in which to conduct its studies, finally contracting with the Los Angeles County/University of Southern California Medical Center. Peter Heseltine, M.D., was selected as principal investigator.

Intravenous administration of peptide T to the first group of six patients in this trial began in November, 1987. NIMH expanded this study in July, 1988 to include 24 patients. They were given the drug by intravenous injection for twelve weeks, followed by a four week "washout" period, during which no antivirals (including peptide T) could be taken. The patients were then given the option of continuing to take the drug intranasally. This study focused on searching for toxic side effects and determining a suitable dose for later trials of the drug's effectiveness.

The first results of human trials came from the Karolinska Institute, where seven patients were given the drug by intravenous injection. Dr. Lennart Wetterberg and others reported, "There was no evidence of clinical improvement in any of the patients except in one case where a remarkable improvement in the patient's psoriasis was observed. From all patients HIV was isolated from peripheral blood mononuclear cells or plasma before and after treatment. However, in three of the seven patients there was a decline of HIV p24 antigen levels in serum.

"During treatment a transient rise in the CD4 (T4) cell count was recorded in two patients. In four of the six treated patients, those who could be evaluated, the area of pathologically altered brain white matter, as estimated by magnetic resonance imaging, was reduced.

"These findings suggest that peptide T may have biological effects in HIV-infected individuals. The results from this small series of patients should be followed by further trials to evaluate the possible therapeutic usefulness of peptide T" (Wetterberg and others, 1988).

Dr. Wetterberg did not respond to requests to reconcile the statement of "no evidence of clinical improvement" with the assertions made in his next two paragraphs.

The Swedish researchers suspended a double-blind, placebo controlled study in 36 patients when Bristol-Myers was granted the federal license in August, 1988. The Karolinska team sought financial assistance as well as clarification of their access to the drug. The study was not resumed.

When Bristol-Myers acquired the license for peptide T some people anticipated the pharmaceutical giant would speed up testing of the drug and resolve the lingering questions about its efficacy. However, the trial's pace was not increased. The company withdrew from the license in May, 1989. Susan Yarin, manager of public affairs for pharmaceuticals at Bristol-Myers, said, "We determined that peptide T's antiviral activity against the HIV-1 virus is limited."

Some of the drug's supporters said the firm's decision had a strong financial component, namely to concentrate the millions of dollars necessary for large phase II trials on ddI. Integra Institute, which had shared the license with Bristol-Myers, recently notified the government it wishes to be the sole licensee, according to Pert, one of Integra's founders. Pert responded to Bristol-Myers' announcement saying, "I think it's an unwise decision. Integra is ready, willing and able to meet all responsibilities of the license to the drug." Bristol-Myers will continue to fund the Los Angeles trial and supply the drug to a phase I trial at the Fenway Community Health Center in Boston (see "Boston, Los Angeles: Peptide T Trials Recruiting," *AIDS Treatment News* # 78).

Reports from the Los Angeles study presented at the Fifth International Conference on AIDS in Montreal concentrated on the drug's ability to improve neuropsychiatric and neuromotor functioning in HIV-impaired individuals. Peter Bridge, M.D., from NIMH reported that peptide T reversed neuropsychiatric problems in AIDS and ARC patients with HIV-related brain and central nervous system impairment.

Dr. Heseltine asserted there were significant improvements in brain function measured by tests of memory, motor speed, attention and cognitive processing. The patients' test scores declined when the drug was withdrawn after 12 weeks of treatment. He said comparisons with other clinical trials that measured the ability of AZT to improve brain function showed peptide T to be twice as effective. Heseltine was associated with early studies of AZT.

Responding to these assertions, Dr. Sodroski said, "It may very well make people feel better or give them better appetites, or do other things because it does have this homology (similarity) with VIP, but in terms of stopping HIV infection in patients, I think peptide T will do absolutely nothing."

Michael Ruff, Ph.D., Pert's associate, reported at Montreal that cerebrospinal fluid "from 9 out of 18 HIV-infected individuals (in the Los Angeles trial) showed significant (>20% of control) in vitro neuronal killing activity which was always blocked by peptide T."

A draft of a letter submitted to *The Lancet* and expected to be published in July, 1989 reports on results of administering peptide T to six patients: "No toxicity was observed. Where HIV-associated deficits (2 Standard Deviations below population norm) had been present at baseline, cognitive neuromotor function returned to normal during drug testing. Similarly, where HIV constitutional symptoms had been present at baseline (weight loss, watery diarrhea, fatigue, anergy, HIV-associated dermatitis), improvement or resolution was observed. Two patients were p24 antigen positive at baseline, becoming negative at follow-up. T4 counts remained stable while T8 counts increased 50% on average (400 to 600). No changes were observed in natural killer cell activity or in delayed hypersensitivity skin testing. . . . Constitutional/neuropsychiatric benefit, absent toxicity, and reduced p24 antigenemia in these patients is encouraging" (Bridge and others, 1989).

A serious snafu at the Los Angeles study occurred this summer. Two volunteers who had gone off AZT for one month in compliance with the protocol were told nine hours after they had entered the hospital that there was no drug for them. They were asked to return a month later. One volunteer came down with PCP and the other was told one month later there still wasn't enough drug. The volunteer said he had great difficulty getting information from officials connected with the study and has decided not to participate in the trial. He says his T4 count decreased significantly while he was off AZT. "I feel helpless and victimized, in addition to fearing for my life more than ever before," said Gordon McMahon, Ph.D., the volunteer.

The third study of the drug began in May, 1989, at the Fenway Community Health Center in Boston. Sixty volunteers will receive the drug intranasally for six months. Seventeen people have enrolled in the trial so far, according to Kenneth Mayer, M.D., the study's research director and an assistant professor at Brown University. "The jury is still out (on the drug's efficacy) and these studies need to be done. . . . We don't have enough data to know the drug's efficacy," Dr. Mayer said.

*David Smyth is a free-lance reporter based in San Francisco who has participated in the peptide T study in Los Angeles. He has reported on AIDS treatments for the* Bay Area Reporter, *the* San Francisco Sentinel, Bay Windows, Frontiers, Health Week *and other publications.*

## REFERENCES

Barnes, D. Debate over potential AIDS drug. *Science*, 237(4811), pages 128-130, July 10, 1987.

Brenneman, D. and others. Neuronal cell killing by the envelope protein of HIV and its prevention by vasoactive intestinal peptide. *Nature*, 335(6191), pages 639-642, October 13, 1988.

Brenneman, D. and others. Peptide T prevents gp120 induced neuronal cell death *in vitro:* relevance to AIDS dementia. *Drug Development Research,* volume 15, pages 361-369, 1988.

Bridge, P. and others. Peptide T: Improvements in phase I trial of AIDS patients. Draft of letter submitted to *Lancet*, July 1989.

Kowalski, M. and others. Functional regions of the envelope glycoprotein of human immunodeficiency virus type 1. *Science*, 237 (4820), pages 1351-1355, 1987.

Lasky and others. Delineation of a region of the human immunodeficiency virus type 1 gp120 glycoprotein critical for interaction with the CD4 receptor. *Cell,* volume 50 number 6, pages 975-985, 1987.

Nygren and others. 95- and 25-kDa fragments of the human immunodeficiency virus envelope glycoprotein gp120 bind to the CD4 receptor. *Proceedings of the National Academy of Sciences U.S.A.,* volume 85 number 17, pages 6543-6546, 1988.

Pert, C., and others. Octapeptides deduced from the neuropeptide receptor-like pattern of antigen T4 in brain potently inhibit human immunodeficiency virus receptor binding and T-cell infectivity. *Proceedings of the National Academy of Sciences U.S.A.*, volume 83, pages 9254-9258, December 1986.

Pert interview, *Science Impact*, pp. 6-7, June 1987.

Ruff, M., and others. Peptide T[4-8] is core HIV envelope sequence required for CD4 receptor attachment. *Lancet,* 2(8561), page 751, Sept. 26, 1987.

Sodroski, J., and others. HIV envelope-CD4 interaction not inhibited by synthetic octapeptides. *Lancet*, 1(8547), pages 1428-1429, June 20, 1987.

Wetterberg, L., and others. Treatment with peptide T in seven immunodepressed HIV infected patients. Draft of paper submitted to *AIDS, Gower Academy Journal*, London, June, 1988.

Wetterberg, L., and others. Peptide T in treatment of AIDS. *The Lancet,* 1(8525), page 159, Jan. 17, 1987.

# SAN FRANCISCO: DHEA STUDY RECRUITING

In January 1988, *AIDS Treatment News* reported on DHEA, a hormone which is already present in the body and is closely related to testosterone, and which was being tested as an AIDS treatment in a small study in Paris (see issue #48). Recently, at the AIDS conference in Montreal, some DHEA studies suggested that the drug might have a protective effect.

A phase I trial in San Francisco is now recruiting persons who have some ARC symptoms (such as thrush, or hairy leukoplakia, or chronic diarrhea, or fevers and sweats) and T-helper counts between 250 and 600. Persons with an AIDS diagnosis are not eligible for this study (because they meet the FDA criteria for AZT, and therefore it would be considered unethical for researchers to keep them off of that drug). Women also are not eligible, because the drug is a male hormone which might be harmful to them. (If the treatment is determined to be valuable it might be usable by women, but researchers are reluctant to take the increased risk before efficacy has been shown.) Patients cannot use any antiviral with known or suspected anti-HIV activity (such as AZT or dextran sulfate) during the study.

Volunteers will take DHEA by mouth for 16 weeks; there is no placebo. Three different doses are being tested; 250 mg three times a day, and 500 and 750 mg on the same schedule. Patients cannot start on the next higher dose until all have completed eight weeks on the lower dose without harm. (Even the lowest dose in this study is higher than any we reported in the Paris study in 1988.) After the study, the sponsor and the FDA have agreed to provide maintenance of the drug, provided that it is well tolerated and appears to be beneficial.

The trial is sponsored by Elan Corporation, which is based in Ireland, and which also sponsored the Paris study. In San Francisco, the principal investigators are Toby Dyner, M.D., and Mark Jacobson, M.D.


# IN MEMORIAM:
## CHARLIE SAMSON AND DON WRIGHT

*AIDS Treatment News* recently lost two friends and former staff members, Charlie Samson and Don Wright. They are remembered for their strong fight to survive with AIDS and their good work for the newsletter.

Charlie was responsible for the painstakingly thorough index found at the end of the collected back issues of *AIDS Treatment News* #1 through #50. He was fluent in treatment information and assisted many subscribers who called the newsletter with related questions. Charlie also stood by very strong political convictions. He fought for social justice before the epidemic, and often protested the homophobic and xenophobic mishandling of the AIDS crisis by the Reagan administration. When his friend Eric died several years ago, Charlie contended that Eric and all people who have died of AIDS were essentially murdered by the purposeful neglect of their own government and a healthcare system which puts profits ahead of people. Charlie was particularly grateful for all the work women have done in the epidemic, and often said so to his supporting circle of friends, which he called his "Helper Cell". Charlie died on May 24th.

Don worked only briefly at *AIDS Treatment News* but in that time he developed a careful and useful method of archiving the vast quantity of periodicals and correspondence we receive. Like Charlie, Don viewed his life and his world through a political perspective which challenged oppression of women, people of color, gay people, and of course people with AIDS. He was familiar with medical terminology and enjoyed discussing the newest developments in AIDS treatments. Don died on July 23rd.

Charlie Samson and Don Wright will not be forgotten, and their fight has brought us closer to the day when AIDS and the injustices it exposed are defeated.

# Issue Number 85
# August 11, 1989

## R-HEV: BETTER TEST FOR NEW AIDS TREATMENTS?

*by John S. James*

A new blood test developed in France may allow testing of proposed AIDS treatments in clinical trials much more rapidly than is now being done—and to give individuals early information about how well a particular treatment is working for them. *AIDS Treatment News* interviewed the test's principal developers, Jacques Leibowitch, M.D. and Dominique Mathez, M.D., clinical immunologists at the Raymond-Poincare Hospital/University Rene-Descartes, Paris-Ouest. Leibowitch stressed that these results must be considered very preliminary as they have not yet been confirmed by peer review. (The work has been submitted for publication, but not yet formally published; a short, early poster was presented at the June 1989 AIDS conference in Montreal.)

A retrospective study using frozen blood samples examined how the test performed in predicting disease progression. Researchers tested 131 samples from 57 HIV+ patients followed over five years; none of the patients received any anti-HIV treatment during this time. Because the test can be run on frozen blood, it is possible to study its prognostic value quickly, without waiting for years to see how AIDS/HIV progresses in the patients tested, as would be necessary if fresh blood were required. The new test, called R-HEV, performed much better than the P24 antigen test in predicting who would do poorly or do well in the future.

In a separate study, the R-HEV test clearly showed the antiviral effect of AZT—an effect which was partial and temporary—and also the effect of alpha interferon. (Some of the 57 patients whose blood was tested in the earlier study were later treated with these drugs, and frozen blood samples collected after treatment began were tested.) These results suggest that R-HEV may allow researchers to determine very quickly whether and to what extent a new drug is working. Also, much might be learned quickly and inexpensively about the efficacy of existing drugs by studying stored blood samples of patients who have already been treated, without needing to wait for new clinical trials to be funded, organized, and conducted.

## What Is the R-HEV Test?

R-HEV, an abbreviation for "radiation-resistant HIV expression ex vivo," is based on a technique which has been used in viral research for over 20 years (Henle and others, 1967), but has not previously been applied to HIV. It basically consists of viral cultures on cells which have been treated with radiation. The goal is to measure the HIV **expression levels** of the patient's virus, on the theory that radiation will suppress cells carrying HIV but not expressing it in the patient, and with the assumption that viral expression in the person is required for HIV disease to progress.

Ordinary viral cultures are unreliable as a measure of disease progression. Part of the reason is that latent virus, which is not causing any immediate problem, can be stimulated to become active by the culturing process itself, causing a positive result which does not reflect disease progression or poor prognosis for the patient.

In the R-HEV test, the radiation treatment causes the cells to die shortly after the time that culturing begins. If the virus was latent at the time the blood was drawn from the patient, the cells containing the latent virus die without being able to infect cells in the culture medium. But if the virus was active in the patient, some of the infected cells will just have time to transmit the infection to cells in the culture medium. Eight separate wells are cultured for each test, and the result reported by the R-HEV test is the percentage of wells which do grow virus.

Hundreds of sites in the U.S. already have the equipment needed to do the R-HEV test. The radiation can be provided by a machine already used in blood banks to irradiate blood before transfusion to persons with immune deficiencies. HIV cultures are somewhat expensive today—just the materials for each R-HEV test cost $40—but the technology is already available to reduce the cost enough to allow regular use of the test in medical practice, not only in research.

## The AIDS Progression Study

Of the 57 HIV+ patients whose frozen blood and five-year followup results were available, 22 already had AIDS or ARC, or T-helper cells under 400, at the time of their first visit. The other 35 had few or no symptoms, and T-helper cells over 550, at their first visit.

Of the latter 35 (the apparently healthy patients), 13 remained well and had T-helper counts which remained above 500. These 13 were called slow progressors. The other 22 had rapid clinical deterioration or rapid fall in T-helper cells (the fast progressors). How well did the R-HEV test do in distinguishing who was already ill, and more importantly, in predicting who would become ill in the future?

Of the 131 specimens available from the 57 HIV+ subjects, 91 tested positive on R-HEV; the other 40 were negative. Of these 40, all but one came from 15 patients with few or no symptoms and high T-helper cells. Among these 15 were ten who remained R-HEV negative for an average of 32 months; all ten of them remained well, and their T-helper counts remained over 500.

On the other hand, 43 of the 44 patients with serious illness or bad prognosis (the 22 with AIDS or ARC, and the 22 fast progressors) tested R-HEV positive. (And the one who tested negative did test R-HEV positive on alveolar lavage cells.)

Of the 22 apparently-healthy patients who were fast progressors, 17 were R-HEV positive at their first visit—an average of one year before clinical symptoms or falling T-helper cells were seen; the others became R-HEV positive eventually (in one case, only when alveolar cells were tested.) By contrast, P24 antigen was positive in only eight of the 22 patients at their first visit. All together, 33 percent of the 44 patients who were seriously ill at some point in the five years were P24 antigen negative, vs. only one of those patients who was R-HEV negative (and that patient was R-HEV positive when alveolar cells were tested).

These results suggest that R-HEV is much better than P24 antigen in correlating with disease state, and in providing early warning of poor prognosis—long before T-helper cells decline. If future work confirms these results, then R-HEV will be the best test available for HIV-disease status, and an excellent HIV-specific "surrogate marker" to use in clinical trials to find out quickly whether or not a drug is working.

## R-HEV and Antivirals

How good is the R-HEV test for showing how well an antiviral is working? The very preliminary results now available appear promising.

Eighteen of the 57 patients mentioned above were later treated with AZT. While we do not have the exact figures, R-HEV scores were greatly reduced in almost all of them within six months of AZT treatment. However, between six and 12 months after the patients started AZT, their R-HEV scores were back to an average close to their original value.

Three patients were treated with alpha interferon; one improved greatly, going into a long clinical remission. Ordinary viral cultures decreased initially, but then produced as much virus as they had before, even though the patient was in remission and did not have P24 antigen—illustrating that R-HEV correlated with this patient's condition, whereas a conventional viral culture did not. (The other two patients treated with interferon did not show as complete or as prolonged a remission.)

## Discussion

The R-HEV test is still very preliminary; until the early results outlined above are confirmed by other researchers, we cannot be sure that the test will prove useful. But if future work confirms the results obtained so far, then this test will have great importance in speeding the clinical trials of new AIDS drugs, by providing an objective, specific measurement of disease status which can be followed to see how well a treatment is working. A few weeks of testing in a small number of patients may provide a better measure of a new drug's efficacy than current trials—which require hundreds of patients and commonly take two years or more, because they do not have a good measure of efficacy and have to wait for deaths or opportunistic infections to accumulate instead.

A detailed report on R-HEV will be presented at a scientific meeting in Bethesda, Maryland, later this month.

On September 11-12, a crucial meeting in Washington, DC will attempt to reach professional consensus on "surrogate markers"—meaning results other than deaths or opportunistic infections which can be used as endpoints of clinical trials to determine whether treatments work. At this time, there is much scientific debate about whether existing blood tests—especially P24 antigen and T-helper counts—are meaningful enough to use as rapid proof of efficacy of a drug, without needing to wait for statistically significant numbers of "clinical events"—deaths and major opportunistic infections—which require the large, slow trials now causing bottlenecks and great delays in AIDS drug testing. While some leading scientists—such as Samuel Broder, M.D., the principal developer of both AZT and ddI—believe that new drugs could be tested using existing measurements such as P24 and T-cell subsets, it appears that most of the scientists involved doubt that those tests are good enough, and that clinical trials must therefore continue to recruit hundreds of subjects and take years to prove efficacy, as they have in the past.

*AIDS Treatment News* has argued that statistical indices of patients' overall health should be used in clinical trials to determine whether drugs are working. But few physicians and scientists have been willing to accept this approach. They argue that measures of clinical condition are often "subjective" and are not HIV specific, and that AIDS does not follow a steady course, with patients' health often improving or deteriorating unpredictably. Because of these concerns, there is no chance that the approach we have proposed will emerge as a consensus from the October meeting.

We also fear that there may be no consensus on existing markers of HIV progression either—that many scientists will not accept P24 antigen, T-helper counts, beta-2 microglobulin, etc., as good enough for proving efficacy in drug trials. In that case we would be left with the current "body count" clinical trials as the only accepted designs—trials which cannot possibly test drugs fast enough to prevent tens of thousands, if not hundreds of thousands, of AIDS deaths.

This is why the R-HEV test, if its early promise is confirmed, would be so important. It is the kind of test which the scientific community might accept, and which could greatly speed AIDS treatment research. It is urgent that this approach to drug efficacy testing get prompt, objective consideration.

## REFERENCES

Henle, W. and others. Herpes-type virus and chromosome marker in normal leukocytes after growth with irradiated Burkitt cells. *Science*, vol. 157, pages 1064-1065, September 1, 1967.

Leibowitch, J; Mathez, D; Cesari, D; Belilovsky, C; Gorin, I; Deleuze, J; and Paul, D. Morbidite systemique et expression retrovirale (infection productive) chez le porteur HIV. V International Conference on AIDS, Montreal June 4-9, 1989, poster number W.C.P.72.

# DDI, PARALLEL TRACK NEGOTIATIONS

*by John S. James*

During the last week a series of meetings and conference calls, arranged by different organizations and individuals, has brought diverse groups concerned with ddI and with proposed "parallel track" treatment access to the discussion table. Part of the urgency of these discussions was the deadline of a meeting on August 17 to advise Assistant Secretary for Health James O. Mason about the parallel track. We have not attended these meetings, but have spoken with some of the participants. Some observations, based on what we have heard:

• A major meeting August 8 in Washington brought together most of the groups involved. Ten persons represented Federal agencies—including Anthony Fauci from NIH, and Ellen Cooper from FDA. Several came from Bristol-Myers, including at least one of the principal writers of the ddI protocol. There were several representatives from patient and advocacy groups, three community physicians, three clinical researchers, and a representative of the Pharmaceutical Manufacturers' Association.

The AIDS patient advocates were Paul Boneberg from Mobilization Against AIDS, Jim Eigo from ACT UP/New York's Treatment and Data Committee, Jay Lipner (who has worked closely with Lambda Legal in New York, and with Martin Delaney of Project Inform), and Earl Thomas of NAPWA (National Association of People with AIDS). The community physicians were Bernard Bihari of New York, Neil Schram of Los Angeles, and Melanie Thompson of Atlanta.

The information below came not only from that meeting, but also from a New York meeting on the following day called by Jay Lipner and attended by physicians from NYPHR (New York Physicians for Human Rights), and by Ellen Cooper, M.D., of the FDA. Later, a conference call coordinated by the American Foundation for AIDS Research (AmFAR) included additional participants in these discussions.

• Despite major unresolved issues (see below), and specific concerns about process in these discussions, the fact that they occurred at all is a major advance. One FDA representative was heard to comment on the advantage of talking to physicians who see many AIDS patients, instead of only to those who are experts in trial design but see few patients.

It appears that until now, protocols for multicenter AIDS trials have not even been seen by the major private-practice physicians (much less by the patients who will put their lives on the line for them) until after the protocols have hardened into concrete—been submitted to Institutional Review Boards across the country, which makes even the slightest change impossible, as it would require re-approval of the study by all these boards. Apparently for the first time, the physicians who must refer patients if the trials will be successful, and representatives of patients themselves, have had a chance to look at a study while changes are still possible, and point out the kinds of practical problems that could make the trial unworkable but often could easily be corrected by the trial designers if they knew about them in time.

• Some examples of the kinds of problems that can be worked out (or at least addressed) by bringing the different parties together:

— PWAs are concerned about what would happen to persons randomized to receive either ddI or AZT, probably for two years, and who then did poorly. Would they be left to get a major opportunistic infection or die, or would they be allowed to try the other drug?

This issue is still unresolved, and apparently was not discussed in the meetings except for one trial—the "AZT worrisome," those who responded well to AZT and can still tolerate the drug, but are showing early signs that AZT is beginning to fail for them. This group is not included in the three trials already planned, apparently because the idea for it came later; but this trial could be very important, because it could obtain statistical proof of efficacy of ddI faster than any of the other trials. And the issue of treatment failures is most important here, because everybody going into such a study would already be starting to fail on AZT, and half of them would be randomized to continue the same drug. There seems to be a developing consensus that criteria could be devised under which the code would be broken for patients who continued to deteriorate, and if they had been receiving AZT, they could change to ddI.

But for the three trials, planned to start in September, this issue of great importance to the PWA community is still unresolved. The question should also be important to the trial designers, because if volunteers who do poorly on the study medication are not allowed to try other options within the trial, they are likely to obtain treatments outside of the trial instead, perhaps without telling the investigators. And patients will be reluctant to volunteer—and physicians reluctant to recommend that they enter trials— if there is no provision for changing their treatment if they do poorly.

— AIDS community representatives insisted on allowing compassionate provisions for persons who clearly need an antiviral but could not use AZT because they are already using ganciclovir, which like AZT has hematologic toxicity. (These persons will not be eligible for any of the formal trials.) Since ddI does not have the same toxicity, there is no reason to think that persons using ganciclovir could not also take ddI. But because no one has yet tried the combination, there is no proof that it is safe.

If ACT UP and Jay Lipner had not raised the issue, these patients would have been told to wait for ddI until a safety study of the combination had been done. But from the discussion which developed in the meeting, it quickly became clear that it would in practice be a long time before this study could be finished. So an alternative, apparently proposed by the FDA and acceptable to everyone, was to allow these people compassionate access to ddI, and also to put a small number (perhaps eight to 15) of such patients into a new trial at one of the ACTG sites which has previously done the phase I study of ddI, to find out quickly about any unknown dangers in the combination. If problems are found, then the compassionate access for persons also using ganciclovir could be re-evaluated.

— Community physicians suggested that useful data could be collected from parallel-track access by community-based clinical trials organizations working together with Bristol-Myers. Bristol-Myers has agreed to supply ddI for at least five thousand people within a year (the number could go higher if justified), in addition to those in the trials; but it has not yet decided how to obtain data from these patients. Community-based research organizations could collect data from about two thousand or more of them; the others (for example, those too far from any such organization) would receive the drug without data collection. The cost would be small, and the data would be collected by organizations with a track record in research, rather than by individual physicians who would usually not be interested. Then later, in case the formal studies were slow in recruiting, data would be available; if, perhaps a year from now, the FDA is willing to accept surrogate markers (blood tests, etc., instead of deaths or OIs) as proof of efficacy, the drug could be licensed much earlier than otherwise.

— One physician was concerned that ddI may be blamed for cases of pancreatitis which have been found in some of the people using it, when the drug might not be responsible. He pointed out that New York physicians have seen increasing numbers of cases of pancreatitis recently, in patients who have never used ddI.

— AIDS activists expressed concern about recent moves to limit parallel track to those who cannot get into **any** trial. There are a number of moribund trials, which fail to recruit patients because they are poorly designed, or because they are testing drugs which do not look good but made it into trials because somebody had the money to pay for them. There is fear that restrictions on access to experimental treatments will be used to blackmail the AIDS community into filling these dead-end trials.

However, Dr. Bernard Bihari of the Community Research Initiative, who attended the meetings, told us that the idea of limiting access in this way was brought up but was clearly rejected, and that it will not happen, at least not for ddI.

• Specifics of the trials—according to the memory of one participant:

— The three ddI trials to start soon—hopefully by late September—will be named ACTG 116, ACTG 117, and ACTG 118. It is hoped that they will enroll 1800 volunteers total.

— The trial considered most important will be ddI vs. AZT, for persons with AIDS or advanced ARC. In some ways this trial will try to replicate the early phase II trial which led to approval of AZT. It hopes to have 400 patients in each arm. Some prior use of AZT (up to two months) is OK.

— Another trial is for persons who have taken AZT for a year or more, and are tolerating it well. This study is to find out whether these people do better staying on AZT, or switching to ddI. It is hoped that this trial will produce the earliest conclusive evidence.

— The third trial is for those who have had to stop AZT due to hematologic toxicity. Since these people cannot be randomized to AZT, and a placebo would not be acceptable, they will be randomized to receive one of two different doses of ddI. The low dose will be the lowest which showed efficacy in phase I (apparently 100 mg twice a day), and the high dose will be the standard ddI dose for all three of these trials, (apparently 375 mg twice a day). There is concern that these doses are similar enough that it will take a long time for this trial to prove that there is a statistically significant difference between them.

— Later, there are plans to organize a trial for the "AZT worrisome," those who are on AZT and not intolerant, but show signs that the drug is beginning to fail, short of a major opportunistic infection. There will also be a pediatric trial.

— Two different existing programs for early access—"compassionate use" and "treatment IND"—for those who clearly need an antiviral and cannot use AZT or enter the trials, should begin at the same time as the trials. The competing "parallel track" concept will not be used for ddI at this time—partly because parallel track is not yet fully defined, and partly because in the turf wars between FDA and NIH, the FDA is in the position to make this decision. Parallel track may be the more far-reaching proposal, returning more choice to patients and their physicians when patients cannot enter trials, whereas compassionate access is for those who clearly cannot use AZT effectively and have no other choice.

• As we went to press, we received a two-page consensus statement on the parallel track prepared by 15 organizations: AIDS Action Council, ACT UP/New York, ACT UP/San Francisco, AIDS Project Los Angeles, American Association of Physicians for Human Rights, American Foundation for AIDS Research, Community Research Alliance, Gay Men's Health Crisis, Human Rights Campaign Fund, Lambda Legal Defense and Education Fund, National Association of People with AIDS, National Gay & Lesbian Task Force, National Gay Rights Advocates, Project Inform, and the San Francisco AIDS Foundation. This statement calls for the creation of an independent panel to make "decisions regarding the definition and implementation of the parallel track." This panel "must include full, voting representation by AIDS primary care physicians, representatives of community-based research groups, and people with AIDS, HIV infection and their advocates"—as well as representatives from government agencies and the pharmaceutical industry. The statement points to the lack of decision-making representation by the AIDS community as a key factor in impeding previous efforts (compassionate use, and the treatment IND) to make AIDS treatments more available.

The statement also calls on this panel to "consider mechanisms for assuring that any person with HIV infection who has a demonstrable medical need for a parallel track treatment could obtain access regardless of economic circumstances."

• A major concern we have heard about the developing program for ddI involves the responsibility of the AIDS community. Bristol-Myers and other participants have taken risks to handle this drug much better than others have been handled, moving very rapidly at this time to get trials going, consulting with community physicians and patients, and planning to make their drug available free. But ddI is not the last drug, and other companies will be watching to see how well this policy works. If it fails, access to other drugs will be harder in the future.

One fear in the AIDS community is that patients who could qualify for the formal trials, or their physicians, may fudge records to get patients ddI through compassionate access or treatment IND instead, in order to avoid the chance of being randomly assigned to AZT, and to be able to receive the drug directly from one's physician and have the physician know which drug it is. On the other hand, the trials will have the advantage of offering excellent testing for free—and none of them will give AZT to patients who clearly will not benefit from it.

We hope that fudging records to stay out of trials will not be a serious problem, as it is important for many reasons that the trials be able to recruit effectively—both to get the efficacy data quickly, and to avoid future restrictions on treatment access.

Another concern, which we have heard from persons in the Community Research Initiative in New York, is that the great attention to ddI is leading to an irrational rush to this particular drug, with people avoiding other trials, or calling off other treatment plans, to get ddI. Not only could a stampede for ddI damage other trials and make it more difficult to get legal access to treatment in the future, but also it does not make sense medically, because the case for this drug is not yet very strong. Only about 90 patients have taken ddI in trials, and there are many questions remaining about risks and benefits. ddI may prove to be more useful and less toxic than AZT—but at this time the uncertainties are much greater. ddI may be especially valuable to those who cannot use AZT effectively, and it is important that the AIDS community make sure they have the option. But those who can use AZT should weigh the choice carefully, and not overemphasize ddI just because it is new or in the news.

Other new drugs now entering clinical trials, such as D4T and AZDU, may be at least as good as ddI. We hope that ddI will show the way to an effective compromise, in which well-designed clinical trials can be quickly enrolled and conducted, while at the same time patients' options are maximized and there is some provision for everybody.

## Major Unresolved Issues:

• How will data be collected when treatments are released for compassionate use or parallel track access?

Ideally, data collection from early access could provide valuable experience about how drugs are working in the real world, outside of the artificial, controlled conditions of the trials. Patients want more data collection, and so do community-based clinical-trials organizations, which see a role for themselves in collecting it.

But pharmaceutical companies often fear that in today's regulatory climate, this data could only hurt a drug's licensing, not help it. The concern is that the FDA is unlikely to take seriously results obtained outside of a rigorously controlled clinical trial, meaning that data from parallel track, treatment IND, or compassionate use could not help the drug be licensed. But adverse effects reports are taken seriously. The fear, then, is that results from early release can only hurt—a fear which makes companies reluctant to allow use of their drugs, no matter how medically justified and urgent the case for doing so.

Unfortunately, many FDA employees do not believe in any early access—perhaps because they fear that exceptions to the regular licensing process cast doubt on the rationale of their work. If their standard drug-licensing procedures are sound, then why are exceptions necessary?

Fauci's parallel-track proposal has added a new element to the debate—an authoritative statement that it is possible to relax some restrictions on treatment access without harming clinical trials. But the FDA has more than research to worry about. Like a circus lion trainer, in a cage with entities more powerful than itself, it must not lose control for a moment. This fight to keep control has led to cruel and irrational outcomes, which are increasingly becoming a mainstream political issue.

This is the basic problem which has stood in the way of earlier access to treatments. The FDA has not wanted to find ways to allow data from pre-licensing use (other than through trials which most patients cannot qualify for) to help a drug get licensed. If early access can only harm their interests, pharmaceutical companies will not provide their drugs for any form of compassionate treatment use. Bristol-Myers may have made an exception for ddI because otherwise it would have faced enormous bad publicity. Instead, by agreeing to provide the drug subject to FDA approval, it put the ball in the FDA's court, where it belongs. But the great majority of drugs do not capture the public's imagination. The only sound solution we see is to insist on a full, ongoing examination of the scientific and public-policy assumptions underlying the drug-approval process.

In addition, pharmaceutical companies are understandably reluctant to have others collecting data about their products outside of their control, because they fear being held responsible for adverse effects which may have nothing to do with their drugs. Most private-practice physicians who are not associated with research organizations do not want to do data collection, either. To them it is just more paperwork.

One possible solution to this problem is for the pharmaceutical company to fund data collection by community-based or other research organizations, under the sponsoring company's control, through negotiated protocols. Data would be collected only for those patients who volunteered (the free blood work would be an incentive), and were geographically convenient to a monitoring organization.

• A major disagreement is what to do for "AZT refuseniks," those who do not want to try AZT but do want access to ddI. Patients and some physicians see it as wrong to force somebody to use a drug they do not want and get sick from it in order to qualify for treatment. But at this time the other side seems to have little sympathy—as if those who refuse AZT are to be punished for their distrust of the system, or as if the doors are to be closed to "economic refugees" who come to ddI because they cannot afford AZT, or as if patients must do their share of sacrificing themselves for some greater good in the future.

One suggestion is to develop standards for documenting who is a "real" refusenik, for example by chart notes over a period of time, so that there will not be a huge number of people who receive ddI this way.

This issue shows that we have a long way to go to reach consensus that treatment decisions should be made by patients and their physicians, on medical grounds, in the patient's interest. There are excellent arguments for being cautious with ddI until more is known, for not using it if other viable options are available. The case against accepting unknown risks as preferable to known ones must be well stated. But when there are legitimate medical grounds for choosing a drug, the ultimate decisions should be made by patients and their physicians, rather than by scientists, officials, or committees who make rules in advance with no knowledge of each specific case.

• All three of the trials currently planned will take a long time to complete—especially since it may be difficult to recruit as many as 1800 volunteers. AZT was approved much faster and with many fewer volunteers, because it could be tested against a placebo instead of another active drug—and a placebo test would not be acceptable today since AZT is available. There is concern that no system of early access will meet all the needs, and many will be denied the treatment until it is licensed and regularly distributed.

## Physician Access

Bristol-Myers has made plans to distribute ddI rapidly. Physicians will be able to call an 800 number, then receive and return forms by fax, or by express delivery for physicians who do not have fax machines. Then a 30-day supply of the drug can be shipped immediately.

## Need for Caution

Persons considering using ddI should realize that not everybody in the AIDS community thinks that this drug is beneficial. There are growing questions and concerns. The history of new drugs suggests caution, as serious side effects of AZT and ddC were not noticed in early trials.

The best information we are hearing at this time is that ddI may add a year of life for persons who are burned out on AZT (or who never took AZT), but that it will not replace AZT. Researchers are finding the same pattern of rising T-helper cells, then a plateau, then falling T-cells, so that after about a year or eighteen months, patients will probably be back where they started. ddI is becoming available underground, but it must not be considered harmless, as there are side effects including rash, rise in liver function tests, pancreatitis, and peripheral neuropathy. So far the neuropathy has caused the most concern, as a few patients have had severe pain in the feet after 30 to 40 weeks of the drug at doses about equal to those which will be used in the trials; in extreme cases the pain can be debilitating and not responsive to opiates, and it can take weeks to recover after the drug is stopped. At higher doses, the neuropathy has occurred as soon as ten weeks; the problem may depend on total cumulative dose. ddI might prove most useful when taken in cycles alternating with AZT, instead of taken continuously.

Questions have also been raised about the evidence for efficacy. Rebecca Smith of the AIDS Treatment Registry in New York pointed to the report that patients on four higher doses did better than those on four lower doses (recent article in *Science*, June 28). But the graphs on page 413 of that article show that patients on the lower doses started with about half the T-cells of those on the higher doses. This difference should be considered when evaluating the fact that all but one of the six opportunistic infections which developed occurred in patients on the lower doses. (Other indications of efficacy are more clear, however, such as the fact that every one of the 13 patients on the four higher doses had T-helper cell increases in the first six weeks.)

This article has looked at the the current status of the negotiations concerning the issues and mechanisms of early access to experimental drugs including ddI, but only briefly at the arguments for or against the drug itself. We plan to follow all of these issues as they develop.

# LOS ANGELES HUNGER STRIKE FOR TREATMENT ACCESS; 28 ORGANIZATIONS FORM COALITION FOR COMPASSION

Hunger strikers urging the Food and Drug Administration to speed the release of safe experimental drugs moved their protest to a site in West Hollywood after 20 of them were arrested "for reasons of encampment" outside the Federal building at the Los Angeles Civic Center.

The strikers are supporting the demands of the Coalition for Compassion, a coalition of 28 gay and lesbian community and AIDS service organizations. The Coalition launched it's "Compassion = Life" campaign "to focus upon responsive use of drugs and to alert the nation to the immediate need to make medical treatment available to people with AIDS."

The hunger strike had been planned to consist of 24-hour shifts of concerned citizens and celebrities at the Federal building, to bring attention to treatment development and access issues. But in addition to the rotating shifts, two persons with AIDS have fasted for three days, and are continuing. They are being monitored by physicians.

The hunger strike began at 10 AM on August 9 outside the Federal Building. Federal officials ordered the people to leave by 6 PM that day. After 20 arrests on August 9 and 10, the strikers were granted sanctuary in the City of West Hollywood and moved to their current location at Crescent Heights and Santa Monica Boulevards, while negotiating to return to the Federal Building site.

The hunger strike is only one aspect of the Coalition for Compassion campaign, a movement which hopes to spark similar organizing in other cities. So far we have seen no press coverage outside of Los Angeles, where the protest has been reported by the *Los Angeles Times* and on local television. But word spread nationally, since AIDS Project Los Angeles is both associated with the Coalition for Compassion and also one of the 15 national organizations which drafted the consensus statement on the parallel track (see "DDI, Parallel Track Negotiations," in this issue).

## UPDATE: COMMUNITY-BASED TRIALS AND SAN FRANCISCO'S COMMUNITY RESEARCH ALLIANCE

*by John S. James*

In a development unprecedented in the history of medicine, persons with AIDS or HIV and their physicians have begun to organize and run their own clinical trials of potential treatments, conducting this human research in ways which meet all FDA and other legal requirements. One of about 20 such organizations is the Community Research Alliance (CRA), which *AIDS Treatment News* covered in issue #70. This writer is one of the founders of the CRA and is currently a member of the board of directors; we chose to focus our report on this particular organization because we are closest to it and know it best.

### What Is Community-Based Research?

Clinical research traditionally takes place in major medical centers, usually academic institutions, and is paid for by pharmaceutical companies or by the Federal government. Some research, especially tests of new chemicals never before taken by humans, can only be done in specialized institutions. But other studies, such as "monitoring" trials designed to collect consistent, reliable data on a new use of a treatment already well known in medicine, can usually be done more rapidly in the less formal setting provided by a community organization working together with front-line physicians in private practice or at public clinics.

Research initiated by persons with AIDS or HIV or their physicians, and conducted under the professional guidance of physicians and scientific specialists, can:

• Test immediately practical treatment options, which otherwise might not be tested at all if they lack commercial incentive or elegant scientific appeal;

• Design trials which will get results quickly (in contrast to the "body count" designs usually used in mainstream research, which usually take two years or more to produce results, due to the wait for persons not being treated to get sick);

• Negotiate trial designs which are attractive to the participants and their physicians, as well as scientifically sound, greatly reducing recruitment delays and the danger of invalid results due to cheating;

• Build an in-depth knowledge base, allowing the PWA community to make sure its interests are represented when decisions are made in mainstream research.

The public has not realized the extent to which the specific interests of institutions and professionals have shaped medical research in ways which differ from patients' interests. One example came to light over a year ago, when Dr. Anthony Fauci, director of the National Institute of Allergies and Infectious Diseases, which runs most of the Federal government's AIDS treatment research, had to tell a Congressional committee that some of the most promising treatments, including aerosol pentamidine prophylaxis, had been delayed for a year or more due to lack of a single staff person to "shepherd" each one through the research and regulatory labyrinth (see *The New York Times*, April 30, 1988, page 1). Because the community-based research movement had been small until that time, no one knew what was happening, except those too dependent on the system to make a public issue. Therefore, nobody raised the warning early, and a year was lost. (Aerosol pentamidine received full FDA approval last month, based on data from studies begun by the two oldest community-based research organizations, the County Community Consortium in San Francisco and the Community Research Initiative in New York. Emergency funding was provided by pentamidine licensee LyphoMed, Inc., after the U.S. National Institutes of Health had unexpectedly refused to fund the study.) This incident illustrates the fact that treatment and prevention of opportunistic infections has often fallen through the cracks of mainstream research, as there are usually too few patients to generate much commercial interest, and government scientists have preferred to study high-tech antivirals which relate to genetic research and the growing biotechnology industry.

Today's movement for community-based research exists to make sure that the interests of patients and their physicians are better represented in the future.

The groups developing today are modeling themselves on one of the two pioneering organizations in the community-based trials movement—the Community Research Initiative in New York, and the County Community Consortium in San Francisco— the same organizations which conducted the studies leading to the approval of aerosol pentamidine. These original organizations developed separately, creating two different flavors of community-based research:

The Community Research Initiative was first suggested in a position paper by Joseph Sonnabend, M.D., Michael Callen of the PWA Coalition, Dr. Mathilde Krim of the American Foundation for AIDS Research (AmFAR) and others. The organization started with a five thousand dollar grant from New York's PWA Coalition—beginning the tradition of extensive PWA involvement. Two more physicians—Bernard Bihari, M.D. and Nathaniel Pier, M.D.—joined the group in its earliest stages, and administrator Tom Hannan did the lengthy paperwork required to establish an organization meeting all legal requirements to conduct human research.

For the first year the group attracted little attention. But after favorable comments by the Presidential Commission on the HIV Epidemic (see *The New York Times*, March 15, 1988), the organization and the concept on which it was based attained wide acceptance. Today the CRI has 190 participating physicians, and a scientific advisory committee headed by Donald Armstrong, M.D., Chief of Infectious Diseases, Director of the Microbiology Laboratory, and head of the AIDS Clinical Trials Group (ACTG) at Memorial Sloan Kettering Cancer Center. (Two other members of the scientific advisory committee are also ACTG researchers.) Nine trials are now underway or completed, with over 500 patients participating; the organization has an annual budget of slightly over a million dollars. (For more background on the Community Research Initiative, see *AIDS Treatment News* #70.)

The other pioneer in community-based research, San Francisco's County Community Consortium (CCC), did not begin as a research organization, but as a forum for communication between physicians with AIDS practices and AIDS researchers at San Francisco General Hospital. Almost all AIDS physicians in San Francisco are members of the CCC, although many are primarily interested in sharing information, rather than conducting research.

In addition to its information-sharing function, CCC now has five clinical trials underway, is building an infrastructure to provide research-nurse support to help physicians throughout the San Francisco area participate in research within their practices, and has published a directory of clinical trials in the San Francisco area (see "San Francisco: New Clinical Trials Treatment Directory," elsewhere in this issue for information about the directory and how to receive a copy). (For more background on the history and development of the County Community Consortium, see *AIDS Treatment News* issues # 54 and # 56).

These two organizations have established two different styles of community-based research:

(1) The Community Research Initiative emphasizes patient involvement, with PWA participation on the governing board and on the institutional review board (IRB), which must review and approve any trial's ethical treatment of human subjects. Studies can take place either in the offices of primary-care physicians or at a central location, with the physician consulted. Much of the CRI's research takes place at its clinical center, however, as physicians are usually too busy to do the additional paperwork required for research.

(2) The County Community Consortium emphasizes technical support to enable primary-care physicians to conduct AIDS treatment research. Physicians with large HIV practices are usually the first to see the potential of available, immediately practical treatment options. But few practicing physicians have the time, training, or inclination to organize their own clinical research projects without assistance. Technical support provided by organizations like the Consortium allows the knowledge and experience of leading physicians to produce credible scientific data which can be used everywhere to improve medical practice. Studies take place within the practices of the physicians, with the Consortium providing technical support and assuring quality control of the data.

The CRI model applies when patients want to be involved not only as subjects, but also in the development and decision-making of research. The Consortium model applies when an existing (or new) group of physicians, in private practice or in a public or private hospital or clinic, want to begin participating in clinical trials. Both models are crucially important for organizing practical research to make new treatments available faster.

## The Community Research Alliance

*AIDS Treatment News* described the formation and early history of the Community Research Alliance last December (issue #70). At that time the scientific advisory committee had not met, and the institutional review board had not been formed. This article will focus on current projects, instead of the details of the rapid organization building which has taken place since then. We should point out, however, that developing an organization which meets all legal requirements for conducting human research is not only a matter of completing paperwork and complying with regulations, but more centrally is a process of developing working relationships with scientific and medical professionals, and with other organizations and community leaders. Over 30 volunteers are involved as members of the various boards and committees.

The Community Research Alliance is currently conducting a hypericin monitoring project which has been running for two months and has 30 patients participating. This study went from proposal to operation in three months. It provides a model for what could become a series of studies by the organization.

Hypericin is a substance found in a plant (St. John's wort) long used in herbal medicine. Recently researchers at New York University and elsewhere have found that hypericin appears to be an excellent antiretroviral, not only active against HIV in the test tube, but also against two other retroviruses in mice. (Since animals do not get AIDS, it has not been possible to run a direct animal test of hypericin as an anti-AIDS treatment.) For more background on hypericin, see *AIDS Treatment News* issues # 63, 74, 75, 77, 79, and 80; the major scientific report so far was published in the *Proceedings of the National Academy of Sciences, USA* in July 1988, and five abstracts were published at the Montreal AIDS conference in June 1989 (including number M.C.P.115, not listed under "hypericin" in the subject index).

But approval and regular human use through the mainstream research system will probably be years away. At this time, chemists are developing better methods for synthesizing large quantities of the pure chemical. Then there must be more animal tests before human trials can begin. The human trials can take years, despite recent efforts to speed the process.

Meanwhile herbal extracts are available. No one is sure if they can be useful. How can we find out?

A randomized controlled trial (today's gold standard of clinical research) would probably be impossible, at least in the United States. Such studies are difficult to run, and expensive—and herbal extracts have very poor prospects for patent protection and therefore do not attract investors. Besides, it would probably be legally impossible to do the study, as the FDA is very unlikely to give an IND (Investigational New Drug approval) for the herbal extracts available. The FDA does not like crude plant extracts since they are not completely characterized chemically, and vary from batch to batch.

The FDA exists to regulate (and protect) the pharmaceutical industry—not herbalists, who are not taken seriously in the U.S. mainstream. Without an IND, it is not legal to give an unapproved drug to people.

What, then, can be done, besides waiting several years for large-scale synthesis of pure hypericin and animal and human tests of the chemical?

One option is to conduct a survey—such as the one *AIDS Treatment News* distributed in our June 2 issue, which we are now analyzing. A survey is better than nothing, but it has the major limitation of having no uniformity in data collection. People get different blood tests, or none at all, and on completely different schedules. Because of such problems, our survey will only be a study of peoples' **beliefs** about whether herbal extracts containing hypericin are helping them. What objective evidence does get reported (such as blood results, or clear appearance or disappearance of symptoms) is so diverse and scattered that it is difficult or impossible to draw reliable conclusions from it.

Between the survey and the randomized controlled trial is the monitoring study, such as the one the Community Research Alliance is doing with hypericin. A monitoring study avoids the need for an IND by not giving anybody a drug. Instead, it only collects data—by doing blood work, physical examinations, and medical histories. But it collects the data under a strict, scientifically designed protocol, to maintain uniformity and quality control.

In the hypericin monitoring study now being run by the Community Research Alliance, patients are not told what kind of hypericin to use, or how much. They are not told to stop or change any other treatment. Of course they are asked to report every treatment they are using.

As we described in our June 2 issue, which announced the start of this monitoring study, baseline (before starting hypericin) and four monthly blood tests are given. Tests (not all given every month) include P24 antigen, T-cell subsets, the CMI skin test, CBC, ESR, and SMA 25. Before and after physical exams are given, and a medical history is taken. All blood work for all patients is done by the same laboratory, to reduce inter-lab variations.

This kind of monitoring study cannot control or standardize the treatments people are using—for both legal and ethical reasons. But it can rigorously control the data collection. As as result, it can quickly collect much better data than is available from any other source about many, if not most, of the non-approved treatments now being used.

Since there is no control group for comparison, this kind of study cannot obtain statistical "proof" of whether the treatment works better than no treatment, or better than some other treatment. Instead of seeking such proof, this study aims to keep very good records of what happens to people who are using the treatment. The rationale is that since every patient's health status going into the study is well documented, any major or dramatic effects should be evident to physicians when they compare the histories of these patients, during the trial or afterward, with the histories of other patients they have known.

Therefore monitoring studies do not aim to prove a drug effective, but rather to produce quality information which can support treatment decisions. Note that almost any result of a well-conducted monitoring study can support such decision-making to some degree. If the treatment shows dramatic effects, of course that would be interesting. But if it shows nothing at all, or only ambiguous, debatable results, this information would also be helpful to patients and physicians, in supporting the case **against** using the treatment.

Monitoring studies are relatively inexpensive and easy to administer, because they do not give treatments, or change what the patient is doing anyway. The main expenses are for blood tests, and staff time. This kind of study can quickly obtain the best information available on treatments which are coming into use but have not been formally studied—either food supplements, etc. which patients can obtain on their own, or drugs formally approved for other purposes and prescribed by physicians.

## Future Prospects

Here are examples of the kinds of projects which the Community Research Alliance may pursue in the future:

(1) The CRA might develop many small monitoring studies, like the hypericin trial currently underway, and focus on doing this particular kind of research well. Funding would come mainly from individual donations, fund-raising events, and foundation or corporate grants, rather than from pharmaceutical company sponsorship of particular projects. The treatments studied would be those already available; and because funding would be from community and other public sources, treatments could be selected only on the basis of medical merit and public-health importance, without regard to their commercial prospects. This research arm of the organization will operate entirely in service to the AIDS community and the larger public.

(2) Some of the most important studies, however, could only be done with pharmaceutical-company sponsorship. Collaboration between pharmaceutical companies and community-based research organizations has worked well in the past, and the companies have been happy with the results. More time may be required up front to negotiate a protocol acceptable to people with AIDS and their physicians, as well as to the other parties involved—a step usually omitted by academic research centers. But the care taken to include their interests is repaid many times over by easier and faster recruiting of volunteers for the trial.

Community-based organizations have a reputation for getting top-quality results much faster and less expensively than other alternatives. And today there are more drugs to test than research facilities available to test them (for background on this problem, see "The Trials of Conducting AIDS Drug Trials," *Science*, May 26, 1989). Therefore community-based organizations not only have opportunities to contribute to the mainstream research process, but by doing so they can help relieve a major bottleneck in the system, in addition to the qualitative contributions they can make by being close to the PWA community.

At this time the two most important drugs which could be studied by community-based research organizations are compound Q and ddI. Genelabs, the developer of compound Q, is exploring the possibility of organizing some phase II trials through community-based groups. For ddI, the phase II trials will be through NIAID's ACTG system, but there may be a role for community-based organizations in collaborating with Bristol-Myers to collect data from patients who receive drugs through compassionate use, treatment IND, or (later) the parallel track.

No final decisions have been made at this point, but these are some of the projects the Community Research Alliance is exploring as possible industry-sponsored trials.

(3) A number of other potential avenues are also being examined, including:

• Studying treatments for opportunistic infections, an area which has been neglected by the AIDS research mainstream. The treatments would be used by physicians in their usual practice, with the Community Research Alliance doing paperwork to facilitate access, data collection, and reporting of results;

• Participating in multicenter community-based trials, carried out by a developing network of community-based research organizations around the country, focusing on prophylaxis of opportunistic infections;

• Opening doors for full participation in clinical trials by people of color and other groups which so far have been under-represented—both in the decision-making process and as volunteers—speeding AIDS trials by reducing recruitment delays, at the same time as the trials are made more equitable.

## How Can You Help?

Community-based research organizations need public support. The biggest immediate need is money. The Community Research Alliance, for example, has had its office space and almost all of its office equipment donated, as well as the efforts of many volunteers, but it must have some paid staff in order to move as rapidly as possible to negotiate future trials, as well as completing the one already going. The hypericin study is completely financed by the CRA itself, as there is no pharmaceutical company sponsor for it.

The Community Research Alliance has received a $30,000 grant from AmFAR (the American Foundation for AIDS Research), and individual gifts totalling over $60,000. But expenses at the current rate of growth and activity are about $12,000 per month. The CRA did not originally ask the public for money, as it wanted to establish a track record first. Now it needs contributions within the next two months, or its growth must be greatly curtailed.

The Community Research Alliance also needs volunteers, especially people with professional skills and/or who can develop or manage long-term projects.

# Issue Number 86
# August 25, 1989

## AZT PROVES USEFUL GIVEN EARLIER, AT LOWER DOSES

*By Denny Smith*

Three separate announcements in less than six weeks may change the course of the AIDS epidemic for thousands of people, and confirm the value of a treatment approach already in use by many with HIV. Reports from three clinical trials, when combined, have shown that AZT (Zidovudine), even at low doses, can slow the progression of HIV infection in people with moderately low helper cells but with few or no symptoms, and may be less toxic the earlier it is initiated. (The indications for AZT therapy approved so far by the Food and Drug Administration have been limited to people with a T4-helper cell count below 200 or a diagnosis of AIDS.) Following is a brief description of the details and sequence of recent developments, and the questions they raise about lack of access to health care for AIDS, and in the U.S. generally.

### Lower Dose Shown Effective

On July 14 *AIDS Treatment News* #83 reported preliminary results of an AZT/acyclovir study still in progress at the University of California in San Francisco. This is a small trial combining a low dose of AZT with two different amounts of acyclovir (Zovirax), testing the possibility that acyclovir enhances the activity of AZT, and simultaneously suppresses the threat of active herpes, shingles and perhaps CMV infections. Several similar studies combining AZT and acyclovir were presented at the V International Conference on AIDS in Montreal last June, most of them suggesting that the combination was better than AZT alone. The anti-clotting drug dipyridamole (Persantine) may also extend the effectiveness of AZT (see *AIDS Treatment News* #79), as well as the anti-gout medication probenecid, but neither has been tested with AZT enough to establish safety.

Although the UCSF study was designed to measure toxicity and not efficacy, we noted that AZT appeared to be more easily tolerated and more effective in reducing HIV activity when initiated **before** helper cells were seriously depleted or symptoms appeared. We added that such results had been predicted by some physicians, and would support the HIV early intervention strategy proposed by Project Inform, a San Francisco-based AIDS advocacy organization.

In the same article, we mentioned the July 12 announcement of results of a much larger trial conducted by the National Institute of Allergy and Infectious Diseases (NIAID) demonstrating that survival rates for people taking a low dose of AZT (100 mg every four hours) were equal to those obtained by a high dose (250 mg at the same frequency). All of the 572 participants had experienced one episode of *Pneumocystis carinii* pneumonia (PCP) prior to entering the study; blood toxicities were less common in those receiving the lower dose. The researchers are continuing to evaluate the trial's data to identify the degree of neurologic improvement and the rate of development for new opportunistic infections. The principle investigator of that study was Margaret Fischl, M.D., of the University of Miami. On August 3 Dr. Fischl announced results of another important AZT trial, known as Protocol 016, which found that AZT delayed progression from the symptoms of ARC to infections of AIDS in a significant number of people.

## Benefits of Treatment Determined For ARC

Protocol 016 began in August of 1987 and eventually recruited 713 individuals who met the study's parameters of a T4-helper count between 200 and 800 and one or two symptoms of ARC. The participants were randomized to receive either 200 mg of AZT every four hours or a placebo on the same schedule. They were followed to observe any progression to "endpoints"—which for this trial were defined as new or worsening ARC symptoms or development of AIDS-defining infections.

By July of this year it was clear that those participants getting a placebo had progressed to endpoints in markedly greater numbers than those getting AZT—36 versus 14. The bulk of progression was concentrated among those participants who entered the trial with helper cells below 500. And within this subgroup the contrast between placebo and active drug outcomes was sharper than in the group who entered with helper cells over 500. Additionally, side effects were experienced by only 5% of the participants, substantially less than the nearly 50% of people with AIDS who cannot tolerate AZT.

The researchers interpreted these results as showing that people who have ARC and who have less than 500 helper cells can benefit from AZT. They felt that the data are not sufficient to show benefit of AZT if helper cell counts are above 500, but nevertheless recommend testing for HIV antibodies to anyone who may be at risk. Those who test positive "should seek early treatment as appropriate."

These studies confirmed the approach used for over two years by many physicians and their patients: if AZT slows HIV activity in people with AIDS, but only for those who can tolerate the side effects, then why not begin the intervention at lower, less toxic doses, and before early symptoms advance to life-threatening infections? The next logical question to ask is whether people without any observable symptoms can intervene in the progression of HIV to prevent deterioration of their immune systems. The most recent AZT developments suggest that the answer is yes.

## Value Seen in Treating Before Symptoms

On August 17 a study known as Protocol 019 of the AIDS Clinical Trials Group (ACTG), conducted by NIAID, was interrupted because it found growing evidence that AZT delayed progression to illness in many people who are HIV+ but asymptomatic. This trial began more than two years ago, in July of 1987, and was still recruiting until July of this year. A total of 3,200 participants were recruited. All of these entered the trial without symptoms, but about 1,300 entered with a T4-helper cell count of less than 500.

The participants were randomized into three arms of the trial: one third received 1500 mg of AZT daily, another third received 500 mg a day, and the remainder got a placebo. Significantly, but to many observers not surprisingly, participants with helper cells under 500 were twice as likely to progress to ARC or AIDS if they got the placebo than if they received AZT. In the same group, disease progression was about the same in patients receiving 500 mg or 1500 mg of the active drug, and side effects of both doses were minimal. The principal investigator, Paul Volberding, M.D., of San Francisco General Hospital and the University of California, said that now all of the participants with fewer than 500 helper cells will be offered AZT. The study will continue for the group of participants with helper cells over 500, since among them the progression to symptoms was negligible. Protocol 019 is the largest AIDS clinical trial ever conducted.

The question of when to begin antiviral treatment if helper cells are declining but remain over 500 is being clarified by the growing refinement of prognostic indicators. In addition to an uneven decline in the number of T4-helper cells, HIV infection over time usually results in anemia (low red cells or hemoglobin), thrombocytopenia (low platelets), and increases in serum neopterin, beta 2 microglobulin, and p24 antigenemia. AZT has been connected with reversals of all of them, but singly they do not always indicate that AZT or any antiretroviral is warranted. When analyzed in combination they provide a more accurate picture from which to consider treatment intervention.

For example, some people may have consistently low helper cell counts (under 500) for several years without any external symptoms. In this situation, many physicians have not initiated AZT therapy unless the level of p24 antigen is high or rising, suggesting that the system may soon be destabilized by current HIV activity. A study at the University of California in Los Angeles found a strong correlation between elevated neopterin levels in HIV+ individuals and their subsequent progression to AIDS, and when neopterin levels were considered together with helper cell counts, the prognosis value was much greater than either gave alone (Melmed and others, 1989). Since helper cells can fluctuate greatly, two or even three counts must be charted over the course of several months to be meaningful. So testing for neopterin levels could hasten the process of identifying viral activity in an individual, or of determining the effectiveness of a new anti-viral treatment.

P-24 antigenemia and helper cell counts may be useful tools for monitoring asymptomatic seropositive people, but a study at the Northwestern University School of Medicine found that these tests did not predict the course of AIDS during treatment with AZT (Steinberg and others, 1989). Instead, decreased hemoglobin and platelets often predicted an increased chance of AZT-related toxicities in people who have had an opportunistic infection. This study suggests that the range of tests useful for predicting or monitoring the course of an HIV infection is narrowed as symptoms progress and immune functions become more impaired. In other words, the sooner HIV is confronted, the more tools may be available to assess questions of when and how much to treat.

One warning offered by Professor David Cooper, Director of AIDS Epidemiology & Clinical Trials at the University of New South Wales, and also by Marcus Conant, M.D., of the University of California, San Francisco, is to avoid swallowing AZT capsules dry, without water or juice, since the drug is caustic enough to create ulcerations in the esophagus, which could then be misdiagnosed. On the other hand, an old caution to avoid combining AZT with acetaminophen (Tylenol) has been largely dismissed.

To improve AZT therapy further, trials continue which combine AZT with acyclovir, alpha interferon, ddC, interleukin II, granulocyte macrophage-colony stimulating factor (GM-CSF), and other drugs. NIAID is also sponsoring trials at the University of Miami and the University of California Los Angeles to determine if AZT given to seropositive women during the last trimester of pregnancy can prevent HIV transmission to their infants.

## Vindication of the Early Treatment Strategy?

When all of these studies are considered together, they support the premise that the benefits of AZT can be obtained with lower, less toxic doses, and that these benefits decrease in proportion to immune deficiency.

Protocols 016 and 019 resulted in real advances for understanding how to interrupt the course of HIV. But they also verified the "underground" strategy of earlier, and therefore easier, treatment for HIV. The idea of intervening early in HIV infection is nearly as old as the epidemic, championed by many long-term survivors with HIV, both symptomatic and asymptomatic, by many progressive physicians, and by the persistent activism of Project Inform and ACT UP. The medical establishment has historically promoted early detection and treatment in other diseases, such as cancer, heart disease, diabetes, hypertension. But for the years preceding these recent announcements, people with HIV were dismissed with false pessimism in the media and inappropriate Federal regulations, and told to wait.

In light of the above studies, the original recommendations for using AZT may have been too much, too late, and too expensive. Now many researchers and activists agree that AZT, at least, is effective earlier, and in lower amounts, than the FDA approval indicated. The controversy regarding the optimal dosage and timing for AZT has long simmered in public discussions as well as medical literature, usually framed in a way which begged the question: "Why should asymptomatic patients be given a drug which may poison and impoverish them?" This view of the issue permitted thousands of asymptomatic people to drift aimlessly into illness.

Others have instead questioned the high cost of the only approved treatment for HIV, questioned the regulatory structure which discouraged the idea of informed choice for people with few choices, questioned a research process which sought recruits for AZT/placebo studies as late as July of 1989, and questioned the continuing dominance of AZT in the treatment landscape.

## REFERENCES

R Melmed, R N and others. Serum neopterin changes in HIV-infected subjects: Indicator of significant pathology, CD4 T-cell changes, and the development of AIDS. Journal of *Acquired Immune Deficiency Syndromes,* volume 2, number 1, pages 70-76, 1989.

Steinberg, J P and others. Predictors of outcome in AIDS patients receiving zidovudine. *Journal of Acquired Immune Deficiency Syndromes*, volume 2, number 3, pages 229-234, 1989.

Jacobson, M. How does zidovudine effect virologic immunologic markers of HIV activity? *AIDS Medical Report*, volume 2, number 2, pages 13-14, 1989.

Oskenhendler, E and others. Zidovudine for Thrombocytopenic Purpura Related to Human Immunodeficiency Virus (HIV) Infection. *Annals of Internal Medicine*, volume 110, number 1, pages 85-86, 1989.

# MAIL-ORDER PHARMACIES: SAVING MONEY ON PRESCRIPTION DRUGS

The new information supporting the value of early treatment with AZT, together with the unconscionable price of that drug, has focused attention on the problems of paying for treatment. We will cover policy questions on cost of care in later issues; this article discusses filling prescriptions by mail to reduce costs—whether or not one has insurance which includes drug coverage.

Mail-order pharmacies are high-volume operations which can locate where costs are low, and can negotiate good prices from suppliers. Also, they compete with each other mainly on price, because location doesn't matter, whereas traditional corner drugstores may have a captive market. Therefore they usually (but not always) have the lowest prices available. *AIDS Treatment News* published price comparisons in issue #64.

For this article we briefly surveyed customer satisfaction, by asking people to tell us their own experiences with mail-order pharmacies. We did not ask the pharmacies to recommend customers for us to interview; instead we called AIDS organizations and spoke to anyone who had information, and also asked physicians and other knowledgeable people whom we were contacting anyway for other reasons. Everyone we talked to who had experience with mail-order pharmacies (about ten people in all) was completely satisfied; most of them only knew about a single one, because they were happy with the first one they tried and did not need to look further.

Yet many of the people we contacted did not know of any source for prescription drugs, even though they had talked with tens or hundreds of persons with AIDS or HIV. It seems that filling prescriptions is usually a solitary or personal activity, one which patients seldom talk about. Therefore, information about money-saving options does not circulate in the AIDS community as freely as it should. We hope this article helps to fill that communication gap.

In our interviews we did not name specific pharmacies, but let the interviewees volunteer the names. Only two mail-order prescription vendors were mentioned more than once: American Preferred Plan (APP), and Family Pharmaceuticals of America. Both had excellent references from customers. Others may be equally good; but we did not have time to make this short article into a complete list.

[Note: Readers should know that several months ago *AIDS Treatment News* received an unsolicited donation of $500. from one of the companies (APP) which appears in this article. We considered returning the money in order to avoid any questions about our objectivity in future reporting. Instead we decided to accept the donation, but use it only for contributions to non-profit AIDS organizations, not for our own operations. Because of the urgent needs in the AIDS community, we felt it was better to handle the contribution this way than to return it. We also felt we should disclose the matter to our readers.]

For most mail-order pharmacies:

• Physicians can call in prescriptions, avoiding the need to wait for the mail, if patients can pay by credit card, or if the prescription is fully paid by insurance (see below). The pharmacies we talked to send the drugs by two-day express, unless overnight delivery is necessary. Delivery can be to a different street address (such as a friend's, or a work address), so that nobody needs to stay home to receive the medicines. (The couriers used, such as UPS and Federal Express, do not deliver to post-office boxes. Also, we have not heard of deliveries outside of the United States and its possession.)

• The pharmacy should bill insurance directly and handle the paperwork. The ones we interviewed seldom or never require patients to front the money which will be paid by insurance. Some other mail-order pharmacies require full payment from the patient, with the insurance company reimbursing the patient for the percentage it pays—a process which can take months. (Fortunately it is only necessary to pick up the phone to reach a mail-order pharmacy which does not require this money up front.)

• Patients can, of course, get price and other information by phone.

• Drugs like alpha interferon which need to be refrigerated can be shipped overnight in insulated containers. Make sure the shipper includes some kind of cold pack, such as "blue ice", able to keep the medicine cold even if a delivery is missed. (While we have heard only good reports about mail-order pharmacies, the fact remains that they are relatively new and not adequately regulated by government agencies; therefore uniform standards about such matters as shipping refrigerated drugs cannot be assumed, and patients and physicians should be vigilant.)

• While prices are usually lower at mail-order than at traditional pharmacies, they are not always lower, and it does pay to shop around.

We called the two companies named by our interviewees and asked them what advantages they offered to customers:

### Family Pharmaceuticals of America, 800/922-3444
### (in South Carolina only, call 803/881-3444):

This mail-order pharmacy has been in business since 1981; we first mentioned it in *AIDS Treatment News* issue #46, December 1987. It is "AIDS sensitive," having long sought business in the AIDS community. It competes mainly on price but also has a good reputation for service.

In our recent interview, president John Richards, M.D., told us about new home services including intravenous medications and TPN (total parenteral nutrition). Family Pharmaceuticals has affiliated with a home-care company to deliver such treatment anywhere in the country, at what it claims are significant savings; Dr. Richards said that the first 20 patients put on this system showed savings totalling $200,000 per year, compared to what they had spent previously. Family Pharmaceuticals provides a "turnkey" system, meaning that it arranges for nursing and other necessary support, so that patients do not need to make these arrangements themselves.

Medications delivered this way can include ganciclovir, intravenous antibiotics, and aerosol pentamidine. The company also supports the "cassette" system for pain-control and other medications. This system uses a small computer-controlled pump to inject medication continuously or on a pre-programmed schedule. The apparatus and medicines can be worn on the arm; the self-contained unit is about the size of a cigarette pack.

Alpha interferon is a special case, in that suppliers have announced a cap of about $9800. that a single patient will have to pay for the drug in one year. Family Pharmaceuticals has made arrangements so that its customers do not have to front the money after this annual limit is reached.

Patients or physicians interested in home care with intravenous medications should call a special number, 800/232-3003 and ask for William J. Taylor, Pharm. D. (Dr. Taylor, incidentally, is also chair of the pharmacology committee of the Physicians' Association for AIDS Care.) Patients calling to fill ordinary prescriptions should call Kim Richardson at 800/922-3444.

**American Preferred Plan (APP), 800/227-1195 (in New York State only, call 800/445-4519):**

This company is technically not a pharmacy but a membership organization; it places orders with a pharmacy, and specializes in covering the 20 percent copayment (which many insurance policies require) for its members. In most cases, APP will accept the 80 percent insurance coverage as payment in full, and the patient does not need to put out any money, or do any paperwork after they have joined the organization. There is no fee to join.

APP is very similar to Preferred Rx, which was covered in *AIDS Treatment News* issue #66. However, Preferred Rx (800/365-2646; in Ohio 216/661-1977) requires a $25 membership fee every 12 months. Both Preferred Rx and APP were started by Ron English, who is also well known as a board member and major fundraiser for the Community Research Initiative in New York.

After our interviews with customers, we interviewed Ron English and Ellie Adiel at APP. This company focuses exclusively on working with people with AIDS; besides filling prescriptions, it can refer callers to organizations, agencies, legal and emotional support services, and sources of free medications.

Patients with insurance which covers 80 percent or more of the cost of pharmaceuticals should be able to fill prescriptions through APP without paying any money out of pocket. Patients without insurance can also use APP, but for them it has no special advantage over other mail-order pharmacies. Patients should compare prices on the drugs they need.

## Other Options

This article does not cover free or subsidized medical care, a very important area which needs to be discussed elsewhere. Also, it does not cover any form of underground market in prescription or other pharmaceuticals.

In some locations non-profit pharmacies have been set up to reduce drug prices for persons with AIDS or other chronic diseases. We did not find any in this brief survey, but patients should know that such organizations exist.

A few traditional pharmacies have sold AZT at cost, as a public service; therefore their price is lower than that of mail-order pharmacies. We do not have a list of these pharmacies; persons should check with local AIDS support groups, which may know any in their area.

One pharmacy in Los Angeles goes beyond paying the 20 percent insurance copayment and offers cash rebates in certain situations. Will Basso at Bob's Pharmacy (6136 Venice Blvd; it also sells by mail, phone 213/838-7292) said that rebates have been as high as $300. per month, but are more typically in the range of $100. to $150., if patients are using full-dose AZT and other drugs in addition. Potential customers can learn by phone what their rebates should be before they place their orders. Basso assured us that rebates are completely legal—"We can do what we want with our profits"—and that they have not had complaints or problems. (*AIDS Treatment News* has not yet interviewed anyone who has used this service.)

This article could not be comprehensive, and obviously many good sources for prescription drugs have not been listed. Instead of providing a list, we gave examples to show some of the options available, and to show some of the creative ways that have been developed to reduce the cost of drugs.

# HYPERICIN NOTES

Our hypericin survey (published in *AIDS Treatment News* # 80) is taking longer than expected to analyze, but we plan to have a report in the next issue. Meanwhile we must pass on recent information about potential side effects.

We previously published reports of several people who had to stop taking extracts of St. John's wort (the herb which contains hypericin) because blood-chemistry panels showed elevated levels of liver enzymes. Recently we heard of three more such cases. The two for whom the best data is available showed gradual rises over a two-month period while they used the herb. There is no proof that the St. John's wort caused the abnormal liver function tests, but until more is known, persons using the herb should have a blood-chemistry panel (such as SMA 25) which includes liver-function tests. Physicians usually recommend that patients stop all medicines, temporarily at least, if these tests become seriously abnormal.

Also, St. John's wort may act like a kind of antidepressant called an MAO inhibitor—although no one knows for sure. MAO inhibitors are dangerous if combined with certain other drugs, and even any of a long list of foods and beverages. In *AIDS Treatment News* #74, we pointed out that this problem was possible, although it seemed remote.

But recently we heard of one case where this interaction might have occurred. The patient combined St. John's wort with a tricyclic antidepressant (a kind of drug which must not be combined with an MAO inhibitor) and suffered rapid heart beats, skipped beats, and anxiety. This is the only case we have heard of such a problem. But since this reaction is dangerous, the physician who brought this case to our attention suggested that St. John's wort extracts should not be combined with prescription antidepressants, and possibly not with certain foods either.

More information can be found in medical reference books, which list foods and drugs which must not be combined with MAO inhibitors, and symptoms which may occur if they are combined.

It is possible that these problems with St. John's wort extracts—if they exist at all—are caused not by hypericin, but by some other chemicals in the plant. In that case, the problems could be overcome by using pure hypericin, from which the other chemicals had been removed.

# REPORT FROM CONFERENCE ON AIDS AND MINORITIES

Washington, D.C. was the site of "Prevention and Beyond: A Framework for Collective Action," a conference August 13-17 sponsored by the Department of Health & Human Services to discuss the impact of the AIDS epidemic on ethnic and racial minorities in the U.S., and to create a plan of action to combat HIV transmission and create access to services and treatment in these communities.

The Black, Latino, Asian/Pacific Islander, and Native American communities were well represented at the conference, with a cross-section of disciplines from each community. The conference addressed issues such as the double and triple oppressions which minorities face, the need for language/culture-specific literature to explain HIV transmission, racist tilting of epidemiological and budgeting statistics, low-income families receiving inferior overall health care (if any at all), and the inadequate access to early diagnosis and treatment options for HIV and AIDS.

A group of concerned attenders interrupted the conference proceedings at one point in an effort to dramatize some of the deficiencies of the conference. The future of the epidemic is bleak unless dramatic changes are made in the manner information is disseminated and the way health care is delivered, or not delivered, in the U.S. Even if an effective treatment and/or vaccine is found, who will get it? Will money or skin color or language or geography or gender decide? Two staff members from *AIDS Treatment News* attended and participated in discussions of these problems and possible solutions. We will report again when the statements from the various conference caucuses are completed.

# Issue Number 87
# September 8, 1989

## ANTIVIRAL FOUND IN BLUE-GREEN ALGAE

Scientists at the U.S. National Cancer Institute and the University of Hawaii have discovered a class of anti-HIV chemicals in certain species of blue-green algae, some of them found in the ocean off Hawaii or off the Palau Islands. This discovery was reported last month in the *Journal of the National Cancer Institute* (Gustafson and others, "AIDS-Antiviral Sulfolipids from Cyanobacteria (Blue-Green Algae)," pages 1254-1258, August 16, 1989). No one yet knows whether these substances can become useful drugs, but they have been selected for high priority for further research by the National Cancer Institute.

### Background

The chemicals, called sulfolipids (or sulfonic acid-containing glycolipids) were previously known, but not known to be antiviral. The recent discovery resulted from a National Cancer Institute program to search systematically for new AIDS and cancer drugs which might be found in algae.

Plants have been used as sources of medicines throughout history, but algae have been largely unexamined, because they are difficult to work with. Now that it is possible to collect and test large numbers of species, researchers may find important medicines which could not have been discovered earlier.

In the current program, the algae species are collected from a research ship, or on land, and grown in the laboratory to assure a future supply. If crude plant extracts show potential value in laboratory assays, then chemical "fractionation" procedures are used to divide the extracts into different groups of compounds. Antiviral assays are used to determine which of the different components includes the antiviral, and this process can be repeated to find the pure chemical(s) which have the desired effect.

After the sulfolipids were identified, researchers spent a year trying to synthesize them, but without success, according to a report in *The New York Times*, August 16. Currently, lack of supply is the major problem delaying drug development, since the laboratory used so far is set up for screening, not mass production. After supplies are obtained, animal studies and other pre-clinical work will be done before human trials.

## Navy Expels Ship

In April of this year, the U.S. Navy interrupted this research program by expelling a Soviet research ship which would have carried U.S. and Soviet scientists searching for algae near Hawaii. Although the project included the National Cancer Institute and had been approved by the State Department, the Navy feared that the ship would spy on U.S. military installations. The captain was given one hour to leave Hilo, where the ship was docked, and was forbidden to enter Hawaiian waters. Some of the U.S. scientists rushed off the ship; others stayed on, but were unable to carry out the 10-day research trip at the planned locations.

This incident was reported by Honolulu newspapers, and also by science writer David Pearlman in the *San Francisco Chronicle* on May 6, but otherwise it had little or no coverage in the U.S. press. (The sulfolipids had already been discovered in algae picked up in an earlier voyage.)

Dr. Gregory Patterson, one of the researchers who found the sulfolipids, told *AIDS Treatment News* that it is impossible to estimate the importance of the cancellation of the planned trip, since the project is looking for completely new drugs from algae. It is impossible to know the value of what might have been found.

## Could Eating Plant Sources Be Beneficial?

Seven different species of blue-green algae—named in the article cited above—were found to inhibit HIV; all contained sulfolipids. In two species, the sulfolipids were about ten percent of the "organic extractables" from the algae. The different sulfolipids tested were all about equally active as antivirals, protecting cells from infection in concentrations of about 1 to 100 micrograms per ml, depending on what kinds of cells were used to grow HIV. Sulfolipids have been known since 1959; the recent article cited earlier published research which found that they occur widely in higher plants, as well as in algae.

*AIDS Treatment News* contacted two of the researchers (one indirectly, through the National Cancer Institute press office) to find out if there was any information about whether the chemicals, related to fatty acids, could be absorbed if taken orally. Both scientists insisted that it is much too early to consider using these chemicals as drugs, before any animal studies have been done. Dr. Patterson pointed out that there is much variation between different species of plants, that the chemicals may be broken down in the body, and that as there have been no toxicity tests, there may be unknown toxicities.

Of course it will be a long time before sulfolipids get through the drug-development process and (if found effective) onto pharmacy shelves. Meanwhile there will certainly be an interest in whether a treatment could be developed using herbal sources.

One way to minimize the risk of any such attempt would be to look for plants which have already been used as human food or medicine, and which also contain high levels of sulfolipids. The plants would not necessarily be algae. The first step in this research would be to search the scientific literature to find what plants are already known to contain sulfolipids; the references in the article cited above would be a place to start. It may also be necessary to chemically analyze likely candidates (the tests required have been published), to determine which plants are the best sources.

At least two species of blue-green algae—spirulina, and a species from Klamath Lake, Oregon—are sold as health foods in the United States. We do not know whether or not either contains sulfolipids.

If there are plants which contain these chemicals and are already used as human food or medicine, a monitoring study could look for any effects of using such plants (together with whatever other treatments each patient was already using) on p24 antigen level, T-helper count, or other laboratory or clinical measurements. Such a project would cost little, and could be conducted by a community-based research organization.

# INTERFERON, HIV, AND KAPOSI'S SARCOMA UPDATE
## by Denny Smith

Alpha interferon, approved by the Food and Drug Administration last November for the treatment of Kaposi's sarcoma (KS), has received more attention lately as a treatment for HIV infection as well as AIDS-related KS. Interferons are naturally occurring proteins secreted by cells in response to infection, and they serve multiple roles as antiviral, antitumor, and immune stimulating agents. The three major classes of interferon (alpha, beta, and gamma) have been synthesized, and each is being studied in various applications for the treatment of HIV and AIDS.

A combination of alpha interferon and AZT was discussed as a possible improvement in HIV antiviral therapy in the May 5 issue of *Science* (Poli and others). The authors, reporting on the results of *in vitro* research at the National Institute of Allergy and Infectious Diseases (NIAID), found that alpha interferon prevented the assembly and release of new virus from cells chronically or latently infected with HIV, interrupting the progress of HIV at a point later in the life of the virus than AZT, which inhibits viral replication within infected cells. Combining the two drugs would theoretically enhance, not just duplicate, their anti-HIV potential.

(Note: For a different viewpoint on alpha interferon, see recent article by Joseph Sonnabend, M.D., cited in references section, below. Dr. Sonnabend, an interferon expert and a cofounder of the Community Research Initiative in New York, points out that alpha interferon levels are already too high in many persons with AIDS, and that high levels might contribute to the disease process.)

A small clinical trial involving asymptomatic seropositive individuals, was discussed at the V International Conference on AIDS in Montreal in June. In this study, 35 million units of subcutaneous alpha interferon given daily for 12 weeks appeared to slow the decline of helper cells and reduce the risk of developing opportunistic infections (Lane and others). The August 15 issue of *Annals of Internal Medicine* published additional findings from NIAID which further support the combined use of AZT and alpha interferon to combat HIV infection and HIV-associated KS. After comparing various pairings of AZT and alpha interferon doses, the researchers found that the maximum dose of both drugs which could be tolerated without serious side effects was 100 mg of AZT every four hours with a single daily injection of 5 to 10 million units of alpha interferon. This was enough to obtain an antitumor and anti-HIV effect in some participants, without an increase in the side effects normally seen separately with higher-dose AZT or interferon. Unfortunately the combination produced some unexpected toxicities: decreased platelets and neutrophils, and liver dysfunction. These generally occurred at the larger AZT doses.

The researchers note that the antiviral and antitumor benefits cannot for certain be attributable to the interferon/AZT combination, rather than to interferon alone. But this combination has the advantage of confronting KS while inhibiting HIV at two different steps in its replication; combined therapies are often better than single-agent treatments. The pattern of these studies is in line with others which found a correlation between a decrease in alpha interferon levels and the depletion of helper cells in HIV infection, suggesting the use of alpha interferon as a marker for monitoring the activity of HIV as well as an agent for blocking it (Rossol and others, 1989). High doses of alpha interferon can cause unpleasant side effects; Dr. Mathilde Krim of the American Foundation for AIDS Research, told *The New York Times* (August 15) that alpha interferon should be tried early in HIV disease, at low doses. Beta interferon is also being combined with AZT in clinical studies, and we hope to report on that in the near future.

In the treatment of KS, AZT has been studied in combination with alpha interferon with more success than the combination of alpha interferon and other chemotherapeutic agents, which seems to increase toxicity more than benefits. In March 1989, the *Annals of Internal Medicine* published a thorough overview of the use of alpha interferon for KS, by Jerome E. Groopman, M.D. and David T. Scadden, M.D. of New England Deaconess Hospital. Among their observations, Drs. Groopman and Scadden noted that alpha interferon's capacity to inhibit the proliferative growth of KS, as well as its stimulation of the immune system's own antitumor activity, may make it an attractive alternative to chemotherapy agents like vincristine, vinblastine, doxorubicin, and bleomycin, which can further impair immune functions with bone marrow toxicity. They pointed out that interferon worked much better when patients had T-helper cell counts over 200.

We spoke with Dr. Scadden, who is now conducting a trial in Boston involving the use of alpha interferon with AZT to treat KS, with the addition as warranted of granulocyte macrophage-colony stimulating factor (GM-CSF), a synthesized product of the immune system which may reverse some of the toxicity of the combination, and which has been speculated to potentiate its activity. This is not a placebo trial. Interested people can call 617/732-8528. Dr. Scadden cautioned that combining interferon with AZT is still an experimental idea, and would be considered a long-range therapy even if it is successful. People who need more immediate treatment for cosmetically or functionally impairing KS lesions would obtain a more short-term response from conventional chemotherapy (see *AIDS Treatment News* #73).

*AIDS Treatment News* #75 also reported on the use of alpha interferon, and on two other relatively new therapies for KS—laser surgery and the Prosorba column. Although interferon has been usually described as a systemic treatment which is administered by injection into muscle tissue or beneath the skin surface, we recently heard of a physician giving alpha interferon intralesionally—that is, small amounts injected directly into the edges of individual lesions. Ostensibly there would be few systemic benefits from this administration, but neither would there be the disadvantage of unpleasant side effects which often accompany the larger injections. Such an approach might be appropriate for small lesions which are few in number and do not need more aggressive treatment. (The official indications for the administration of alpha interferon are described on the product insert.)

Earlier, in issue #73, we described some standard chemotherapy for KS, both intravenous and intralesional, and radiation therapy. The ratio and frequency of the drugs described in that article had been refined to minimize the side effects usually seen with chemotherapy. The substances used in chemotherapy are usually caustic and must be handled with plastic gloves by the health care workers involved. Sometimes during the administration of intravenous medication, some of the I.V. fluid escapes from the puncture site (extravasation) into surrounding tissues. If the I.V. needle is withdrawn as soon as this is noticed, it is not ordinarily a serious problem. However, in the case of chemotherapeutic agents, it means that the surrounding tissue has been exposed to a drug designed intentionally to kill cancerous cells, and which can also have a corrosive effect on many healthy cells.

The ulcer resulting from this mishap can take weeks or months to heal, as well as make an important I.V. site unavailable. Several years ago researchers at the University of Alabama discovered that butylated hydroxytoluene (BHT) greatly reduced the progression of necrosis (dead and dying tissue) in doxorubicin-induced skin ulcers in mice (Daugherty and others, 1985); they suggest its evaluation in modifying skin necrosis from doxorubicin.

In addition to interferon, radiation, lasers, chemotherapy, and the Prosorba column, other possible treatments for KS under investigation include bropirimine ABPP, CL246,738, IMREG 1 and 2, and interleukin II. Tumor necrosis factor (TNF) is a substance naturally produced by macrophages and is active against a variety of tumors, but a study at the University of California in Los Angeles found multiple toxicities and no obvious antitumor or anti-HIV effect with TNF administered intravenously (Aboulafia and others, 1989). Another study at the University of California San Francisco Medical Center obtained some reduction in lesion size and number, but not without side effects, by administering TNF intralesionally (Kahn and others, 1989). Finally, cimetidine, a common prescription drug which has been shown to have immune stimulating and antitumor properties, may be a complementary treatment possibility for KS (see *AIDS Treatment News* #80). We will follow new treatments as they progress.

## REFERENCES

Aboulafia, D and others. Intravenous recombinant tumor necrosis factor in the treatment of AIDS-related Kaposi's sarcoma. *Journal of Acquired Immune Deficiency Syndromes,* volume 2, number 1, pages 54-58, 1989.

Daugherty, JP and Khurana, A. Amelioration of doxorubicin-induced skin necrosis in mice by butylated hydroxytoluene. *Cancer Chemotherapy and Pharmacology,* pages 243-246, Spring 1985.

Groopman, JE and Scadden, DT. Interferon therapy for Kaposi's sarcoma associated with the acquired immunodeficiency syndrome (AIDS). *Annals of Internal Medicine,* volume 110, number 5, pages 335-337, March 1, 1989.

Kahn, JO and others. Intralesional recombinant tumor necrosis factor-alpha for AIDS-associated Kaposi's sarcoma: A randomized, double-blind trial. *Journal of Acquired Immune Deficiency Syndromes,* volume 2, number 3, pages 217-223, 1989.

Kovaks, JA and others. Combined zidovudine and interferon-alpha therapy in patients with Kaposi's sarcoma and the acquired immunodeficiency syndrome (AIDS). *Annals of Internal Medicine,* volume 111, number 4, pages 280-287, August 15, 1989.

Poli, G and others. Interferon-alpha but not AZT suppresses HIV expression in chronically infected cell lines. *Science,* volume 244, pages 575-577, May 5,1989.

Rossol, S and others. Interferon production in patients infected with HIV-1. *The Journal of Infectious Diseases,* volume 159, number 5, pages 815-821, May 1989.

Sonnabend, JA. Fact and speculation about the cause of AIDS. *AIDS Forum* volume 2, number 1, pages 2-12, May 1989.

# Issue Number 88
# October 6, 1989

## NAC: BRONCHITIS DRUG MAY SLOW AIDS VIRUS

*by John S. James*

Stanford University researchers reported last week that a drug widely used in Europe to treat bronchitis inhibits HIV in laboratory tests. They are developing plans for clinical trials of the drug, called n-acetylcysteine (NAC). No human results for AIDS/HIV have been published, but *AIDS Treatment News* has learned that at least ten people are using NAC for this purpose, at least one of them for almost a year.

Dr. Leonard Herzenberg and Dr. Leonore Herzenberg, who are husband and wife and both professors of genetics at Stanford University and well known for developing the Fluorescence-Activated Cell Sorter (FACS), a machine widely used to count T-cells, conducted the laboratory studies, together with other researchers at Stanford. Last week Dr. Leonard Herzenberg reported on their work with NAC at a scientific conference in Geneva, Switzerland. The Herzenbergs credited a German immunologist, Dr. Wulf Droge at the German Cancer Research Center in Heidelberg, for first suggesting the potential use of the drug in AIDS.

In laboratory experiments, NAC increased the level of the chemical glutathione in HIV-infected blood cells. Glutathione is necessary for life, as it is needed for energy generation and other cell functions. It also protects cells against oxidizing agents. Dr. Droge had discovered that glutathione levels were too low in persons with AIDS, and fell as the disease progressed. He also knew that NAC had increased these levels when it was used to treat bronchitis.

NAC is also believed to counter some effects of excessive levels of tumor necrosis factor (TNF), which often occur in AIDS. TNF is believed to increase the production of HIV, to cause wasting syndrome in some cases, and to cause production of more TNF. (Paradoxically, other reseachers are testing TNF as part of a combination treatment for KS.)

The Herzenbergs' laboratory at Stanford is supported by the U.S. National Institutes of Health. The NAC research received support from the Zambon Group of Italy, which markets the drug.

In a Stanford University press release, the Herzenbergs stressed that NAC is not a cure for AIDS, but that laboratory results suggest that it might be a useful treatment. "Our studies show we can block the TNF activation of HIV with increased thiol levels in models of HIV-infected cells. We propose that by administering NAC we can augment thiol levels, and neutralize TNF activity and production which will slow or stop the virus from going into an active stage."

## Comment

AIDS drugs are usually classified either as antivirals or as immune modulators. NAC appears to be an antiviral, but it may be better to consider it an example of a third class of potential treatments—those which intervene in the pathogenesis of AIDS.

Pathogenesis has been defined as "the origin and development of a disease." In AIDS research, a remarkable ignorance of pathogenesis has been widely tolerated, probably because of an unbalanced research focus on HIV and the search for a magic bullet to kill it. NAC appears to work (if it does) not by killing the virus directly, but rather by correcting biochemical imbalances which occur in the course of the illness, and which then cause other problems, including further viral growth.

## Human Experience with HIV

We interviewed one person who is using NAC, and several others familiar with the drug or with the laboratory results suggesting its possible use as an HIV treatment. This is what we learned:

- At least ten people have tried NAC, and no side effects have been reported. (The drug is generally considered very safe in its standard use, treating bronchitis and other lung problems by reducing the thickness of mucus. However, there is little experience with long-term use by persons with AIDS.)

- Those most likely to benefit seem to be persons with cachexia (wasting syndrome). Early reports are that these patients feel better quite quickly, and then regain weight.

- Two persons with KS are using the drug. Both are said to be doing well, but we do not have detailed information.

- There are also reports of improvement in T-helper cells and p24 antigen levels. However, we do not have any detailed information at this time.

- Almost everyone who has started the drug is continuing on it, as they believe it is helping.

## Availability

NAC for oral use is available in most of the world, but not in the United States. It usually requires a prescription, but it might be sold over the counter in some countries; we could not find out by press time.

**October 6, 1989**

In the U.S., NAC is available only in a liquid form intended for aerosol, not oral use. The liquid can be diluted and given orally—and is FDA-approved for such use, for treatment of poisoning caused by overdose of acetaminophen, the painkiller in Tylenol and some other over-the-counter medicines. But it would be difficult to use this liquid as an HIV treatment. This formulation was not made for oral use, and often causes vomiting; many patients have trouble keeping it down. As an HIV treatment, the drug would have to be taken three or four times a day indefinitely.

Most people so far who have tried this drug for HIV have used a brand named Fluimucil, which is available in Italy, Switzerland, Germany, The Netherlands, and Spain, and perhaps elsewhere. One person who has used it told us that Fluimucil comes in two forms; an effervescent tablet containing 600 mg, and a packet of powder with 200 mg. Both forms need to be dissolved in a glass of water or fruit juice (not milk or hot drinks) before being taken. NAC should not be heated above body temperature. The drug will not keep after it has been dissolved, so it has to be mixed shortly before use, not stored and taken later. Most people have taken 600 mg (one tablet) three times a day, or 400 mg four times a day, using the packets of powder. We have heard that the drug is inexpensive in Europe.

There is much concern that in the U.S., where NAC for oral use is not available, people will use chemicals not intended for human consumption, resulting in unknown risks. To prevent this from happening, some way of obtaining the pharmaceutical products (through buyers' clubs or otherwise) will need to be set up.

There is also concern that people who try this drug may stop taking other treatments. NAC is not a substitute for any other drug. There are no known harmful interactions with other drugs commonly used in treating AIDS; however one medical reference warns that "some antibiotics including amphotericin, ampicillin sodium, erythromycin lactobionate, and some tetracyclines are either physically incompatible with or may be inactivated on mixture with acetylcysteine (NAC)."

It is too early to tell if NAC will be useful. But certainly it is important to find out quickly. It is easy to call for controlled clinical trials, and of course such trials are necessary. The problem, however, is that there seems to be no way for the drug to become available quickly through trials in the United States (elsewhere it is already available). NAC has been discussed among scientists as a potential AIDS treatment for over a year; six months ago a protocol for a trial had been written. The new attention resulting from recent public knowledge about the drug may help to speed the process.

## *AIDS Treatment News* Seeks Information

If you have any information about use of NAC for AIDS or HIV, we would appreciate it if you would contact *AIDS Treatment News* at the above address or phone 415/255-0588 (or fax at 415/255-4659). We will, of course, keep your identity confidential.

Persons planning to start taking NAC should get blood work done first—including T-cell counts and p24 antigen level—and also record their weight, so that later they can tell whether or not these measures improved after treatment. Asymptomatic patients, in particular, will have no other way to judge whether the drug is working for them.

## Disclaimer

This article is **not** intended as instructions for using NAC. It may omit necessary information; for example, we have not yet seen the European product literature or instructions for physicians, nor have we talked to U.S. physicians whose patients have used the drug. Information for HIV-positive persons and their physicians on how to use NAC still needs to be prepared.

# DDI TRIALS, ACCESS ANNOUNCED

On September 28 the U.S. Department of Health and Human Services announced that the antiviral ddI would be tested in three clinical trials, and also be made available to some people who have no other option and cannot participate in the trials. There has been some confusion as the details of this important, urgent, and flawed program are worked out. This article reports what we have learned about the present status of ddI; there will be changes, probably for the better, in the future.

## Background

ddI is an antiviral in the same class as AZT. Early human trials suggest that it will probably be about as effective as AZT, perhaps somewhat less. The immediate importance of ddI is that it provides a different treatment option which may be effective when AZT is not. Persons who cannot tolerate AZT will probably be able to use ddI. And persons for whom AZT has stopped working (probably because the AIDS virus has become resistant to the drug) will probably also be able to benefit. Virus which has become resistant to AZT is usually not resistant to ddI.

This drug is no cure. Like AZT, it must be taken indefinitely, and it has toxicities which limit the dose which can be used. (They are different from AZT toxicities, however.) ddI might also lose its effectiveness in many patients after a year or two—it is too early to tell. For these reasons, persons who are now using AZT successfully will probably want to stay with what is working for them, and not start DDI until they need it, or until more has been learned about it.

The new ddI program consists of three different formal clinical trials, plus two other studies intended primarily to make ddI available to some persons who cannot join the trials. Persons not eligible for some of these programs might be eligible for others.

In the discussion below, we include the most important (but not all) of the inclusion and exclusion criteria—the details of who can or cannot qualify to get ddI. Patients can get some sense from this article of whether and how they might qualify. But we did not include all the rules, because they are long and confusing and might change in the future.

Some patients—and certainly any physicians who want to get ddI for their patients—will want to obtain a current copy of the full inclusion and exclusion criteria. Physicians will probably receive a copy when they register with Bristol-Myers for the ddI program (see phone number below); patients can probably receive a copy from the Clinical Trials Information Service, a hotline on clinical trials run by the U.S. Public Health Service; call 800/TRIALS-A. It is likely that various AIDS organizations will also have copies. (This hotline, incidentally, can provide information about clinical trials of ddI, as well as other experimental AIDS drugs, in your area.)

As we show below, the current rules for access to ddI are much too restrictive. Hundreds if not thousands of people will be denied the treatment when they have no other alternative. To prevent rejection, either patients and/or their physicians must know the rules, in order to direct each patient to the right program, put his or her best case forward, and submit an application likely to be successful.

## The Three Trials

The three trials starting now or expected to start soon will compare ddI with AZT in two different groups of patients, and also compare different doses of ddI in patients intolerant to AZT. These trials are:

• **ACTG 116—comparing ddI with AZT in patients with AIDS or advanced ARC.**

To be accepted for this trial, patients must be ages 12 through 99, and have either an AIDS diagnosis, or under 300 T-helper cells and one of a number of ARC symptoms. They may have taken AZT already; for the "116" study they cannot have used it more than 48 weeks (but those who have used AZT for over a year may qualify for ACTG 117, described below). If they have used AZT, they must have been able to take at least 500 mg per day (a low dose) without major intolerance.

Those who have taken AZT for over eight weeks and have ARC must have met the entry criteria (under 300 T-helper cells and one or more of certain symptoms) when they started AZT, but not necessarily when they enter the study. But those who have taken AZT for eight weeks or less can only enter the study with an AIDS diagnosis, which must be due only to a single instance of PCP; they cannot enter the study if they only have ARC. (Presumably persons with ARC who are otherwise qualified could keep taking AZT until the eight weeks are up, and then apply.)

There are many other exclusion criteria, such as KS requiring chemotherapy, grade 2 neuropathy, past or present heart disease, seizures within the last six months, certain liver enzymes more than five times normal, or hemoglobin, neutrophils, or platelets too low. A few prior or concurrent medications are not allowed. Patients should check with their physicians, or obtain a copy of the full criteria as described above. The entry criteria we listed above are the ones likely to affect the most people.

Fifteen hundred patients will be enrolled in this trial. For those receiving ddI we do not know the dose, but it will probably be 375 mg or less taken twice per day. Neither the patients nor their physicians will be told which drug they are getting.

All persons in this trial must be on aerosol pentamidine, and they can use most other treatments for opportunistic infections as required, without being dropped from the study. We do not know who will pay for the required aerosol pentamidine.

ACTG 116 will take place at about 50 different sites in the U.S. Persons can call 800/TRIALS-A to find out if one is located in their area.

• **ACTG 117—comparing ddI with AZT in patients who have taken AZT for a year or longer.**

The purpose of this study is to see if ddI is better than AZT for patients who have already taken AZT for a long time, and may have developed resistant virus.

To enter, volunteers must have AIDS or advanced ARC, as defined above, and have taken AZT for at least 12 months. They must at least 12 years old. Again there are many other entry criteria, so potential volunteers should ask their physicians, or obtain the full eligibility information thenmselves.

- **ACTG 118—test of ddI in patients who cannot tolerate AZT.**

For this study patients must be ages 12-99, have AIDS or advanced ARC, and have shown hematologic intolerance to AZT at least twice—at least one of those times at doses of 500 mg per day or less. Intolerance must be documented by specified decreases and levels of either hemoglobin or neutrophils. AZT must have been taken for at least 10 weeks but not more than a year, at doses of 500 mg per day or more. There are various other entry criteria, much like those of the other two studies.

ACTG 118 will take place at about 50 sites around the United States. 350 patients will be enrolled.

For more information on any of these studies, call the U.S. Public Health Service information number, 800/TRIALS-A.

## DDI Availability for Persons Who Cannot Enter the Above Trials

Persons who do not meet the criteria for any of the three trials, or who live too far away from any of the trial sites, may be able to receive it through one of two other programs. Unfortunately many others will be excluded from these programs by their restrictive entry criteria—criteria which might be relaxed in the future.

- **"Treatment IND" for people who cannot tolerate AZT.**

Patients must be 12 or older, have a diagnosis of AIDS or be symptomatic, and have a T-helper count of under 200. They must be intolerant to AZT in any one (or more) of seven ways: decrease in hemoglobin at a rate of at least 2 grams/month, a decrease in neutrophils to less than 750, severe nausea or vomiting, intractable headaches, acute psychosis, severe agitation, or loss of muscle strength. Any of these except the hemoglobin must have happened at least twice (i.e., happened again on rechallenge with AZT), and patients must have remained intolerant even when the AZT dose was reduced to 500 mg per day or less.

In addition, patients who are too sick will not be allowed in this program. At least for now, patients must have hemoglobin of at least 8.0, platelet count at least 50,000, neutrophils at least 600, bilirubin, SGOT, and SGPT within 5 times upper limit of normal, creatinine less than 2.5, alkaline phosphatase within five times the normal limit, uric acid less than 7.5, and amylase less than or equal to twice the normal upper limit. These lab criteria must be met within 14 days prior to initial ddI dosing. Patients cannot require systemic chemotherapy in the first three months of ddI treatment, or have acute pancreatitis, a poorly controlled seizure disorder, or grade B or greater peripheral neuropathy. Women cannot be pregnant or breast feeding. Patients cannot concurrently take AZT or phenytoin (Dilantin), and they will also be excluded if they have taken any antiviral except AZT within 15 days. Extra tests are required for the first four months of ddI use if patients are concurrently using any of a number of drugs, including ganciclovir, acyclovir, ketoconazole, or sulfa drugs, or if patients have intractable diarrhea or are following a low sodium diet. Certain other patients considered at high risk for side effects of ddI must have tests every ten days while they are using the drug; these patients are those with "peripheral neuropathy, pancreatitis,

seizure disorder, cardiac abnormalities, gout, and significant elevations of liver function tests results."

Patients who meet these conditions may receive one of three different doses of ddI,
probably about 375, 250, or 167 mg twice daily; the exact dose may depend on body
weight. Physicians will have to submit the required data to Bristol-Myers every 30
days to receive the next 30-day supply of the drug. The ddI will be free, but patients
will apparently be responsible for payment for the required laboratory tests and
medical care.

- **Open label use of ddI for patients for whom AZT is not working.**

To qualify, patients must have AIDS (not ARC), have used at least 500 mg of AZT
for at least six months, and be at least 12 years old. Despite AZT, they must have had
any one of the following: specified weight loss, marked neurological deterioration,
AIDS-defining opportunistic infections at least three times in the last six months, T-
helper count under 50 on two occasions at least a month apart, or Karnofsky score 40 or
less due to AIDS. As with the treatment IND above, they cannot take AZT together
with ddI, cannot take Dilantin, and cannot use chemotherapy in the first three months
of ddI treatment. There are other criteria like those of the treatment IND, above.

There are other exclusion criteria not mentioned here. Do not rely on this outline of
some of the rules for access to ddI, but consult a full and current copy, obtained as
described above.

## Comment

The program outlined above will clearly exclude many people who might be helped by
ddI, have no other viable treatment options, and cannot get into any of the clinical
trials. Excluded patients include:

- Children under 12;

- Persons who are too ill to pass the laboratory criteria required, some of which do
not seem to have any relationship to known risks of ddI;

- Persons who would be on AZT except that they need ganciclovir or other
incompatible treatment;

- Persons with ARC who are failing on AZT but not intolerant to it;

(These people might be able to enter a trial where they could be randomly assigned
to receive AZT, known not to be working for them. Are they being excluded from
access in order to force them into a trial which will make AZT look bad and therefore
ddI look better in comparison?)

- Persons who cannot afford primary care, cannot afford a physician willing to fill
out the required forms, or cannot afford the required laboratory tests. This may be the
largest excluded group of all. We urgently need workable procedures to extend access
to ddI (and other "parallel track" experimental drugs) to patients who use public
clinics—perhaps by letting a panel of physicians in each clinic decide locally who
should be given the drug, without the expensive laboratory tests and paperwork
required by the present system.

According to the September 28 press release from the U.S. Department of Health
and Human Services, the treatment IND and open label use are "consistent with the

parallel track concept and (is) an interim measure to make a promising investigational therapy available for people with AIDS who do not have satisfactory treatment options." It is likely that less restrictive access will be allowed in the future. Under the current rules there will be many extreme cases of people who clearly should have access to ddI but are denied it. As a result there will be much pressure to make access less restrictive.

The basic concept of "parallel track" is that after an experimental drug has passed initial safety tests and shows some evidence that it works, persons who cannot get into the formal efficacy trials should be allowed access to the drug, while the trials are going on, if they have no other treatment options. Ultimately, we believe that this concept does not go far enough. It is wrong to force people into trials by denying them other treatment options. Instead, trials should be better designed to take patients' needs into accounts. And if necessary, subjects should be paid for participation in trials; everyone else involved in the drug-approval process is paid, as are most healthy volunteers in medical-research studies.

But politically there is not now enough support in the AIDS scientific establishment for patient-physician choice and truly voluntary participation in trials. Instead, the AIDS community and part of the scientific community have in effect reached a compromise—that parallel track treatment access should be available, but only to those who could not enter the formal trials, so that their access to treatment does not reduce the number of volunteers and therefore delay completion of the scientific studies. Many hard-liners in the scientific community do not accept this compromise, however, and are waiting for the current effort (to allow limited access to ddI outside of trials) to fail.

Our immediate task concerning access to ddI is to support the formal trials, and also to push to expand the parallel access so everyone who needs an antiviral and cannot use AZT will have the option to use ddI, if the best available information suggests that this drug is appropriate for them.

# "COMPOUND Q" RESULTS RELEASED

*by John S. James*

On September 19 Project Inform presented the results to date of its study of the treatment use of trichosanthin, commonly known as "compound Q." This controversial project organized nine physicians in four cities (San Francisco, New York, Los Angeles, and Miami/Ft. Lauderdale) to employ a very extensive and rigorous data-collection protocol to obtain good-quality information on the results of treatment with trichosanthin. Patients had obtained the drug from China, where it is used to induce abortions and to treat certain cancers.

Trichosanthin is not a cure for AIDS, and it can be very toxic for certain patients. Project Inform has urged that no one use it without expert medical supervision—and that if, after careful consideration, anyone does decide to use this treatment, their physician should first consult with other physicians who have experience in using the drug and managing its side effects.

**October 6, 1989**

But although it is dangerous, this drug is also potentially very important. *AIDS Treatment News* interviewed Martin Delaney of Project Inform, who helped to coordinate the study, to learn more of what is known about this treatment today.

*Note:* Of the four cities mentioned above, Project Inform has reported detailed efficacy results from only two, San Francisco and New York. The Florida arm, which pioneered this treatment program, used a different protocol, different laboratories, and sometimes a different route of administration; its results are not entirely comparable, and they have been reported separately (see below). The Los Angeles results are not complete at this time. However, Project Inform's report on toxicity and safety-related information includes what was known from all four of the centers.

## Toxicity of Compound Q

Two kinds of toxicity were found. One appeared to be dose-related. The other did not seem to depend on the dose, but rather on the condition of the patient.

The most important toxicity was central nervous system effects, which were seen in six of the 52 patients reported on by Project Inform. Three cases were especially serious, involving a coma, severe dementia, or seizure. Two of these patients have died, and while the deaths did not appear to result from the drug, there is controversy over whether or not the drug might have contributed.

The other four had disorientation or confusion lasting for hours or days. The longest-lasting case occurred before the researchers knew about the use of Decadron (dexamethasone) to control these side effects.

These neurological effects (which often start 30 hours or more after use of the drug) did not appear to be dose related, as the doses had varied by three fold (10 to 30 micrograms per kilogram). Instead, the problem appeared to depend on the condition of the patient. Their T-helper counts were very low, an average of 23. Four of the seven patients who experienced neurological effects had had an MRI scan; in three of these four the scan was suspicious. Every patient who has had a suspicious MRI scan has had problems.

Mr. Delaney knows of two different theories of what causes these neurological side effects in some persons with HIV who are treated with trichosanthin. (In China, where the drug is used for people without HIV infection, such effects are rare.):

• One theory is that the drug kills HIV-infected glial cells in the brain. Glial cells can be replaced. But there may be problems if too many are killed at once.

• Another theory is that HIV dementia can be caused by a toxic protein which is released by infected macrophages, without any brain infection. Suddenly killing these macrophages releases more of this protein into the bloodstream.

It might be possible to control these side effects by better testing to tell which patients are at high risk, by treatment with Decadron or other drugs (perhaps before the symptoms start), or by beginning trichosanthin treatment with very low doses in certain patients. But at this time no one is sure that the danger can be controlled. Persons with very low T-helper cells, or with any evidence of dementia, seem to be at highest risk.

A different and less serious kind of side effect does seem to be dose related. Most patients have some degree of muscle aches, especially of the back and shoulder, relatively minor fevers, joint pains, irritability, and/or rashes. Various drugs are being used to prevent or relieve these effects.

There are also other dangers. Trichosanthin can cause temporary immune suppression, making existing infections more severe. Antibodies can develop against the drug, which may limit future use; test doses must be used to avoid the danger of severe reactions. Only one such reaction has been seen in the Project Inform study (in a patient with high T-helper cells), and it was easily controlled by the immunologist who administered the trichosanthin.

On September 24 Project Inform distributed a warning which listed the kinds of patients at greatest risk for a bad reaction to trichosanthin. Those at high risk include:

- Persons near death, as very ill patients have not done well with this treatment.

- Those with low T-helper counts, less than 100 and especially less than 50, and with any indication of neurological damage by HIV.

- Those with low T-helper counts and no evidence of neurological problems are also at some risk.

- Persons currently fighting any active infection (since trichosanthin causes temporary immune suppression which can make the infection worse).

- Patients with a history of allergy to other drugs.

- Patients with KS. (Two persons with KS may have had their lesions worsen.)

## Potential Benefits

With these dangers and side effects, trichosanthin might be discarded if it were only another drug like AZT or ddI. But unlike other treatments, trichosanthin kills HIV-infected cells, so it might be able to reduce the total amount of infection, rather than just slowing its spread. What do we know from the Project Inform study about potential benefits?

- P24 antigen level—a measure of HIV viral activity—was greatly reduced, although later it started to rise again. This test could not be given in New York, because a state law there prevented physicians from using it. But in San Francisco, of 15 patients who were p24 positive and evaluable, 9 still had a sustained drop two or three months after administration of trichosanthin. No other antiviral had been used in this period. The mean p24 level dropped 66 percent after the treatment, a drop sustained for at least two months.

Those who had high p24 levels (over 100 by the Coulter assay) were most likely to improve. Most of these patients had been on AZT for one to two years when their baseline (pre trichosanthin) p24 levels were measured. Then they had been off AZT during the two to three months before their last p24 measurement.

- T-helper cells improved. In San Francisco, where five of the patients were healthy and 14 very ill, T-helper cells showed a 12 percent gain. In New York, where the patients where healthier over all (mean T-helper count was 129), there was a 42 percent gain. Patients with under 100 T-helper cells did almost as well (22 percent increase) as those with over 100 (27 percent).

Separate averages were computed for various subsets of patients. Those who took lower doses (less than 20 micrograms per kilogram) had a 52 percent T-helper gain, while those with high doses had a 14 percent gain. The lower dose may have been more beneficial.

A more detailed breakdown shows that those with high T-helper cells seemed to do best with a low dose, but those with low counts to start did best with a higher dose. Those who started with high T-cells and used a high dose had only a seven percent gain. But those with high T-cells who used a low dose had a 188 percent gain. Those with low T-helper counts did better on the high dose, however, with a 201 percent gain; those with low T-helper counts who used the low dose had only a 19 percent drop.

One week after the last infusion, T-helper counts were often down by five to 15 percent, possibly because some of the T-cells were infected and killed by the drug. This drop was temporary.

•   The sedimentation rate (a measure of overall inflammation or infection) improved 47 percent in the San Francisco group, 15 percent in New York (where the patients were not as seriously ill).

•   There was no important change in liver enzymes or other blood chemistry. Total white counts went up after treatment, but in two months they were back to near baseline levels.

•   Patients who were AZT resistant appear to be benefitting from AZT again. They had stopped AZT during the trichosanthin treatment, but have now started it again. Typically, p24 values had remained high despite use of AZT. After treatment with trichosanthin, the p24 declined sharply, then started to move back up. At this time AZT was effective in lowering p24 levels, when it had not been effective before.

•   In the San Francisco group, six of 19 patients had weight gains over five pounds. Twelve of the 19 reported substantial improvement in energy, or improved in their Karnofsky performance rating. In one patient with documented dementia, there was mental clearing; one is now able to work after being unable to do so for over two years (and spending 16 to 18 hours a day in bed). One tested negative for cryptococcus for the first time in two years; besides trichosanthin, his only other treatment was garlic.

The physicians involved in the study have come to feel that they need this tool (trichosanthin), in certain circumstances. But because of its serious dangers, the drug must be used carefully. Physicians still need to learn much more about the best ways to administer this treatment.

A more detailed report of the results of this trichosanthin treatment protocol is being prepared for publication in a medical journal.


## Florida Study Report

As mentioned above, this treatment program involved physicians and patients in four locations. One of them, Miami/Ft. Lauderdale, started earlier and used a somewhat different protocol, so its efficacy results were not included in the Project Inform report above. Instead, results have been published in a 27-page document, *Trichosanthin Treatment of HIV Induced Immune Disregulation* (final report, September 20, 1989) by Robert A. Mayer, M.D., Paul A. Sergios, and Kathy Coonan.

This report, describing the treatment of 20 patients, is hard to summarize. It does reinforce the suggestion of the Project Inform report that trichosanthin might be a valuable drug, but that it also can cause serious side effects which need proper medical management.

# HYPERICIN NOTE

On June 2, *AIDS Treatment News* published a survey asking our readers to let us know about their experiences with herbal extracts containing hypericin, an antiretroviral which has proven effective in animal tests, but not yet been tested in humans. It has taken longer than expected to analyze this survey and prepare a complete article for publication. This note will outline what we have learned so far; we will publish a full report later.

A total of 101 people responded to the survey by the time of our deadline. (Those who replied after the deadline will also be counted, but they will be analyzed separately.) Of the 101, 24 reported side effects and 77 did not. 57 reported benefits, 35 did not, and 9 were asymptomatic and did not have blood work available, so they had no way to tell whether or not they had any benefit.

Almost all of the side effects were minor, such as loose bowel movements, minor drowsiness or fatigue, or increased appetite (unwanted). Only one person reported rising liver enzymes; most of the respondents apparently had not been tested. Several people reported increased sun sensitivity, usually minor.

The benefits believed to be due to hypericin were more dramatic. Of the 57 who reported benefits, 20 named increased energy; 14 others listed improved well being, feeling better, etc. Nine had T-helper cell increases, and three had p24 antigen go negative. (Few respondents had been p24 positive, and few had test results before and after using hypericin). Several listed clearing or improvement in chronic opportunistic infections.

It is hard or impossible to get definitive information from such a survey, because of unknown biases due to self-selection of those who responded, lack of uniform clinical evaluation or laboratory testing, and the lack of objective evidence of whether a benefit or side effect was due to the treatment. Nevertheless this survey does suggest that hypericin herbal extracts may be helping at least half of the people who are using them, and that no serious problems have appeared so far.

# PML TREATMENT UPDATE

*by Denny Smith*

Two Los Angeles activists, Peter L. Brosnan and Lisa A. Muller, have compiled an exhaustive report on the treatment of progressive multifocal leukoencephalopathy (PML). *AIDS Treatment News* mentioned this report in issue #79, and since then Lisa and Peter have added new information to the list of possible treatments for PML. The report includes all referenced articles from medical journals, making it useful for AIDS clinics and physicians as well as individuals.

PML is caused by the JC papovavirus, which infects much of the population but is ordinarily controlled by an intact immune system. An inflammation of JC results in progressive neurological impairment which might resemble that of some other HIV-related infections: toxoplasmosis, herpes encephalitis, or cryptococcal meningitis. Any of these can be life-threatening, so someone who is experiencing neurological symptoms like unusual vision problems, arm or hand uncoordination, difficulties with balance when walking or standing, confused speech, or disorientation should be seen by an AIDS-knowledgeable physician immediately.

A diagnosis of PML is very serious, and a completely effective therapy has not yet been found. Several experimental approaches are now obtaining some success, so no one facing PML should be denied an informed attempt at treatment, as has often happened in the past. The address listed in *AIDS Treatment News* #79 for ordering the report has changed. Interested people should now write to: Lisa A. Muller, 3031 Angus St., Los Angeles, CA 90039. For urgent requests, call 213/666-0751. Indicate if only the recently added information is desired. For both the update and original report, a donation of $10 (or $15 for overnight delivery) is appreciated to help pay for copying and mailing.

## BUYERS' CLUB IMPORTS LOW-COST AEROSOL PENTAMIDINE

On September 22 the PWA Health Group in New York announced that it will help people import pentamidine from England, where it costs about a fifth as much as in the United States.

In the U.S., a 300 mg vial of the drug, enough for one month's treatment of aerosol pentamidine, costs $99. wholesale. In England, the same drug sells for $26. retail. There are also great variations in the prices which U.S. physicians and hospitals charge to administer the drug.

Pneumocystis is still the leading cause of death from AIDS, despite an effective (and now approved) treatment to prevent it. A major reason for these preventable deaths is that many people cannot obtain preventive treatment because of inability to pay. Much less expensive treatments, such as bactrim or dapsone, are available, but many patients cannot tolerate them.

The PWA Health Group pentamidine project is endorsed by ACT UP/New York, Body Positive, Community Health Project (CHP), the Community Research Initiative (CRI), Gay Men's Health Crisis (GMHC), Lambda Legal Defense and Education Fund, New York Physicians for Human Rights, People With AIDS Coalition, and Project Inform.

# Issue Number 89
# October 20, 1989

## MOBILIZING FOR EARTHQUAKE RELIEF: THE CONTRAST WITH AIDS

*by John S. James*

The October 17 earthquake killed 10 people in the city of San Francisco; the AIDS epidemic has killed over 400 times as many here. Yet in two days, national institutions mobilized as they have never done in eight years of AIDS. For example:

- No one imagines that when an earthquake or hurricane strikes one part of the United States, other parts would turn their backs and say it isn't their problem. Yet with AIDS, impacted cities like San Francisco and New York are left to cope on their own, largely without Federal help.

- When a mile-long section of Interstate 880 collapsed in Oakland during the earthquake, killing dozens of people, no one dreamed of delaying rescue efforts until someone could make money off them. Yet when a life-threatening virus has infected *hundreds of thousands* or more in the U.S., and millions in the world, practically nothing moves in AIDS research until corporations smell profits, or academics get grants. Not five years ago, not last year, not today.

We do not object to people being paid for their work, or making reasonable profits. We do object to the nearly universal practice of delaying critical research a year, two years, or more, for the sake of financial arrangements—and to the lack of leadership which allows this practice to continue.

For over three years, *AIDS Treatment News* has pointed to obvious, inexpensive, and critical steps needed to save lives. Usually we knew that nothing would be done. Therefore we have had to focus on what people could do for themselves, with or without institutional support.

The city official who called the earthquake the worst disaster to strike San Francisco since 1906—overlooking the epidemic which has killed 400 times as many—inadvertently illuminated the crucial but overlooked fact that AIDS has not been treated as a disaster. Outside of the immediately affected communities, there isn't even a pale shadow of the mobilization that the far less deadly earthquake has called forth.

How can we address the fundamental lack of national will to save lives? Clarifying and explaining what should be done can help. Protest and political action can help. But ultimately the AIDS community cannot create mobilization which is not there, so we will have to wait for people to become ready. We can only continue to do our work as best we can, for as long as necessary.

# SAN FRANCISCO, SAN DIEGO: ORAL GANCICLOVIR STUDY

An oral form of the anti-CMV drug ganciclovir (DHPG) will be tested in patien.. in a phase I clinical trial. The trial will take place in San Francisco and San Diego, and is now recruiting volunteers. Until now, ganciclovir has only been given intravenously— a serious drawback since use of the drug must be continued indefinitely.

One arm of the study will recruit 12 people with stable CMV retinitis, to see if they remain stable when switched from IV to oral ganciclovir. However, this part of the study may be filled by patients already at the institutions running the trial.

The other arm needs 36 volunteers who are HIV positive, are not now taking AZT, and do not have any symptoms of CMV infection. They will be tested for CMV in the urine, which they must have in order to enter the trial. Then they will be given one of three different doses of oral ganciclovir for 28 days, to see if the drug can eliminate or reduce the virus in the urine. (The 12 patients with stable retinitis will only be given the highest dose, to minimize the danger that the retinitis might progress. For those who have no sign of infection except CMV in the urine, however, it is safe to test lower doses.)

Volunteers may have used AZT before, but not during the last 28 days; they should *not* go off AZT in order to enter this study. The reason for excluding AZT is that it usually cannot be combined with ganciclovir, because both can cause bone-marrow toxicity. Volunteers must not now have active PCP, cryptococcal meningitis, severe diarrhea, or certain other conditions. They must have over 1000 neutrophils and over 50,000 platelets, and must be between 18 and 60 years old. There may also be other conditions.

The study will last 28 days. Volunteers will spend the first two days in the hospital for tests, then come in for daily visits for one week. There will be one whole day of hospitalization after 2 weeks, and 24 hours at the end of the trial. There is no cost to participate in this study.

## Historical Note

Oral ganciclovir has existed for years, but has not been developed, apparently because of the confusion over the official status of the intravenous form of the drug (see "CMV

Retinitis—Ganciclovir, Foscarnet, and Other Treatments: Background, History, and Emerging Controversy," *AIDS Treatment News* #71). Intravenous ganciclovir was officially approved for marketing as a treatment for CMV retinitis on June 26. Before then, it had been given free to thousands of patients under compassionate use.

A study published over two years ago showed that the drug could be given orally and produce a high enough blood level to inhibit CMV (Jacobson, M.A. and others, "Human Pharmacokinetics and Tolerance of Oral Ganciclovir," *Antimicrobial Agents and Chemotherapy*, August 1987, pages 1251-1254). However, only about three percent of the drug is absorbed, and it is not clear that oral use will be feasible; that is the question the current study seeks to answer.

At least two other oral drugs to treat CMV—FIAC, and HPMPC—are being developed. (For background on HPMPC, see *AIDS Treatment News* #76).

Oral ganciclovir could have been developed any time during at least the last two years, and probably much longer. Approval of the intravenous drug, plus the development of potential competitors, provided a motive for it to be developed now. As in almost all such cases, no one represented the patients' interest in the matter, as both AIDS organizations and practicing physicians chose not to involve themselves in treatment research and development issues.

# DEXTRAN SULFATE NOT ABSORBED, STUDY FINDS

A small trial at Johns Hopkins University found that less than one percent of dextran sulfate taken orally by healthy volunteers was absorbed into the bloodstream— suggesting that taking the drug orally is unlikely to be useful. This information, published October 1 in the *Annals of Internal Medicine*, is not new, but was announced in February by Frank Young, M.D., Commissioner of the Food and Drug Administration. It took until now to be formally published.

The research team used three different tests to measure the level of dextran sulfate in the blood. Only one of the methods detected any of the substance after oral use, and the amount was small. By contrast, all three methods showed large amounts of dextran sulfate after intravenous administration.

After the early announcement by the FDA that oral dextran sulfate was probably not absorbed, sales fell greatly. One buyers' club reported a drop in total sales of 80 percent. Some people have continued to use dextran sulfate, however, and some of them are convinced that it is helping.

## Comment

To us, the history of dextran sulfate shows that the AIDS community can respond appropriately and very rapidly to new information when it is made available in a useful way—in this case, by an authoritative announcement from the FDA. Persons who were interested in the drug learned immediately that serious doubt had been raised about its value.

But some people have chosen to continue using dextran sulfate, even though they know about the absorption results, because they believe that the drug is helping them.

This action seems sensible, too. Much is still unknown; for example, it is conceivable that the drug might help some people even if it does not get into the bloodstream, by coming into direct contact with HIV infection in the gastrointestinal tract. Theories are only guides, which may be more or less helpful; ultimately what is important is what works.

Unfortunately a very different conclusion was drawn by one of the researchers who did the absorption study. Paul S. Lietman, M.D., Ph.D., criticized the FDA for allowing patients to obtain unapproved drugs for persons use—both in an Associated Press story October 2, and in a Johns Hopkins University press release issued a few days later. He called such access "a step backward," saying that "it is wrong to provide drugs of unproven value to patients with devastating diseases."

The AIDS community first learned about dextran sulfate over two years ago, when laboratory results suggested that it was one of the best anti-HIV substances yet found. Patients knew that millions of people had used it orally in Japan, where it had been found safe enough to have been sold for 20 years without a prescription. There were doubts about absorption, but it seemed unlikely that millions of Japanese had fooled themselves for 20 years and taken a useless drug. Patients also knew that if the drug did work, it would probably take years to be approved in the United States (in fact it did take two years just for a test for absorption, and for an intravenous trial to start). And with the drug's extensive safety record, the AIDS treatment community knew that the consequences of using it and being wrong would probably be small—whereas not using it and being wrong could easily have cost tens of thousands of lives.

Based on what was known at the time, the decision to obtain dextran sulfate from Japan and use it seems clearly to be the rational one. Conversely, the decision to wait for approval might have been suicidal.

We now know that dextran sulfate when taken by mouth is not promising. But decisions must be made on what was known at the time, not what is known two years later. By this standard, we think that the AIDS community has handled dextran sulfate well—and that calling for police power to prevent people from making rational and compelling decisions about their health care is not helpful.

# AMFAR WILL FUND AIDS PROJECTS IN DEVELOPING COUNTRIES; DEADLINE NOVEMBER 30

The American Foundation for AIDS Research (AmFAR) announced a new program to fund AIDS projects carried out in the developing world by non-governmental organizations. Areas of interest include educational projects for professional or lay audiences carried out by local service providers, and small-scale projects to facilitate communications and information exchanges on AIDS.

The deadline for letters of interest (not longer than two pages) is November 30, 1989. Letters may be sent by fax to (U.S.) 212/719-0712.

For a copy of the September 26 announcement of this program, or for other information, contact Mervyn F. Silverman, M.D., M.P.H., Chairman, International Committee, at the above fax number. Or phone AmFAR at 212/719-0033.

# HEMOPHILIA GROUPS MAY BOYCOTT OR MOVE U.S. CONFERENCE

On September 15, the UK Hemophilia Society wrote all member organizations of the World Federation of Hemophilia that it could not participate in the biannual hemophilia conference planned for August 1990 in Washington, DC, because of the exclusion of persons who are HIV positive from entry to the United States. Most persons with hemophilia are HIV positive, because they were infected by blood products years in the past before blood was screened for HIV.

In May of 1989 the U.S. Immigration and Naturalization Service (INS) instituted a 30-day waiver to allow HIV-positive persons to visit the United States for purposes including attending conferences, obtaining medical treatment, and visiting family members (not for tourism). The UK Hemophilia Society is concerned that to obtain this waiver, persons must declare their HIV status and can then be singled out for discrimination. And "people with hemophilia are immediately identifiable as potential targets" because they are carrying supplies of blood products. The letter urged that the conference be moved out of the U.S. unless the law was changed.

It is generally believed that there is no chance that Congress will repeal the provision in the foreseeable future.

For HIV-positive persons visiting the United States, the National Gay Rights Advocates in San Francisco has published a 62-page guide on how to obtain the waiver. The INS wants applications 30 to 60 days in advance, but may accept an application after an attempt to enter the United States if the applicant can establish that he or she did not know about the need to apply. There is no routine testing at the border, but the INS can require testing for entry if it has reason to suspect that a person is HIV positive—for example, if AZT or medical records suggesting HIV are found in a search of the luggage.

Obtaining the waiver is burdensome. Applicants must show that they are not a danger to public health and can pay for any medical care they may need in the United States, so that there will be no cost to any government here. Extensive documentation is suggested for supporting the application, and anything not in English must be translated and properly certified by the translator. The National Gay Rights Advocates urges anyone to obtain legal advice before submitting an application, because applying can affect all future entry into the United States, whether the waiver is granted or not.

## History

The law excluding persons with HIV was passed in 1987. It was introduced by Senator Jesse Helms (Republican, North Carolina) as an amendment to the bill to pay temporarily for AZT for persons with AIDS who had no other way to afford it. The exclusion law was passed almost unanimously by Congress, in part as a political trade to obtain the funds for AZT.

In April 1989, Dutch AIDS educator Hans Verhoef was jailed for several days in St. Paul, Minnesota when he tried to enter the United States to attend a medical conference in San Francisco. The local INS granted a waiver, but the Washington, DC, office overruled the local and denied it. An immigration judge then overruled the national office and granted the waiver, and Mr. Verhoef arrived at the conference as it was ending.

Before the Verhoef case, the law had not attracted attention in the United States. But in a bizarre incident several months earlier, at least one Canadian had been turned back when trying to enter the United States to obtain medical treatment. This case was front-page, mainstream television news in Canada, but completely blacked out in the United States; as far we can determine, no U.S. news organization reported the story, despite the fact that it very much concerned this country.

The Verhoef case led to widespread concern that the international AIDS conference scheduled for June 1990 in San Francisco would be disrupted by detention of persons trying to attend. Conference organizers pressured Washington for some way to keep that from happening. The result was a May 25, 1989 INS memo intended to codify a waiver policy. This is where the matter has stayed since.

Very few people have yet applied for the waiver, so there is little precedent to indicate what documentation the INS will and will not accept as sufficient, or how much the decision will depend on individual officials.

## Comment

Foreigners are justifiably outraged by the U.S. exclusion policy because the U.S. is a net exporter of HIV—and also is violating World Health Organization principles which the United States itself agreed to.

Perhaps the greatest harm from the exclusion of HIV-positive visitors is that it creates an incentive all over the world for people not to step forward for testing within their own countries if they suspect that they might be HIV-positive. Because of the potential economic, personal, and medical importance of being able to enter the United States, and the difficulty and uncertainty of the waiver process, many people will find a clear advantage in not knowing their status and ignoring the issue as long as possible. Therefore many people will not know to obtain early treatment if they need it, and not interact with public-health authorities on how to avoid further transmission.

The June 1988 report of the Presidential Commission on the Human Immunodefi-ciency Virus Epidemic—the famous "Watkins Commission" report, probably the most authoritative recommendation on U.S. AIDS ever written—made nondiscrimi-nation protection a cornerstone of efforts to control the epidemic, so that citizens would come forward and cooperate with public health programs. But now the United States itself is threatening citizens of all other countries with potentially serious consequences for doing just that. Its discriminatory policy creates a hidden disruption in the public health program of every country on Earth whose citizens are free to visit the United States.

## DDC: THE LOW-COST ANTIVIRAL

ddC is an antiviral closely related to ddI, which is widely considered to be one of the most promising new AIDS treatment. ddC may be as effective as ddI, and is currently undergoing large-scale clinical trials sponsored by Hoffmann-La Roche (see two articles in *AIDS Treatment News* #81). And ddC costs hundreds of times less than ddI to manufacture, meaning that its potential cost, pennies a day, is within reach of every person in the United States, and of every government in the world.

About two years ago, ddC was found to cause serious peripheral neuropathy in some patients, and therefore many people gave up on the drug. But now it appears that ddC may be effective in doses much lower than were previously used, and that at these low doses, the toxicity may be rare, and easily manageable when it does occur. We may not have an ultimate answer until the current large-scale trials are completed; these trials are expected to take two years (see "Why No Antivirals: A Case History of Failed Trial Design," in *AIDS Treatment News* #81, cited above). But at least 300 people have so far taken ddC in clinical studies—and others have used "underground" ddC—and there appears to be enough information available now to make practical decisions. Since most of the world's people with HIV have no access to treatment because of economic obstacles, a drug which eliminates these obstacles deserves careful attention.

The true cost of a drug must include not only the cost of manufacture, but also any other costs of appropriate use, including detection and management of side effects. For example, the cost of using AZT must include the cost of blood tests for hematological toxicity, of transfusions when needed, and of the Western medical infrastructure which makes this technology available. But with ddC, the management of toxicity consists largely in not exceeding the proper dose, and stopping the drug immediately if neuropathy does develop (treatment may be resumed later at lower doses). The management of toxicity, therefore, has little or no economic cost. And this drug does not require the expensive infrastructure of Western medicine; instead, it might be delivered through the traditional healers which are already in place in most cultures.

In the United States, the government has claimed exclusive worldwide rights to ddC as an AIDS treatment, and licensed these rights to Hoffmann-La Roche. We checked with a patent attorney, and learned that patent rights are in fact highly geographical, and that it would probably be entirely legal to manufacture ddC for medical use in many countries. In addition, ddC can only be covered by a "use patent" (the weakest of all patents), since the chemical has been commercially available and has been known for over 20 years. A use patent for a drug is violated only at the time of ingestion.

In the United States, ddC was available as an "underground" drug over a year ago, but few people used it because of fear of its toxicity. The most serious side effect is peripheral neuropathy, often noticed first as pain in the feet. However, the new clinical trial is using a very low dose, .01 milligram per kilogram of body weight three times a day. This dose is less than a quarter of what the U.S. "underground" has been using even recently, which itself is much less than the doses which caused serious side effects in the first clinical trials, before it was known how little of the chemical was effective. This .01 dose—which has enough preliminary evidence for efficacy that a major corporation is willing to test it in hundreds of people—is so low that for persons of average weight, a single gram of ddC will last for well over a year.

In the U.S., both ddC and ddI have sold for about the same price, about $30,000 per kilogram. For ddI, this price translates to hundreds of dollars a month. But ddC is used in such small doses that it will usually cost under 10 cents a day. (Note: the ddC which has been on peoples' shelves for the last year or more may have deteriorated, and must be tested before use.)

The official trials of ddC will probably take at least two years to complete. Meanwhile, the AIDS community may want to develop ddC as a treatment for those who have no other option. The whole continent of Africa has been written off, ignored in drug-development decisions because it cannot pay what U.S. companies want to charge for their drugs. Within the U.S., minority groups are also likely to be written off—and many people from all social classes who cannot use AZT will fall through the cracks of the ddI trials and parallel-access system.

ddC *might* be as good a treatment as any that exists today; and it is readily available and there are no economic barriers to its use. But it is also dangerous, and successful ways of using it will not happen automatically; they must be systematically developed. In different countries, for example, the drug would need to be integrated differently into existing health systems.

We published this article to point out these possibilities. We call on development experts, AIDS organizations, and others to examine new systems for providing state-of-the-art treatment now, without waiting for bureaucracies to move, for corporations to find profit, or for the time required for national health care to be established, or for a Western medical infrastructure to be created where it does not now exist.

# Issue Number 90
# November 3, 1989

## U.S. VIDEOTAPE EXPLAINS COOKING, FOOD PREPARATION FOR PERSONS WITH AIDS

Persons with immune deficiencies are in serious danger of food-borne diseases. Proper selection, cooking, and handling of food can greatly reduce the risk. Now two Federal agencies—the Food and Drug Administration, and the Centers for Disease Control—have produced the first videotape to alert people to this danger, and explain how they can protect themselves.

The 15-minute videotape includes information on foods to avoid, proper cooking, avoiding contamination in the kitchen, eating in restaurants, and travel abroad.

Individuals and organizations can obtain the tape without charge from the CDC's National AIDS Information Clearinghouse (NAIC). To order a copy, call NAIC at 800/458-5231; or send a written request to NAIC, P.O. Box 6003, Rockville, MD 20850.

## HYPERICIN STUDY NEEDS HELP TO FINISH

*by John S. James*

The hypericin monitoring study by San Francisco's Community Research Alliance has enrolled 33 patients, and is collecting some of the best data anywhere on anti-HIV use of hypericin, which may be one of the most promising antivirals. (For background see *AIDS Treatment News* #63, #74, and later issues.) Now we need the community's help to finish the study, and to start other rapid, low-cost trials of promising treatments.

The Community Research Alliance (of which this writer is a co-founder) is not the only group researching hypericin, but it was able to begin its study early. The leading academic team studying the drug is now planning animal toxicity tests required for

FDA approval before its human trials can begin. But the Community Research Alliance could start its study last June, because people with HIV were already trying hypericin, found in herbal extracts which have been in human use for years for other medicinal purposes. Because the organization does not give anybody a drug, but is only doing blood work and other data collection on patients who obtain their own treatment from buyers' clubs or health-food stores, the study could proceed immediately. Data is being collected as in university clinical trials, under a protocol designed in advance and approved by the organization's scientific advisory committee and institutional review board. It took only two weeks to recruit enough study volunteers, partly because the Community Research Alliance was created by the PWA Coalition and other grassroots AIDS organizations in San Francisco, and partly because this study does not ask patients to give up any other treatment or otherwise change what they would be doing anyway.

The Community Research Alliance helped pioneer this kind of prospective monitoring study. While this study will not obtain the more definitive data of a randomized controlled trial, it has the advantage of taking weeks instead of years to get into operation. And because all patients have blood work and other tests under a protocol designed in advance to answer important questions—and all are tested at the same intervals and by the same lab, to obtain comparable results—this trial can produce far better information about an available treatment (in this case, hypericin-containing herbal extracts) than anecdotal reports, or any data collected from patients who were not following a uniform protocol. In short, this low-cost, rapid, and flexible kind of trial, which does not ask patients to make any sacrifices in their treatment, can produce the best data available for years—and if it shows promising trends, it could stimulate interest in more formal trials, so that they would be organized sooner than if the observational study had not been done.

In New York, the Community Research Initiative plans a similar study of hypericin. It will be larger and better funded, but it has not started yet. The importance of the San Francisco study is that it started in June and its data collection will be finished next month.

## What We Need Now

The hypericin study needs your help. The Community Research Alliance needs $10,000 to finish it—for laboratory costs, data entry and analysis, and to pay the principal investigator and a staff assistant. Few foundations have ever funded any AIDS project—and of those who have, almost none will touch research. (The one major exception, the American Foundation for AIDS Research—AmFAR—has already given $30,000 to the Community Research Alliance.)

In the future, the Community Research Alliance hopes to conduct similar studies of treatment possibilities which may be important, but will not otherwise be researched promptly. For example, when a potentially important antiviral might be obtained from an edible plant (such as the sulfolipids in blue-green algae—see *AIDS Treatment News* #87) academic and commercial researchers spend the time to prepare the pure chemical, with associated laboratory and animal tests, before any human trial can start. Only pure chemicals, not plant products, have academic and commercial value in the United States. But in appropriate cases, a prospective monitoring trial of a natural product could begin very quickly, avoiding years of delay. The Community Research Alliance has already done one such study, and is well positioned to do others.

The government will not pay for this kind of research, foundations will not pay for it, the pharmaceutical industry will not. Unless the community supports this work, it will not happen. In the future, we hope to find one or more sponsors for each study— a community-minded individual or business who could contribute the relatively small amount, usually under $20,000, required for this kind of trial. People are more willing to contribute when they know exactly what their money will pay for, what they will make possible that would not happen otherwise.

The Community Research Alliance has shown that it can organize studies very quickly. But at least for now it gets little support from established research institutions, which have their own ways of doing business, ways which cannot respond quickly to the AIDS emergency. The work of this organization, and of other community-based AIDS research, depends on you.

## AZT NOW AVAILABLE FREE FOR CHILDREN

Until recently, it has been very difficult for physicians to give AZT to children, for two reasons. First, the drug was not approved for children, as the early dosage, safety, and efficacy trials only recruited adults. Physicians could legally prescribe AZT for children, but without official guidance, most were reluctant to do so, and if they did, insurers were unlikely to pay. Also, the drug only came in capsules designed for adults; these had to be opened and their contents divided to obtain the right dose for a child.

On October 4, Burroughs Wellcome announced that AZT would be available in syrup form in a few weeks—allowing dose adjustment for children, and also making the drug more accessible to adults who cannot swallow capsules.

On October 26, the Department of Health and Human Services announced that the FDA had approved a "treatment IND" application from Burroughs Wellcome, allowing the company to distribute the drug free for children who meet certain medical requirements. AZT had already been given to at least 200 children in clinical trials; it seemed to be no more or less toxic to them than to adults, and it seemed clearly beneficial in some cases, especially in treating dementia. For more information about the treatment IND, physicians can call Burroughs Wellcome at 800/829-PEDS.

While the drug is free, we do not know how associated costs will be paid— especially the cost of blood tests to detect toxicity, and of any treatment required for side effects. Many children with AIDS come from poverty backgrounds and are unlikely to have insurance. State Medicaid programs ought to cover these costs, but we do not know if they will do so.

## INFORMATION ON HIV IN PREGNANCY AND PEDIATRICS

The standards of medicine applied to children, infants and pregnant women are often different and more complex than those for other populations. Some treatments which are ordinarily safe can be dangerous during pregnancy, and drugs approved by the Food and Drug Administration are assigned a rating according to the Pregnancy Risk Category. Drug doses for newborns and pediatric patients are not arrived at by simply lowering the recommended adult dosage, because the mechanisms through which children's bodies absorb, metabolize and excrete drugs are qualitatively different. Consequently, when questions of treatment for HIV and AIDS have been addressed for non-pregnant adults, they have remained largely unanswered for children and women in pregnancy.

The October issue of *Focus*, published by the AIDS Health Project in San Francisco, contained two good overviews of these questions: "Pregnancy and HIV," by Laurie B. Hauer, R.N. who is the Coordinator of the Bay Area Perinatal AIDS Center at San Francisco General Hospital, and "Caring for Children with HIV Infection," by Ellen R. Cooper, M.D., Medical Director of the Pediatric AIDS Program at Boston City Hospital. To obtain a copy of this issue, (volume 4, number 11, October 1989), write to *Focus* , UCSF AIDS Health Project, Box 0884, San Francisco, CA 94143. Single issues are $3.

The Children's Hospital AIDS Program (CHAP) of Children's Hospital of New Jersey published a useful guide for families with HIV+ children called *The Child with AIDS*. The guide discusses blood tests, opportunistic infections, medications, nutrition, and emotional dilemmas for parents, siblings and legal guardians. CHAP also houses the National Pediatric HIV Resource Center. The Center provides telephone consultations to health professionals regarding drug trials, home care, school issues and child welfare agencies. Both CHAP and the Pediatric HIV Resource Center can be reached at 201/268-8251.

We will report on more resources for parents and children with HIV in an upcoming issue.

# GERMANIUM DANGER: BRITISH GOVERNMENT WARNS PHYSICIANS

In an unusual letter dated October 10, the British government warned all doctors in England of health risks from use of germanium compounds, which have been widely sold in health-food stores. The warning followed an article on germanium toxicity by well-known investigative reporter Duncan Campbell, published September 8 in *New Statesman & Society*, London. The official letter to physicians begins as follows:

"The purpose of this letter is to alert you to a potential health hazard caused by germanium, found in certain dietary supplements which can cause nephropathy, leading in some cases to renal failure and death. Other complications include cardiomyopathy and peripheral myopathy. (The letter references T. Matsusaka and others, "Germanium-induced nephropathy: report of two cases and review of the literature," *Clinical Nephrology* (West Germany), December 1988, volume 30 number 6, pages 341-345.) In a review of 10 cases, pathological changes occurred following ingestion of germanium, 50 to 200 mg per day, for periods of four to 18 months. Death occurred in two cases."

The letter went on to express concern that persons with AIDS and chronic fatigue were especially likely to use germanium. It said that the Department of Health had no evidence that the substance had any nutritional value or health benefit, and urged physicians to have their patients stop using it.

Except for occasional mentions in lists of treatments, we have not previously covered germanium in *AIDS Treatment News*.

## Another View

We spoke with Parris Kidd, Ph.D., founder of the Germanium Institute of North America (which he has since closed). Dr. Kidd told us that there are no published cases of toxicity from the germanium compound which is supposed to be in the capsules, namely germanium sesquioxide, also called Ge-132. He believes that the toxicity is due either to another compound, germanium dioxide, or to an unknown contaminant. (This information is consistent with what we have seen in the published literature; however, we know of no proof that even the pure product would be safe.)

Dr. Kidd explained that it is difficult and expensive to test for potentially dangerous contaminants—and that because of lack of uniform testing, no one can be confident of the safety of germanium compounds.

He also told us that while there were no controlled human trials, he has heard many anecdotal reports suggesting that germanium sesquioxide might be helpful in treating various conditions, including chronic viral infections. He also told us that germanium is not known to be a nutrient, as no deficiency condition has been established.

There has been a little research published in medical journals on possible medical uses of germanium sesquioxide; we have not seen any related to AIDS. (A different compound, spirogermanium, has been widely tested as a potential cancer treatment.)

Our conclusion, based on the evidence we have seen so far, is that germanium compounds available today may be dangerous, and that no benefit has been proven.

# PROPOSAL: AN OMBUDS OFFICE FOR PROMISING TREATMENTS AND PUBLIC POLICIES

*by John S. James*

Note: We submitted this suggestion to the Mayor's HIV Task Force, San Francisco, which requested our comments on clinical trials and the parallel track. One of the other invited speakers challenged our characterization of ddI as a relative success in drug development. He pointed out that the anti-HIV activity of ddI was discovered at almost the same time as that of AZT, and that if ddI had been developed promptly the clinical trials could have been finished, and ddI approved two years ago. (We should note that Bristol-Myers Squibb and others now working with ddI were not involved at that time.)

We left the statement below as we submitted it, but the point is a good one.

## The Problem

The mainstream, national response to the earthquake shows what can and should be done in responding to a disaster. But AIDS has killed hundreds of times as many people, both in San Francisco and nationally, without calling forth even a shadow of the response to the earthquake. The Federal failure to support San Francisco's model AIDS programs illustrates the lack of national mobilization, the fact that the United States has backed into the epidemic and still does not have a coherent, rational AIDS program.

How can San Francisco increase its impact on national policy?

## Lost Opportunities: An Example

Our three and a half years of publication has documented a catalog of lost opportunities—both particular treatments, and broader public policies—largely neglected when they clearly deserved feasible, cost-effective research or other followup.

The example of ddI shows that while Federal policies have significantly improved, they are still unable to respond effectively to the epidemic:

• ddI has been handled with unprecedented speed and unprecedented communication between AIDS advocates, industry, and the FDA—all very much for the good.

• But this rapid mobilization applies only when the public's imagination is engaged. For example, the related antiviral ddC appears to be about as good as ddI, but costs hundreds of times less to manufacture. It could be developed as a treatment available to all, anywhere in the world, regardless of ability to pay. But our initial inquiries indicate that no one anywhere is developing this treatment option—a critical lack when many people have no treatment available at all, and little prospect of treatment in the future, since only the expensive treatment possibilities are being developed.

• The current clinical trials of ddI will probably take over two years to complete—obviously not acceptable for the purposes of public health. Clinical trials are still being designed under business as usual, without mobilization of top scientific and statistical talent to re-examine the underlying assumptions of trial design in view of the current emergency.

Questions about the two-year delay are usually dismissed with the comment that those who need the drug in the meantime can get it through parallel access. But—

• The parallel-access system now developing for ddI will work only for those who have aggressive primary-care physicians, and who can afford the extensive paperwork and laboratory tests required. Insurance will probably refuse to pay for these costs, meaning that we will have parallel access only for those with money.

Yet ddI is the success story. Hundreds of promising treatment and policy options have been overlooked for lack of attention and advocacy. One systematic problem is that the interests and views of impacted jurisdictions like San Francisco, which are called on to provide medical care of last resort when other institutions have walked away, are not represented when decisions are made.

## What Can San Francisco Do?

Inadequate national response to the AIDS/HIV epidemic is creating intolerable burdens in impacted areas. The recent earthquake will make the financial strain even worse. How can San Francisco affect national policy through programs which cost little or no money?

One way would be to apply the concept of an ombuds office—which usually serves individuals—to serving **proposed policies** instead.

**November 3, 1989**

The traditional ombudsman hears problems from individuals, and helps get these problems addressed as well as possible by existing agencies or other institutions. The ombuds office may advise the individual on how to proceed, or may call officials and others to help clear up snafus; but it does not substitute for the agencies, or do their work itself. Therefore a small effort can have a great impact, by overcoming just those problems which the experienced ombuds office can easily deal with, and getting the existing system to work as well as it can. Later, statistics generated by the ombuds program can be used to guide legislation or other institutional improvements.

San Francisco could develop a highly leveraged impact on national policy by creating an ombuds function which receives **promising public policies** instead of individuals—and helps shepherd them through existing systems, as the traditional ombudsman helps individuals. The proposed ombuds office would receive complaints or suggestions from anyone, then investigate and prioritize the problems and decide which ones it might handle most effectively. It could help to resolve simple snafus through telephone calls to Federal, state, local, or other government officials, to corporate officials, to the media, etc. It could make recommendations to City departments, but would have no power except persuasion. And of course it could refer persons who brought problems, complaints, or suggestions to anyone else they should be talking to.

A key to the success of such an ombuds office is that it could address any problem that impacts on San Francisco's ability to respond to the epidemic—medical research, standards of care, insurance reimbursement (private, Federal, or state), funding for services, organizational snafus. Some problems can be resolved quickly by bringing the right people into communication. Problems which cannot be resolved easily can be articulated with cogent analysis and well-justified recommendations.

# Issue Number 91
# November 17, 1989

## HYPERICIN SURVEY REPORT

*by John S. James*

On June 2, *AIDS Treatment News* published a survey asking readers about their experience in using hypericin, an antiviral which is available in extracts of St. John's wort, a plant which has long been used as a medicinal herb. 101 people returned questionnaires by the deadline, which was extended to July 15; eleven others returned theirs later, and we decided to report on all 112 together. We published a brief overview of some of the results on October 6 (issue #88).

For the scientific background on laboratory and animal studies of hypericin as an antiretroviral, see Lavie and others, 1989, and Meruelo and others, 1988 (references below).

Note: The survey presented here should not be confused with the ongoing monitoring study by the Community Research Alliance (CRA) in San Francisco, which was described in our last issue; the two projects are entirely separate. In the CRA study, the 33 volunteers are all following a common protocol—with the same baseline tests before anyone started using hypericin, the same scheduled followup for medical examinations and blood work, and all testing done at the same laboratory. The survey reported in this article, however, could not collect systematic information; it could only obtain whatever information the respondents had available. Surveys can be done rapidly and at low cost, but their limitations must be considered.

We designed our questionnaire to be as easy as possible to use; for example, it was only one page long, including space for replies. To obtain better information, we asked people to reply in their own words, rather than using multiple-choice or similar questions often chosen for easy statistical tabulation. Statistics would be unreliable in this case, because such an uncontrolled survey could not possibly hope to "prove" that hypericin does or does not work. Instead, we asked people to let us know what possible side effects they found—and similarly, what possible benefits.

Instead of giving statistical tabulations, we decided to approach this survey as journalists, reporting the results as we might report any other news. But if we only gave a summary, readers would have no way to check our judgment. Therefore we decided to list the benefits, side effects, and other results reported in people's own words, deleting any identifying information, of course. We will give our interpretations, but readers can check our conclusions or draw their own (see the lists below, on pages 3 through 8).

The bottom line, in our view, can be seen in the lists of side effects and the benefits. 27 of the 112 respondents reported side effects, but most of them were minor; very few required stopping the hypericin. But the benefits—reported by 65 of the 112—are usually significant. Some directly affect quality of life, and others suggest improvement in underlying health. Most are benefits that persons with HIV would want to have. (And the 47 who did not report benefits do not all represent failures of the treatment, as some of them were asymptomatic and had no way to register a benefit because there was nothing to improve.)

56 of the 112 respondents reported symptoms which failed to improve while they used hypericin. This list shows that despite reports of benefits, the hypericin-containing herbal extracts are far from the whole answer.

The list of general comments gives a sense of what people felt about this treatment after using it. And the appendix gives information about preparations and doses used, how long people had been using hypericin extracts, and what other treatments they were using.

## Details

Over 5,000 copies of the survey were mailed with our June 2 issue. As stated above, 112 completed questionnaires were returned.

Replies to the open-ended questions could be any length, and a few were many pages long, but most fit into a single typed line. We abbreviated or selected from the longer ones, to fit them into a one-line format for the lists below. In these lists, the replies which were shortened are usually indicated by lines of the maximum length, as we tried to fit in as much material as possible; the short replies are usually reproduced verbatim.

We corrected spelling and did minor editing for clarity, but did not try to correct any substantive errors.

## REFERENCES

Lavie, G. and others. Studies of the mechanisms of action of the antiretroviral agents hypericin and pseudohypericin. *Proceedings of the National Academy of Sciences, USA*, volume 86, pages 5963-5967, August 1989.

Meruelo, D. and others. Therapeutic agents with dramatic antiretroviral activity and little toxicity at effective doses: Aromatic polycyclic diones hypericin and pseudohypericin. *Proceedings of the National Academy of Sciences, USA*, volume 85, pages 5230-5234, July 1988.

# WORLD AIDS DAY, DECEMBER 1

Executive directors and board presidents of dozens of AIDS organizations plan to risk arrest at a White House demonstration on World AIDS Day. Protesters—not all of whom plan civil disobedience—will gather at 11 AM, December 1, at Lafayette Park, across the street from the White House.

The purpose of the action is "to call attention to the continuing failure of the Federal government to respond to the AIDS epidemic and to call for more direct and assertive leadership by President Bush." AIDS cases in the United States are expected to double in the next two years, and the community organizations which have created a model of how to respond effectively cannot continue to do the job without support. Government attention, leadership, and resources are needed now to prevent many thousands of unnecessary deaths.

Organizations involved include AIDS Action Council, Dallas AIDS Resource Center, Gay Men's Health Crisis, Lambda Legal Defense and Education Fund, Mobilization Against AIDS, National Association of People With AIDS, National Gay and Lesbian Task Force, Project Inform, San Francisco AIDS Foundation, and ACT UP/NY.

Besides protests, World AIDS Day is marked by ceremonies, conferences, speeches, and other events in almost every country in the world. In Washington D.C., the Pan American Health Organization will sponsor talks by leading experts and government officials. The American Association for World Health, also in Washington, is coordinating events throughout the United States. Every major city is planning some kind of observance, usually focused on Youth, this year's theme for World AIDS Day.

World AIDS Day was first officially observed on December 1 of last year.

---

## Hypericin Survey Replies: Benefits Reported

The following table shows the benefits that people believed might have been due to hypericin (in St. John's wort extract). Most are in the respondents' own words; we abbreviated a few so that they would fit into one line of the table below.

The sequence number ("Seq"), on the left, can be used to connect these reports of benefits with the reports of side effects, other drugs taken, etc., in the tables below.

65 out of the 112 who completed the survey reported benefits. The actual picture is brighter than this proportion suggests, because some of the 47 remaining were asymptomatic, and not candidates for this table because they had nothing to improve. The list below also excludes those who only reported stable health; it only includes those who listed an improvement.

The 112 completed questionnaires were given sequence numbers arbitrarily, so they are in no special order. Those returned first tend to have the lowest sequence numbers. We did not read the questionnaires, or sort them in any way, until after the sequence numbers were assigned.

| Seq | Benefits |
|---|---|
| 4 | Some reduction of recurrent skin rashes. |
| 5 | 24 percent increase in T-4 count over 5 weeks 2 days. |
| 6 | Symptoms went away, feel better. |
| 8 | Initial 10 percent increase in T-4 cell. |
| 11 | More energy, feeling of well being, decrease in skin and oral problems. |
| 12 | T-helper count. |
| 15 | Slight increase in T-cells, feel better, have more energy. |
| 18 | MAI coughing and mucus virtually gone, less fatigue, more energy, lymph glands normal. |
| 21 | More energy, loosened phlegm, sense of well being, reduced toxicity of AZT. |
| 22 | Weaned myself off anti-depressants. |
| 25 | Fewer anger attacks, improved mental view, increased white and neutrophil counts, feel good. |
| 26 | T-cells stay on plateau (400-600), no excessive fatigue. |
| 27 | T-4 cells up, T-4/T-8 ratio improved; after first month back to original. |
| 31 | Brighter, return of sense of humor, less tired, desire to do more. |
| 32 | Feel good, tested antigen negative, T-4 cells doubled (24 to 56). |
| 33 | Initial burst of energy, positive view until present, no medical benefit. |
| 34 | Improved T-cell counts: 620 to 1000 to 1100. |
| 35 | Higher energy, sense of well being. |
| 39 | Skin condition improvements, lupus in upper arm is gone. |
| 44 | Feel better, blood work up, platelets increased. |
| 45 | Feel better overall. |
| 46 | More energy, sense of well being. |
| 50 | Initial increase in energy, then back to baseline. |
| 52 | T-4 went from 268 to 386. |
| 53 | Improved energy level, hairy leukoplakia and oral thrush gone overnight after 6 weeks. |
| 54 | No severe headaches since a week after I started taking. |
| 55 | Increased feeling of well being; no tests done yet to see physical benefit. |
| 57 | White blood count increased from 5.4 to 5.8, firmer stools. |
| 58 | Improved sense of well being, faster recovery from problems. |
| 59 | Drop in p24 and beta 2 microglobulin, increase in white blood count. |
| 61 | Increase in energy and mental clarity. |
| 62 | Feeling better; herpes simplex improving, but also taking large dose acyclovir. |
| 64 | T-4 from 400 to 600, red blood count 4.0 to 8.4, white blood count 4.0 to 11.0. |
| 66 | Leveling off of T-cell drop. |
| 67 | 33 percent rise in T-cell count. |
| 69 | 8-10 lb. weight gain, T-4 cells from 18 to 54. |
| 71 | Overall energy better, some weight gain. |
| 75 | Maintenance of good health, p24 went negative. |
| 77 | Dramatic increase in energy, cleared oral thrush and folliculitis. |
| 78 | More energy, higher libido. |
| 79 | Lower temperatures, 7 lb. weight gain, better attitude. |
| 80 | Stomach symptoms may have improved slightly. |
| 81 | T-4 improvement. |
| 83 | Increased energy, increased appetite. |
| 84 | Energy increase, fewer infections, p24 has gone negative. |
| 85 | Feeling better. |
| 86 | Increase in T-4. |

| | |
|---|---|
| 88 | Increased energy, less opportunistic infections. |
| 90 | T-cell increase, swollen glands decreased. |
| 91 | Increased energy, feeling well, chronic cough almost gone after 4 years, p24 to 0. |
| 93 | Headaches and sore throat gone, hairy leukoplakia is improving. |
| 94 | Slight improvement in mental outlook. |
| 95 | Improved T-cells, SGOT, SGPT, platelets. |
| 97 | More energy, less mouth sores and thrush, less skin dryness. |
| 98 | Less winded, more energy, better sense of well being. |
| 99 | More energetic, generally feel better. |
| 101 | More energy. |
| 102 | Increased energy and sense of well being. |
| 103 | More energy, decrease of hairy leukoplakia, lymph node improved. |
| 105 | Skin rash disappeared. |
| 106 | Beta-2 microglobulin went from 4.7 to 3.2. |
| 108 | Increase in T-cells, improvement in mood. |
| 109 | Some increase in energy levels initially. |
| 111 | Less swelling in lymph nodes, elimination of chronic 6-month sinus infection, more energy. |
| 112 | Increased energy, increased appetite, decreased lymphadenopathy, less night sweats. |

## Side Effects Reported

27 of the 112 questionnaires reported side effects (below). Few were serious enough to require stopping the treatment.

| Seq | Side Effects |
|---|---|
| 2 | Perhaps dizziness, fatigue; liver tests always normal. |
| 6 | Sleepiness. |
| 9 | Drowsiness. |
| 11 | Minor sunburn on short exposure. |
| 17 | Severe rash, itching, skin blotches. |
| 18 | Sluggish on 2nd day of 5cc dosage each week. |
| 21 | Occasional nausea (mild). |
| 22 | More susceptible to sunburn. |
| 23 | Fullness in head, emotionally volubility for few hours after taking hypericin. |
| 32 | Had possible skin allergy after taking capsules. |
| 36 | Farting—stops within 24 hours of taking the pill. |
| 47 | Swallowing pills makes me choke and throw up. |
| 50 | Occasionally feel pain in liver; not verified by blood work. |
| 51 | Bowel movements chalk color; maybe photosensitivity, ok with #20 sunscreen. |
| 56 | Diarrhea (corrected by using "colon conditioner" fiber supplement), lower T-4. |
| 59 | Minor drowsiness. |
| 77 | Very hyper, bitchy mood, edgy and irritable after 5 weeks of daily use. |
| 78 | Loose bowel movements in afternoon/early evening, following normal one in morning. |
| 93 | Fatigued at 40 drops twice daily, increase in liver enzymes. |
| 94 | Tinnitus, possibly antagonist of Xanax, sleeplessness. |
| 95 | Increased appetite. |
| 96 | Nausea, lack of appetite, chest cold and diarrhea; not sure if hypericin. |
| 97 | Nausea and dizziness, possibly liver related, then went away; liver normal 2 weeks later. |

| | |
|---|---|
| 101 | Some fever, oral dryness. |
| 102 | Elevated liver enzymes; hypericin discontinued. |
| 107 | Purple rash (failed to recur when hypericin resumed). |
| 111 | Mild diarrhea, altered taste sensation—metallic taste. |

## Symptoms Which Failed To Improve

56 of the 112 reported the following symptoms which failed to improve while they were using hypericin.

| Seq | Failed To Improve |
|---|---|
| 2 | Fatigue, T-4 counts, diarrhea. |
| 8 | Fatigue. |
| 10 | Fatigue, nausea. |
| 11 | Foot and other fungal problems. |
| 14 | Neuropathy in feet, fatigue. |
| 16 | Weight loss. |
| 18 | Neuropathy—foot numbness and calf pain. |
| 19 | T-cells decreased. |
| 20 | P24 still positive, declining T-cells. |
| 22 | Joint pain continues when symptoms flare. |
| 24 | Muscle aches and joint pain. |
| 25 | T-4, p24. |
| 26 | Lymphadenopathy. |
| 27 | Hairy leukoplakia. |
| 30 | Impetigo, psoriasis. |
| 33 | Thrush, neuropathy, low counts due to bone marrow TB. |
| 37 | Skin rashes. |
| 39 | Seborrhea, lymphadenopathy, fatigue. |
| 41 | Hairy leukoplakia seems even worse. |
| 42 | Skin rash around waist. |
| 43 | Diarrhea, weight loss, malaise, fever. |
| 45 | Rash. |
| 50 | Fatigue back after first week. |
| 51 | White blood count low, problems sleeping all night. |
| 54 | Peripheral neuropathy. |
| 56 | No increase in energy t-counts. |
| 57 | Neuropathy in legs. |
| 59 | No rise in T-4 or T-4/T-8 ratio, rise in killer T-8's. |
| 61 | T-cell count remained same slightly lower. |
| 66 | Acute lymphadenopathy, OHL. |
| 68 | Recurring herpes simplex and zoster. |
| 71 | KS, thrush. |
| 72 | Glands still swollen periodically. |
| 73 | Beta 2 microglobulin. |
| 74 | Antigen positive, fatigue, skin infections, diarrhea. |
| 76 | Sore throat which has been intermittent for 2 years. |
| 78 | Oral thrush. |
| 79 | Weakness after modest exertion. |
| 80 | T-cells 330 to 136, night sweats, low fever, fatigue. |
| 81 | Loose stool. |

| 84  | Skin problems, blood work. |
| 85  | KS spots. |
| 86  | Haven't gained weight. |
| 88  | T-cell count. |
| 90  | Loose bowel movements which I attribute to dextran sulfate. |
| 91  | T-4 cell. |
| 92  | Too early to tell yet. Weight loss, fever, sweats, thrush. |
| 93  | Low T-cells. |
| 95  | Seborrhea. |
| 99  | Fevers and lymphadenopathy. |
| 101 | Fatigue, some nausea. |
| 104 | T-4 count varied. |
| 105 | T-cells decreased. |
| 106 | Thrush, fevers, occasional night sweats. |
| 109 | KS, possible MAI, wasting syndrome. |
| 112 | Chronic diarrhea, skin problems when bitten by insects. |

## General Comments

All but seven of the 112 who replied included comments, which we asked for on the questionnaire. As in the other tables, we selected or abbreviated when necessary to fit each comment into one line. This table provides an overall sense of what people thought of the treatment.

| Seq | Comments |
|-----|----------|
| 1   | Probably not toxic, can't tell about efficacy, may increase dose. |
| 2   | Wish I saw better results, white cell count from 4.6 to 5.2, though. |
| 3   | Dramatic T-cell increase, very good health, can't tell what treatment is working. |
| 4   | Optimistic, appears to be safe and without side effects. |
| 5   | Optimistic, appears to be safe and without side effects. |
| 6   | (8 pages, cannot summarize). |
| 7   | Just started at low dose, too early to say much. |
| 8   | Not noticed increased sensitivity to light, liver panel normal. |
| 9   | T-helper and suppressor cells both down, ratio the same. |
| 10  | Ineffective so far. |
| 11  | Feel positive, in better health, blood tests next week. |
| 13  | No clinical test results, or side effects, so far. |
| 14  | Doubtful, though treatment may not have been long or strong enough. |
| 15  | Keeps me on more even emotional keel, feel well with good energy. |
| 16  | No difference so far; other treatments, diabetes may interfere. |
| 18  | I don't understand it, but it's working. |
| 19  | Good health all along, T-cell decline continues. |
| 20  | I think it has some value, but not sure what that is. |
| 21  | Seems beneficial. |
| 22  | Have chronic fatigue, not HIV; thought it would help joint pain, it has somewhat. |
| 23  | Jury still out though I'm hopeful. |
| 24  | Willing to give it time, hope it will be backup for AZT. |
| 25  | Improved mental outlook, white count 1.6 to 2.7, neutrophils 800 to 1404. |
| 26  | Believe works synergistically with medications to keep T-cells stable, prevent OIs. |
| 27  | Still have faith in it, feel fine, convinced four friends to try it. |
| 28  | Don't know, haven't felt different. |

29   Too soon to say.
30   Easy to take with no apparent adverse reactions, had to stop AZT earlier.
31   Look forward to higher T-cells, feeling of well being has increased.
32   Think hypericum has had a positive effect; hard to know, with other treatments.
34   Surprised at jump in T's when taking the tea, now on tablets, so far excellent.
35   Too short a time period to draw any further conclusions.
36   No opinion at this time.
37   Too early to tell, will continue, hope t-cells improve.
38   Not sure, waiting on blood tests.
39   I hope it helps.
40   Unsure of effectiveness but had no major problems since started.
41   It seems only to be like a vitamin.
42   Some promise based on anecdotal reports, not enough personal data to assess.
43   Not sure what to think, no change apparent yet.
44   Blood work has improved.
45   I'm positive about hypericin, don't know if it is reacting to the virus.
46   I like it and feel positive about using it; what do I have to lose?
47   Hope it will help p24 and T's, wish it were easier to swallow.
48   Too soon to tell, was attracted by the few reports of p24 antigen going negative.
49   No effect, I'm asymptomatic except reduced energy.
50   Taking hypericin for three weeks, feel no different.
51   Easy to take in pill form, confusion on dose, cannot get liver tests paid for.
52   I have no idea (whether it works or not).
55   Think it's great so far; just about to take tests to see if any benefit.
56   Too early to tell, have not had increase in energy level.
58   Too early to tell, subjectively seems worthwhile.
59   Potentially promising therapy which needs critical investigation.
61   Surprised by how good I felt, more energy for work, mental attitude.
62   Seems to be helping, but I increased acyclovir at the same time.
63   Honestly I cannot tell, but I am an experimenter.
64   Blood values improved, feel better, less fungal skin infections.
65   I have no opinion other than what I read.
66   Convenient and cheap, don't think Herb Pharm is efficient enough.
67   T-count increase could have been from stress relief, or Carrisyn.
68   Not sure about hypericin, but feel good about it.
69   After PCP in Oct 1986, last thing I expected was significant weight gain, T-cell increase.
70   Unsure to date.
71   Seems to be helpful but hard to separate specific effects.
72   I feel it's working, so I continue to take it with supervision of doctor.
73   After last blood test (6/21/89), increased hypericin dose from 2 to 3 tablets/day.
74   Easy, fairly inexpensive, it hasn't seemed to do much for me.
75   Believe it does work against HIV, but needs more study on dose, much potential.
76   Simple to use, low cost.
77   I'm very positive about hypericin, problem of dosage to prevent bitchy, nasty, hyper mood.
78   Impressed with increase in energy; can't be sure it's hypericin.
79   It may be helping a little, is cheap, no side effects; can't be sure, PATH helped before.
80   No clear benefit for two months—until started AZT and acyclovir.
81   Firming of stools, increase in energy; believe due to hypericin, can't be sure.
82   Health continues to be good, but may be due to diet, vitamins.

83   My experience with it was good, and I don't think it can hurt.
84   Not seen increases in blood work, it has given boost of energy, less infection.
85   Seems very worthwhile to try, I feel better than during last weeks on AZT.
86   Haven't taken it long enough to have an opinion, feel good, no side effects.
87   Too early to say.
88   Nontoxic, relatively harmless, may be contributing to my sense of well being.
89   Too early to tell, feel neither better or worse.
90   Believe definitely helped, T-helpers not so high since starting AZT 18 mo ago.
91   Think hypericin tablets very valuable, major difference in 4 weeks of 3 or 4/day.
92   Too early to tell, if nothing happens in 1 month will increase dose.
93   Think hypericin helped, headaches stopped, sore throat not recurring.
94   At present in available form not helpful, blood tests worsened.
95   T-cell counts (74 to 120) speak for themselves.
96   Nausea, lack of appetite, bad cold, diarrhea after starting hypericin.
97   Also use St John's wort oil to rinse tongue 3 times/day, useful to decrease thrush.
98   Feel much better, almost like new, more energy, stools normal.
99   Feeling better, improved lifestyle makes drug worthwhile even if markers do not improve.
100  I don't think it's doing anything.
101  Reduced HIV neuropathy, doctor recommended discontinue due to liver function tests.
102  Less tired, in better state of mind, discontinued due to liver function tests.
103  Not harmful, possibly beneficial, more energy, T-cells up.
104  Unknown, my p24 has always been negative.
105  Inexpensive, accessible, may be most useful synergistically with other therapies.
106  Doesn't seem to hurt, might even be helping.
107  Just started, no conclusions.
108  I like it.
109  So far seems moderately effective, no harm.
110  Not sure, may prevent deterioration.
111  Pleased with the results based on subjective feelings.
112  Hypericin a great help to me, best with 1/4 dose AZT (AZT alone no longer worked).

## Appendix: Dose, Length of Use, Other Treatments

This table has most of the other information of the questionnaire. It is provided mainly for readers interested in further research.

*State:* Two-letter postal codes for states are included. This field was left blank for respondents outside the U.S.

*Prep:* The next column, containing only a 'Y' or 'H', is the preparation used. We only coded 'Y' for Yerba Prima brand tablets, and 'H' for Hyperforat brand tincture, as other preparations were reported infrequently, and it is easier to examine the forms manually than to computerize the information.

*Dose:* This column was only entered for the Yerba Prima tablets. These were used by the large majority of respondents, and we did not want to risk introducing errors by converting doses between different formulations.

*Weeks:* The number of weeks using hypericin is reported.

*Other Treatments:* If AZT was included, we listed it first, followed by dosage information if given. A number of respondents named more treatments than we could put in one line; in these cases we listed the ones we considered most important for the purposes of this survey, and ended the line with a '+' to show that there were others in addition.

| Seq | State | Prep | Dose | Weeks | Other Treatments |
|---|---|---|---|---|---|
| 1 | NJ | Y | 2 | 1 | AZT 600, Bactrim, prednisone |
| 2 | NJ | Y | 3 | 11 | De Veras beverage, acyclovir |
| 3 | AK | | | 6 | AZT 300 mg, acyclovir, aloe, LEM |
| 4 | PA | Y | | 14 | dextran sulfate, supplements |
| 5 | PA | | | 20 | dextran sulfate, supplements |
| 6 | NY | H | | 10 | vitamin C, vitamin a, carrot juice w avocado, others |
| 7 | NY | Y | 2 | 1 | AZT low dose, acyclovir, naltrexone |
| 8 | TX | Y | 2 | 6 | AL 721, naltrexone |
| 9 | CA | Y | 2 | 8 | acyclovir, naltrexone, Antabuse |
| 10 | VA | | | 4 | AZT low dose, acyclovir |
| 11 | NY | | | 14 | vitamins, homeopathic remedies |
| 12 | CA | Y | 1 | 16 | |
| 13 | CA | Y | 2 | 8 | AZT 1/3 dose, acyclovir, Bactrim, naltrexone |
| 14 | CA | | | 3 | AZT low dose, acyclovir, transfusion |
| 15 | TX | Y | 2 | 15 | iscador |
| 16 | | Y | 2 | 10 | AZT 800, acyclovir, aerosolized pentamidine, Nizoral, Megace |
| 17 | CA | Y | 2 | 2 | dextran sulfate, acyclovir, Gamimune, ozone, transfer fact. |
| 18 | MA | H | | 5 | AZT, astra 10+, isatis, ganoderma, shiitake, healthy diet, + |
| 19 | CA | Y | 6 | 6 | AZT low dose, acyclovir, Antabuse, dextran sulfate |
| 20 | FL | Y | 2 | 15 | AZT, acyclovir, dextran sulfate |
| 21 | | | | 12 | AZT low dose, acyclovir, shark oil |
| 22 | CA | Y | 2 | 11 | (used for chronic fatigue not HIV) |
| 23 | GA | Y | 3 | 10 | acyclovir, dextran sulfate, vitamins, herbs |
| 24 | LA | Y | 3 | 10 | AZT low dose, aerosolized pentamidine |
| 25 | IL | | | 7 | AZT low dose, acyclovir, beta interferon placebo study |
| 26 | OR | Y | 3 | 13 | dextran sulfate, acyclovir, iscador, transfer factor, DNCB |
| 27 | TX | Y | | 10 | multivitamins |
| 28 | NY | | | 5 | dextran sulfate, Imuthiol |
| 29 | | Y | | | AZT low dose, acyclovir, Nizoral, astragalus 8, + |
| 30 | | H | | 10 | Quan Yin herbal treatment, homeopathic remedies |
| 31 | CA | Y | | 6 | AZT low dose, acyclovir, fluconazole |
| 32 | | | | | AZT low dose, foscarnet, acyclovir, fluconazole |
| 33 | NY | H | | 12 | cipro, acyclovir, pyrazinamide, Myambutol, Lamprene, Nizoral + |
| 34 | MA | Y | | 11 | AZT triple blind |
| 35 | NJ | Y | 2 | 5 | AZT low dose, acyclovir, dextran sulfate |
| 36 | CA | Y | | 4 | acyclovir, AL 721 |
| 37 | NY | Y | 2 | 4 | AZT low dose, acyclovir, sulfoxaprim, dipyridamole |
| 38 | NY | H | | 8 | naltrexone |
| 39 | CA | Y | 2 | 5 | AZT low dose, acyclovir, naltrexone, lysine |
| 40 | CA | Y | | 3 | pentamidine |
| 41 | CA | Y | 2 | 8 | dextran sulfate |
| 42 | CA | Y | 2 | 4 | AL 721 |
| 43 | CA | H | 4 | | AZT |

| 44 | LA | Y | 4 | 18 | AZT |
|---|---|---|---|---|---|
| 45 | PA | H | | 8 | acyclovir, Mycelex troche, acupuncture, vitamins |
| 46 | | | | 2 | peptide shots, Chinese herbs, vitamins, toxo drugs, echinacea |
| 47 | NY | Y | 2 | 4 | AZT low dose, acyclovir, fluconazole |
| 48 | CA | Y | 2 | 3 | BHT, vitamins, minerals |
| 49 | NY | Y | 2 | 9 | naltrexone |
| 50 | NY | H | | 3 | vitamin C, multivitamin, Prevention Plus |
| 51 | NY | Y | | 7 | AZT low dose, acyclovir, folic acid, pentamidine, Nizoral |
| 52 | FL | Y | | 7 | ozone, typhoid injections |
| 53 | PA | Y | 2 | 8 | herbs, Ri Shi Gen mushrooms |
| 54 | | H | | 2 | AZT low dose, acyclovir |
| 55 | AZ | Y | 6 | 16 | AZT low dose, acyclovir, lithium, dextran sulfate |
| 56 | CA | Y | 4 | 6 | AZT low dose, acyclovir, Antabuse, Zantac, interferon |
| 57 | IL | Y | 3 | 8 | AZT low dose, Chinese herbs |
| 58 | CT | H | | 5 | AZT, acyclovir, Zantac |
| 59 | CA | Y | 3 | | |
| 60 | CA | Y | 4 | 4 | AZT low dose, acyclovir |
| 61 | CA | Y | 2 | 13 | AZT low dose |
| 62 | FL | H | | 3 | AZT low dose, acyclovir |
| 63 | NY | Y | | 12 | AZT low dose, acyclovir |
| 64 | CA | Y | 2 | 8 | AZT low dose, acyclovir, vitamin B12 |
| 65 | CA | | | 10 | acyclovir |
| 66 | WY | | 16 | | |
| 67 | TX | Y | 2 | 6 | Carrisyn |
| 68 | CA | | | 12 | AZT low dose, dextran sulfate, acyclovir, Chinese herbs |
| 69 | CA | Y | 2 | 16 | AZT low dose, acyclovir, doxycycline, vitamins, BHT, lysine |
| 70 | CA | Y | 4 | 10 | AZT low dose, acyclovir, Septra, Antabuse |
| 71 | NY | Y | 1 | 14 | AZT low dose, acyclovir, bleomycin |
| 72 | NJ | Y | 3 | 14 | Antabuse, Humilin |
| 73 | CA | Y | 2 | 8 | Jarrow HNLEL, Antabuse, naltrex., acyclovir, BHT, dextran |
| 74 | NY | H | | 16 | AZT low dose, acyclovir, aerosolized pentamidine |
| 75 | CA | Y | 2 | 8 | |
| 76 | NY | | | 11 | Antabuse |
| 77 | NY | | | | AZT, acyclovir |
| 78 | CA | Y | 2 | 4 | AZT low dose, acyclovir, aerosolized pentamidine |
| 79 | NY | Y | | 10 | AZT low dose, passive immunotherapy, Nizoral, Megace |
| 80 | CA | | | 18 | AZT low dose, acyclovir, isoprinosine |
| 81 | NY | | | 32 | dextran sulfate, AL 721 |
| 82 | CA | Y | 2 | 20 | vitamin C, multivitamins, vitamin E, selenium, iron, zinc, + |
| 83 | CA | Y | 2 | 6 | compound Q protocol, aerosolized pentamidine |
| 84 | WA | | | 22 | acyclovir, aerosolized pentamidine, ginseng, estagar, + |
| 85 | | | | 10 | AZT low dose, iscador, naltrexone, Antabuse, aerosol pentam. |
| 86 | OH | Y | 2 | 7 | AZT |
| 87 | GA | Y | 3 | 3 | vitamins, herbs, aerosolized pentamidine |
| 88 | WI | Y | 2 | 6 | AZT low dose, acyclovir, lithium, prosac |

| 89 | NY | Y | 3 | 7 | dextran sulfate, Caiazza's syph. tx, vitamin C, herbs, + |
|----|----|---|---|----|----|
| 90 | NY | Y | 3 | 10 | AZT low dose, acyclovir, dextran sulfate |
| 91 | NJ | Y | 4 | 10 | dextran sulfate, shiitake mushroom, AL 721, Antabuse |
| 92 | NC | Y | 2 | 2 | AZT low dose, aerosolized pentamidine |
| 93 | OH | | | 7 | multivitamins, vitamin B, vitamin C, lysine, Resist, + |
| 94 | HI | Y | 3 | 12 | |
| 95 | CA | | | 4 | aerosolized pentamidine, factor VIII |
| 96 | CA | Y | | 3 | AZT, acyclovir |
| 97 | | | | | vitamin A, vitamin C, lysine, arginine, selenium, + |
| 98 | PA | | | 3 | Tagamet, naltrexone |
| 99 | | Y | 4 | 4 | ddI, compound Q |
| 100 | CA | H | | 12 | AZT, acyclovir, aerosolized pentamidine |
| 101 | CA | Y | 2 | 4 | AZT low dose, aerosolized pentamidine |
| 102 | PA | Y | 2 | 6 | Mycelex troches |
| 103 | NY | Y | 3 | 18 | AZT low dose, acyclovir, dextran sul.., lipids, aerosol pentam. |
| 104 | CA | Y | 2 | 16 | dextran sul., AL 721, naltrex., lentinan, Chinese herbs, homeop. |
| 105 | CA | Y | 4 | 3 | aloe vera, ddI, acyclovir, Bactrim, Aralen |
| 106 | CA | Y | 2 | 10 | DHPG, pyrimethamine, leucovorin |
| 107 | CA | Y | 2 | 4 | AZT, aerosolized pentamidine |
| 108 | CA | Y | 2 | 12 | vitamin C, multivitamin |
| 109 | MD | Y | 2 | 10 | AZT, acyclovir, Seldane, Zantac, Megace |
| 110 | NY | Y | 2 | 9 | dextran sulfate, naltrexone |
| 111 | NY | Y | | 5 | |
| 112 | NJ | Y | 2 | 12 | AZT, acyclovir, Nizoral, Lomotil, Imodium, Antabuse, + |

# Issue Number 92
# December 1, 1989

## NAC: NEW INFORMATION

*by John S. James*

On October 6, *AIDS Treatment News* reported that a prescription drug commonly used in Europe to treat bronchitis (N-acetylcysteine, or NAC), might also be useful as an HIV treatment. New information continues to suggest that NAC might be valuable. While the drug is far from proven, the growing evidence in its favor—as well as its relative safety and availability, and the short time needed to see whether it is working—suggest that this potential treatment belongs among the top priorities of the AIDS community.

This article reviews a major academic study, published December 2; the study did not directly involve NAC, but it confirmed the existence (in symptom-free persons with HIV) of the serious biochemical defect which this drug has been found to treat. In addition, we interviewed an activist in Florida who has followed 24 people who are using NAC; he told us that all of them seemed to benefit.

### Background

Use of NAC for HIV infection was first suggested by a German immunologist, Dr. Wulf Droge. Dr. Droge knew that levels of a chemical called glutathione were abnormally low in persons with AIDS; these levels fell further as the disease progressed. He also knew that NAC increased glutathione levels to normal or almost normal values (within a few hours in the two HIV-positive people who tried the drug), and that proper glutathione levels are important for immune functions and for other reasons.

In October 1988, Dr. Droge sent a cover letter and unpublished manuscript to colleagues in various countries, urging that they give appropriate attention to this information, which "may be life-saving or life-prolonging for many AIDS patients." The manuscript had been submitted to *Nature*; it was later published, but in a journal not well known to U.S. AIDS researchers or physicians (Eck and others, 1989). The cover letter had pointed out that pharmaceutical companies were unlikely to pursue NAC aggressively, because it was already widely available and would be difficult to protect by patent.

NAC first came to public attention in October 1989, after news reports that two professors of genetics at Stanford University (Dr. Leonard Herzenberg and Dr. Leonore Herzenberg) told a scientific conference in Geneva of laboratory results suggesting that the drug might inhibit the AIDS virus. At that time we also reported that at least ten people were using NAC as an HIV treatment, apparently with good results.

In the United States, NAC has been available only in an aerosol form, which is not suitable for oral use for treating HIV. Buyers clubs are now beginning to obtain oral forms of the drug.

(For more background information, see "NAC: Bronchitis Drug May Slow AIDS Virus," *AIDS Treatment News* #88.)

## New Scientific Study: Glutathione Deficiency Confirmed

A study by seven researchers at the National Heart, Lung, and Blood Institute of the U.S. National Institutes of Health, and an eighth at Universitaire Sherbrooke, Quebec, was published in *The Lancet*, December 2, 1989 (Buhl and others, 1989). The researchers reported that glutathione levels in blood plasma of symptom-free HIV-positive subjects were found to be only 30 percent of those of uninfected controls. (The 14 HIV-positive subjects, all symptom-free, had an average T-helper count of 346; four were taking AZT and the other ten were untreated.) Fluid from the lungs, obtained by bronchoalveolar lavage, was also tested for glutathione, and persons with HIV were found to have 60 percent of normal levels.

The paper listed many important functions of glutathione. It is believed to protect cells from oxidation injury, aid in synthesis of proteins and DNA precursors, and serve as a cofactor for certain enzymes. It also has direct effects on the immune system:

"Glutathione is also believed to be important in the initiation and progression of lymphocyte activation, and thus essential for host defense. Furthermore, depletion of intracellular glutathione inhibits lymphocyte activation by mitogens, and glutathione is critical for the function of natural killer cells and for lymphocyte-mediated cytotoxicity."

In short, this paper confirms and extends the pioneering work of Droge, two of whose papers are cited in its references.

On December 1, *The New York Times* published an article on this work ("New Research Suggests Underlying Factor in AIDS"), and interviewed one of the researchers, Dr. Ronald G. Crystal. According to the *Times* article, the researchers have developed an aerosolized glutathione (not NAC) to spray directly into the lungs to see if it will correct the deficiency there. Several months will be required just to find the right dose of this chemical.

## Question

Why develop a new drug to restore glutathione levels only in the lungs, when NAC has already been found to do so systemically? We could not reach the researchers by press time to answer this question. Another scientist familiar with the subject pointed out that this research team consists of pulmonary specialists and experts in aerosol medication; their interest is studies of the lungs. The paper seems to go out of its way to avoid mentioning NAC, especially in the short section at the end where less promising methods of raising glutathione levels are discussed.

## The Florida Study

The Fight for Life Committee, an AIDS activist organization in North Lauderdale, FL, is collecting information from 24 people who are using NAC as an HIV treatment. (The Fight for Life Committee is described by chairman Lenny Kaplan as a "Southern-style ACT UP"—one which works through court challenges and the media more than through demonstrations. For example, the organization has successfully gone to court to obtain AZT for prisoners with AIDS. It is also working through the state legislature and otherwise to reduce the cost of aerosol pentamidine treatment in local hospitals.)

When we interviewed Mr. Kaplan on December 3, the 24 people had used NAC for between 10 and 45 days. All of them are keeping diaries. All of them have ARC or AIDS. Interpretation of results is complicated by the fact that 12 of the 24 are also using Compound Q; but those involved attribute the following benefits and side effects to NAC. (Mr. Kaplan told us that the NAC seemed to work better and sooner for those who had also used compound Q; he felt there should definitely be a clinical trial to test the combination.)

Everybody reported increased energy, often greatly increased; persons who once needed naps during the day have become able to work full time without them. Only a few have blood work results available after using NAC; their T-helper counts were up by an average of about 75.

The two who showed the most benefit both had wasting syndrome. One gained 12 pounds, and his physician found no new growth of KS. The other gained 10 pounds.

Some people had headaches or dizziness during the first week. The dose had to be reduced to 1000 mg per day (500 mg after breakfast and 500 mg after dinner) after three of the first five had stomach upset on a higher dose. These side effects may have been due to the formulation of the drug (see below).

## Drug Formulation Issues

Many brands of NAC are sold in different countries in Europe for oral use. As far as is known, any of these brands would be satisfactory; however, most contain large amounts of sugar or other sweeteners to cover the bad taste of the NAC; some patients might not want the sweeteners. Prices vary as much as 3-fold between expensive countries (such as Germany or England) and inexpensive countries (such as Spain). Persons with HIV are using somewhat more of the medication than persons with bronchitis; as a result, NAC costs about $2. per day even from the less expensive countries, with doses of 1600 mg per day (400 four times per day) or 1800 mg per day (600 three times).

Meanwhile, the chemical NAC has been pressed into tablets and sold at prices much less than the European brands. Because these tablets are not regulated as drugs, there is widespread concern that they might not be safe. Some of the concerns we have heard are:

• Customers can only trust that the manufacturer used a grade of the chemical intended for human use;

• According to one chemist, the European products are packed in foil because they oxidize rapidly when exposed to air. The other tablets are just put into bottles. They may have a short shelf life, especially after the bottles have been opened. The shelf life needs to be checked.

• All or almost all of the European brands are intended to be dissolved in water outside the body before being taken. Usually the drug is provided as a single-dose packet of powder. These packets are not as convenient as pills, especially since NAC has an unpleasant taste; presumably the packets are provided for a reason, possibly to reduce stomach irritation.

To avoid such problems, the PWA Health Group in New York is planning to obtain one of the European NAC preparations. For more information, call them at 212/532-0280. The PWA Health Group is also planning to do its own chemical testing and other research on the suitability of the various formulations.

It may be possible to create a very inexpensive product which is satisfactory-perhaps by putting pharmaceutical-grade NAC into capsules to be opened before use, and dissolved in water. Some research — for example, checking with pharmacologists in Europe — would be necessary.

There are efforts to organize a formal clinical trial of NAC as an HIV treatment. These efforts are moving slowly, and it will probably be years before the drug is officially approved. NAC is not a high priority for any organization. Meanwhile the AIDS community must organize itself to obtain proper supplies, and to collect the best information possible about this potential treatment and its uses.

## REFERENCES

Buhl, R and others. Systemic glutathione Deficiency in Symptom-Free HIV-Seropositive Individuals. *The Lancet*, pages 1294-1297, December 2, 1989.

Droge, W and others. Glutathione augments the activation of cytotoxic T lymphocytes in vivo. *Immunobiology*, volume 172 number 1-2, pages 151-156, August 1986.

Eck, HP and others. Low concentrations of acid-soluble thiol (cysteine) in the blood plasma of HIV-1 infected patients. *Biol Chem Hoppe Seyler*, volume 370 number 2, pages 101-108, February 1989.

# DDI ACCESS IMPEDED; PROTESTS PLANNED DECEMBER 14

New restrictions on access to the antiviral ddI, imposed under pressure from Federally-funded principal investigators (PIs) in the AIDS Clinical Trials Group (ACTG) system, are leading to a bitter dispute over patients' access to experimental treatments. The PIs say that allowing patients to use ddI outside of formal trials is harming their research, by making it difficult to recruit subjects. Patient advocates say that the recruiting difficulties are not due to the expanded access, but to poor design and administration of the trials.

We do not know how many of the PIs oppose expanded access. But it is clear that many have strongly fought against Fauci's "parallel track" proposal, against the current system of expanded access to ddI under existing regulations (technically different from "parallel track," which has not yet been officially defined), and also against the FDA's liberalized rules for patients seeking medicines approved abroad for personal use. In short, some of the PIs have consistently fought against patients' access to treatment options—both openly and (more importantly) behind the scenes—on the grounds that if patients have more options, they will not volunteer for their studies.

Now some patients requesting ddI are unexpectedly being denied it, and there is widespread suspicion that pressure from PIs is to blame. For example, Bristol-Myers was expected to drop the requirement for an AIDS diagnosis for access to ddI by patients who are failing AZT, allowing patients otherwise qualified to enter this program even if technically they only have ARC. Now it appears that this restriction will not be dropped, although exceptions might be considered on a case-by-case basis. We are also hearing reports of a general slowdown in the system, with patients who are eligible under all the rules being told that there is not enough drug—when before we had heard that there was no problem with supply.

Arguments against allowing wider use of the drug were stated in a much-criticized article on page 1 of *The New York Times*, November 21, 1989. Headlined "Innovative AIDS Drug Plan May Be Undermining Testing," this article reported that "almost 20 times as many people have flocked to free distributions of the new drug ddI than have signed up for the clinical trial, leaving researchers in despair over whether they will ever be able to complete the formal study." But a closer look shows a very different picture:

• According to Bristol-Myers, available data on the patients who have "flocked" to ddI distribution outside of the trials show that 60 percent of them would not be allowed into any of the three ddI trials because they do not meet medical criteria, and another 30 percent live too far from the nearest trial site to participate. Well under 10 percent could possibly have entered a formal study.

Some principal investigators have dismissed these numbers by saying that doctors lie to get ddI for their patients, and therefore some of those counted as ineligible for the formal studies may really have been eligible. But they have not presented any evidence to show whether significant number of patients are lost to the study this way.

• At some of the sites where the study will be conducted, no one can enroll because the local institution is not ready for them. Often the local Institutional Review Board has not yet given its approval. The program to allow expanded access to ddI to patients ineligible for the trials cannot be blamed if low enrollment totals result from the fact that some centers are not ready.

• Some of the study sites only have enough staff to enroll a few patients a week.

For these and for other reasons, patients are on waiting lists at some of the centers—in some cases, for months. And most centers have done little or nothing to tell the public about their studies.

- In addition, there are concerns about the studies themselves. In two of the them, patients may be randomized to 1200 mg of AZT per day—the dose which is officially approved but which the medical community is rapidly coming to consider too high. Attempts to change the trial to use a lower dose have not yet succeeded. Other concerns include the appropriateness of randomizing patients to AZT when those patients were selected to be ones for whom that drug is likely to be losing effectiveness (study number ACTG 117). Such concerns about study design create disincentives for patients to enroll.

- Despite all these problems, the ddI studies have actually recruited *faster* than most ACTG trials in the past (when there was no system for access outside of trials), according to Jim Eigo of ACT UP/New York, who for months has been one of the principal patient advocates in the ddI negotiations.

## Demonstration December 14

ACT UP/New York is planning protests on December 14 against denial of treatment to patients who have no other alternatives. Protests are also being planned in other cities. These demonstrations are being called on very short notice.

## If You Have Trouble Getting ddl

David Barr of Lambda Legal is collecting information about people's experiences when they try to obtain ddI, either by volunteering for a trial or by trying to enter the expanded access program. Anyone who has difficulty should call him at the above number. Many of the access problems have not been announced, but have been discovered by comparing notes of persons who have been turned down.

## For More Information

For more information about the controversy over access to ddI, see the column by Mark Harrington and letter by Jim Eigo in *Out Week* magazine (New York, December 10 issue date). There is also an unpublished November 21 letter to *The New York Times* from David Barr and Jay Lipner of Lambda Legal, and a November 21 press statement by Project Inform, both written in response to *The New York Times* article of that date.

## PASSIVE IMMUNOTHERAPY: PATENT DISPUTE IMPEDES RESEARCH

An important study of passive immunotherapy by Marcus Conant, M.D. in San Francisco may be halted by a patent dispute between two rival companies. Recently Medicorp, of Montreal, Quebec, obtained a broadly-worded patent for passive immunotherapy—a treatment consisting of plasma transfusions from selected donors with high levels of anti-HIV antibodies, to recipients who need the antibodies. In a November 28 letter from its attorneys, Medicorp refused a request from Immutech, a small

Solano Beach, CA company working with Dr. Conant, for permission to use passive immunotherapy. After months of preparation, Dr. Conant had obtained California approval and was ready to begin the trial, designed to treat 40 people, some who are very sick. There is no placebo arm in this study.

AIDS activists are considering a legal challenge to the patent through the patent office. They may also prepare a wrongful death lawsuit, to be brought against Medicorp if anyone dies while waiting for treatment.

## ISCADOR: PROMISING EXPERIENCE TO DATE

*by Denny Smith*

An extract from mistletoe which has been used for more than sixty years in Europe to treat certain solid-tumor cancers has been studied in the U.S. recently for immunomodulatory and anti-viral activity against HIV. *Viscum album*, or European Mistletoe, is the species from which an aqueous extract is produced by the Institut Hiscia in Switzerland, under the trade name Iscador.

The most extensive HIV-related clinical work with Iscador has been conducted by two physicians in San Francisco; both are European-educated. Immaculada Marti, M.D., from Spain, is a staff physician at Davies Hospital in San Francisco, and treats many people with HIV in her practice. Robert Gorter, M.D., from The Netherlands, is an Associate Professor at the University of California in San Francisco.

We asked Dr. Marti to share her impressions of Iscador's usefulness. Although her experience, and Dr. Gorter's as well, has been encouraging, she feels that it cannot be described as conclusive. The last report of their work appeared a year ago, in the November 1988 issue of *BETA*, the treatment bulletin of the San Francisco AIDS Foundation.

At least 37 different components have been isolated from *Viscum album*, characterized as polysaccharides, viscotoxins and lectins. The latter two are under study for anti-tumor and immunomodulatory properties. Iscador is available in two preparations: the useful lectins are preserved in unfermented extract of *Viscum album*, while the fermented version loses an important lectin. As a semi-parasitic organism, mistletoe requires life on a host plant, often apple, oak, elm, or pine trees. Interestingly, the chemical properties of the parasite plant vary somewhat depending on which host tree it grows on.

Dr. Taseem A. Khwaja, Director of the Comprehensive Cancer Research Center of the University of Southern California, has observed that Iscador blocks *in vitro* syncytia formation, the clumping of cells which provides HIV an efficient passage from cell to cell. He suggests that Iscador may also inhibit the binding of free virus to the receptors of uninfected cells, as well as inhibit reverse transcriptase within infected cells. In spite of its apparent potential, *Viscum album* actually demonstrates little ability to directly harm HIV particles, but Dr. Khwaja is investigating another species of mistletoe, *Viscum coloratum*, which may be superior in this regard.

In her clinical experience, Dr. Marti has seen Iscador enhancement of five specific immune responses:

- An increase in the number and activity of neutrophils;
- Increase in T4-helper cells;
- Increased number and activity of natural killer cells;
- Enhanced anti-body dependent cell-mediated cytotoxicity (ADCC);
- Increased lymphocyte mitogenicity, or immune cell-multiplication.

Some of these responses are similar to those obtained with alpha interferon treatments, and in fact Iscador appears to facilitate the immune system's own production of interferon. Related improvements in Dr. Marti's patients included weight gain, reduction of KS lesions, decreased lymphadenopathy, increased hemoglobin, and decreases in beta 2 microglobulin and p24 antigenemia. She notes, however, that the positive KS response does not appear to result directly from the effect of *Viscum album* on KS lesions, but rather from an indirect enhancement of the body's immune response to KS.

Iscador is administered by subcutaneous injection two or three times a week, beginning with a low dose, 0.01 mg. As it is presently formulated, Iscador is less effective taken orally, since some components are inactivated in the gastrointestinal tract. The dosage is gradually increased, and doses approaching 15 to 20 mg resulted in blood work improvements for asymptomatic patients. However, people who are currently fighting an opportunistic infection or who have low helper cell counts seem to have a lower dose tolerance, above which the drug may become useless or detrimental. The dosage must be tailored to take these factors into account. (A similar observation was made in the results of Project Inform's recent study of Compound Q.) Many people experience redness and tenderness at the injection site, but no serious or permanent toxicity has been attributed to Iscador. Reactions in some people to high doses caused fever, insomnia, fatigue and loss of appetite. Temporarily discontinuing the injections resolved the reaction.

No other medications are contraindicated with the use of Iscador, and in fact Dr. Marti has combined it successfully with AZT, chemotherapy and ddI. She has found that Iscador helps counter the bone marrow suppression induced by long-term use of AZT. In addition to the objective improvements in blood markers, her patients have reported improved appetite and sleep, vivid dreams, and relief from HIV-associated fatigue and depression.

All of these observations would seem to make Iscador, or some future *Viscum* preparation, a very pursuable treatment possibility. As a prescription drug in Switzerland, Iscador costs about $4 an ampule, or $12 a week, and personal use requests can be sent with a physician's prescription directly to the manufacturer: Institut Hiscia, CH-4144 Arlesheim, Kirschweg 9, Switzerland. Drs. Gorter and Marti continue to monitor their patients' response to Iscador, and are interested in conducting formal trials to expand their study.

## REFERENCES

Holtskog, R and others. Characterization of a toxic lectin in Iscador, a mistletoe preparation with alleged cancerostatic properties. *Oncology*, volume 45 number 3, pages 172-179, 1988.

Kuttan, G and others. Isolation and identification of a tumor reducing component from mistletoe extract (Iscador). *Cancer Letters*, volume 41 number 3, pages 307-314, 1988.

Hamprecht, K and others. Mediation of human NK-activity by components in extracts of Viscum album. *International Journal of Immunopharmacology*, volume 9 number 2, pages 199-209, 1987.

Metzner, G and others. Effects of lectin I from mistletoe (ML I) and its isolated A and B chains on human mononuclear cells: mitogenic activity and lymphokine release. *Pharmazie*, volume 42 number 5, pages 337-340, 1987.

*Oncology*, (entire issue devoted to *Viscum album*) supplement 1 of volume 43, 1986.

# Issue Number 93
# March 24, 1989

## 1989/1990: WHERE ARE WE NOW?

*by John S. James*

1990 begins at a time of confusion about research and new-treatment issues. Much is happening, and the year ahead could develop in any of a number of different ways. Here is one area we believe will be important next year.

## From Access to Oversight?

Last January we predicted that **access** would be the major treatment issue of 1989. At that time it was already clear that no major treatment advance would be approved in 1989; one could know that by looking at the drugs in the clinical-trials pipeline. Therefore, the issue would be whether people could use promising treatments while they were still experimental—treatments like ddI which probably work but will take years to acquire statistical proof that they do.

Great progress on access was made last year, thanks largely to two key events: Fauci's proposal for a parallel track, and the ddI program developed by Bristol-Myers in cooperation with the FDA, AIDS activists, front-line physicians, and others. Major problems remain, and questions, issues, and conflicts around access will be very much with us in 1990. But we think that another issue may become central next year—the need for better definition, design and management of the clinical trials, so that they can respond better to the needs of the public-health emergency.

We see **resources** as the most important single issue of 1990—money for prevention, research, treatment, and other care. Since we are not experienced in financing issues, we will follow the lead of service organizations and others. We are familiar with research, however, and here we believe that effective scientific and administrative oversight of the trials will become a critical issue. It has been the most important issue all along, but until now little has been said about it. Pressures are building to end the silence:

• **No major approvals in 1990.** It is already clear that no important HIV treatment will be approved in 1990 under current procedures. ddI and ddC are now farthest ahead, but approval for each must wait for (among other things) trials which will probably take two years. And neither of these clocks has started yet, because each only starts when the last patient called for by the respective protocol has been recruited and entered into the study.

As we will show below, this problem does not arise from any law of nature, but from unexamined assumptions in an overlooked meeting place between scientific study design and public policy. Critical options have been ignored because policy makers lack the scientific background to develop them, scientists lack the authority, and institutions lack the incentive. The growing AIDS case load and continually worsening emergency are increasing the pressures to bring the light of public examination and debate into some previously dark corners.

• **Parallel track limitations.** A pivotal event of 1989 was the proposal by Anthony Fauci, M.D., Director of the National Institute of Allergy and Infectious Diseases (NIAID), for "parallel track" access to promising treatments while they are still being tested in clinical trials. Until Fauci's proposal, the dominant idea had been that no early or compassionate access should be allowed for AIDS treatments, because otherwise people would not volunteer for clinical trials. Much of this thinking had been based on a misreading of the case of the drug ganciclovir, made available for compassionate use to thousands of people over a several-year period to prevent blindness from AIDS-related cytomegalovirus (CMV). The pharmaceutical industry wrongly assumed that ganciclovir's developer, Syntex Corporation of Palo Alto, CA, was being punished by the FDA for making an AIDS drug available through compassionate use.

Since an analysis of the new drugs in the pipeline showed that no important HIV treatment would be fully approved for several years, this prevailing mindset was a death sentence for tens of thousands of people. Fauci's parallel track proposal broke this mental logjam and opened a door for new thinking throughout government and industry. The head of the world's largest AIDS trials program had proposed that some early access could be allowed without damaging the trials. The new openness allowed the development of the system for early access to ddI—a development unprecedented both in its speed, and in its bringing together of many different interests, getting some of the people involved talking to each other for the first time, to produce results.

Parallel track is urgently necessary. But it will not solve all the problems:

(1) Parallel track requires the good will of the company which has the exclusive rights to each new drug. The company must spend money to save lives, with no certainty of reward. Many will be unwilling to do so.

(2) Individuals receive the drug without charge but pay for required physician time and laboratory tests. Third-party payers will probably learn to identify these expenses and refuse them as "experimental," meaning that parallel track may be even more limited by social class than standard medical care. It will be difficult to define standards of care if crucial parts of care come to be delivered on an optional, "experimental" basis.

(3) The most important question is what drugs to use and how to use them. Clinical trials are supposed to help answer these questions. But there are no trials designed to address the needs of parallel track. Parallel track lives only on the crumbs of knowledge which happen to fall out of trials designed for something else. (This isn't as bad as it sounds, however; clinical-trial design has so lost its way that standard medical practice lives largely on such crumbs, also.)

Despite these reservations, we totally support the parallel track. It is a life and death issue and there is no alternative ready to go. Sometimes a second-best solution is infinitely better than no solution at all. Parallel track is an emergency stop-gap until the entire system of clinical trials can be rethought and redesigned.

• **The clinical-trials logjam.** Those who run the major Federal system of AIDS clinical trials, the AIDS Clinical Trials Group (ACTG) system in NIAID, are quick to admit that the system is overloaded and cannot keep up with the important new drugs coming out of the laboratory. People are tired from overwork due to inadequate staff; tasks which everyone agrees are important are postponed or eliminated. The problems only look worse in the future as there will be more people with AIDS, more new drugs to try, but no more and maybe even less support from Congress.

Behind this problem is the fact that new-drug approval in the United States has become so elaborate and inefficient that it costs an average of $120 million for each new drug approved. The ACTG system, started from scratch to provide grants for testing AIDS drugs, cannot be expected to test dozens of new drugs under these rules with the limited resources available.

• **Serious administrative problems.** At a closed ACTG meeting on November 6-8, 1989, it was announced that no major new trials could start for six to nine months—an estimate which may be optimistic. The reason is that the statistical and data-processing center for the ACTG system was being moved from Triangle Research Institute to Harvard University, and the new center would not be ready until then. This delay most seriously impacts trials for opportunistic infections, since other trials were not ready to go anyway.

In any system adequate to meet the needs of the emergency, no such delay would be tolerated.

• **Questions about lack of results.** A December 12 memo from ACT UP/New York to Federal agencies and others begins with the sentence, "After three years supported by hundreds of millions of public funds, the AIDS Clinical Trials Group (ACTG) has yet to develop data leading to a single new treatment for any HIV related condition."

We are not close enough to the ACTG to evaluate its performance independently. But ACT UP's Treatment and Data Committee is very well informed about the ACTG system and its problems.

## Needed: Effective Oversight

It seems clear that some capable and independent oversight body needs to examine and analyze the record, point out problems or improvements needed, and see that the changes are made.

The National Commission on AIDS will not do this job. It is working in other areas and has no interest in oversight of research.

The well-regarded Institute of Medicine of the National Academy of Sciences has a committee to investigate the ACTG system. It remains to be seen whether this group will be effective.

The entire area of clinical research needs a thorough examination by top scientists and top administrators, with the staff, resources, authority, and independence to do the job.

## THE WRONG NIGHTMARE: THE WORST DELAY OF CLINICAL TRIALS

*by John S. James*

The clinical trials of ddI and ddC both illustrate what we believe is the worst bottleneck delaying AIDS treatment research. The problem, which affects any HIV treatment but is usually less severe with other diseases, is largely responsible for the fact that hundreds of millions of dollars have gone into AIDS trials and produced few useful results. This lack of productivity is not due to any law of nature, but to a widespread misjudgment. Physicians, scientists, and regulators have marched into a morass because they have chosen the wrong nightmare.

The clinical trials of ddI need hundreds of volunteers and will probably have to run for two years after the last subject is recruited. The same delay applies to all HIV treatments, and therefore becomes a death sentence for tens of thousands of people— although some of them will be saved by the parallel track. (The public does not realize that the faster approval of AZT cannot be repeated, because today it would be unethical to give research subjects only a placebo when an approved treatment is available, and it is much harder to get definitive results when comparing a new treatment to an active control than to a placebo.)

In the design of the ddI trials, statisticians computed the numbers of subjects needed, assuming a two-year study. The fact that the numbers came from mathematical computations gave them an aura of infallibility, unchallengeable by ordinary mortals. But we can and must examine what these trials are trying to do, and why.

The trial design—including the two years, the hundreds of subjects, and the consequent need for time-consuming and expensive coordination of many widely distant medical centers—was created to produce a single bit of information, one yes-or-no answer. The question to be answered is whether, if the drug really does nothing at all, the chance of the trial falsely concluding that the drug does work (just by chance alone) is less than a given probability (usually five percent).

Is this the question that most needs answering? Should this question be allowed to add two years or more delay to every new HIV drug? Should this question serve as a gatekeeper which prevents other research from starting until it is answered? Should it be allowed to make research so costly in money, facilities, and (most importantly) qualified personnel, that it limits the trials to a handful of new drugs, when there will soon be dozens that clearly deserve followup?

The real issue with ddI is not whether it works. A growing working consensus holds that it probably does. And drugs do not begin multimillion dollar clinical trials unless pharmaceutical companies, which are in the business of evaluating drugs, believe in them. The most important questions now are long-term toxicity, and when and how to use ddI most effectively in various groups of patients.

Some of this information will come out of the ddI trials—but only by accident. Because the trials will take so much time, long-term toxicity data will be produced. And restrictive entry criteria will assure us much information about using ddI in certain groups of patients, and none about using it in other groups. The whole structure of the trials is built around the need to get that one statistical bit of information, to be able to walk away with that single yes-or-no answer—not to answer the questions which are most important now to patients and physicians.

Trials which studied long-term toxicity by design instead of by accident could be started much sooner, probably as a continuation of phase I, and could use many fewer patients. The time and money saved could be used to test several other drugs which otherwise will be neglected.

The medical world today is obsessed with one nightmare—that a worthless drug will come into widespread use. This danger is real, as such cases have occurred many times in the past. The problems come from using this nightmare as the sole gatekeeper which controls everything else, regardless of all other elements in the real-world situation.

## A Better Way

A rational program for clinical testing and early use of new drugs would probably involve an expanding circle of research and treatment, starting with dose and toxicity studies and, depending on results obtained, moving continuously into wider use in appropriate groups of patients. The research aspect would be most intensive at first; then gradually the treatment aspect would predominate.

This expanding circle of use, with research most intensive at first, is what already occurs with conventional phase I, II, III, and IV studies. But today's process is not rational or planned as a whole. It is full of arbitrary discontinuities, prohibitively burdensome requirements derived from theories, and deliberate, studied blindness to the actual questions, issues, knowledge base, and opportunities of the specific drug, in its social and public-health context.

Note that we are not suggesting dropping the legal requirement that drugs show efficacy before they are marketed. That is a different issue. We are saying instead that narrow efficacy testing should not completely dominate clinical trials, should not be applied blindly and rigidly in ways that straightjacket and paralyze the entire research enterprise.

A coherent, rational design for an integrated research and treatment process, using to advantage the specifics of each situation and addressing the actual questions at issue, could get the most important answers far faster than the present system, and at a fraction of the cost. It could bring many more drugs into trials than the present system, which is seriously overloaded with unnecessarily costly trials. It could bring us years closer to better treatments for AIDS, thereby saving most of the lives which otherwise would be lost.

This is one of the central research issues we intend to address in 1990.

# NAC: "NO MIRACLES"

In our issues of December 1 and October 6, *AIDS Treatment News* reported on indications that NAC (N-acetylcysteine), a drug widely used in Europe to treat bronchitis, might be useful in treating AIDS or HIV infection.

Since publishing those articles we have talked with Barbara Starrett, M.D., who sees many AIDS patients in New York. About ten of her patients have used the European form of the drug, some starting as early as December 1988.

Dr. Starrett is confident that the drug has not hurt anybody, and thinks that it may work as a stabilizer or mild immune modulator. Her patients have remained stable. But she has seen no great improvements, and has no definitive proof that the drug helped. Most of her patients had chosen to stop taking the drug, because it did not seem worth the expense. (Prices vary greatly, and her patients had been using one of the most expensive brands, from Switzerland.)

Dr. Starrett is concerned that people may have expectations which are too high. But she says there is no question that the drug should be available.

## NAC Survey

In New York, the PWA Health Group, in association with ACT UP's Treatment and Data Committee, will conduct a survey of people using NAC, to ask about short-term subjective benefits and risks. They hope "to gain some practical information about 'real-world' use of NAC now, years before the projected clinical trials yield results."

Registration forms and baseline questionnaires will be available at the PWA Health Group; followup surveys will be mailed for at least three months. Buyers clubs in other cities might also join this study.

# SAN FRANCISCO: CHINESE HERBAL
# PROGRAM DEADLINE JANUARY 5

The Quan Yin Healing Arts Center in San Francisco continues to sponsor HIV treatment and research studies for seropositive people, whether symptomatic or not, through its Chinese Herbal Treatment Program.

## Results of Earlier Programs

We asked Quan Yin about results of their earlier programs. A summary appears in "The Role of Chinese Herbal Medicine in the Defeat of the AIDS Epidemic," by Subhuti Dharmananda, Ph.D., published by his Institute for Traditional Medicine and Preventive Health Care, Portland, Oregon. Two groups of patients were reported. In the first, with 93 participants completing the study, "40 felt more healthy at the end of the program, 47 felt about the same, and only 6 reported feeling less healthy. White blood cell counts increased by an average of 2.85 percent and hematocrit increased by an average of 1.08 percent. T-cells were measured in 26 participants. Fifteen showed an increase, 10 showed a decrease, and one had no change. Individuals who were categorized as HIV+ indicated better response overall, and by blood tests, than those with ARC or AIDS. . . Of the 93, six changed diagnosis from HIV to ARC and two from ARC to AIDS.

Besides the 93 who completed that study, 54 dropped out (including two who died); a total of 147 had started. Many were listed as dropping out only because they failed to provide the last report at the end of the three months.

In the next group, 164 participants began the protocol and 127 completed it. "Fifty nine of the individuals completing the study reported feeling more healthy and 58 reported feeling about the same, while only 10 individuals considered themselves to be less healthy at the end of the three-month period. White blood cell counts increased by an average of 5.8 percent and hematocrit increased by an average of 2.1 percent. T-cell counts were available for 12 participants; of these, six showed an increase, one stayed about the same, and five experienced a decrease. . . Four individuals changed diagnosis from HIV+ to ARC and one from HIV+ to AIDS during the course of the study."

Another group began in September, 1989, but results are not yet available.

# LYMPHOMA: A CURRENT LOOK AT THERAPIES

*by Denny Smith*

Lymphoma is a diagnosis facing at least 5% of people with AIDS. The term lymphoma refers to a number of malignancies in which various cells of the body's lymph system have proliferated out of control; those most commonly seen in the presence of HIV are of B-cell origin, and are classified as high and intermediate grade, large cell immunoblastic or small non-cleaved Non-Hodgkin's lymphomas (NHL). They may develop in lymph nodes, but are more commonly found at extra-nodal sites such as the central nervous system (CNS), bone marrow, the bowel, liver, or lungs. The other major malignancy identified with AIDS is Kaposi's sarcoma (KS—see *AIDS Treatment News* #73, 75, & 87), which has probably gathered more attention than lymphoma from the treatment establishment. Fortunately the rate of new KS diagnoses has slowed since early epidemic years; however, the incidence of lymphoma appears to be on the rise.

Like KS, lymphoma occurring as a consequence of HIV infection is considered an opportunistic neoplasm, or cancer, rather than an infection caused by organisms. In spite of that distinction, however, the development of some lymphomas has been linked to infections of a herpes-family virus, Epstein-Barr (EBV). This virus can cause infectious mononucleosis, and is implicated in the development of lymphomas in people who must take immunosuppressing transplant medications. For similar reasons, an HIV-impaired immune response may allow a latent EBV infection to reactivate, and theoretically provoke lymphoproliferations. EBV is already known to be implicated in hairy leukoplakia, and has been much discussed as a possible cofactor in HIV immune deterioration—each virus has been observed *in vitro* to activate the other. However, EBV is not always present in people with HIV, nor uniformly evident in AIDS-associated lymphoma tissue. In data collected at San Francisco General Hospital, EBV was identified in only about a third of lymphoma biopsies, suggesting that EBV could be a passenger virus which coincides with but is not the cause of AIDS lymphoma.

Diagnosing lymphoma can involve several complications. The symptoms of CNS lymphoma in adults might resemble other, more common AIDS-related neurological problems such as toxoplasmic encephalitis. By contrast, CNS lesions in children with AIDS will much more likely prove to be lymphoma than otherwise. The non-invasive tests for diagnostic purposes, CT or MRI scans, are not usually dependable for distinguishing infections from lymphoma in the brain. A conclusive diagnosis can be made by biopsy, but antibiotic therapy may be tried first in adults to rule out infections, and if the symptoms fail to respond then presumptive treatment can begin for lymphoma. For children that approach could represent a dangerous delay in appropriate treatment, given the probability of finding lymphoma behind these symptoms.

Symptoms of lymphoma in the rest of the body may resemble lymphadenopathy but are easily verified with a biopsy. Obtaining a sample of tissue through a fine-needle aspiration is less invasive than a surgical biopsy, although needle aspirations produce a somewhat higher rate of false-negative results.

Standard treatments for lymphoma have involved radiation or chemotherapy, or both. These and a few experimental therapies are briefly discussed below. The occurence of AIDS-related lymphoma, like any consequence of HIV, warrants the start or continuation of an anti-HIV agent such as AZT to address the underlying problem. A review of patients treated for CNS lymphoma at three Los Angeles medical centers pointed to concurrent opportunistic infections as a factor diminishing the rate of survival following otherwise successful lymphoma treatments. The report suggests that an HIV therapy would affect positively a course of treating lymphoma. Ironically, the underlying problem can be exacerbated by treatments for secondary infections. Radiation and chemotherapy, for example, each suppress bone marrow production of blood cells (myelosuppression) independently of HIV or AZT. We spoke to several AIDS-experienced physicians about refinements in lymphoma therapy which, like new approaches to KS, attempt to minimize this danger.

CNS lymphoma usually develops as small, individual lesions on the brain, and can be treated with a series of localized, low-volume doses of radiation over a period of 5 to 7 weeks. If the lymphoma is disseminated, present at multiple sites within the central nervous system, radiation treatment alone is not advised and is augmented with a chemotherapy agent, such as methotrexate, administered intrathecally (injected into the cerebrospinal fluid) since many drugs given intravenously fail to penetrate the blood-brain barrier. William Wara, M.D., of the Department of Radiation Oncology at the University of California in San Francisco, described his modification of the treatment for AIDS-related CNS lymphoma. By irradiating lesions with larger dose volumes and shortening the duration of the total therapy to 3 weeks, Dr. Wara obtains an optimum tumor response while minimizing the trauma of a longer course of therapy. He found this more intensive regimen improved on previous practice without increasing immunosuppression, because the field of radiation remains very small and specific.

Treatments of peripheral lymphomas, those diagnosed at sites outside the CNS, are relieved of the challenge of crossing the blood-brain barrier; therefore the diseases can be addressed with a wider spectrum of treatments. The first line of options consists of various chemotherapy combinations, both with and without radiation.

A list of chemotherapeutic agents tried against lymphoma, in addition to methotrexate already mentioned, includes bleomycin, cyclophosphamide, daunorubicin, dexamethasone, doxorubicin, etoposide, ifosfomide, prednisone, procarbazine, and vincristine. Apparently no consensus regarding the choice of agents or degree of treatment aggressiveness has been established. Physicians at San Francisco General Hospital noted shortened survival rates among patients who were treated with high-dose cyclophosphamide, and they suggest that lymphoma regimens be designed to control toxicity or to include agents for reducing bone marrow and immune suppression. Another report at the Montreal Conference described a decision by clinicians at the Los Angeles Oncologic Institute and Baylor University Medical Center in Dallas to decrease the aggressiveness of lymphoma chemotherapy. They then obtained excellent results in five patients with cautious use of bleomycin, vincristine, and prednisone combined with acyclovir and low-dose AZT (abstract B.588).

The investigational agent called granulocyte macrophage-colony stimulating factor (GM-CSF) may prove useful for protecting the bone marrow from damage associated with chemotherapy, and permit the addition of other valuable but potentially suppressive therapies, such as AZT and interferon. Researchers at the Centro di Riferimento Oncologico in Aviano, Italy, presented a report at the International Conference on AIDS last June finding GM-CSF effective for reversing myelosuppression due to chemotherapy and AZT in some people with KS or lymphoma (abstract M.C.P.103). GM-CSF is available in the U.S. only through clinical trials.

Refractory lymphomas, those which resist other treatment attempts, have been affected by mitoxantrone with cytarabine. Researchers at the Johns-Hopkins University describe a man successfully treated for AIDS-associated NHL with a bone marrow transplant from his sister (Montreal abstract W.B.P. 319). Anti-idiotype antibody therapy and chlorodeoxyadenosine (CDA) are both currently pursued in clinical trials in the U.S.

We spoke to Lawrence Kaplan, M.D., an oncologist at San Francisco General Hospital and principle investigator for five trials there involving some of the potential treatments mentioned above. These trials are all still in progress, and we hope to report any conclusive results in the future. Dr. Kaplan was willing to share some early positive impressions:

CDA, a novel drug used with success in treating another diagnosis, has been helpful for some patients with NHL which was unresponsive to previous treatments.

Anti-idiotype antibody therapy, also for relapsed lymphoma, is a strategy which borrows functions ordinarily employed by natural immune defenses. This treatment appears useful in about 25 percent of certain lymphomas.

In a randomized study, GM-CSF is being administered to two of every three participants, all of whom receive chemotherapy for NHL. Dr. Kaplan is optimistic for the potential of GM-CSF to reduce the neutropenia following chemotherapy, and shorten associated hospitalizations. For this trial and two others at San Francisco General Hospital which include chemotherapy, the particular agents used are cyclophosphamide, doxorubicin, vincristine, and prednisone. These trials are open for recruitment, and persons interested in participating in any of them should call 415/821-5531.

## REFERENCES

Epstein, L G and others,"Primary Lymphoma of the Central Nervous System in Children With Acquired Immunodeficiency Syndrome," *Pediatrics* volume 82, number 3, September, 1989.

Formenti, S C and others, "Primary Central Nervous System Lymphoma in AIDS-Results of Radiation Therapy," *Cancer*, volume 63, number 6, pages 1101-1107, March 15, 1989.

Ho, A D and others, "Mitoxantrone and High-Dose Cytarabine as Salvage Therapy for Refractory Non-Hodgkin's Lymphoma," *Cancer*, volume 64, number 7, pages 1388-1392, October 1, 1989.

Kaplan, L D and others, "AIDS-Associated Non-Hodgkin's Lymphoma in San Francisco," *Journal of the American Medical Association*, volume 261, number 5, pages 719-724, February 3, 1989.

Lang, D J and others, "Seroepidemiologic Studies of Cytomegalovirus and Epstein-Barr Virus Infection in Relation to Human Immunodeficiency Virus Type 1 Infection in Selected Recipient Populations," *Journal of Acquired Immune Deficiency Syndromes*, volume 2, number 6, pages 540-549, 1989.

Rahman, M A and others, "Enhanced Antibody Responses to Epstein-Barr Virus in HIV-Infected Homosexual Men," *The Journal of Infectious Diseases*, volume 159, number 3, pages 472-479, March 1989.

## CHRONIC FATIGUE ORGANIZATIONS SEEK COALITION WITH AIDS EFFORTS

A major advocacy group for persons with Chronic Fatigue Immune Dysfunction Syndrome (CFIDS) wants to contact AIDS activists and organizations to discuss coordination of our efforts to advance prevention, research, and patient care.

CFIDS, like AIDS, is an infectious disease that causes serious immune-system malfunction. In 1984-1985, a major outbreak among residents at Incline Village, Nevada, affected 300 people; since then the disease has become a widespread epidemic, with thousands of cases.

While few people die from CFIDS, about a third become seriously disabled, often for months or years. CFIDS, like AIDS, can also cause neurological symptoms, or lead to lymphomas. CFIDS is more contagious than AIDS, although most people exposed do not become ill. The illness appears not to be sexually transmitted. It affects women two to three times as often as men. Treatments, including acyclovir, ketoconazole, and gamma globulin, may be helpful in some cases.

As with AIDS (although for different reasons) government agencies and medical professionals have been slow to respond to CFIDS. Recently, however, important progress has been made. Milestones include publication by the U.S. Centers for Disease Control of official criteria for diagnosis, and a major scientific conference in San Francisco in April 1989.

The best single information source on CFIDS (also called CFS, for Chronic Fatigue Syndrome) is *The CFIDS Chronicle*, published by Community Health Services, P.O. Box 220398, Charlotte, NC 28222-0398, phone 704/362-CFID.

## COMMUNITY RESEARCH ALLIANCE HYPERICIN FUNDING

Our issue number 90 included an appeal to help San Francisco's Community Research Alliance finish its hypericin observational study. Readers contributed $3049. in response to this appeal. In addition, the Community Research Alliance received two other contributions of $5,000. each.

The total is more than enough to complete the study. Data collection is being finished this week, and there is also a budget for a statistical consultant to help in interpreting the results.

While the hypericin study is proceeding well, we do not have funds to continue the operation of the organization itself beyond the end of January. The Community Research Alliance was started primarily by persons with AIDS. It represents the patient's perspective and interests, but has always been weak on fundraising. Anyone who could help in developing an ongoing fundraising program could contact John James at *AIDS Treatment News*.

# CAUTION: MALICIOUS "AIDS" COMPUTER DISK

Widespread news reports have warned that an "AIDS Information Diskette" mailed to thousands of computer users actually contains a malicious program to destroy other data in the computer. The disk is for IBM PC-compatible personal computers.

The disk was mailed from "PC Cyborg Corp.," a company which may not exist. A Panama City address included with the program was fictitious.

The malicious program is not technically a computer virus, because it does not spread from computer to computer. The program appears to involve no great technical sophistication. What is unusual about this case is that someone appears to have spent over a hundred thousand dollars to package and promote a destructive program, with no apparent motive. The disk was sent primarily to mailing lists of computer users, and to health professionals.

Anyone who receives a copy of the disk should destroy it, so that it is not accidentally installed in any computer.

# SULFADIAZINE TEMPORARY SUPPLY PROBLEM

A temporary interruption in the supply of sulfadiazine, one of the most common drugs used to treat toxoplasmosis, occurred last week when Eli Lilly Co. discontinued manufacturing it. Physicians learned about the supply problem only after patients could not get their prescriptions filled.

At least two other companies are now manufacturing sulfadiazine. Pharmacies should be able to get the drug through their regular wholesalers. Wholesalers can buy sulfadiazine from either Consolidated Midland, in Brewster, NY, or from Lannett, in Philadelphia. Pharmacies can also order directly from Lannett.

# Issue Number 94
# January 5, 1990

## PLANS FOR 1990

*by John S. James*

A year ago, *AIDS Treatment News* published a list of treatments to watch in 1989 (see "Last Year's Predictions," below). This year we are less confident about which treatments may be important—although there are some clear candidates, including ddI, ddC, AzdU, compound Q, and hypericin, among the antivirals. We are less confident than last year about predicting for the year ahead, because so much is happening that it is impossible to follow all relevant developments.

We did select three developments which, in addition to the resource problems we outlined in our last issue, we believe will be important in 1990:

### (1) Viral Tests for Rapid Drug Trials

Existing clinical trials for antivirals (ddI, ddC, and others to follow) are typically planned to run for two years, but may take much longer because they must recruit hundreds of people before the two-year timer begins. These study designs are highly inefficient because they rely on body counts—deaths or other serious events—in those *not* being treated. Therefore the pace is set by the slow progression of AIDS, regardless of how well the new drug works.

We are now on the verge of having better blood tests which will allow researchers to get the same level of statistical proof (of antiviral efficacy in humans) in weeks instead of years, and with far fewer subjects—probably less than a tenth as many as needed today. Such trials could be done now. The tests required are somewhat difficult and expensive; better ones should become available in the future.

The AIDS community must follow this development closely, because the normal forces of inertia which slow the acceptance of any new way of doing things could in this case cost many lives. Federal officials or others may insist that body counts are still necessary to be absolutely sure that the drug, combination or other treatment improves survival, even after safety and antiviral efficacy in patients are well established. No proper weighing of costs and benefits could justify delaying all new antivirals for years because of the small chance that one of them might not save lives even after it shows clear antiviral activity in humans.

For more information about new viral tests for rapid drug trials, see the article below.

## (2) Affordable Treatments for the Third World

Almost no research anywhere in the world is developing treatment options for Africa or elsewhere (including the Third World nation of poverty within the United States) where people cannot afford AZT-scale drug prices. Most of the world is being written off.

But occasionally an affordable treatment possibility accidentally appears. The most important example today is ddC (2',3'-dideoxycytidine—see "ddC: The Low-Cost Antiviral," in *AIDS Treatment News* #89). Now in major U.S. trials in very low doses, ddC may be at least as valuable as AZT or ddI—but it costs pennies a day, is widely available from chemical supply houses throughout the world, and can be taken by mouth with little or no medical technology needed. The drug is dangerous if misused, but traditional healers in any culture could be trained to use it properly, whether or not Western medical infrastructure is available.

No organization in the world is developing ddC as a Third World treatment possibility. Therefore *AIDS Treatment News* will help interested people find each other. To keep informed, write to: ddC Project, *AIDS Treatment News*, P.O. Box 411256, San Francisco, CA 94141.

ddC is only one example. What is needed is an ongoing organization to find and develop the best possible treatment options for those who are otherwise excluded from AIDS/HIV treatment for economic reasons.

## (3) The Sixth International Conference on AIDS, June 20–24 in San Francisco

Each year many if not most of the scientific papers on AIDS are presented at a giant international conference in June. Each January scientists rush to finish work and submit abstracts before the deadline (January 22 this year). The 1990 meeting is in San Francisco; previous meetings were in Montreal, Stockholm, Washington, Paris, and Atlanta. In San Francisco there may also be a meeting of NGOs (non-governmental organizations) before the conference, as there was last year in Montreal.

To avoid overcrowding, the international conference will only admit 12,000 paid registrants; to be sure to get in, persons should register early.

This year's international conference differs from the previous ones in that it is not co-sponsored by the government of the host country. The School of Medicine of the University of California San Francisco is responsible for planning, funding, and conducting the event.

This year's conference also differs from all previous ones in that it is threatened by U.S. government rules which make it difficult and possibly dangerous for persons with HIV to enter the United States, even for a few days for a scientific conference. They must apply for a special waiver, a difficult procedure as there are no clear standards of what constitutes an acceptable application, and therefore no clear end to the work needed to gather supporting evidence. In addition, persons will have their passport stamped with a code which identifies them as HIV-positive, and may subject them to discrimination in their own countries or elsewhere.

Organizations which have withdrawn from the conference as a result of this policy include the European AIDS Service Organizations, the League of Red Cross and Red Crescent Societies, the Scandinavian AIDS and HIV organizations, British Hemophilia Society, Canadian Hemophilia Society, British Frontliners, British Red Cross, Norwegian Red Cross, several member organizations of the UK NGO AIDS Consortium, and in the U.S., the National Association of People With AIDS.

It is commonly believed that the travel restrictions which already are disrupting planning for the conference were imposed by an act of Congress in 1987. But according to Steve Morin, legislative assistant to Congresswoman Nancy Pelosi (Democrat, San Francisco), the documentary history clearly shows that the intent of Congress was to restrict only permanent or long-term residents, not short-term visitors. Apparently the law passed by Congress was misinterpreted by Federal officials who wrote the regulations.

## Last Year's Treatment Predictions

A year ago, *AIDS Treatment News* #72 listed the following nine treatments to watch in 1989:

- ddI
- passive immunotherapy
- hypericin
- compound Q
- Chinese anti-infection herbs
- FLT (fluorodeoxythymidine)
- AzdU
- D4T
- Soluble CD4

To evaluate our predictions in detail would require researching the current status of all these treatments—research effort which we would rather spend on other matters. Two of the treatments—ddI and compound Q, both largely unknown a year ago—did receive major attention during 1989 and are still promising. We do not know of any of the nine which has been eliminated from consideration. But overall, we may have been too optimistic in expecting more in 1989 than would be accomplished.

In 1990 we hope that new methods of quantifying virus in the blood will allow rapid determination of whether proposed antivirals do or do not work—and if so, how well they work—during actual use by patients.

**January 5, 1990**

# NEW VIRAL MEASUREMENT FOR RAPID DRUG TESTING

*by John S. James*

On December 14, 1989, *The New England Journal of Medicine* published an editorial and two articles on measuring the amount of HIV in blood. Since then we have heard that many AIDS experts consider this work among the most important of the year. At first it was not clear to us why a new blood test should be so important, when what we need are treatments.

The new tests are important because they tell researchers quickly and accurately which antivirals are working in actual human use—and how well they are working. It should now take weeks, instead of two years or more, to obtain statistical proof that a treatment does have efficacy in patients.

The new tests could break the logjam of promising drugs waiting for clinical trials. Also, they should make it possible to find the best doses quickly, to develop drug combinations rationally, and even to tell individuals whether a particular treatment regimen is working for them, and when it has stopped working and should be changed.

In the past, the only rapid test for antiviral activity was in a laboratory dish. Even if the drug worked and was known to be safe, many questions remained. Would enough of the drug be absorbed? Would it get to the virus in the body? Could high enough concentrations be achieved? Would the drug remain in the body long enough to have the desired effect? The new tests bypass these questions by directly measuring whether or not patients' viral levels have decreased. They quickly measure antiviral effectiveness of treatments in actual use, not of chemicals in test tubes.

The biggest bottleneck to making new drugs available is the time taken by very slow, cumbersome, and expensive clinical trials. For example, since hundreds of volunteers are needed to prove that each antiviral works, each trial must run at many different sites, requiring time-consuming coordination among institutions in distant cities; for example, dozens of different IRBs (institutional review boards) must approve any change in the protocol of a major trial. By contrast, the new tests can show a clear, unambiguous antiviral effect in a handful of patients in a few weeks.

There are several different approaches to quantifying HIV levels in blood plasma or blood cells. The ones described last month in *The New England Journal of Medicine* have the most visibility and professional momentum at this time; they are the ones ready for use now. We will focus on them in this article, but also mention alternative approaches.

## Background: Viral Cultures

Most (although not all) methods for quantifying HIV in blood use viral cultures; in other words, they determine if the virus is present by attempting to grow it in the laboratory. HIV cultures have been used for several years, but until now they have not proved very useful for measuring the effects of antivirals. The fundamental problem is that cultures remained positive even after treatment, and therefore they did not show how well the treatment worked. No drug yet known can kill all the AIDS virus in patients; therefore, to evaluate a drug today, we need a quantitative test—one that shows how much virus is present, not just whether or not any is there.

In addition, there are practical difficulties with using viral cultures—and these remain today. The tests are more expensive than routine blood work like T-cell counts, and they require special laboratory facilities to protect lab workers from exposure to virus. Also, it is difficult to get consistent results with viral cultures—partly because the tests must use human blood cells as "food" for HIV, and since everyone's cells are different, it is difficult or impossible to reproduce a test exactly. Fortunately the ACTG (AIDS Clinical Trials Group) of the U.S. National Institute of Allergy and Infectious Diseases has certified certain labs as able to perform viral cultures competently. At this time, because of the difficulty of doing viral cultures, the best way to get them done for clinical trials is probably by collaboration between researchers doing the trials and those developing testing methods. The latter usually need more blood samples for their research—especially samples collected under the controlled, well-documented conditions of clinical trials.

## Measuring AIDS Virus in the Blood

The most important new development for faster testing of new treatments was the publication last month of a means for measuring the amount of HIV in blood (Ho and others, 1989). Two different tests were reported: one for blood plasma, and the other for certain blood cells.

The basic idea of the new tests is so simple that it is surprising no one tried it before. The sample of blood plasma (or blood cells) is successively diluted to lower and lower concentrations, until finally the solution is so dilute that usually there is no virus left in the small amount of the solution which is tested. Ordinary viral cultures are run at all the different dilutions, and the researchers merely note the amount of dilution beyond which the cultures stop being positive. From this information, the amount of virus in the original blood serum or cell sample can be estimated.

Since it is not known how many viral particles may be needed to make a culture become positive, the test does not estimate the actual number of particles, but rather gives results in units called "tissue-culture-infective doses" (TCID) per milliliter of blood. For example, patients with asymptomatic HIV infection were found to have 30 TCID per milliliter of blood plasma—meaning that one thirtieth of a milliliter was enough to infect a viral culture and make it positive, while less than that amount was not enough.

Dr. Ho and his team found virus in the plasma and blood cells of every one of 54 HIV-positive persons who were not receiving antiviral treatment—and from none of 22 HIV-negative subjects used as controls. While persons who were asymptomatic had only 30 TCID per millimeter of plasma, persons with AIDS and ARC had over 100 times as much virus, 3500 and 3200 TCID respectively. Blood cells from persons with AIDS or ARC were also found to be more than 100 times as infective as cells from asymptomatic seropositives (20 TCID per million cells for asymptomatic patients, 2200 for AIDS, and 2700 for ARC).

How well do these tests show whether a treatment is working? Seven patients were tested before and after four weeks of AZT; the amount of virus in plasma dropped 94 percent, although unfortunately the level of virus in blood cells did not change greatly. In contrast, in four persons with ARC who were not receiving antiviral treatment, the viral levels in plasma remained stable during the 12 to 20 weeks they were tested.

These results clearly showed antiviral effectiveness of AZT in human use, in a four-week test with only seven patients. In six of the seven, plasma viral levels decreased more than ten times; in the seventh, they decreased almost ten times. But in clinically stable, untreated patients, the levels stayed the same. This complete separation between treated patients and controls suggests that statistical proof of antiviral efficacy could be obtained with a small number of volunteers; and the short time required (four weeks to prove efficacy of AZT, for example) might allow placebo trials to be ethically conducted in clinically stable patients who agreed to risk being untreated for that time (some patients cannot tolerate standard treatment anyway). Placebo trials can usually get results much faster than trials which use an active control such as AZT.

A well-designed, focused program of small, rapid clinical trials could screen the most attractive of the many safe, available, but so far unproven treatment possibilities, and provide numerical measures showing which ones do or do not work to reduce the AIDS virus in actual use by patients. Such a program could quickly and inexpensively test ddI, ddC, compound Q, hypericin, very low doses of AZT, etc., as well as drug combinations, or even proposed diet or lifestyle changes. Some immune modulators might also be found to reduce viral levels indirectly, by helping the body control HIV, even if there is no direct antiviral effect. Such a testing program could give much better guidance for making treatment decisions than any information now available, and greatly reduce the time now taken for clinical trials and new-drug approval.

(Note: Part II of this article will examine other new evidence that plasma viral level is the best marker available to show the stage of HIV infection. It will also discuss other approaches to measuring HIV in the blood, including R-HEV and quantitative PCR.)

## REFERENCES

Ho, DD and others. Quantitation of Human Immunodeficiency Virus Type 1 in the Blood of Infected Persons. *The New England Journal of Medicine*, volume 321, number 24, pages 1621-1625, December 14, 1989.

# CMV/HERPES THERAPIES– SCANNING THE NEWS

*By Denny Smith*

The story of treatments for cytomegalovirus (CMV) infection contains more than its share of chapters on intrigue and neglect. When CMV was first recognized as an AIDS opportunistic infection, no drug was yet available to treat it effectively. Slowly the AIDS community became aware of ganciclovir (see DHPG, *AIDS Treatment News* #44) and then of Foscarnet (*AIDS Treatment News* #71), as effective but limited therapies for CMV retinitis or colitis. Ganciclovir was begrudgingly approved last year by the FDA; but Foscarnet, which could save the eyesight of many PWAs who cannot continue with ganciclovir, remains unapproved and generally unavailable.

CMV belongs to a viral family which includes the cause of cold sores and genital lesions (herpes simplex 1 and 2, or HSV), the cause of chicken pox and shingles (varicella-zoster virus, or VZV), and one source of mononucleosis and certain lymphomas (Epstein-Barr virus, or EBV). These viruses are commonly latent in the general population, but can re-emerge as an active infection for people who are HIV-positive or who must take immunosuppressive drugs to protect transplanted organs.

Fortunately, the "herpesvirus" family is well-studied and some FDA-approved drugs, as well as several investigational agents, appear to have overlapping activity against more than one herpesvirus. Acyclovir (Zovirax), can be administered orally for mild herpes simplex flareups, or intravenously for severe episodes. Acyclovir is relatively non-toxic, and may suppress latent CMV as well as HSV, and is often prescribed in conjunction with AZT (*AIDS Treatment News* #86).

Unfortunately, certain toxicities may pose limits on the duration of other drugs, or their safety in combination with AZT and other treatments. Prolonged treatment with ganciclovir often results in neutropenia (low neutrophil counts), and Foscarnet can be toxic to the kidneys. Vidarabine as well as Foscarnet has been used successfully to treat herpes simplex which will not respond to acyclovir, but vidarabine can suppress bone marrow, making it a questionable choice to replace ganciclovir for treating CMV. Since ganciclovir and Foscarnet pose different toxicities, people who cannot tolerate ganciclovir should have unqualified access to Foscarnet, in our opinion. In terms of therapeutic value against CMV, however, Foscarnet is not considered to be superior to ganciclovir.

We spoke to Shelley M. Gordon, M.D., an infectious disease specialist who said early trial results indicate that granulocyte macrophage-colony stimulating factor (GM-CSF) can counter the neutropenia of ganciclovir, allowing extended use of that treatment. Dr. Gordon also described laser treatments as a successful way to correct retinal detachment caused by CMV, although they would be a complementary treatment and not a replacement for anti-viral drug maintenance therapy. Laser therapy is available already for many other indications, but GM-CSF is accessible only through participation in clinical trials.

In September *AIDS Treatment News* #87 reported the early success with GM-CSF for controlling the toxicity of AZT and alpha interferon, a combination approved to treat KS and which may also prove synergistic against HIV. Dr. Gordon mentioned that interferon has been discussed as a possible agent for treating CMV as well.

Ganciclovir is presently administered intravenously, but studies are under way testing the effectiveness of an oral formulation, as well as intraocular injections. *In vitro* studies suggest that DFMO (Eflornithine) has a synergistic effect with ganciclovir, implying that lower, less toxic doses might be possible in the future to control retinitis.

We spoke to Danny King, a researcher who has studied a drug called FIAC at Oclassen Pharmaceuticals in San Rafael, California. He said that FIAC is active against all the herpesviruses, as well as the hepatitis B virus. Although FIAC is a nucleoside analog like AZT and ddI, it has no effect on HIV. One early advantage seen with FIAC is its ability to be administered in an oral form. FIAC was first studied in the early 1980s at Memorial Sloan-Kettering Hospital in New York for treating severe VZV and CMV infections, and demonstrated some bone-marrow toxicity and gastro-intestinal upsets.

FIAC is now entering additional phase one (toxicity) trials at four sites: the University of Alabama, the University of Washington in Seattle, the University of California in San Diego and the National Institute of Health in Bethesda. For information about local clinical trials involving FIAC, GM-CSF, and Foscarnet, interested persons can call 800/TRIALS-A.

In the interest of renewing the discussion of CMV treatments and questions of promising but neglected options, we want to bring attention to a list of possibilities for treating CMV or herpes infections which are still in laboratory or animal studies or known to us anecdotally: aphidicolin (APH); BHT (see *AIDS Treatment News* #10);

capsaicin; decyclovir; dextran sulfate; HPMPA and HPMPC (see *AIDS Treatment News* #76); hypericin; pentosan polysulfate; SQ 32,829 and SQ 33,054; and tumor necrosis factor. Many of these were discussed at the Interscience Conference on Antimicrobial Agents and Chemotherapy last September in Houston. Some of them were discussed a year earlier at the same annual conference. At least five CMV possibilities have demonstrated *in vitro* activity against HIV as well as against the herpesviruses: APH, dextran sulfate, pentosan polysulfate, foscarnet, and hypericin.

The question now is how long these possibilities will remain on the drawing board, and why Foscarnet, GM-CSF and FIAC are usually not available to many people who need them. Compassionate use or parallel track access does not seem too much to ask for people who stand to lose first their sight and then their lives.

# IN MEMORIAM: NATHANIEL PIER, 1952–1989

Nathaniel Pier, M.D., one of the strongest advocates for faster development of AIDS treatments, died of AIDS complications on December 27, 1989.

We first spoke with Dr. Pier in 1986, while researching lentinan. He had long urged trials for this drug, an immune modulator derived from the shiitake mushroom and widely used in Japan in treating cancer. In February 1988 Dr. Pier presented the history of his four-year efforts to spark research on lentinan to the Presidential Commission on the HIV Epidemic. (Recently clinical trials of lentinan were conducted at San Francisco General Hospital, and at New York's Community Research Initiative.)

Dr. Pier, who had a large AIDS practice in New York, was also a founder of the Community Research Initiative, a model organization for conducting clinical trials outside of the usual research centers, through the help of practicing physicians. Dr. Pier and the other founders carried the organization through the first difficult year before it was popular, and stayed with it afterwards.

*AIDS Treatment News* published interviews with Dr. Pier on January 1, 1988 and August 12, 1988. The conclusion of the August interview suggested the "parallel track" later proposed by NIAID director Anthony Fauci, M.D., as well as the criticism of mainstream clinical AIDS research which is now becoming more common:

"The current system simply has not produced the goods. And if Dr. Frank Young's prediction [of few new drugs approved by 1991] is any indication, it will not produce the goods for a long time to come. This consigns large numbers of people to death without giving them a dignified chance to fight back. It is not an acceptable human or reasonable approach to doing research in this epidemic.

"After five years of being on the front lines, my heartfelt feeling is that the top priority for people with AIDS and people who care about AIDS is to demand access to experimental therapies to try to save their lives.

"I appeal to people to organize this effort immediately, to bring it forward in their local groups, then present the case to their political people, and to the people who are running the present medical system of testing drugs. It's time we told them that the emperor has no clothes, that the current system is not working. It's time to insist on wider access to promising therapies, and rapid testing of existing drugs to develop better treatment options."

In our last conversation, shortly before his death, Dr. Pier told us that hypericin herbal extracts appeared disappointing to him and other New York physicians—they were not seeing the results that had been hoped. Earlier, Dr. Pier had been the first to tell us that AL 721, and later dextran sulfate, appeared disappointing.

Dr. Pier graduated summa cum laude from the University of California at Berkeley in 1974, and received his M.D. from the Albert Einstein College of Medicine in 1977. He is survived by his lover, Michael Hannaway.

# Issue Number 95
# January 19, 1990

## MYCOPLASMA INCOGNITUS: NEWLY DISCOVERED TREATABLE OPPORTUNISTIC INFECTION?

*by John S. James*

Researchers at the U.S. Armed Forces Institute of Pathology (AFIP) in Washington, D.C., and the Warren Grant Magnuson Clinical Center at the National Institutes of Health, have found compelling evidence that a previously unrecognized opportunistic infection—one potentially treatable with antibiotics—may be a major cause of illness in people with AIDS. Many infections of organs including the brain, spleen, liver, or lymph nodes—as well as some systemic infections—might be caused by the newly-discovered organism, called *Mycoplasma incognitus*. Until now, these infections would be counted among the many which cannot be diagnosed.

While the first report of the organism now known as *Mycoplasma incognitus* was published over three years ago, most of what is now known was learned later and published last year. And only in the last few weeks has the AIDS research community paid serious attention. Until recently the new organism was mistakenly believed to be a virus, and its discovery seemed to have little immediate relevance to treatment.

Then a series of five articles by Shyh-Ching Lo and others in the *American Journal of Tropical Medicine and Hygiene*, between February and November 1989, showed:

(1) The new organism is a mycoplasma—which is potentially treatable. Mycoplasma, a form of life between bacteria and viruses in complexity, was discovered about 100 years ago. Some species are known to cause human diseases.

The published articles only hint that the new organism might be treatable with antibiotics. But scientists at AFIP tested 15 common antibiotics against the *Mycoplasma incognitus* in the laboratory. A detailed report is being prepared for publication, but because of the public-health importance of the information, AFIP released a list of the drugs and their effective concentrations in a separate document. Doxycycline, tetracycline, clindamycin, lincomycin, and ciprofloxacin were found to be effective against *Mycoplasma incognitus*. But erythromycin, the antibiotic most commonly used to treat mycoplasma infections, was not effective—and penicillin, streptomycin, gentamicin, and others also had no effect.

(2) *Mycoplasma incognitus* was found in the thymus, liver, spleen, lymph node, or brain of 22 of 34 persons who had died of AIDS. The patients who were selected for this autopsy study had all had evidence of organ failures.

(3) In a separate study with different patients, the mycoplasma was found in seven of ten persons with AIDS. Also, a much earlier study had found *Mycoplasma incognitus* in blood lymphocytes of 12 of 23 living persons with AIDS—but in none of 22 healthy blood donors used as controls.

(4) The mycoplasma was also found in six HIV-negative patients (with no sign of AIDS) from different parts of the world, who had died in one to seven weeks of an undiagnosed infection.

No one knows how the organism spreads, but evidently it is not by casual contact, as family members of infected persons have not become infected themselves.

(5) Four monkeys were injected with *Mycoplasma incognitus*; all died in seven to nine months. The organism was found in the spleens of all the monkeys, and in some other organs as well. It was not found in a fifth monkey tested as a control.

(6) Extensive evidence from electron-microscope examinations, from specially designed PCR tests to look for the DNA of *Mycoplasma incognitus*, and from immunologic tests, showed that the organism was concentrated in lesions in affected organs. *Mycoplasma incognitus* is unusual in that it often infects and kills tissue without causing an inflammatory reaction, suggesting that it disables or evades part of the immune system.

The publication of this evidence, much of it in November 1989, led to a meeting between Dr. Anthony Fauci, director of NIAID (the National Institute of Allergy and Infectious Diseases) and other AIDS experts, with Dr. Lo and his colleagues at AFIP. The meeting, on December 14, 1989 in San Antonio, was chaired by Dr. Joel B. Baseman, chairman of the Department of Microbiology at the University of Texas Health Sciences Center in San Antonio, an expert on mycoplasma. An article in *The Washington Post* (January 5) quoted Dr. Baseman as saying that Lo's mycoplasma "might be a significant agent for many infectious diseases, not just AIDS. There is enough information to say that this agent is real." The same article quoted Dr. Fauci as saying that *Mycoplasma incognitus* "may be an important opportunistic infection . . . If it's real, it could have an important impact on how doctors look at AIDS patients with unexplained problems."

An in-depth history of the discovery of *Mycoplasma incognitus* and its early dismissal by parts of the scientific community was published in *The New York Times*, January 16, 1990.

## What Should Be Done Now?

Awareness of the new importance of *Mycoplasma incognitus* has not yet spread far in the medical community. The biggest problem is that there is no readily available test for the organism; at this time, there may be only one research lab which can do the test reliably. Other mycoplasmologists are becoming involved, however, and a much easier blood test is being developed. In addition, clinical trials are now being planned.

The AIDS physician and patient community should help make sure that trials proceed quickly. There may also be immediate uses of the new information, for example:

## (1) Empirical Use of Antibiotics

Several months ago, before *Mycoplasma incognitus* was known, Dr. Nathaniel Pier mentioned that he had found good results trying doxycycline for patients who had an apparent infection which could not be diagnosed. (Doxycycline is the antibiotic most often discussed as a possible treatment for *Mycoplasma incognitus*; however neither it nor any other antibiotic has yet been tested for treating this infection in humans.) Incidentally, the next physician we asked about empirical use of antibiotics preferred erythromycin, which would *not* be effective against the mycoplasma.

The discovery of *Mycoplasma incognitus* provides an additional rationale for trying doxycycline (or one of the other antibiotics found effective against this organism in the laboratory) for certain patients, such as those with signs of undiagnosed infection, especially in the central nervous system, spleen, or certain other organs. Patients should know that antibiotics can cause side effects—some of which, such as over-growth of *Candida*, might be more severe in persons with HIV. Physicians and patients must use appropriate precautions.

Physicians' groups could make a major contribution by developing interim guide-lines for empirical use of antibiotics—guidelines to use now before a blood test for *Mycoplasma incognitus* is available. It may seem premature to develop guidelines with no diagnostic test and no trial results. But physicians are already using antibiotics empirically to treat undiagnosed infections in persons with AIDS or HIV. Instead of waiting months or years for definitive information, it would be helpful to collect reports of such clinical experience with the drugs known to be active against the organism, detailed information about the symptoms of persons who have already been found to be infected, and any special precautions necessary when using the antibiotics to treat persons with AIDS or HIV.

## (2) A Rapid Clinical Trial Research Design

The usual kind of clinical trial—randomly treating some patients and leaving others untreated, then waiting to see which group does better—would create some unusual ethical, practical, and scientific problems in this case. Therefore we are suggesting a possible alternative, which research groups, including community-based research organizations, might want to consider. Readers not interested in clinical trial design might want to skip this section. We included it because some of the ideas are not obvious, and we believe they might contribute to discussions of clinical trials.

The *scientific* problem with the common trial design—selecting patients who test positive for *Mycoplasma incognitus* and randomly treating part of the group with a broad-spectrum antibiotic like doxycycline—is that AIDS/HIV patients have many undiagnosed infections, so patients might improve even if mycoplasma is not what is being treated. We propose the following design which not only overcomes this problem, but also answers the ethical concerns about leaving patients untreated, and at the same time makes a trial much less costly and easier to administer. This design would be especially suitable for community-based research. And it should prove definitively whether or not a given test for mycoplasma is relevant to the decision to use or not to use a particular treatment.

Before beginning the trial, it would be necessary to negotiate arrangements to get blood samples tested for mycoplasma. At this time, AFIP may be the only organization which could do this work.

When the trial begins, the physicians involved would continue their usual treatment, making decisions strictly for their patients' benefit, not for research. Those patients who met clinical criteria suggesting possible *Mycoplasma incognitus* infection could be enrolled in the trial. A blood sample would be taken before antibiotic treatment began, and sent to the lab for the mycoplasma test. Later, the physicians would rate how well the patients had responded to the treatment.

The research organization would "blind" both parties. The physicians would not know which patients' blood samples had tested positive for mycoplasma. And the lab which tested the samples would not know which patients had responded to the treatment.

The results would be analyzed by a two-by-two table, or similar statistical technique. One dimension of the table would divide patients who did or did not respond to the antibiotic; the other dimension would be whether or not the patients tested positive for mycoplasma. A statistically significant relationship between the two variables would prove that it is possible to use the blood-test information to help predict who is likely to respond to the therapy. Such a result would strongly support the hypothesis that the mycoplasma was causing human disease, although academic scientists could still argue that the mycoplasma might only be a marker for some other organism which was the real target of the treatment. (Even if this possibility were true it would have no practical effect, as it would not diminish the usefulness of the test for predicting which patients would respond to the treatment.)

Note that the trial we propose would *not* prove that treatment was better than no treatment for any particular group of patients, since no one is randomly assigned to be deliberately left untreated. In theory, this question of whether treatment or no treatment is best is the key issue which trials are designed to address. But in the situation here, after a successful trial as outlined above, that question would not really be the point at issue. For the patients would clearly have needed treatment and have a poor prognosis without it; they would have responded to a generally safe and very well known treatment, and the trial would have generated strong evidence that *Mycoplasma incognitus* did cause human disease (in addition to the strong pathology evidence already available). The issue of whether the patients would have been better left untreated would only be academic.

One apparent problem with this proposed design is that it would be difficult to calculate in advance the number of patients needed (to prove statistically that the test for *Mycoplasma incognitus* would be useful for guiding treatment decisions). If the two-by-two table turned out to be strongly unbalanced on either of its dimensions—for example, if 99 percent of the clinically-selected patients tested positive for the mycoplasma, or if 99 percent tested negative—the number of patients required for proof would be very large. But again this problem is more apparent than real. For if the table is highly unbalanced, then the result of the study would not only be more expensive to obtain, it would also be less valuable, as it would affect few treatment decisions.

Therefore if the first group of patients tested were to show that either dimension of the table was strongly unbalanced, the study could be aborted at that point and redesigned. Therefore, a worst-case maximum number of patients (and cost estimate) could be prepared in advance for planning purposes.

Most observational studies—those which simply record results of patients' treatment, without randomly assigning patients to receive different regimens—cannot produce statistical proof of any hypothesis. We believe that the design proposed above is an exception. It avoids the usual constraints by asking a different question: not "does the drug work," but "can information from the test help determine which patients will or will not respond to the drug." By addressing this question instead of the usual one, the proposed trial allows treatment to proceed totally in the patients' interest, without any compromise for research purposes—while at the same time rigorously proving (or failing to prove, or even disproving) a medically relevant hypothesis.

## Summary

The organism previously called a "virus-like infectious agent," discovered by Dr. Shyh-Ching Lo and colleagues at the Armed Forces Institute of Pathology, has been found to be a mycoplasma which is susceptible to several common antibiotics. Even before a blood test is widely available and clinical trials have been done, physicians may want to consider this new information when choosing empirical antibiotic treatment for patients with certain undiagnosed problems. We will report further as more information becomes available.

## REFERENCES

Altman LK. Unusual microbe, once dismissed, is now taken more seriously. *The New York Times*, January 16, 1990, page B6.

Booth, W; Specter, M. Microbe may play role in AIDS, other diseases. *The Washington Post*, January 5, 1990, page A3.

Lo SC; Dawson MS; Wong DM; Newton PB 3d; Sonoda MA; Engler WF; Wang RY; Shih JW; Alter JH; Wear DJ. Identification of Mycoplasma incognitus infection in patients with AIDS: an immunohistochemical, in situ hybridization and ultrastructural study. *American Journal of Tropical Medicine and Hygiene*, November 1989, volume 41, number 5, pages 601-616.

Lo SC; Shih JW; Newton PB 3d; Wong DM; Hayes MM; Benish JR; Wear DJ; Wang RY. Virus-like infectious agent (VLIA) is a novel pathogenic mycoplasma: Mycoplasma incognitus. *American Journal of Tropical Medicine and Hygiene*, November 1989, volume 41, number 5, pages 586-600.

Lo SC; Dawson MS; Newton PB 3rd; Sonoda MA; Shih JW; Engler WF; Wang RY; Wear DJ. Association of the virus-like infectious agent originally reported in patients with AIDS with acute fatal disease in previously healthy non-AIDS patients. *American Journal of Tropical Medicine and Hygiene*, September 1989, volume 41, number 3, pages 364-376.

Lo SC; Wang RY; Newton PB 3d; Yang NY; Sonoda MA; Shih JW. Fatal infection of silvered leaf monkeys with a virus-like infectious agent (VLIA) derived from a patient with AIDS. *American Journal of Tropical Medicine and Hygiene*, April 1989, volume 40, number 4, pages 399-409.

Lo SC; Shih JW; Yang NY; Ou CY; Wang RY. A novel virus-like infectious agent in patients with AIDS. *American Journal of Tropical Medicine and Hygiene*, February 1989, volume 40, number 2, pages 213-226.

In addition, the *New York Native* has published frequent and sometimes controversial coverage of this research.

# CRYPTOSPORIDIOSIS NEWS

*by Denny Smith*

Infections of the intestinal parasite *Cryptosporidium* can be extremely debilitating, causing abdominal cramping, watery stools, weight loss and fatigue. A recent report from Columbia University (Roberts, 1989) describes *Cryptosporidium* in patients who did not have any symptoms, suggesting that some people might be carriers, and the possibility that even if the protozoan is found in people with HIV who have diarrhea, cryptosporidiosis might not necessarily be the cause.

Last June, *AIDS Treatment News* published a report on the drug diclazuril, a possible treatment for cryptosporidiosis (issue #80). Diclazuril is available for agricultural use under the trade name Clinicox, and human trials have been proceeding to determine efficacy and toxicity.

We contacted each of the three diclazuril study sites in New York, and found results which are preliminary yet hopeful. Douglas Dieterich, M.D. of New York University, Rosemary Soave, M.D. of Cornell University and Donald Kotler, M.D. at Columbia University St. Luke's/Roosevelt Hospital Center have found that so far the drug has reduced *Cryptosporidium* oocyst counts in some participants at doses ranging from 200 mg to 400 mg, given daily for one week. No side effects have been noted; doses below 200 mg did not affect cyst counts. Some participants also reported a reduction in the frequency and volume of diarrhea, but this observation is not yet statistically significant. They plan to initiate a 600 mg dose as well as a 28-day protocol, with the rationale that a higher or longer dose regimen may improve the results.

They are also recruiting for a study of hyper-immune milk to treat cryptosporidiosis. In addition, Dr. Kotler's office is conducting a study of a salicylic acid compound called asacol to treat non-specific HIV-related bowel inflammation, and Dr. Soave is studying the efficacy of the investigational antibiotic spiramycin, given intravenously.

Researchers at the University of Texas in Houston have proposed that eflornithine (DFMO), which is active against *Pneumocystis*, may alleviate some of the symptoms of cryptosporidiosis, and might work especially well if tried in conjunction with hyper-immune colostrum. The use of antibody-rich milk or colostrum from cows or goats which have been inoculated with *Cryptosporidium* has long been discussed as a possibility for treating such infections in people with HIV. In January of 1988 *AIDS Treatment News* #49 mentioned this idea along with several other promising approaches to cryptosporidiosis, including AZT, trimetrexate with leucovorin (sometimes discussed as a treatment for PCP), spiramycin, somatostatin, Artemesia annua (an herb reportedly used successfully to treat malaria which will not respond to antibiotics), and garlic.

Spiramycin is available on a compassionate use basis and has been shown to reduce cyst counts and the severity of diarrhea in some people. Somatostatin and AZT can also relieve some diarrhea but can not eliminate the infection. We have not heard any substantial news regarding the other treatments, except for scattered rumors that large amounts of garlic may help control both cryptosporidiosis and toxoplasmosis (each is caused by protozoa).

*AIDS Treatment News* has received anecdotal reports of another treatment for cryptosporidiosis which is available in Mexico and now used by some PWA's in the U.S. The treatment is named mebeciclol, although it is not just one drug but actually three separate agents combined in one tablet.

We spoke to Ronald Woodroof, director of the Dallas Buyer's Club which has informally monitored people who have tried mebeciclol. The Dallas club has also monitored a French product called roxithromycin (see *AIDS Treatment News* #75 for background information) used by its members who were looking for new treatments for cryptosporidiosis. Mr. Woodroof described to us anecdotal reports which suggest that neither mebeciclol nor roxithromycin alone were very effective at ridding the body of the parasites or even controlling the profuse diarrhea associated with cryptosporidiosis. But a specific combination of the two has apparently helped some people.

The combination as it has evolved so far concurrently applies roxithromycin twice a day for four weeks, and mebeciclol three times daily for two weeks. Roxithromycin comes in tablets of 150 mg, and mebeciclol, also in tablets, is composed of 60 mg of mebendazole, 200 mg of niclosamide, and 300 mg of tinidazole. The first two of these three are already approved in the U.S. to treat certain parasites. Mr. Woodroof noted that the combination usually increased diarrhea initially, possibly due to successful killing of the parasite colonies, but that within several days the diarrhea improved.

We want to emphasize the speculative nature of this treatment combination, yet make the information available to physicians and PWA's who have not had success otherwise dealing with this debilitating infection. As with any experimental therapy, we strongly advocate the supervision of a physician for administering and monitoring roxithromycin or mebeciclol.

Anyone who has had significant experience involving mebeciclol, roxithromycin, spiramycin, hyper-immune milk, diclazuril or other attempts to treat cryptosporidiosis is encouraged to write to *AIDS Treatment News* or call Denny or John at 415/255-0588.

## REFERENCES

Roberts, W G and others. "Prevalence of cryptosporidiosis in patients undergoing endoscopy: evidence for an asymptomatic carrier state." *American Journal of Medicine*, November 1989, volume 87, number 5, pages 537-539.

Rolston, K V I and others. Intestinal cryptosporidiosis treated with eflornithine: a prospective study among patients with AIDS. *Journal of Acquired Immune Deficiency Syndromes*, October 1989, volume 2, number 5, pages 426-430.

# AZT LOWER DOSE APPROVED

During the last several months there has been a strong movement among physicians to prescribe lower doses of AZT for most patients—not the 1200 mg per day which has been officially recommended. While there is still difference of opinion in the medical community, the standard of care seems to be moving toward 500 mg per day—a dose which appears to be just as effective as 1200, and less toxic. Physicians could legally prescribe the lower dose all along; but because many will follow the official recommendation, there was much pressure on Burroughs Wellcome to apply to the FDA for a change in the official "labeling" of the drug, and to provide the data to support the change. The FDA could not make the change on its own, without an application and data from the company.

Recently this work has been accomplished, and the labeling now includes an optional dose reduction, to 600 mg per day, after one month of 1200. (There is still some question of whether the lower dose will work as well as the 1200 mg dose for treating patients with neurological complications, and this uncertainty is reflected in the official language.)

One major benefit of the labeling change is that some of the new clinical trials anticipated the movement to the lower dose; their protocols allowed the AZT dose to be reduced as soon as the FDA changed the labeling. Since those protocols had already been approved by the Institutional Review Boards (IRBs) of the different institutions which will run the trials, the change to low dose can be made quickly, without waiting for all the IRBs to meet again to approve the new dose. The high AZT dose has seriously slowed recruitment for some of the trials, because patients have been unwilling to risk receiving that much AZT.

Why does the official labeling specify 600 mg, instead of 500 which was becoming medical practice? The 600 mg dose implies that patients will wake up in the middle of the night to take a pill; the 500 dose does not. Also, why does the official labeling specify at least one month at 1200 mg? This month of high dose may cause some patients to discontinue the drug, due to side effects such as headache and nausea.

We have heard repeatedly from AIDS experts that there is no medical reason for the choice of 600 mg per day, or for the recommendation of 1200 for at least the first month the patient is on the drug. The official recommendation came out as it did because the data Burroughs Wellcome submitted to support the change came from one study (ACTG 002). About three years ago, when this study was being designed, there was much less experience with AZT. The regimen for the low-dose arm of the trial was selected as a compromise among the study designers. The FDA had to decide the new labeling based on the data submitted. Therefore the new labeling, while a great improvement over the old, may have been outdated on the day it was issued.

# FLU SHOTS RECOMMENDED

A major influenza epidemic is developing in the United States this year, and it is not too late to get the flu shot. It takes about two weeks for the immunization to provide protection.

Persons with AIDS or HIV should check with their physician; those we have heard from are recommending the shots. In some areas they are available without charge through public-health clinics.

# Issue Number 96
# February 2, 1990

## FLUCONAZOLE: IMPORTANT ANTIFUNGAL APPROVED

*by John S. James*

On January 29, the U.S. Food and Drug Administration (FDA) approved fluconazole (brand name Diflucan), a major broad-spectrum antifungal especially important for treating cryptococcal meningitis. Fluconazole, which has long been approved in England, is about equally effective as amphotericin B, but has much less toxicity. Also, fluconazole can be taken by mouth, while amphotericin requires intravenous infusions, often every day in a hospital.

Fluconazole should be available to pharmacies by late February. If local pharmacies cannot get it quickly, patients or physicians could check availability with a mail-order pharmacy such as American Preferred Plan, 800/227-1195 (in New York State the number is 800/445-4519). Until the drug is actually delivered, the PWA Health Group in New York will continue importing it from England, which takes about a week.

We do not know the price, but fluconazole will be very expensive. If price is an obstacle, people should know that another drug itraconazole (brand name Sporanox) may be almost as good as fluconazole and is available in Mexico at a fraction of the fluconazole price (see *AIDS Treatment News* #80).

### History and Comment

Physicians familiar with fluconazole agree that it should have been approved long ago, probably well over a year ago. No one seems to know why it took so long for this drug to become widely available in the United States.

*AIDS Treatment News* published an in-depth article on fluconazole over two years ago ("Fluconazole: A Major Advance for Cryptococcal Meningitis and Other Systemic Fungal Infections?" issue #41). At that time the drug was already in widespread use in Europe, where over a thousand people had taken it, mostly for relatively minor infections. In addition, about 150 persons with AIDS had been treated with fluconazole for serious or life-threatening fungal infections. But few U.S. physicians knew about the drug at that time; one leading AIDS specialist told us he had heard about fluconazole but could not follow up because he did not know how to get more information about it. (*AIDS Treatment News* had also given up on an earlier attempt to cover fluconazole, because we could not find information.)

The fluconazole history illustrates once again how much U.S. medicine could improve if it could take advantage of important treatment successes in common use elsewhere in the world. In this age of rapid globalization of business and communication, why is medicine such a major exception to the trend? The answer is that the corporate/regulatory dynamic creates business, regulatory, professional, political, and media empires which are threatened by the free flow of medical practice into the United States from other countries. Medicine will be the last refuge of protectionism, to the great detriment of the health of the American people. Progress in solving this problem could make solid contributions to better quality, less costly health care.

While fluconazole was unapproved in the United States, it was made available through studies and/or compassionate use in life-threatening emergencies for people who could not tolerate amphotericin and had no other alternative. We do not know how many fell through the cracks of this system. For example, although the drug was free, did grotesquely underfunded public clinics have the physician time to do the paperwork required? What happened when their clients needed the drug to save their lives?

Of all drugs in history, fluconazole may be the most precisely targeted to matter least to those who in the United States matter most—HIV negative white men. For aside from AIDS, the drug will be especially important to Blacks and members of some other races for treatment of valley fever (coccidioidomycosis), a disease much more serious for them than for whites. (Valley fever is endemic in certain geographical areas, including parts of the Southwestern United States, and the San Joaquin Valley in California.) And in Europe, fluconazole has been used primarily for treating women with vaginal candidiasis. We do not know whether this demographic profile of the drug allowed it to remain unavailable for so long.

*AIDS Treatment News* did not investigate these particular questions about fluconazole because of repeated rumors that approval was imminent. And after mailing our 1987 article to thousands of people, we thought that followup could be left to others. In retrospect, we made a mistake in not pursuing this drug aggressively.

The shallow press coverage of this shameful chapter in U.S. medicine shows that history laundering is well advanced.


# AZT: FDA COMMITTEE RECOMMENDS EARLY USE

On January 30, an advisory committee of the FDA unanimously recommended that AZT be officially approved for treating persons with T-helper counts of 500 or less, even if they have few or no symptoms. Approval is not yet official, but the agency almost always follows such recommendations of its advisory committees.

Physicians already can legally prescribe AZT for any patient, without specific FDA approval. But more physicians will prescribe it for early HIV infection when the drug's official "labeling" suggests that they do so. And when the new recommendation becomes official, it will be much easier than now to get insurance companies to pay for AZT for those patients. Hundreds of thousands of patients could be affected by the new recommendation—but probably most of them do not know that they are HIV positive and will not be receiving medical care.

In the past, the main arguments against early AZT use have been fear of side effects, and fear that the virus might become resistant to the drug. But now it is clear that side effects are much less of a problem if patients are healthier when they start AZT— especially with the lower doses which are increasingly being used. There seems to be less concern about early use causing viral resistance, and more thinking that the drug might be even more effective at slowing the development of the disease if given early than if given late.

Much is still unknown about long-term effects of AZT. The advisory panel decided that it was better to take the risks of using it earlier in HIV infection, than to take the risks of leaving the infection untreated.

# HYPERICIN RESULTS: COMMUNITY RESEARCH ALLIANCE STUDY

*by John S. James*

## Background

Hypericin is an antiviral found in St. John's wort, a plant long used as a medicinal herb. AIDS researchers at New York University have studied hypericin's activity against HIV, and also against other retroviruses in animals (Lavie and others, 1989; Meruelo and others, 1988). Hypericin works in an entirely different way than AZT, and was better than AZT against the retroviral infections in animals.

The researchers have now developed methods for synthesizing large amounts of hypericin; with luck they will begin early "phase I" human trials next summer. Meanwhile the Community Research Alliance, a San Francisco research organization started by San Francisco's PWA Coalition, began its own observational study of hypericin herbal extracts as an AIDS/HIV treatment *last* summer. Because the study volunteers obtained their own extracts from buyers' clubs or health-food stores, the Community Research Alliance did not administer any drug and therefore did not need to go through the FDA to obtain an "IND" (Investigational New Drug approval), which for various reasons would have been impossible in this case. The study complied with legal and ethical requirements by being approved by an Institutional Review Board, which the Community Research Alliance had previously organized in accordance with Federal regulations. The organization's Scientific Advisory Committee had also approved the study.

For more information on the Community Research Alliance, see *AIDS Treatment News* #85. This writer is a co-founder of the Community Research Alliance, and co-author of the formal report of the study, which has been submitted to the Sixth

International Conference on AIDS. The study's principal investigator, and principal author of the report, is William C. Cooper, M.D.

## Methods

The Community Research Alliance study lasted four months; a total of 33 volunteers were enrolled. The only entry criteria was to be HIV positive, and not to have used hypericin extracts within the last six months (so that baseline data could be obtained). Extensive blood tests were given at baseline and at four additional monthly visits; other data collected included medical history, physical examinations before and after the four-month test period, and the Merieux Multitest of skin immune response. All testing and other expenses (except for the cost of the herbal extracts, which the research organization could not legally provide) were paid by the Community Research Alliance, which financed the study primarily through donations from individuals; a grant from the American Foundation for AIDS Research (AmFAR) paid salary for a medical director.

While four months of data were collected, the study actually ran six months, as resource limitations prevented enrollment of all the volunteers at once. There was no problem recruiting people to join the study. Volunteers were not asked to use any particular brand or dose of hypericin extracts, and they were not asked to make any changes in the treatments they would have used anyway, for the sake of the study. They were, of course, asked to report all treatments they used. All volunteers kept daily logs, and compliance with the protocol is believed to have been very good.

A separate treatment database now being developed may be able to collect long-term followup information from the volunteers in the future.

## Results

Of the 33 patients enrolled, 26 completed the four months. Of the seven who did not complete the study, six were hospitalized for AIDS complications and had to drop out; one was dropped for non-compliance with the protocol.

A first look at the data showed no clear trends. About as many of the volunteers had T-helper decreases as increases. But a closer look showed a pattern which had not been expected. Of the 26 volunteers who completed the study, ten had never used any AZT, while ten others had been on AZT throughout (the remaining six had either started or stopped AZT during the four months). Of the ten "AZT virgins," eight had T-helper increases; the mean increase for the ten was 12 percent, which occurred in the first month and was sustained for the four months for which data are available. But of the ten on AZT throughout the study, eight had T-helper decreases, with the mean decrease for the ten of 13 percent. (The mean T-helper count increased nine percent in the first month, then declined.)

These results do not show that AZT worked poorly with hypericin. Those who were on AZT were more seriously ill, with mean T-helper count of 189 at baseline (before they started hypericin) than those who had never used AZT (mean T-helper count 558 at baseline). The difference in outcome is not surprising, since other anti-HIV treatments, such as AZT and ddI, are known to work better in patients who begin with higher T-helper counts.

The 12 percent T-helper increase in the ten who had never used AZT may be a meaningful trend, since without any treatment the average T-helper count would tend to decrease. However the increase in this small group was not enough to be statistically significant, meaning that it might have occurred by chance. The fact that the increase occurred in the first month, and then was sustained for several months, is consistent with results of other antivirals.

P24 antigen test results were inconclusive—although they did show that there was no dramatic antiviral effect of the hypericin-extract treatment. Only six of the 26 who completed the study were p24 positive at the beginning. Two became p24 negative, but they were on AZT throughout the study, so the improvement might have been due to AZT. Of the other four, two went up and two went down. No one changed from negative to positive.

What about safety? There have been several anecdotal reports that some people's liver enzyme values have risen after use of St. John's wort, suggesting possible toxicity. In this study, five of the 26 volunteers showed rises in liver-function test values, and were advised to discontinue the herbal extract. All returned to normal after 30 days off the treatment, except for one who had earlier liver problems and high liver-function values before starting the study. This effect (rise in liver function tests in some patients) is suspected to be due not to hypericin but to some other component in the herbal extract, since animal studies have shown no effect on liver enzymes even when very large doses of pure hypericin were given.

Much other data was collected and has not yet been analyzed. But principal investigator Dr. William Cooper has not seen anything striking or unusual in a first look.

## Comments

A small, uncontrolled observational study like this one is not designed to prove that a treatment does or does not work. This study provides no proof either way, although the trends observed were in the direction which would be expected if there was some effect.

One reason for doing this study was the hope that there might have been benefits dramatic enough (for some groups of patients at least) that they would be unmistakable even in this limited trial. No such benefits were found. We should remember, however, that the available herbal extracts contain only small amounts of hypericin, and there have been doubts as to whether there is enough to be effective. It is still possible that pure hypericin, or perhaps better extracts, could be of major benefit.

Even before this study began, it was clear that the chance was slight that the herbal extracts would have so dramatic an effect that a small observational study would show it unmistakably. But the chance was not zero; and a positive result would have been of such great importance that we believe the chance justified doing this study, and justifies future studies of other available treatments which have a good scientific rationale.

## REFERENCES

Lavie, G. and others. Studies of the mechanisms of action of the antiretroviral agents hypericin and pseudohypericin. *Proceedings of the National Academy of Sciences USA*, volume 86, pages 5963-5967, August 1989.

Meruelo, D. and others. Therapeutic agents with dramatic antiretroviral activity and little toxicity at effective doses: Aromatic polycyclic diones hypericin and pseudohypericin. *Proceedings of the National Academy of Sciences USA*, volume 85, pages 5230-5234, July 1988.

# CMV UPDATE

*by Denny Smith and John S. James*

*AIDS Treatment News* #94 carried a brief report on the latest developments in the treatment of herpes and CMV infections. Recently we spoke with knowledgeable people who had additional information.

Our article had suggested that ganciclovir, approved last year by the FDA, may be at least as good a treatment as Foscarnet, which remains experimental. But some people cannot use ganciclovir because of its toxicity—especially those who are also using AZT, which has similar toxicities—and therefore they should have access to Foscarnet.

Dale Henderly, M.D., who practices ophthalmology at Northwestern University and has treated many people with CMV retinitis, suggested some other approaches for these patients. He pointed out that the new anti-HIV drug ddI can be administered simultaneously with ganciclovir in many patients, since the drugs have different toxicities. He also feels that if neutrophil counts are within normal limits during treatment with ganciclovir, the patients may be able to tolerate the newly lowered dose of AZT, 500 mg a day.

If ganciclovir cannot be used with either ddI or AZT, then theoretically no obstacles would prevent access to Foscarnet, through a clinical trial or compassionate use. But Dr. Henderly urged people newly diagnosed with CMV to seek the care of a physician experienced with AIDS treatment, so that all the options for dealing with both HIV and the opportunistic infection will be explored. One example is the possibility of entering a clinical trial of granulocyte macrophage-colony stimulating factor (GM-CSF), an agent which looks promising as a control for bone-marrow suppression induced by AZT or ganciclovir.

An experimental use of ganciclovir which may avoid the systemic toxicities involves intraocular administration of the drug. This method uses a small needle to inject the ganciclovir directly into the eye, which delivers the treatment to the specific site of the infection. Although this mode appears to be successful for stabilizing the retinitis, it is not especially practical or safe, as the injections must be repeated twice a week indefinitely, and they risk introducing other eye infections. However, intraocular injections remain a potential "salvage" option if other attempts to treat CMV fail.

Dr. Henderly also told us that laser therapy should not be construed as a treatment for retinitis. Rather, lasers have been used to correct a complication of treating retinitis—the detachment of a retina which has become thin and fragile *because* of prolonged treatment. Even in this context, lasers have been only moderately useful, and only for detachments which were not severe. Dr. Henderly added that lasers have also been tried as attempts at "sealing off" the retina to prevent detachment, but results were unconvincing.

For retinal detachments which are too severe to correct with laser surgery, Dr. Henderly suggests the use of silicone oil to replace the vitreous interior of the eye; this treatment usually works to hold the retina in place again. The silicone oil, like laser treatment, has no therapeutic effect on the CMV infection.

## Future Possibilities

The antiviral HPMPC is looking especially promising in animal studies for treating CMV and perhaps other herpesvirus infections. But as far as we know, it has never yet been tried in humans; therefore it is too early to know whether it will ever be a useful drug. An early report on animal studies was published as an abstract at the Interscience Conference on Antimicrobial Agents and Chemotherapy (ICAAC), September 17-20, 1989, abstract number 751; for other background see *AIDS Treatment News* #76.

Other potentially important CMV treatments are FIAC and oral ganciclovir, both now in small-scale clinical trials. For more information on FIAC, see *AIDS Treatment News* # 94. We do not know how well this drug is working. For more information on oral ganciclovir trials, see *AIDS Treatment News* #89. Oral ganciclovir has the same toxicity as the approved intravenous treatment; its advantage is avoiding the need for intravenous infusion.

*AIDS Treatment News* believes that the most important action to improve treatment for CMV and other herpesviruses would be to speed the development of HPMPC. Apparently this potential drug works very well in the well-established "animal model" for CMV infection; if it passes standard toxicity tests, there would be no shortage of volunteers willing to try it as a therapy. When a new drug is potentially so important to so many people, its development should be treated as an emergency, not business as usual.

# Issue Number 97
# February 16, 1990

## TIBO DERIVATIVES: MOST SELECTIVE ANTIVIRAL?

Researchers in Belgium and the U.S. have developed a new antiviral which appears to act more selectively against HIV than any other known chemical. Early results were published February 1 in *Nature*, which is widely considered to be the world's most prestigious scientific journal.

In an important departure from research procedures enforced in the United States, this early report includes not only laboratory results but animal and human safety information as well. After developing a drug (so far known only as R82150), researchers gave dogs a thousand times the dose likely to be effective, with no adverse effects. Then six healthy volunteers took a single 200 mg dose orally; blood levels sufficient to inhibit HIV were maintained for over 24 hours, with no toxicity. No test with persons with AIDS or HIV was reported. But this initial human experience could greatly speed future development of the drug, because a huge psychological and legal barrier — the reluctance to try a new chemical in humans for the first time — has already been crossed.

In the laboratory, R82150 inhibited HIV in concentrations about 31,000 times less than those toxic to cells; a comparable value for AZT was about 6,200. The drug was effective against five different strains of HIV-1, but was so selective that it did not act against HIV-2, or against any other virus tested. R82150 is believed to inhibit reverse transcriptase, like AZT; but unlike AZT, it is not a nucleoside analog. R82150 is difficult to manufacture in quantity by currently known techniques.

R82150 was developed in Belgium, at the Katholicke Universiteit in Leuven, and the Janssen Research Foundation in Beerse. The drug-development strategy was to start with 600 basic molecules, and then use intelligent trial and error to synthesize related chemicals to find ones which are more effective in laboratory assays. 'TIBO' is an abbreviation for the name of one of the chemicals.

Until the drug is tested on persons with AIDS or HIV, it is not possible to know whether it will be effective. We do not know what clinical trials are planned.

# NEW THREATS TO AIDS RESEARCH FUNDING

*by John S. James*

A growing chorus of voices in Washington and in the media is saying that AIDS has unfairly been given special treatment, that the epidemic is not as serious as had been believed, and that money should be taken away from AIDS research and distributed to other diseases or other purposes.

*AIDS Treatment News* focuses mainly on scientific and medical information about treatment, and on how to design and administer research to get results, rather than on funding issues. But many arguments now being circulated to support reduced AIDS funding are one-sided or worse, and so far the other views are not being widely heard. This article outlines some of the issues in the current funding debate, in order to provide a more balanced view and help our readers support attempts to deal with AIDS through effective research, prevention, and treatment, instead of by writing off certain populations and dismissing the epidemic as not a concern to the majority.

## The Case Against Research Funding

Much of the case for reducing AIDS treatment research was summarized in an article published last month in *Time* magazine ("The AIDS Political Machine," January 22). It made the following arguments:

• The Federal AIDS budget of $1.6 billion is greater than that for cancer ($1.5 billion), although cancer killed 12 times as many people last year. The article also quoted without challenge a statement by Michael Fumento, author of *The Myth of Heterosexual AIDS*, that AIDS would never kill more than 35,000 to 40,000 people a year.

• Twice as much money is being spent on drug development as on prevention of transmission, although experts believe that prevention, not treatment, should be the key to stopping the epidemic.

• Money targeted to AIDS reduces funding for other diseases.

• Traditional principles of drug approval are being "distorted." The article's prime example: that AZT was approved in less than four months, compared to an average of two years. The article invoked the memory of Laetrile, a discredited cancer treatment, to suggest that changes to speed FDA drug approval threaten to leave the public vulnerable to quack cures.

• "AIDS has a far greater impact than the number of its victims [sic] would dictate" — implying it has been overemphasized—because of the money, organization, and articulateness of the gay community.

Another common argument against AIDS funding, which did *not* appear in the *Time* article, is that the public need not pay for AIDS because it was acquired by people's voluntary behavior and therefore is their fault. This argument ignores the fact that the average time from infection to AIDS is about nine years, and highly variable, while the disease was unknown until 1981, the virus not announced until 1984, and prevention information was not widely disseminated until later. Most of those now ill were infected before they had any warning of how to protect themselves. Much of the public does not know that persons now ill were infected years ago, but those quoted as AIDS opinion leaders almost certainly do. Apparently this argument against paying for AIDS has been spread even when it was known to be false.

## The Other Side

Here is some of the information omitted from the *Time* article and from similar attacks on AIDS funding:

•   The comparison of the money spent for AIDS and cancer is misleading. According to a fact sheet prepared by the Human Rights Campaign Fund in Washington, D.C., the $1.5 billion for cancer only includes the spending of the National Cancer Institute, part of the National Institutes of Health (excluding spending for AIDS-related cancer research). But the $1.6 billion AIDS figure includes not only the entire National Institutes of Health (including the NIAID clinical trials, AIDS spending in the National Cancer Institute, and much basic biomedical research sometimes arbitrarily counted under AIDS), but also the Centers for Disease Control, the Food and Drug Administration, the Health Resources and Services Administration, and the Alcohol, Drug Abuse, and Mental Health Administration. If cancer spending in the National Cancer Institute alone is compared with AIDS spending in the entire National Institutes of Health—a comparison which still exaggerates the relative money spent on AIDS—then cancer receives twice as much money as AIDS, $1.5 billion vs. $750 million.

•   The cancer infrastructure has been built over decades, whereas the AIDS infrastructure had to be created from scratch during the last few years in which funding was available. It is unfair to ignore this difference when comparing recent funding only. And cancer is really many different diseases; comparing cancer with AIDS can obscure more than it reveals.

•   Spending on AIDS is comparable to that for other diseases in research dollars spent per year of life lost.

•   The four months to approve AZT vs. two years average for drugs refers to the time taken for government paperwork, not scientific research. Although figures are not available, it is likely that most of the cited two years is due to inadequate staff at the FDA, causing drugs to wait in line while nothing happens. Until staff shortages can be corrected, it is essential to give vitally important new drugs for any disease priority over marginal or "me too" product introductions. This kind of reform does not weaken the approval process or threaten to introduce quack remedies.

•   AIDS is spreading rapidly in many communities and will certainly kill more people in the future than it is killing today. Research funding should consider not only today's deaths, but the future as well.

•   Aside from all these specifics, the thrust of some current efforts to compare dollars for cancer vs. AIDS is to get the different disease lobbies fighting among themselves, when everyone would benefit if we could work together better as a coalition. We should remember that the entire budget of the National Institutes of Health, for *all diseases combined*, is $7.6 billion, less than the current year's cost of only two military systems, the Strategic Defense Initiative ("Star Wars," at $3.8 billion), and the B-2 bomber ("Stealth," at $4.3 billion). Which effort is more cost-effective in saving the lives and protecting the quality of life of U.S. citizens? Which is the better use of the same tax dollars—Star Wars and the Stealth bomber, or all Federal biomedical research on all diseases conducted by the National Institutes of Health? This country can afford adequate medical research; the real issue is national priorities, not whether money is available.

• The *Time* article suggested that money should be spent on prevention rather than drug development. It quoted an ACT UP member to portray the AIDS movement as focusing on treatment instead of prevention, implying that people with AIDS or HIV by trying to save their own lives are distorting the national response to the epidemic, thereby threatening the lives of "blacks and Hispanics of the inner cities of the East." But in fact the gay community has long been in the forefront on prevention, and the AIDS movement has emphasized prevention far more than treatment, which only recently became a priority. The scandalous delays in prevention have not resulted from money being spent on drug development, and are not at all the fault of the (mostly gay) AIDS movement, which the *Time* article has framed as a threat to the lives of members of other groups. Anyone involved in prevention knows that the bottleneck has resulted from consistent, long-standing political obstructionism by certain conservatives and fundamentalists. But those unfamiliar with the history of what is actually happening could take from the *Time* article images divorced from the facts.

• Another argument for reducing AIDS funding is that the epidemic is not affecting as many people as had been predicted. For example, new AIDS cases reported in 1989 to the Centers for Disease Control were only nine percent above the total reported for 1988—a much lower rate of increase than in previous years. And according to another recent report, an unexpected change for the better seems to have started in mid 1987.

But much is still unclear. For example, nobody knows for sure why the improvements have occurred; there are at least five different theories, each with its own proponents (safer sex, availability of treatments, underreporting, changes in the definition of AIDS, or estimates not being comparable because the original ones were erroneous). This good news does not justify seizing on new and uncertain information, sometimes before it is even proofed and published, in an unseemly rush to take money away from AIDS.

• Another argument (not in the *Time* article) for de-emphasizing AIDS is that the disease is not spreading rapidly in the heterosexual community—meaning white, middle class heterosexuals in the United States. Aside from the ethical objections to writing off other populations, there are epidemiological reasons to be careful of telling the white middle class that it has little to worry about. In Africa AIDS is spread almost entirely by heterosexual contact, including in the middle class. In parts of Latin America, AIDS is in transition from the U.S./European pattern (gay men and IV drug users) to the African pattern (heterosexual transmission), showing that this change can happen. And in the U.S., syphilis has reached its highest rate in 40 years, mostly among heterosexuals—showing that people are not being careful, and also providing genital sores which are believed to facilitate epidemic heterosexual transmission. A major heterosexual epidemic in the United States cannot be ruled out, and after it starts, it may be too late to stop. Now is not the time to encourage people to let down their guard by telling them that AIDS is someone else's problem.

## Toward Coalition and Consensus—And a Demographic Obstacle

The current push to de-emphasize AIDS research is objectionable not only for its factual distortions, but for what it is trying to do. It is seizing every excuse to try to write off and abandon people with AIDS or HIV, divide the spoils among other interests, and dismiss what AIDS has taught us about weakness in the health-care and research/approval system, and about how to begin to change them. Instead of encouraging disease groups to fight each other, we should be working together to improve health care for all.

One demographic obstacle to building such coalitions has not, we believe, been pointed out before. It appears that almost everyone working in AIDS is under 40. A major underlying problems in mobilizing public support and understanding for AIDS may stem from the tendency of older people not to listen to younger people or take their concerns seriously. And AIDS organizations had to be created from scratch, without benefit of the leadership of those who were older and more experienced, as the older people were not there. The result may have been the development of organizations which are not comfortable for the senior people who are usually the leaders in U.S. institutional life. These leaders are used to being in charge. They are not inclined to learn the ropes from younger activists, as may be necessary in AIDS since usually older people are not involved.

This same dynamic may also explain failures of mobilization within the medical community. Most physicians involved in AIDS are too young to have major influence in the medical profession as a whole. They could not speak out effectively to correct such problems as unworkable clinical-trial designs, irrational barriers to access to necessary treatments, and national research programs which could not possibly save their patients' lives. The senior physicians who could have provided this leadership were not involved in AIDS.

One pioneering effort to bring in leaders from other fields is the Mayor's HIV Task Force in San Francisco. It spent a year investigating AIDS here, and then produced a short report with no surprises. The real significance of the project is that it involved leaders from the business and religious community who had not been familiar with AIDS before, and then developed consensus on needs and recommendations.

Those of us who work constantly with AIDS may not realize how extensive a subculture has developed. This writer, for example, had thought that a few meetings and a little reading would be enough to bring leaders from other fields up to speed in AIDS. Instead it took more than a year, in a specially-designed project sanctioned by San Francisco's mayor.

We hope that the identification of this problem of the absent older generation in AIDS will contribute to the creative thought and experimentation which will be needed for its solution.

**February 16, 1990**

# NEUROPSYCHIATRIC EFFECTS IN AIDS

*by Denny Smith*

A wide range of mental status changes has been attributed directly or indirectly to HIV. Several recent studies have shown that asymptomatic people with HIV **do not** have deficits in cognitive or physical skills when compared to control groups without HIV. Some instances of disorientation, short-term memory loss, diminished motor coordination and withdrawal or personality changes can be symptoms related to HIV disease, and all are potentially treatable given an accurate diagnosis.

Joyce Seiko Kobayashi, M.D., addressed the neuropsychiatric aspects of AIDS at the Fifth Annual Rocky Mountain Regional Conference on AIDS, February 2-3 in Denver. Using a tree-like graph to rule out unlikely causes for a given symptom in order to isolate the source of the problem, Dr. Kobayashi distinguished several symptom categories to consider—depressed emotional frames of mind, delirium episodes from acute illness or drug reactions, AIDS-related dementia, and opportunistic tumors or infections in the central nervous system.

Depression in people with **or** without HIV can be an appropriate reaction to anxiety surrounding a health crisis, or grief for the loss of lovers and friends, or fears of powerlessness over the future. Dr. Kobayashi facilitates discussion groups for HIV positive people to deal with these emotions and seek solutions with the validation of peers.

Mental status changes resulting not from social but from organic reasons may be imminently life-threatening, and should be diagnosed and treated as soon as possible. These include cryptococcal meningitis (see *AIDS Treatment News* #49 and 96); encephalitis or swelling of the brain due to toxoplasmosis (issue #79), herpes or CMV (issues #94 and 96); or lesions in the central nervous system including PML (issue #88), KS (issues #73, 75, and 87) or lymphoma (issue #93).

Cognitive problems which are not a result of opportunistic tumors or infections, but from direct HIV invasion of the central nervous system, are defined as "dementia," or AIDS Dementia Complex (ADC). One theory suggests that HIV damages microglial cells in the brain. Unlike neurons, which are the irreplaceable reservoirs of memory and consciousness, microglial cells function primarily as connections between neurons and can regenerate if the source of their destruction is controlled. A different theory says that HIV-infected cells produce toxins which cause the dementia. AZT, proven to cross the barrier between the bloodstream and the central nervous system, can reverse the dementia caused by HIV, although the new, reduced doses might not be sufficient. Dextroamphetamine and Ritalin are also used to treat mental effects of HIV.

In addition to depression, organic diseases and dementia, some transient mental states are considered a "delirium." Side-effects of some toxic drug reactions, as well as prolonged, high fevers, can alter lucidity and lead to a delirium. Because many of these symptoms and their origins may mimic or overlap each other, Dr. Kobayashi noted that reliance on an AIDS-knowledgeable physician is crucial for determining a diagnosis and therapy.

A doctor who is unfamiliar with a newly symptomatic patient or current HIV care may not accurately distinguish whether memory gaps and lethargy are stemming from demoralization or a rapidly progressing brain infection, whether an apparent motor control deficit is due to cerebral KS lesions or a recent change in medications, or whether Xanax or a new living situation are in order for a long-depressed person. Mutual trust developed between an HIV-experienced physician and an HIV-positive patient can offer each a background familiarity from which to weigh confusing situations.

For an audiotape of Dr. Kobayashi's presentation, call "Sounds True," 303/449-6229. The tape number for her presentation is AP-27.

# NEWS NOTES

• **San Francisco study shows longer life expectancy for people with AIDS.** A study by epidemiologist Dr. George Lemp and others at the San Francisco Department of Public Health, published January 19, 1990 in the *Journal of the American Medical Association*, showed that by 1987, median survival for all patients diagnosed with AIDS had increased from 12.5 to 15.6 months from time of diagnosis; patients with pneumocystis had a median survival of 17.9 months. (Later data is not available, because of the time required for survival trends to become known.) Median survival of patients treated with AZT was 21.3 months, compared to 13.9 months for those not on any anti-viral therapy.

San Francisco is generally agreed to have the most accurate data anywhere on the HIV epidemic.

• **The rate of increase of AIDS in the United States slowed last year.** The U.S. Centers for Disease Control reported that new cases of AIDS in the U.S. increased only nine percent in 1989, compared to a 34 percent increase in 1988 and 60 percent increase in 1987. Experts attributed the slowing increase to reduction in new cases among gay men (probably due to prevention education of years ago), and also to the use of treatments, such as AZT and aerosol pentamidine, which are preventing some infected persons from progressing to AIDS. Cases due to heterosexual transmission rose much more rapidly, however, showing a 27 percent increase last year. The region with the most new AIDS cases was the South, with 31 percent of the cases.

• **Fluconazole will be donated to AIDS and cancer centers.** Pfizer Pharmaceuticals, the developer of the antifungal fluconazole, announced that it would donate 6,000 bottles of the drug to over 200 cancer and AIDS treatment centers in the United States. According to the February 6 announcement, the drug should be available now.

• **Researchers in Kenya claim success with new drug.** The director of the Kenya Medical Research Institute, Dr. Davy Koech, told a Nairobi press conference that a drug called Kemron, a form of alpha interferon, had been given to 101 patients with AIDS or HIV infection. Only one (apparently out of the first 40 for whom the longest followup is available) failed to show improvement. The drug is supposed to reduce or eliminate symptoms of AIDS, usually within four weeks, but not cure the disease. No independent confirmation of its effectiveness is yet available.

Amarillo Cell Culture Co. in Amarillo, Texas collaborated in this study, which used a natural interferon manufactured by Hayashibara Biochemical Laboratories in Japan, where it is approved for treating certain cancers. The drug was given orally but not swallowed. Very low doses were used, 50 to 150 IU; as a result, the treatment is inexpensive. This therapy was suggested by veterinary experience in the U.S. and in Africa.

The Kemron story was carried by Reuters news service, February 7, and was reported in Japan and other countries, but apparently not in the United States.

# Issue Number 98
# March 2, 1990

## SCABIES INCREASING, DIAGNOSIS OFTEN MISSED

Marcus Conant, M.D., a dermatologist and a leading AIDS expert in San Francisco, alerted patients at his February monthly public meeting that he has seen a major increase in scabies in the last few months, with 20 cases since Christmas. Scabies is caused by a mite, a small spider which burrows into the skin. It is very contagious, often transmitted by sexual contact, and often particularly severe in persons with immune deficiencies.

Scabies is not difficult to treat. The biggest problem is getting it diagnosed, as physicians often do not look for it. Historically, scabies becomes widespread periodically; clearly a major increase is starting now, at least in San Francisco. (We do not know about other cities.)

Symptoms include severe itching, which may be worse at night. Itching and rash often start in the web between the fingers. Other areas likely to be affected include the genitals, underarms, elbows, and buttocks. Usually the head is not affected—but it may be in people with immune suppression.

Treatment requires a prescription cream or lotion (such as Kwell), often applied everywhere from the neck down and left on overnight, then washed off in the morning, for four successive nights. Instructions must be followed carefully; sometimes, for example, physicians forget to tell patients *not* to wash their hands at night, after they have applied the medication. The mites are often found on the hands, and they can survive there and re-infect the rest of the body if the hands are not treated.

In addition, clothing and bedding must be collected and properly cleaned, and all sexual contacts must be treated simultaneously, to avoid reinfection.

## FDA APPROVES, NIH RECOMMENDS
## AZT FOR ASYMPTOMATICS

On March 2 the U.S. Food and Drug Administration (FDA) formally approved a change in the labeling of AZT, expanding the indications for use of the drug to include all adults with HIV and a T-helper count of 500 or less. For asymptomatic individuals, the dose recommended was 500 mg per day (100 mg every four hours while awake). For those with symptoms, the recommended dose was higher, the same as for persons with AIDS—1200 mg per day for one month, which may then be reduced to 600 mg per day.

Then, during the next two days, a panel of 19 clinical researchers, community physicians, and others met at a conference organized by the U.S. National Institute of Allergy and Infectious Diseases (NIAID) to prepare recommendations for early use of AZT. This panel made similar, though not identical, suggestions, recommending 500 mg per day for both asymptomatic and symptomatic individuals. The executive summary from that conference also includes recommendations on how often to check T-cell counts for different groups of patients, and on how to manage persons on AZT.

Both of these government actions have been expected, and the recommendations are not surprising. A number of physicians, especially in cities such as San Francisco, have already been providing early AZT treatment to private patients. The importance of the FDA and NIAID actions is that it should now be much easier to get government and private third-party payors to cover early use of AZT, making early intervention available to many who otherwise could not obtain it.

About 600,000 people might benefit from early HIV treatment in the United States alone. Many of them, however, do not even know that they are infected.

# DRUG DEVELOPMENT: WHAT'S NEEDED NOW?

*by John S. James*

For those familiar with clinical trials and drug development, the last few months have been particularly difficult. Aside from ddI, where the research and distribution programs have essentially worked and much of the news at this time is good, research on new treatments appears to have greatly slowed. We have been unable to confirm that the situation is really as bad as it appears, however, because of the widespread confusion; no one seemed to know what was happening. We could not find a vision or direction for AIDS treatment research, a plan with a reasonable chance of success.

Now the outlines of how to overcome the current obstacles and to make research productive again are becoming visible. Scientifically, what needs to be done is already fairly clear. In the past, however, the dismal political landscape ruled out any possibility that what should be done would be done, and led to the current paralysis. Today elements are in place for new consensus, new social contracts among the parties involved. This article describes key elements of consensus which we believe could and should develop.

## What's Wrong Now?

The basic problem has been the expectation that all new antivirals must go through huge trials, usually scheduled for two years and requiring hundreds of carefully selected volunteers who are willing to have their treatment selected at random, before any drug can be recognized as effective. In practice, enormous administrative, financial, proprietary, scientific, ethical, and personnel-shortage problems make these trials take much longer than two years, and guarantee that the great majority of drugs worthy of human testing will not be in trials at all.

Early-access arrangements, such as the current test with ddI or the proposed "parallel track" to provide treatment during the trials for persons with no other medical options who do not qualify for trials, can save many lives; these vital efforts must be supported. But early access only works when there is a public-spirited and well-financed drug company, willing to spend money to save lives when sales of the drug may be years away. It does not address the shortage of researchers and facilities caused by the resource demands of the "dinosaur" (large and slow) trials—demands which in practice prevent drugs from being tested, approved, or considered for early access. In short, while we continue to work for early access, we must also develop more fundamental reforms to improve the productivity of the drug testing and approval system.

## What's Needed, And Why It Hasn't Happened Already

The reason for the "dinosaur" trials in the first place is that disease progression in AIDS is highly variable, and the laboratory tests to measure progression (such as T-cell count and p24 antigen) have drawbacks; many researchers have not been willing to trust these tests to tell whether drugs are working. The two-year trials with hundreds of patients, comparing deaths and serious infections in those who do and do not get the new drug, are used to obtain definitive statistical proof that the drugs are helping people. The problem, of course, is not only that these trials take a long time to get results, but also that they are so unwieldy that in practice they seldom happen at all.

The most important new technology for potentially changing this situation is the development of better tests of disease progression, especially plasma viremia (see "New Viral Measurement for Rapid Drug Testing," *AIDS Treatment News* # 94). A small experiment using AZT showed that it was possible to get definitive statistical proof in a few weeks, with only a small number of volunteers, that an antiviral is working in humans to reduce the level of infectious HIV in the blood. If this kind of test could be used instead of the huge two-year trials required until now, the logjam of AIDS clinical trials could be broken, and all the important drugs could be tested quickly.

At this time the plasma viremia test is gaining widespread professional acceptance. The only objections we have heard are that some researchers question whether the test is quite ready, and some want to wait for future tests which will be more economical. And some leading experts believe that plasma viremia isn't really necessary, because rapid drug testing could have been done all along, using p24 antigen, despite its drawbacks. The big problem now with plasma viremia is that it is very expensive, costing over a thousand dollars per test. Few labs have experience doing this test, which is not available commercially.

The professional consensus now developing sees plasma viremia as something useful to do. But should it be used only to select interesting candidate drugs for the two-year "dinosaur" trials, or can it be accepted as the proof of efficacy required for marketing approval? Could a drug be approved with official labeling stating that it reduces HIV levels in blood, although clinical benefit has not yet been proved? On this question, consensus has not yet developed either way.

**March 2, 1990**

Here is why we believe it is vitally important that the answer to the latter question be "Yes":

• Avoiding the need for two-year, several-hundred-patient multicenter efficacy trials could quickly end the current drugjam, and allow all important antivirals to be tested.

• Additional safety information could be obtained from trials (or supervised access programs) *designed* to answer safety questions—not dredged as a by-product out of trials structured primarily to get statistical proof of efficacy.

• A major study by the FDA found that all five vitally important anti-infective drugs recently approved for marketing were approved based on pivotal clinical trials *none of which* used survival as an endpoint. At least some of these trials did use reduction in microbial levels, instead. AIDS drugs should not be bottlenecked by unworkable requirements which are not applied to other drugs.

• Doctors and patients considering using antivirals which had been proved to reduce HIV (but not proved to increase survival or reduce opportunistic infections, because those studies had not been done) would also have other options available, including AZT, about which much more is known. They can and should be trusted to decide among these options.

• Further clinical research could be required after marketing approval, when necessary.

• Companies with a promising drug would have a realistic chance to get it to market in the foreseeable future, and make an attractive but fair profit. (Today, only companies with great resources and the right connections can seriously hope to do so.) Incentive would stimulate AIDS drug-development projects throughout the clinical-trials pipeline, all the way back to the laboratory, and could get many more companies involved in AIDS research (only a few are today).

• Competition between drugs would help to control runaway prices, potentially saving billions of dollars for governments, other third-party payors, and individuals.

• Faster development of improved treatments could save additional billions of dollars in hospitalization and other expensive care—as well as saving lives.

• The alternative—continuing to require huge, two-year trials before drug approval—is exceptionally grim. U.S. AIDS drug development is now close to a standstill, and there are no prospects for finding enough resources to get it going again under current procedures.

But what if the AIDS researcher establishment will not support plasma viremia or any other alternative to the years-long, "dinosaur" trials for meeting the efficacy requirement for marketing approval? If that happens, then the AIDS community should use the consensus it can get—that plasma viremia is worth doing to help prioritize drugs—and push for parallel track access to the drugs which this test shows works best. And also, we would have to examine how much of the objection to a workable approval system stems from scientific concerns, and how much stems from the empires which have been built under the present system. How much results from the influence which Burroughs-Wellcome (which stands to lose most if alternatives to

AZT are approved for marketing) has purchased throughout the AIDS research community?

In the past, AIDS researchers were inadvertently given incentives to build empires, not to get practical results. No one spoke out when existing procedures, policies, regulatory standards, and scientific conventional wisdom virtually guaranteed that no new drugs would be developed. Today there is much more pressure for results. All the parties involved have a common interest in improving the productivity and efficiency of drug development and regulation.

## Price Vs. Incentive: Toward A New Social Contract?

Recently we have heard concerns that pressures from the AIDS community to lower drug prices will deter companies from engaging in research. We do not know how serious this problem is, but it is hard to see how price will cease being an issue. Usually those who want to let companies charge anything, to give them maximum incentive to develop new drugs, are those who will always get the treatments they need at any price. But for the great majority, the price issue will not go away.

Another approach to improving incentives is to make potential profits more likely, and not as far away in time—instead of insuring the right to make exorbitant profits in some hazy, distant future when the drug in question will probably be obsolete anyway. Consider the following proposed three-way understanding between government, industry, and the AIDS community:

• In an emergency, the FDA would develop standards designed to be feasible for pharmaceutical companies to meet, to promote two public purposes: getting drugs approved sooner, and giving pharmaceutical companies more incentive to be involved in research. The FDA is already moving in this direction. It should explicitly recognize that part of its job is to develop regulations which stimulate commercial development when required to meet a national emergency.

• Companies which respond to an emergency must be able to recover their research costs and make a profit. Some would say the profit should be above industry average, because of the extra  risks and expenses for an accelerated or even crash program. But also there must be some restraint. In return for government assistance, through financing of research, streamlining of regulations, or otherwise, companies with a unique product for a life-and-death emergency must not be allowed to profiteer and charge whatever the market will bear. Companies can no longer take advantage of the bigotry toward AIDS to pioneer unconscionable policies, which they then apply to other diseases later.

• The AIDS community should accept reasonable profits (but not profiteering) for drug companies as a requirement for making the system work. We cannot wait for a new economy—either for socialism or for libertarian free enterprise—but must make the existing system work now. We should continue to support companies which are willing to consider the public interest and work together in mutually beneficial public-private partnerships. Also, the AIDS community will need to communicate and negotiate with the consumer-protection movement, and with advocates and organizations for other diseases, more than it has in the past.

**March 2, 1990**

Until last summer, government-funded researchers and FDA officials had little contact with "front line" private or clinic physicians with large AIDS practices; now there is much better communication. This improvement should make the government-funded research more responsive to practical needs.

Patients and researchers often have different interests; until recently there was little communication, and often hostility, between them. Now both groups are learning that they need to work together.

Today all parties involved in AIDS treatment development realize that there are serious problems in the current system, and that consensus and collaboration are necessary to overcome them. The elements of a new consensus are now taking shape.

## Japanese Company Develops New AIDS Antiviral

Mitsubishi Kasei Corporation, together with the Katholieke Universiteit Leuven (Belgium), the University of Birmingham (England), and Showa University in Tokyo, has developed an AIDS antiviral which, according to a February 16 Reuters report, the company hopes to enter into U.S. clinical trials before the end of 1990.

A technical report on the potential drug, called HEPT (hydroxyethoxy methyl phenylthiothymine) appeared in *Biochemical and Biophysics Research Communications*, December 29, 1989, pages 1375-1381. The antiviral worked in both T-cells and macrophages infected with HIV-1, but did not affect HIV-2 or other viruses. How it works is not known.

## Salk Vaccine Company Sells Foreign Rights

In an agreement announced on February 28, two major medical research institutions in France, the Institut Merieux and its subsidiary Pasteur Vaccins, have jointly purchased rights to market the Salk HIV vaccine outside of North America. (The U.S. company developing the treatment, The Immune Response Corporation of San Diego, CA, has arranged separate North American marketing with Rorer Group, Inc.)

Unlike most vaccines, the Salk HIV vaccine is intended to be used after persons are already infected. This treatment, called AIDS Immunotherapeutic, is currently in clinical trials in the United States.

Despite the reputation of Dr. Jonas Salk, who developed the first polio vaccine, his HIV work has been slow to receive support in the U.S. AIDS research establishment.

Institut Merieux is the leading marketer of vaccines in the world.

## Koop Calls U.S. AIDS Policy "Almost Ten Years Overdue"

On February 27 C. Everett Koop, former U.S. Surgeon General, told Congress that "We don't have a Federal policy on AIDS, period," and that unless Congress intervenes, the situation will only get worse. Dr. Koop was speaking to the House Subcommittee on Health and the Environment, in support of a bill to expand Medicaid coverage for persons with AIDS or HIV.

Dr. Koop called it "incredible that the Federal government has not had a dialog with the states, and with certain municipalities," about how the costs of the epidemic will be paid.

Representative Waxman (D-California) commented that "Having missed the opportunity to get the ounce of prevention, we now have to pay for pounds and pounds of cure."

## Centers for Disease Control Urges End to HIV Border Exclusion

On March 1 the U.S. Centers for Disease Control recommended that all diseases except one be removed from the list of conditions used to exclude persons from entering the United States. Only tuberculosis would remain grounds for exclusion.

However, HIV differs from all the other diseases in that it is the only one added to the list by Congress. (The others were added by public-health professionals.) U.S. officials believe that since Congress specifically put HIV on the list, only Congress can remove it. It may not be possible to do so in time to avoid disrupting the major AIDS scientific conference of 1990, scheduled for June 20-24 in San Francisco.

## Senators Propose AIDS Disaster Relief for Cities and States

On March 6 Senators Edward Kennedy (D-Massachusetts) and Orrin Hatch (R-Utah) introduced a bill to provide $500 million disaster relief to areas heavily impacted by AIDS. The bill is patterned after relief programs for areas hit by disasters like earthquakes and hurricanes—for example, the $3 billion appropriated by Congress for the recent earthquake near San Francisco. Both California senators, Alan Cranston and Pete Wilson, are among 18 co-sponsors of the bill.

About half of the money will go to 13 cities which together have about 60 percent of the U.S. cases of AIDS: Atlanta, Boston, Chicago, Dallas, Houston, Los Angeles, Miami, Newark, New York, Philadelphia, San Francisco, San Juan, and Washington, D.C. The rest of the money would go to states, depending on their numbers of AIDS cases. Different areas will be able to use the money to develop the kinds of programs most suitable for them.

If the bill becomes law in its current form, San Francisco will receive about $40 million for AIDS disaster relief.

## Project Inform and Community Research Alliance Will Merge

Two San Francisco community-based AIDS research organizations, Project Inform and Community Research Alliance, have voted to merge in order to carry out research more effectively. Project Inform, active since 1985, provides AIDS treatment information through a hotline (see phone numbers in the other Project Inform article in this News Notes section) and publishes a newsletter (*PI Perspectives*); last year it organized a study of the Compound Q being imported by patients from China. Community Research Alliance, founded in 1988 as a project of San Francisco's PWA Coalition, organized an institutional review board and scientific advisory committee, and took other steps legally or otherwise necessary to carry out clinical trials. It conducted the hypericin monitoring study reported in *AIDS Treatment News* issue #96.

This merger was consistent with the widespread belief that AIDS organizations should consolidate to provide services more efficiently. In this case, the savings is not in staff or facilities, but in avoiding the need to duplicate the building of a public identity and funding base for separate organizations with the same purpose.

# Issue Number 99
# March 16, 1990

## DDI RISKS: PERSPECTIVE AND PRECAUTIONS

*by John S. James*

Recently there has been much publicity about the risks of using the experimental AIDS treatment ddI. Some of the reporting has been misleading and unnecessarily frightening. But some risks are real, and experts recommend simple precautions that anyone using ddI should begin immediately.

### Background

ddI is an antiviral in the same general class as AZT. It may be about equally effective, although no one knows for sure until trials are completed. There is much interest in ddI, not because it is believed to be better than AZT, but because the toxicities of the drugs are different, and also because ddI may work even after AZT has become less effective, as it does for some patients after a year or two of use. ddI is important because it provides another therapeutic option, with its own profile of risks and benefits.

Three major clinical trials (named ACTG 116, ACTG 117, and ACTG 118) are now testing ddI. In addition to these formal trials, Bristol-Myers, the company developing the drug, has made it available without charge through an expanded access programs to patients who cannot enter the formal trials and cannot use AZT—persons with no other treatment options. At this time, about 700 people are in the formal trials, and about 8,000 additional people are receiving the drug through the expanded access program.

On March 4-7, hundreds of AIDS researchers from around the country met near Washington, DC, at a conference of the AIDS Clinical Trials Group (ACTG). This quarterly meeting is closed to the press and the public, but important news gets out. At this meeting, physicians heard the latest safety reports on the ddI trials and expanded access program, and exchanged information about their own experience with the drug. They learned that at least one patient in the formal trials and six in the expanded access program have died of pancreatitis, believed to have been caused by ddI. This death rate is about one in a thousand for both programs. (Over 30 non-fatal cases of pancreatitis have also been reported.)

The total deaths from all causes (including the pancreatitis) is 2 of the 700 in the formal trials, and 290 of the 8,000 in the expanded-access program. While the data has just begun to be analyzed, this difference in death rates between the formal trials and the expanded-access program is almost certainly caused by the fact that many of the patients receiving the drug through expanded access were more seriously ill. Patients selected for trials are usually well enough to be expected to survive the trial, whereas many enter the expanded-access program as a last resort. There is no evidence that ddI contributed to these deaths (other than those caused by pancreatitis), and no reason to believe that receiving the drug was any more risky in the expanded-access program than in the trials. The safety monitoring is similar in both programs.

Researchers suspect that ddI did contribute to the pancreatitis deaths, because the very severe and rapidly developing pancreatitis had not previously been expected with AIDS. Other drugs or diseases may also have contributed; intravenous pentamidine, for example, can also cause pancreatitis. All data from these cases will be analyzed to determine (1) if there is a dose-response relationship, with those receiving more drug per body weight at greater risk, and (2) if any cofactors, such as other drugs, were present more often in those patients who did get pancreatitis than in those who did not. If the answer to either question is yes, then ddI could be used more safely by adjusting the dose, or by stopping or not using the drug if any dangerous cofactor is present.

The much larger number of deaths from other causes will also be investigated, especially to see whether ddI may have contributed to any of them.

## Precautions

The FDA has asked Bristol-Myers to write to all physicians who are using ddI, to inform them of recommended precautions. Meanwhile, the *Los Angeles Times* quoted Robert Yarchoan, of the U.S. National Cancer Institute, on precautions patients should take now. Dr. Yarchoan has run the longest clinical trial of ddI, at the National Cancer Institute, and is probably the world expert on use of the drug.

"Patients receiving ddI who develop abdominal pain [which can be the first symptom of pancreatitis] should probably stop the drug immediately and consult their physicians as soon as possible. They should also not drink alcohol, and their physicians should try to avoid prescribing medications that might cause pancreatitis." (Dr. Yarchoan, quoted in the *Los Angeles Times,* March 10, 1990.) Other experts have noted that anyone on ddI who develops pneumocystis and must be treated with intravenous pentamidine should stop using ddI while on the pentamidine.

A major problem in treating the pancreatitis believed to be caused by ddI is that it can progress so rapidly that it is difficult to diagnose in time. Other researchers have recently made progress in diagnosing serious pancreatitis, for example by testing for trypsinogen activated peptide in the urine. We do not know if this test is yet available, or if it would be useful in the ddI trials or expanded-access program.

## Perspective

Before the above information about the risk of ddI was available, *AIDS Treatment News* had heard both good and bad reports about the drug, but mostly good. ddI seems to have made a dramatic difference for many people; we suspect that many who are now alive would not be without it. We had also heard of a number of cases where people had to stop using this drug because of side effects.

Dr. Yarchoan told *The Wall Street Journal* (issue of March 12) that it was "absolutely necessary to go forward with phase 2, or effectiveness studies," the formal clinical trials mentioned above. "Only then can you put the toxicity in the context of benefits and go on."

Drug-development experts consider this finding of toxicity with ddI not at all unusual, except for the fact that this drug trial is being conducted in a fishbowl of public attention. Initial studies gave the drug to only a few dozen people. Problems which rarely occur would not be likely to show up until later trials, when more patients are receiving the drug.

News of the deaths in the ddI program was published in the *Los Angeles Times* on March 10, and in *The New York Times*, *The Wall Street Journal*, and the *Washington Post* on March 12. These four newspapers are especially important, because most of the press follows their lead in selecting and framing the news. The coverage in *The New York Times* was more negative and alarming than that in the other three, and it has been widely criticized. Later articles, in *The Wall Street Journal* on March 13, and *The New York Times* on March 19 put the risks in better perspective.

Despite the new information about the risks of ddI, we still consider ddI to be one of the most important new treatment possibilities. It would be tragic to lose this drug—or to lose the concept of parallel track or early access to treatment—due to hasty decisions not based on careful assessment of all the facts.

*NOTE:* The related drug ddC has *not* been found to cause pancreatitis.

## COMPOUND Q: NEW PROJECT INFORM COMMUNITY RESEARCH ALLIANCE STUDY

*by John S. James*

On March 8 the U.S. Food and Drug Administration approved a re-treatment study of compound Q (also called GLQ223, or trichosanthin), to be administered by the Project Inform Community Research Alliance and conducted by physicians in four cities: San Francisco, Los Angeles, Miami, and New York. This trial is for patients who have been treated with the drug previously.

One hundred volunteers will be randomized into two groups, one to receive compound Q every three weeks, the other every six weeks, for up to six months. The dose will be 16 mcg/kg per administration. Unlike most clinical trials today, this one will allow patients to continue using other medications considered important for their health—both for ethical reasons, and to obtain information about use of the drug under realistic conditions, not in a highly restricted test environment. This study, for example, will be the first to obtain practical knowledge about the combined use of compound Q and AZT.

A third group of patients, who meet the identical entry criteria (including previous use of compound Q) but do not choose to continue treatment at this time, can volunteer for a self-selected no-treatment group, which will also be followed under the protocol. (Note: as we go to press, the Institutional Review Board is still reviewing the study; there could be changes in the above design.)

The study director is Larry Waites, M.D., M.P.H., of San Francisco; the four principal investigators are Lysette Cardona, M.D., M.P.H., Los Angeles; Barbara Starrett, M.D., New York; Paula Sparti, M.D., Miami; and Alan S. Levin, M.D., San Francisco. Others, including Vera Byers, M.D., Ph.D., an expert in protein drugs, also contributed to the study design. The trial is financed in part by a grant of $250,000 from Sandoz, U.S.A.; some community fundraising will also be necessary, as Project Inform and the local sites will have to absorb part of the cost. The drug is being contributed by Genelabs Inc., the biotechnology company in Redwood City, California, which developed the U.S. version of compound Q.

## Comment

This study will not by itself be enough to lead to FDA approval of compound Q; other studies are now being run or designed by other researchers. The Project Inform Community Research Alliance study does, however, serve the following purposes:

• Many patients who have already used compound Q want to continue their treatment, and would do so with or without this program. The formal study provides the treatment without charge. At the same time, it collects systematic data which otherwise would be lost.

• Scientists usually want data from "randomized" trials—that is, those which assign patients at random to two or more different treatment groups, which are later compared. Without randomization, it is impossible to be sure that all biases due to self-selection are accounted for, or even known. But randomization raises ethical concerns, as patients and their physicians often have good reason to choose one treatment or another, based on specifics of the individual case which are often not accounted for in the study design.

This trial provides a compromise. Volunteers who want to continue using the drug will be randomized between receiving treatment every three weeks or every six weeks. But the study designers could not have asked these volunteers, who had used compound Q before and had a very good idea of whether or not they wanted to continue, to be randomized between treatment and no treatment.

Having a self-selected no-treatment group is better than having none at all. Not only will it allow an admittedly imperfect comparison with the treatment groups, it will also provide systematic monitoring of long-term results of the compound Q which these volunteers had taken previously. And it will keep faith with those who volunteered for the original Project Inform compound Q study, by providing extensive monitoring free to them even if they do not want to continue the treatment.

• This study will not by itself lead to FDA approval, because it does not address the question of whether treatment or no treatment is best for patients who have never taken the drug before. But it will provide information on use of compound Q in real-world conditions—unlike academic studies, which test drugs under conditions which seldom correspond to how patients are actually treated. For example, this study will allow volunteers to also use AZT, other antivirals, immune modulators, or other treatments which they and their physicians believe they should use. Therefore, it will provide information on the use of compound Q in combination with AZT.

# KS NEWS AND CONFUSION

*by John S. James*

Several different news reports on Kaposi's sarcoma (KS) may have much long-term importance. Unfortunately they have little immediate relevance to treatment—and they have caused some confusion.

## New Treatment in Japan?

On February 22 Robert Gallo, M.D., of the U.S. National Cancer Institute, presented an overview on AIDS to an academic meeting at Fordham University. A short section of the talk implied that a much better potential treatment for KS has been developed in Japan—but did not say whether there had been any human test:

"We have compounds from a company in Japan that wipe out the Kaposi's sarcoma in a way I have never seen before. That is, no toxicity, and the tumor's gone, and never reappears.

"So now comes the politics of forming the collaboration, getting the compound, and all these things that are the most confusing things about recent science, I would say."

Such a statement might normally have been ignored by the academic audience. But the *New York Native* published a transcript of the talk in its March 12 issue, with part of the above quote on page one. A number of people have called the National Cancer Institute, but little additional information has been released.

In response to an inquiry of Congressman Sidney R. Yates (D-Chicago), the National Cancer Institute released the following statement:

"The compounds to which Dr. Gallo referred are under preclinical development. Any activity seen to date is based on laboratory observations and should not be construed as implying that these compounds are cures for Kaposi's sarcoma. Further testing will be required before it may be determined whether these compounds would be effective or safe for use in patients. Dr. Gallo has indicated that his laboratory will pursue establishing collaboration with this company to further investigate these compounds."

Even a successful animal test would be important, however, because there is a good "mouse model" for KS. In the same talk, Dr. Gallo summarized some of the most important animal work, which has been published. When certain cells which cause *human* KS are injected into immune-deficient mice, they caused a KS lesion to form within 10 days. But the cells in the lesion turned out to be *mouse* KS cells. Apparently certain abnormal cells cause KS by secreting a chemical, apparently a kind of growth factor, which causes abnormal growth of blood vessels, resulting in KS lesions. The fact that the same chemical causes human KS in humans and mouse KS in mice suggests that the mice with KS could be used to screen various substances (some of which might already be available in familiar drugs or even in foods) to find ways to destroy the unwanted growth factor or block or reduce its effects. Dr. Gallo's remark quoted above suggests that a good candidate has already been found. (For background on the KS tests in mice, see Nakamara and others, 1988, and Salahuddin and others, 1988.)

We do not have any more information at this time. We are checking a rumor of a successful human test in Japan, but have not been able to substantiate it.

One AIDS research physician guessed that the compound might possibly be beta-cyclodextrin tetradecasulfate or a chemical relative, used in combination with certain steroids. This anti-angiogenic substance (one which prevents unwanted growth of blood vessels) is being tested as a possible cancer treatment, because solid tumors must stimulate growth of blood vessels in order to nourish themselves if they grow beyond a certain size.

For more information on this chemical, which U.S. researchers obtain from Japan, see Folkman and others, 1989, and Folkman, 1989. The latter, an editorial in *The New England Journal of Medicine*, is especially important because it mentions a number of approaches to control of abnormal blood-vessel growth, approaches which may not yet have been investigated for KS. (However, the unprecedented single case of successful treatment of pulmonary-capillary hemangiomatosis, described by White and others and discussed in Folkman's editorial, used alpha interferon, which is already used for KS. We do not know of any human use of beta-cyclodextrins.)

Scientists often discuss the appropriate time to release their findings, and they usually conclude that the right time is after the work is "finished," i.e. well-packaged for publication or presentation to a scientific meeting. Sometimes this approach works badly. U.S. institutional leadership has been slow to mobilize to treat AIDS seriously as an emergency, and therefore the pace of progress is unduly influenced by "the politics of forming the collaboration, getting the compound, and all these things." The public cannot trust that major opportunities will automatically be followed up vigorously. But when even a member of Congress gets the brush-off (the reply to Congressman Yates above could loosely be translated as "get lost," as it leaves no role for his further involvement), the public and its representatives are denied the opportunity to bring attention and resources to bear to overcome the mindless delays which usually set the real pace of research, in AIDS and other diseases as well.

Among many ways to seek one's place in the world, public service usually works better than possession and control of secrets. But too often, career structures encourage the latter.

## KS Is Not Cancer; Is It Also Not AIDS?

While KS is often called a cancer in the general press (and sometimes even in technical papers), experts have long realized that it is not really a cancer (as first suggested by Costa and Rabson, 1983). Biologically, the cells in KS lesions do not behave as cancer cells. Clinically, there are many differences also; San Francisco physician Marcus Conant summarized some of them in a recent public meetings on AIDS. It is generally believed that KS is caused by one or more growth factors. If so, it should potentially be easier than cancer to treat.

Is KS really AIDS? Researchers have long noted that it has a very unusual epidemiology, very different from AIDS itself. For example, it is about 20 times as common in gay or bisexual men with AIDS as in hemophiliac men with AIDS. Women infected with AIDS through heterosexual contact are more likely to have KS if their partners are bisexual than if they are IV drug users. KS is 300 times more common in people with AIDS than in people with other immune deficiencies; by contrast, the incidence of non-Hodgkins lymphoma is about the same. Children are unlikely to have KS—but all 12 children younger than 5 years who have KS are from Florida, and 11 of the 12 have Haitian mothers. This epidemiology has led researchers to suggest that KS may be caused by a yet-unknown infectious disease, usually transmitted sexually (Beral and others, 1990).

Many minor epidemics are always occurring, in the modern, cosmopolitan world at least, and usually they pass without being noticed. Some experts believe that KS might have been another hardly-noticed disease, except that many people also had immune deficiencies due to HIV, and as a result the KS was much worse than it otherwise would have been.

This theory suggests that some persons who were HIV *negative* would also have been likely to get KS, although probably a mild form. Such cases have now been found (Friedman-Kien and others, 1990). Unfortunately, only a small percentage of persons with KS were HIV negative; the researchers had to test 349 people with KS to find the six. These six had a very mild disease, with complete or almost complete recovery, after a median time of five years since diagnosis.

Since KS has by definition been classified as AIDS, due to decisions made early in the history of the epidemic when much less was known, many people diagnosed with KS never took the HIV antibody test; they were assumed to be positive since they had AIDS by definition. Now it appears that a few patients with KS may be HIV negative and not really have AIDS at all (except by the old definition, which is still in force). These people may be able to live for a normal lifespan, with little or no treatment.

Researchers would like to get in touch with anyone who is HIV negative but has or has had KS.

# REFERENCES

Beral V and others. Kaposi's sarcoma among persons with AIDS: a sexually transmitted infection? *The Lancet*, volume 335, page 123-128, January 20, 1990.

Costa J and Rabson AS. Generalized Kaposi's sarcoma is not a neoplasm. *The Lancet*, page 58, January 1/8, 1983.

Folkman J. Successful treatment of an angiogenic disease. *The New England Journal of Medicine*, volume 320 number 18, pages 1211-1212, May 4, 1989.

Folkman J and others. Control of angiogenesis with synthetic heparin substitutes. *Science*, volume 243, pages 1490-1493, March 17, 1989.

Friedman-Kien AE and others. Kaposi's sarcoma in HIV-negative homosexual men. *The Lancet*, volume 335, pages 168-169, January 20, 1990.

Nakamura S and others. Kaposi's sarcoma cells: Long-term culture with growth factor from retrovirus-infected CD4+ T cells. *Science*, volume 242, pages 426-430, October 21, 1988.

Salahuddin SZ and others. Angiogenic properties of Kaposi's sarcoma-derived cells after long-term culture in vitro. *Science*, volume 242, pages 430-433, October 22, 1988.

White CW and others. Treatment of pulmonary hemangiomatosis with recombinant interferon alfa-2a. *The New England Journal of Medicine,* vol. 320 number 18, pages 1197-1200, May 4, 1989.

# PEOPLE OF COLOR CONFRONT HIV, HEALTH SYSTEM

*by Denny Smith*

In less than ten years the AIDS epidemic has highlighted many failings of health care and social programs in the U.S. These include gaps in education and earnings which guarantee lives of poverty and poor health for disproportionate numbers of Blacks, Latinos, Asians and Native Americans; the inconsistent and often nonexistent health care allotted to working-class people in general and women in particular; academic research geared to favor the needs of business at the expense of taxpayers and consumers; and an ongoing barrage of discriminatory legislation aimed against gay people, immigrants, and anyone suspected of being either.

These failings and the prospects for correcting them were among the issues addressed at the Third Annual National Black Gay and Lesbian Leadership Conference and Health Institute in Atlanta, February 16-19. *AIDS Treatment News* attended the conference with a particular interest in discussions of HIV treatment access for HIV positive people of color.

The U.S. government and medical complex was neglectfully slow to respond to the AIDS crisis when the epidemic was considered, incorrectly of course, to be a threat mostly for white gay men and intravenous drug users. To compensate for the lack of concern and urgency, activists of all colors in the lesbian and gay community mobilized their political skill, called on the help of affluent friends of the community, and mounted a strong, compassionate response to AIDS both locally and nationally. Explicit information generated from a community perspective produced a sharp decline in the rate of HIV transmission, and campaigns urging early treatment intervention are now extending health and survival.

The information from the AIDS service community, as well as from the mainstream media, has frequently been designed to target the white, gay male population. The epidemic is expanding rapidly outside of this arbitrary limit, and outside of its network of information and practical resources. People who acquired HIV through heterosexual contact, or contaminated needles or blood products, generally haven't benefitted from the organized community support which helped gays and their families endure the past decade.

A new awareness of these factors is evident in the growing network of organizations and information forums for minority HIV concerns. This network shares much overlap with the older AIDS establishment, particularly for gay and bisexual people of color. Important and unique issues for these communities have frequently been overlooked by the larger gay and minority organizations, but their multiple perspectives are critical to planning for the future.

The largest program offering HIV prevention information to gay and bisexual men of color is the National Task Force on AIDS Prevention, a project of the National Association of Black and White Men Together (NABWMT). This task force is based in San Francisco but operates HIV/safer sex workshops around the nation. Other examples of San Francisco's well-organized multicultural gay and lesbian communities include the Community HIV Project of the Gay Asian Pacific Alliance (GAPA), and workshops for men who have sex with men conducted by the American Indian AIDS Institute. (Supporting early HIV treatment and intervention, the San Francisco

Department of Public Health recently awarded $115,000 to the Gay Men of Color Consortium, and $35,000 to the Mission Neighborhood Health Center.)

A particularly urgent situation is now facing African American and Hispanic communities, where longstanding deficits in community health are now compounded by the new crisis. Current assumptions regarding the epidemic's future could be deceptive unless planners factor into their projections the specific variables in given populations. Some examples:

• Public health information on HIV transmission and treatment often does not take account of differences in language and culture, or for lack of a community's access to printed media. If a community relies on television and radio for news, it will probably receive information that is missing large portions of reality, like the importance of condoms, realistic discussions of sex and drugs, and the optimism around early treatment for HIV.

• Access to quality healthcare in the U.S. is hit and miss to begin with, and low-income or underemployed people are essentially thrown scraps by Federal programs, and patchy supplements from particular states and cities. Scraps do not encourage regular check-ups and aggressive, preventive health care. If medical help is sought only when symptoms appear, treatment for many illnesses, including HIV infection, is more difficult.

• The health of someone using intravenous drugs is often compromised by poor nutrition and infrequent health exams. If HIV is factored into the situation, the prospects of monitoring one's health and obtaining early diagnosis or treatment are hindered from the outset.

• Some occupations which are filled predominantly by minorities, such as migrant farm work, may pose increased exposure to sources of opportunistic infections. Toxoplasmosis, Valley Fever and MAI are all caused by microbes commonly found in soil. Even aside from occupational exposure, Filipino, Native American and Black people are already at higher risk for Valley Fever, or Coccidioidomycosis (Bronnimann and Galgiani, 1989).

These situations help explain why Blacks represent 27.7% of all people diagnosed with AIDS, though only 11.5% of the U.S. population, and Latinos account for 15.6% of AIDS diagnoses, but only 6.4% of the general population. In addition, 75% of all children with AIDS and 71% of all women are Black or Latina. Behind these statistics hides a larger impending disaster, given the delay between the initial infection and the appearance of symptoms, and additional delays in antibody testing or early treatment intervention.

Information on HIV prevention may decrease new infections among people who know their antibody status, yet miss people who are already infected and have not been tested. While they remain asymptomatic, these people may not feel the need to observe safer sex or needle precautions, and can unwittingly transmit HIV to their partners and possibly to future children. Unfortunately, sexually transmitted diseases run highest in the age group least receptive to health cautions—teenagers from 12 to 15 years of age. An HIV infection occurring in adolescence may not cause obvious symptoms until the mid-twenties, well into child-bearing years.

The future success of efforts to stop HIV transmission may depend heavily on parallel efforts to offer testing and treatment. And successful treatment for over a million Americans with HIV will absolutely require a more rational, equitable system of delivering health care.

NABWMT's National Task Force on AIDS Prevention can be reached at 415/255-8378.

## REFERENCES

Bronnimann, D A and Galgiani, J N. Coccicioidomycosis. *European Journal of Clinical Microbiology and Infectious Diseases*, volume 8, number 5, pages 466-473, May 1989.

# GRASSROOTS LOBBYING AND ORGANIZING OPPORTUNITIES

*by John S. James*

Last month, *AIDS Treatment News* examined the arguments now being heard to reduce Federal AIDS research ("New Threats to AIDS Research Funding," issue #97). This article briefly describes some options by which you can make your voice heard in Congress.

There is a widespread myth that an "AIDS lobby" is already highly effective. The fact is that while AIDS organizations have been effective in other ways, much less has been done to reach Congress than most people realize. The great majority of members of Congress are uninformed on AIDS, and have no staff member following it, because they have never heard from voters or opinion leaders in their districts that AIDS matters to them. Only a few members of Congress are carrying all the weight on AIDS—and they need to be supported.

Do not think that Congressional funding for AIDS research proves that lobbying is already being taken care of. Most members of Congress basically want to avoid AIDS. By voting for research money, they can tell themselves that they have done their duty and then forget about AIDS; they can hope that if they propitiate the monster, maybe it will go away. The political organizations we do have deserve much credit for what progress has been made, but there is only so much they can do unless they get more support from the public. It would be a great mistake to complacently assume that our own efforts have been powerful, when in fact the glaring reality is how *little* Congress has heard from the public, compared to the importance of AIDS.

The essence of lobbying today consists of mobilizing public support, letting members of Congress know that voters, opinion leaders, and campaign contributors in their state or Congressional district care enough about an issue to visit their offices, write, call, send Mailgrams, etc. Usually it is not necessary for an organization to address everybody in Congress at once, because a few strategically-placed or swing votes will be crucial at a particular time. But an organization working on AIDS needs to have an ongoing presence among the voters of as many districts as possible, because today power in Congress is decentralized, meaning that a group may need the active support of dozens of Senators or Representatives to get something done. It is no longer enough to convince just two or three chairpersons of key committees, as was often the case 20 years ago. And as battles in Congress develop, organizations may need to mobilize audible public support within days or sometimes hours as new districts suddenly become strategic. But today, unfortunately, many of even the most important members of Congress have nobody in their districts working with their offices on AIDS.

The next few months will be especially important in developing next year's budget, aid to areas heavily impacted by AIDS, funding for early treatment, passage of the Americans with Disabilities Act, and perhaps removing travel restrictions for persons with HIV entering the United States.

If you have only a little time or money to contribute toward Congressional lobbying, then you can work with organizations that will help you be heard by your Congressman or Senators at the most important times. If you can contribute more effort, then you can help by organizing others in your area. In either case it is important to find one or more organizations that you are comfortable working with, as it would be very difficult to follow the details of what is happening in Washington on one's own.

Here are some groups which have, or are developing, programs for involving individuals who want to work directly with their representatives in Congress on AIDS issues. Our list, which is in alphabetical order, is not complete; these are the ones we reached before press time. We would like to hear about others. (Note that this list does not include some very important organizations, such as the American Civil Liberties Union AIDS and Civil Liberties Project, which work directly with Congress or with other aspects of AIDS lobbying and public policy, but do not focus on organized programs directed to the general public to help individuals communicate with their representatives in Congress about AIDS. Also, we did not include those directed to state or local governments, such as the California AIDS Life Lobby in Sacramento.)

• **AIDS Action Council.** This group, whose mission is to lobby for sound Federal AIDS legislation, works primarily with community-based organizations across the United States. Any individual or organization which would like information about lobbying can contact the Council at 2033 M St. NW, Suite 801, Washington, DC 20036, phone 202/293-2886.

Note: AIDS Action Council also convenes the National Organizations Responding to AIDS (NORA), a group of 140 national organizations which meet regularly in Washington.

• **American Foundation for AIDS Research (AmFAR).** AmFAR is beginning to develop a lobbying program targeted to a specific purpose—supporting funding for community-based clinical trials organizations. About 40 such research groups already exist; only a few have Federal funding, and there is no guarantee that this component of Federal research will be continued. The lobbying program aims to help these groups let their Congressional representatives know that they exist, what they are doing, and why community-based research is important. AmFAR has prepared an information packet on lobbying. For more information, contact Bill Flanagan at AmFAR, 212/719-0033.

• **Gay and Lesbian Political Action Committee (GALAPAC).** This group includes a number of elected officials in Congress and local offices; it is a supporting member of five major AIDS or gay political organizations (National Organizations Responding to AIDS, AIDS Action Council, and National Gay and Lesbian Task Force in Washington, D.C.; California Life AIDS Lobby in Sacramento; and the International Lesbian and Gay Association in Stockholm, Sweden.) Its program includes encouraging citizen lobbying for AIDS action, including a national telephone campaign to increase AIDS funding.

Now through the end of April, it is especially important to lobby six Representatives, who are swing votes for AIDS funding in the House. They are Leon Panetta (D-CA), Frank Guarini (D-NJ), Anthony Beilenson (D-CA), Bernard Dwyer (D-NJ), Willis Gradison (R-OH), and William Thomas (R-CA). If you live in their districts or know anyone who does, have them contact GALAPAC.

For more information, contact GALAPAC at P.O. Box 46577, West Hollywood, CA 90046, or call 213/931-6195.

• **Human Rights Campaign Fund (HRCF).** This gay rights political organization, the largest in the country, runs a very effective program called "Speak Out," which sends pre-authorized messages from constituents to their representatives in Congress at critical times. About 70 percent of the issues they select concern AIDS. About 20,000 people throughout the United States have participated. Persons in the program also receive a newsletter, *Capitol Hill Update*, several times a year.

Congress is very much aware of the difference between orchestrated and unorchestrated mail. Letters written spontaneously by constituents are better indicators of public opinion than mail generated by organized campaigns. But orchestrated mail does show how well organized a constituency is in a state or Congressional district. In the past, the HRCF would sometimes find that the majority of the public was on its side of an issue, but there was no mail on its side and an avalanche on the other, orchestrated by conservatives and fundamentalists. The Speak Out program helps redress that imbalance.

Persons can also earn money by signing up new members for this program— sometimes $15 to $25 an hour, especially while working at public events and demonstrations.

Besides the messages to Congress, the HRCF also encourages people to visit their representatives at their local offices, and organizes parties in peoples' homes to discuss how to assure a better Federal response to AIDS. When elected officials visit Washington, HRCF gets them in touch with the important people on Capitol Hill. And anyone visiting Washington can call HRCF to make arrangements for meeting with their representatives—and to be briefed on what is happening on the Hill with AIDS.

For more information, write to Steve Endean, Human Rights Campaign Fund, P.O. Box 1723, Washington, DC 20013, or call 202/628-4160.

• **Mobilization Against AIDS (MAA).** MAA, best known for organizing the international candlelight memorials and for its work on Federal-budget and on treatment issues, is starting a new lobbying effort which so far is fully active only in California. People who join this program agree to write at least four personal letters a year to their Congressional representatives. Meanwhile, MAA follows all the (California) representatives and the AIDS issues in Congress, and lets people know when it is most important for them to write.

Persons in other states can join the program, but they will be contacted infrequently because MAA does not have the resources at this time to keep track of all Congressional districts in the country.

Mobilization Against AIDS can be contacted at 1540 Market St., Suite 60, San Francisco, CA 94102, phone 415/863-4676.

• **National Gay and Lesbian Task Force (NGLTF).** This organization, a leader in the gay rights field but not primarily focused on AIDS, is planning an AIDS and gay rights lobbying month in June. For more information, call 202/332-6483.

## For More Information

For background on how organizations can influence Congress in today's environment, see:

• *How to Win in Washington*, by Ernest and Elisabeth Wittenberg, Basil Blackwell, Cambridge, MA 1989. This is a short (about 150 pages) and very practical book by two Washington, D.C. public-relations professionals. It describes many examples of successful lobbying campaigns, and points out that they all follow similar patterns. This book may be hard to find in stores outside of the Washington area, but it is worth ordering if necessary. It can be ordered through bookstores, or from the distributor at 800/445-6638.

• *The Power Game: How Washington Works*, by Hedrick Smith, Ballentine Books, Random House, New York, 1988. The author, former Washington bureau chief of *The New York Times*, wrote a much longer (almost 800 page) book on how Congress works—and doesn't work.

Neither book has any information about AIDS.

# NEWS NOTES

## Median AIDS Incubation Period Now Eleven Years

The San Francisco Department of Public Health, which maintains the oldest and probably the most accurate data on AIDS epidemiology, has published a study of HIV positive gay and bisexual men showing that the median incubation period from seroconversion to AIDS is eleven years. Dr. George Lemp is the principal author of the report, "Projections of AIDS Morbidity and Mortality in San Francisco," published March 16 in the *Journal of the American Medical Association*. The results were collected in collaboration with the San Francisco City Clinic Cohort Study and the University of California at San Francisco and Berkeley.

Dr. George Lemp, Chief of Surveillance for the AIDS Office, said that "We anticipate the incubation period will become even longer as a result of earlier intervention with new treatment modalities." He also said that projections of the future of the AIDS epidemic—essential for accurate planning for early intervention and other services—have been hampered by lack of information on the distribution of HIV in the population.

## Blue-Green Algae Production Contract from NCI

On February 28 Martek Corporation of Columbia, Maryland, a specialist in commercial production of algae under controlled, closed-culture conditions, announced that it has been awarded a contract by the U.S. National Cancer Institute (NCI) to scale up production of two strains of algae which produce sulfolipids, a class of chemicals found to have anti-HIV activity in the test tube. (For background information, see "Antiviral Found in Blue-Green Algae," *AIDS Treatment News* # 87.) Martek will initially provide four kilograms of algae to the NCI, and it can provide much larger quantities if needed. The two species of blue-green algae are *Lingbya lagerhemii* and *Phormidium tenue.*

*NOTE:* In our September article, we suggested library (and possibly some laboratory) research to quickly determine whether it might be possible to obtain a significant dose of sulfolipids through blue-green algae or other plants which are already in use as food. Someone with a scientific background and no relationship to companies selling algae is needed. We have been unable to take on this project ourselves, and hope that someone can do so.

## Jonathan Mann Forced Out at W.H.O.

Jonathan Mann, M.D., who built the Global Program on AIDS in the World Health Organization (W.H.O.) of the United Nations, resigned effective in June, citing policy differences with Hiroshi Nakajima, M.D., who has been director-general of W.H.O. since 1988. A March 17 *New York Times* report quoted officials as saying that Dr. Nakajima wants to de-emphasize AIDS to focus more on other diseases, and had vetoed Dr. Mann's staff appointments, transferred staff out of the AIDS program, delayed critical decisions for months, and prevented Dr. Mann from attending an AIDS conference he had organized in Eastern Europe.

The Global Program on AIDS, with a staff of 220, raises most of its $109 million annual budget itself, instead of taking the money from W.H.O. This fundraising had given it more autonomy than other programs within the health agency. Dr. Mann has concluded agreements to establish AIDS programs in 155 of the 166 countries in W.H.O.

Dr. June Osborn, chair of the National Commission on AIDS, called the resignation "a world tragedy": "From July 1986, when he didn't even have an office, to more than 150 useable, constructive agreements on such a sensitive issue is the most brilliant job of international creative work that I know of." (Dr. Osborn, quoted in *The New York Times,* March 17.)

## California AIDS Office Leaves Money Unspent?

According to a March 10 story in the *San Francisco Examiner*, California's Office of AIDS has spent only $8 million out of $50 million available, in the first three quarters of its budget year. The article quotes experts and officials in other agencies as saying that excessive bureaucracy and other administrative problems have kept the office, with a staff of 143, from responding effectively to the epidemic. For example, a study by two associations of health officials found that a typical contract can be 60 pages long and take six to eight months for paperwork.

The office says that it has approved contracts worth $35 million, but that much less has been spent so far because requests for payment often come in months later.

# Issue Number 100
# April 6, 1990

## HIV PHYSICIANS—ON THE FRONT LINE

*by Denny Smith*

In the course of pursuing information which could be of use to our readers, *AIDS Treatment News* frequently calls on the experience and expertise of doctors who are familiar with the latest consensus of care for HIV and related diagnoses. For nearly ten years, AIDS-knowledgeable physicians have been facing problems never encountered before, and have been working with their patients to create solutions with and without the benefit of clinical studies.

Unfortunately, we hear from many people with HIV or AIDS whose healthcare providers are apparently not current with diagnostic or treatment information. On the one hand, it is easy to understand the difficulty everyone has with absorbing the avalanche of AIDS developments today. On the other, people facing any serious health crisis are entitled to the most precise and comprehensive medicine available. The rights of a patient do not need to conflict with the responsibilities of a physician. But when there seems to be a conflict, each party might consider whether the difference is one of opinion, or of accurate information.

We discussed some common questions of HIV diagnosis and treatment with two respected San Francisco physicians—Drs. Lisa Capaldini and Larry Waites. Dr. Capaldini is an Assistant Clinical Professor of Medicine at the University of California San Francisco, and cares for many people with HIV in her practice on Castro Street. Dr. Waites is a staff physician at Byers, Levin, Santiago and Waites Medical Group, and currently directs a national clinical trial of compound Q for the Project Inform Community Research Alliance.

## Diagnosing: A Discussion with Lisa Capaldini, M.D.

The causes of symptoms related to an HIV infection can often be difficult to diagnose quickly and accurately. There may be several reasons for this difficulty: HIV is a relatively new medical challenge; AIDS functions as an umbrella for a wide spectrum of illnesses; the immune deficiency sometimes allows for infectious agents to colonize unexpected sites (such as *Pneumocystis carinii* in the gastrointestinal tract). *AIDS Treatment News* asked Dr. Capaldini to share some of her clinical diagnostic experience. Following are some highlights of her remarks.

Generally, Dr. Capaldini likes to schedule visits with her asymptomatic patients about every three to six months. These visits include a T-4 helper cell count as well as a brief physical exam. Like most HIV-knowledgeable physicians, she recommends considering AZT therapy for patients with helper cell counts below 500.

Symptomatic patients should be seen more frequently, usually once a month. Because several symptoms can occur simultaneously or intermittently, Dr. Capaldini encourages her patients to make a list of problems to bring to the appointment. If medications seem to be causing a problem, she asks that they bring the drug packaging with them, to avoid confusing names like ansamycin and ampicillin, and to verify the dosage.

The first consideration in targeting the cause of a new symptom is determining whether a disease process or drug reaction is more likely. Many people are already familiar with past allergic reactions to certain drugs, and they should always make such allergies known to all of their healthcare providers. In addition to the common allergies to the penicillin and sulfa family drugs, Dr. Capaldini notes that some AIDS-related drugs, like rifampin for MAI, can provoke reactions which may not look typical, such as fevers and vomiting without a rash.

Some drugs may cause side effects which are acceptable temporary risks if both the patient and physician are prepared for them. Aerosol pentamidine treatments, for example, can produce an unpleasant cough which is easily controlled with a bronchodilator. Intravenous pentamidine, on the other hand, has been associated with low blood pressure and low blood sugar during infusion, and transient diabetes in some people after prolonged I.V. therapy.

If reactions to medications have essentially been ruled out, then specific possible physical causes are investigated. Generally, physical symptoms are more specific than drug reactions, but also may not present themselves characteristically. Someone with pneumonia may be fatigued but not, as would be expected, short of breath. Unless the attending physician orders a chest x-ray or tests for oxygen saturation in arterial blood gases, a *Pneumocystis* infection could be overlooked.

Fatigue as well as headaches may be due to sinusitis, even without any discharge. Sinus films can help rule out this possibility. Headaches and any focal neurologic symptoms such as confusion or loss of motor skills deserve quick attention; a delay in diagnosing cryptococcal meningitis, or encephalitis caused by *Toxoplasma*, herpes or CMV infections, can be life-threatening. Other neurologic diseases such as PML infections, KS lesions or lymphoma of the central nervous system may progress more slowly but also present grave consequences without treatment.

Some neurologic symptoms are due to primary HIV infection and may respond to AZT alone. Patients whose symptoms evade diagnosis with MRI or CT scans or lumbar punctures should be given a trial of AZT, regardless of their helper cell levels. HIV neurologic symptoms and subtle dementia can occur in some people even in the face of relatively high helper cell counts, although asymptomatic patients should be reassured not to overinterpret isolated moments of forgetfulness.

In any event, fatigue and headaches are commonly reported symptoms of HIV infection, and if the urgent critical possibilities have been discarded and AZT alone hasn't helped, Dr. Capaldini considers depression as a cause. She feels that depression as well as panic attacks are much more frequently experienced by HIV+ people than is generally thought. Neuropsychiatric exams can help identify the problems, which in turn often respond to counseling and/or medication.

The sight-threatening infection known as CMV retinitis is not necessarily identifiable with the resources of a general practitioner. When patients report floating spots or changes in their field of vision, Dr. Capaldini promptly arranges a consultation with an ophthalmologist, even if a cursory exam appears normal. A delay of just a few days can result in irreversible retinal damage. Toxoplasmosis is another, less frequent cause of vision problems.

Skin rashes are often the first signs of an HIV infection progressing to symptoms. Dr. Capaldini suggests to her patients with dermatitis that they use lotions to keep their skin moist, and sometimes offers topical steroid creams for serious problems. Other possibilities to be aware of are eosinophilic folliculitis, scabies, and flare-ups of the herpes zoster virus, or shingles. HIV-related shingles may produce severe pain at nerve endings in the skin, but no rash, and if prescribed early enough, acyclovir is usually effective for preventing the flare-up from getting worse. Skin problems may be misdiagnosed more frequently in people of color, since medical pathology texts are often written and illustrated with a Caucasian bias.

Pain in nerve endings, or neuropathy, can also be due to HIV itself, or toxicity from anti-HIV drugs like ddI or ddC. Drug-induced neuropathy may be reversible if the dosage is reduced or put on hold. Dr. Capaldini has obtained some relief for HIV-neuropathy with non-sedating anti-depressants, like nortriptyline. If the neuropathy is affecting the feet, she suggests that they be kept warm.

Muscle aches and weakness, or myopathy, may also be due to HIV, or prolonged use of AZT. Discontinuing the drug may clarify the cause of myopathy, which incidentally can be improved or exacerbated by physical exercise.

Yeast infections, also called thrush or candidiasis, are frequent problems in people with ARC and AIDS. For women, chronic vaginal yeast infections are often the first symptoms related to HIV, but are often not diagnosed as HIV-related. A *Candida* infection which has invaded the esophagus is a serious situation, causing pain with swallowing. Dr. Capaldini notes that heartburn *per se* is not usually due to candidiasis, but rather medications or excess stomach acid. Ulcers in the mouth not related to thrush can be extremely painful but usually respond to elixirs. Extensive ulcers may require a short application of oral prednisone.

Diarrhea and weight loss are common HIV-related problems. Diarrhea can be caused by a number of intestinal pathogens, including *Mycobacterium avium*, *Isospora belli*, *Giardia lamblia* and *Cryptosporidium*. When a stool specimen is sent for standard parasite tests, labs do not always check for the same set of organisms, so the physician may need to specify "Cryptosporidia," for example, on the lab requisition.

Unfortunately, some microbes may be present in the intestinal tract without causing symptoms. The isolation of one microbe would not preclude the possibility that the diarrhea is actually resulting from some other infection. In addition to the above organisms, HIV and CMV can both cause colitis. One distinction from viral infections in the intestine is the rapid onset of fevers associated with bacterial infections. HIV can also decrease a tolerance for lactose, so dairy products may complicate a bout of diarrhea. Nausea and weight loss which often are associated with gastrointestinal infections may actually be caused by HIV-impaired motility. Dr. Capaldini suggests Reglan to counter this.

Age can influence or disguise symptoms. For example, children with AIDS are prone to recurrent ear infections, but very young children usually cannot articulate the source of their pain. Older people with HIV may already be dealing with health problems which are not necessarily related to the HIV infection. In light of these and many other diagnosis pitfalls, people with HIV need and deserve healthcare provided by HIV-knowledgeable physicians, or physicians willing to learn. Treatment decisions are difficult enough without compounding delays in making a diagnosis.

## Treatment: Interview With Larry Waites, M.D.

**DS:** How early would you intervene in an HIV infection?

**LW:** I feel that the 019 (AIDS clinical trials conducted by the NIH) study clearly showed what I've been saying for over two years, which is that asymptomatic people should be treated—after reviewing the lab data, patient history and physical exam, we start very commonly at 500 T-cells with low-dose AZT, 300 to 600 mg a day. That seemed to be the most effective according to the 019 study. I believe people can often tolerate AZT for more than 18 months, even over two years. Some people are showing signs of resistance after that, but we now have ddI and ddC to go to, so we will be able to leapfrog medicines one after another as resistance develops to any one medicine. There are suggestions as well that we combine some of these drugs, but only limited research has been done on that yet.

**DS:** What about physicians who, in spite of the 019 and 016 studies, continue only to prescribe AZT to people with T-cells under 200 or who have had an opportunistic infection?

**LW:** I think that not giving AZT until the cells are that low is like telling someone with high blood pressure not to get treated until after their first stroke.

**DS:** I'm amazed that some doctors will even state their hesitation publicly.

**LW:** I fully believe that HIV is no different than any other disease, and we've shown over and over that early intervention and prophylactic measures in any chronic illness saves money and saves lives. It boggles my mind that we have to go through this again with HIV disease. This is just a viral illness like any other chronic illness and should be approached the same way.

**DS:** If someone was holding steady at say, 700 helper cells, would you advocate intervention as early as that point?

**LW:** We may come to the point that we treat someone from point zero, as soon as they test positive for HIV, and that the earlier you intervene, the better. Right now, the medicines are so toxic, that I generally do not start people in the 700 range . . . I just have to balance the risk and benefit.

**DS:** What kind of blood markers are now useful?

**LW:** Watching the T-cells, and the percent of T-cells, the helper-suppressor ratio, the beta-2 microglobulin, the p24 antigen as well as the p24 antibody. You know the antigen did not previously seem much of a help; not because it didn't measure viral activity, but because the test then wasn't sensitive enough. Now that, for instance, Immunodiagnostic Laboratories has a test which measures down to 10 micrograms per ml, most people who were originally "negative" are now showing up positive; the older tests just weren't sensitive enough. So now with new tests it will be a better marker to watch. I think the p24 antibody (Editor's Note: do not confuse p24 antibody with p24 antigen) probably decreases between 18 months to two years before people get really sick, so we may actually be able to follow the antibody levels in people who are asymptomatic, and identify who should be treated. I had a half-dozen patients whose T-cells were above 400, and were completely asymptomatic, but whose antibodies had dropped to zero. I started them on AZT and their antibodies went up, so my impression is that they were producing both virus and antibodies, and although their antigen levels remained negative, the antibodies were depleted by trying to keep up with the virus. By using an antiviral, we slowed the replication of the virus, and their antibodies increased again because they were less stressed keeping up with the virus.

**DS:** What about neopterin as a marker—the studies showing a correlation between increases in serum neopterin and disease progression.

**LW:** Oh, we go back and forth about the neopterin; most people aren't taking it seriously because you can find just as many studies which claim there is no correlation.

**DS:** I'm curious to know if you think immune modulators are as useful as antivirals, and if so, when.

**LW:** I think we have to treat HIV disease with a multi-pronged approach, with immune modulators as well as antivirals. The search is on for a good immune modulator. Certainly we know from the research at Stanford that interleukin 2 is a powerful immune stimulant, and I'm very interested in getting involved in some research on that myself. I think the answers are not in yet on Tagamet or Antabuse.

**DS:** Do you share the worry sometimes voiced about immune modulators that taking an immune booster without an antiviral may unwisely promote needless viral replication?

**LW:** If that were true, we'd be seeing more viral replication associated with things like transfer factor; some very elegant Paris studies showed absolutely no signs of stimulating viral replication with transfer factor, yet were able to increase T-cell numbers. So I think that worry has fallen by the wayside.

**DS:** For people in the 500 helper cell range, do you feel that any prophylactic measures, such as against CMV, PCP, *Toxoplasma*, are worth considering?

**LW:** No. I think the likelihood of them developing those illnesses are so low then, less than 5-10%. But between 200 and 400 helper cells, we administer a skin test to look for immune-cell dysfunction. If the person is anergic, we begin aerosolized pentamidine to protect against *Pneumocystis*. I believe the reason people get PCP in the higher helper cell ranges is because they have dysfunctional immune systems, and we can select those people without having to treat everybody prophylactically. But I commonly put people who have less than 100 helper cells on clofazimine to see if I can lower the incidence of MAI. Most recently, there has been a movement to try persons with low T-cells on fluconazole as a prophylaxis against cryptococcal meningitis.

**DS:** Anything for toxo or CMV?

**LW:** Other than environmental precautions, no. I check people for toxo titers to see if people have antibodies from a previous exposure. When helper cells get really low, we feel these illnesses are reactivations more than new exposures. But we should, again, say "get tested, get treated, get followed" . . . if you find you have a high toxo titer then maybe we should think about putting you on some prophylactic program. There is a wonderful report from Montreal which I know has helped me save a dozen people. It described how survival with toxo is much improved by giving the medicines just twice a week instead of every day, since many people have been lost not to toxo but to the drug toxicity. Just that has been very helpful to me.

**DS:** That reminds me of a letter in the *Lancet* which suggested that the idea of pulsing AZT once a day might be similarly effective for treating HIV, since bone marrow cells need about 24 hours to generate, so you allow alternating generations of cells to escape some of the damage of AZT.

**LW:** In a sense I've been pulse-dosing AZT every day, having many patients on every 8 hour doses instead of every 4. I really believe that the body needs to recover from the AZT. Unfortunately, studies have shown that even after stopping AZT, bone marrow suppression continued for six weeks.

**DS:** For opportunistic infections, what's new? PCP seems under control . . .

**LW:** PCP is well under control, but we have to answer the question of whether oral medications are as effective or more effective than aerosol pentamidine. Toxo is getting good results with pulse-dosing twice a week. MAI may be preventable with clofazimine, 50 mg a day. KS, still a big problem.

**DS:** Really? The options for KS seem so wide-ranging, although that doesn't spell effectiveness.

**LW:** The incidence of KS has dropped, except in the low T-cell ranges, when it is difficult to treat. Even all the options don't necessarily make us more effective.

Interferon has a 50-50 chance of working, although higher T-cell counts get a better response to interferon.

**DS:** Anything new for lymphoma or PML?

**LW:** Ivan Silverberg (M.D., of Davies Hospital in San Francisco) has been getting very good results with his chemotherapy, using shorter courses, low doses. He's obtaining good survivals for lymphoma.

**DS:** I spoke to someone at UCSF who was increasing the volume of radiation for treating lymphoma so that the duration of therapy could be shortened.

**LW:** Silverberg has done both with chemo—decreased the duration and decreased the dose.

**DS:** How about PML? I heard that heparin might be effective, for reasons that are obscure to me.

**LW:** Yes, I heard about that too, at the NIH. Well, heparin keeps coming up—you know it's a sulfated polysaccharide, like dextran sulfate. It was thought for a while that heparin also would be able to prevent viral (HIV) attachment. I followed some patients who wanted to be treated with heparin, and I didn't see any significant changes. But it keeps coming back, such as this possibility for PML.

**DS:** Something we hear a lot of at *AIDS Treatment News* is instances of people diagnosed with an opportunistic infection, and they or their physician drop the idea of any anti-HIV strategy. Sometimes people will stop AZT for more than six months while they're on Septra, or MAI drugs. If someone is diagnosed with an opportunistic infection, do you stop treating HIV temporarily or do you keep them on an anti-HIV therapy no matter what?

**LW:** I keep them on an anti-HIV therapy. It's important, very important to continue antiviral therapy during treatment for an OI.

**DS:** I'm sure you agree that a lot of things are missing in the world-at-large concerning AIDS treatments, but are there specific glaring gaps that you wish were addressed?

**LW:** Yes. I'm very disturbed that except for the work with compound Q, most of the work seems to be focusing on nucleoside analog therapy. Fine—we have ddI, ddC, etc. But who is developing ways to kill this virus? Compound Q is a good candidate, but it's only one of six compounds from that family.

**DS:** Given the hubbub over Q, do you think it worthwhile for individuals to consider trying it outside clinical trials, symptomatic or asymptomatic people?

**LW:** Well, I think it will prove to be safe to use for people with over 100 T-cells. With less than 100 there is a great risk of developing disorientation and coma, and they need to be followed very closely by a physician. I have worked on an altered-dosing regimen for those people and have successfully treated about 20 with less than 100 T-cells. We'll need to follow larger numbers to really see if this is true.

**DS:** If you were approached by someone who wanted to try Q, someone who's asymptomatic, with bloodwork relatively stable yet showing some signs of HIV progression, would you . . .

**LW:** Give me three months. I think I can answer that question when our new program is under way. The first program addressed dosage and toxicity. Now we need to answer how we use Q over time.

## PML TREATMENT SURVEY

Last year *AIDS Treatment News* (issues #79 & #88) reported the efforts of two activists in Los Angeles to compile a list of possible treatments for a serious AIDS-related viral infection called progressive multifocal leukoencephalopathy (PML). Lisa Muller and Peter Brosnan have sent this list, with periodic updates, to many interested people, and now they are circulating a "PML survey" to collect anecdotal data regarding the effectiveness of various treatments.

Peter described some early results of the survey, results which verify what they suspected: "PML is frequently misdiagnosed as Toxo or other central nervous system disorders. Valuable treatment time is thereby lost. Moreover, the actual incidence of PML is, we suspect, vastly underreported and underestimated. Treatment can work—those people who have received early, aggressive treatment are, in many cases, doing very well. Those people who were sent home to die have done as they were told. We continue hearing good things about both NAC and heparin in the treatment of PML. NAC, especially, seems useful. We have also learned that intrathecal interferon is being tested, but the M.D.'s running the study refuse to comment."

Anyone who has PML treatment experience to share can ask for a blank survey by writing Lisa Muller, 3031 Angus St., Los Angeles, CA 90039. Of course, the PML treatment report is still available by sending a request to the same address, or for urgency's sake, by calling 213/666-0751. A donation of $15 helps to pay for copying and express mailings. We commend Lisa and Peter for their ground-breaking work on an infection which has been widely, and wrongly, considered to be untreatable.

## EMPRISE: CONTROVERSY OVER UNORTHODOX-TREATMENT DATABASE

*by John S. James*

On February 14, ACT UP/New York sent AIDS organizations an "Open Letter to the AIDS Community: Stop the Insurance Industry's Blacklist of Unapproved AIDS Treatments," together with a cover letter and five-page background paper by its

Alternative and Holistic Treatment Subcommittee. Later, Grace Powers Monaco, president of Emprise, Inc. which is developing the database, sent a 16-page response. The immediate issue is whether the U.S. National Institute of Allergy and Infectious Diseases (NIAID) should give Emprise a grant to compile the computerized listing of "questionable and unproven" AIDS treatments. (NIAID has already given Emprise a $47,000 start-up grant for the project. In 1988, the National Cancer Institute had given Emprise $315,000 to compile a similar database—not yet available— of cancer therapies.)

We cannot fully cover this complex dispute in a short article. We will provide an outline and brief comments, then refer readers to the organizations involved.

The following passages give an example of what the controversy is about. The first is from the ACT UP open letter to the AIDS community, which is currently endorsed by about 20 organizations:

"Monaco describes the Emprise project as an effort to warn doctors and patients against 'the dangers and general worthlessness of unproven approaches'—not to objectively determine which may have merit and are worthy of scientific study. She and her insurance consultant friends will handpick 'expert panels' to 'evaluate the efficacy' of major treatments and practitioners. The cancer panels, already selected, are stacked with sworn enemies of what they label 'health fraud' and 'quackery'—by which they generally mean: 1) non-FDA approved treatments not produced by the largest, high-profit drug corporations, and 2) doctors who differ from orthodox, 'approved' treatment approaches. An analysis by an advocacy organization from people with cancer concluded that 'serious ethics violations, severe conflicts of interest and a systemic negative bias...permeate this entire project.' In short, the clear goal is to compile a blacklist.

"This blacklist will be put on every major medical database used by doctors, and leased to insurance companies to 'assist' them in determining which reimbursement claims to deny. As a federally-funded project, it will also greatly influence Medicaid/Medicare policies and future NIAID/NCI priorities on AIDS clinical trials. Indeed, Emprise explicitly told NIAID, 'The proposed grant will provide sufficient critical and evaluative data to demonstrate which AIDS dubious therapies can be expected to be nonproductive and a bad buy for patients without the expenditure of scarce government resources in a clinical trial to 'disprove' a therapy.'"

The ACT UP open letter calls for treatment information developed by community-based clinical trials organizations, not by Emprise.

Here is the Emprise response to the section quoted above. It refers first to the cancer database now being developed:

"The cancer monographs are now under peer review. If the evaluations by the scientific reviewers hold true through peer review, there are a number of herbal and botanical products and two drugs classed in the 'alternative' category that this research suggests could be safely used adjunctively in cancer treatment and should be put through efficacy screens and potentially studied on clinical trials. The same conclusion was reached about some dietary approaches. Not as cures but as helpful adjuncts.

"Although it is not possible to list those products until peer review is finished, as soon as it is, Ms. Monaco will be communicating this information to the *Townsend Letter for Doctors*, which is a publication for 'alternative' physicians.

"Does this sound like a blacklist?

"Do you want AIDS patients exposed to true quackery? By shutting Emprise down are you saying that you don't want your constituency to be informed about the scientific misrepresentations by commercialized unproven methods purveyors?

"Insurers don't pay for 'worthless' products—do you want them to? Don't you want to keep scarce resources in 'helpful' treatments or for CRI trials? Emprise will enhance the process of finding potentially productive adjuncts to care—not interfere with it."

## Background

Grace Powers Monaco, an attorney and the president of Emprise, lost a daughter to leukemia in 1970. She is a founding member of Candelighters, a support organization for parents of children with cancer.

Ms. Monaco has been one of the most prominent opponents of "health fraud" and "quackery" in cancer, and more recently in AIDS. Since 1978, she "has acted as consulting counsel for insurance companies concerning claims made for treatments which are nonstandard, alternative, unproven, questionable, or experimental, primarily advising on the merits of the claim." She had also been a paid consultant to Aetna Life Insurance Company in a racketeering lawsuit against Stanislaw Burzynski, M.D., developer of the "antineoplaston" cancer drug, but has recused herself from contining that relationship until the antineoplaston monograph (for the cancer-treatment data-base) has been peer reviewed. But despite these ties to the insurance industry, in her volunteer work for Candelighters, Ms. Monaco has strongly criticized insurance companies for denying reimbursement for treatment such as certain "off-label" uses of chemotherapy which are in fact the accepted standard of care—a serious problem for persons with cancer, as for persons with AIDS, even when they are seeking only accepted, conventional medical care.

Recently some of the alternative-treatment cancer activists who have long been fighting Ms. Monaco met with holistic-treatment AIDS activists to form a coalition to oppose Emprise. A recent meeting (organized by Bob Lederer, co-chair of the Alternative and Holistic Treatment Subcommittee of ACT UP/New York and columnist for *Out Week* magazine, and Ralph Moss, author of *The Cancer Industry*) brought together 35 activists from both groups, and laid the groundwork for the ACT UP letter quoted above. Journalists in the cancer group had obtained the Emprise application for the AIDS database pilot study through the Freedom of Information Act; NIAID has not released the application which is now pending. Without the investigation by these journalists, the public would know little about Emprise, as this particular project has had little if any coverage in the general press.

Good friends of the AIDS community have spoken out on both sides of this dispute. A recent editorial in *PAACNOTES*, the newsletter of the Physicians Association for AIDS Care (PAAC), defended the proposed Emprise database because it "could, if funded, provide physicians with peer-reviewed assessments of all available scientific data on the potential value of nutritional supplements, herbals, biologicals and other therapeutic adjuncts, such as imaging and biofeedback. PAAC has supported the need of such a database for physicians who generally have no scientific source to refer to when answering questions from patients on whether these agents or therapies are helpful or harmful. Information about potential drug interaction with alternative therapies is also a critical need of physicians."

(Gordon Nary, the author of the above editorial, is well known for his advocacy with the John Alden Life Insurance Company to set up a model program which will pay for care not usually covered by insurance, for example acupuncture or biofeedback for pain control, and nutrients, food, and food preparation for patients at risk for malnutrition. The program saves money for the insurance company by paying for home care, including transportation or reimbursement for care from family members or significant others, when other companies would refuse to cover these expenses and instead pay much more for hospitalization.)

But Bernard Bihari, M.D., medical director of the Community Research Initiative in New York, is concerned that the Emprise project could "create a climate in which it is harder to raise money for research, in which researchers are reluctant to test a treatment associated with the label of 'quackery.' The media picks up the most dramatic stories. The result could stifle scientific inquiry and the development of knowledge." Dr. Bihari noted that an early list of potential AIDS treatments attacked by Ms. Monaco was oriented against substances of natural origin—even while the pharmaceutical industry itself often turns to natural products to find substances which it develops as drugs. (Dr. Bihari does not see insurance as the problem, however, as companies seldom reimburse anyway until after treatments have official sanction.)

## Comment

We are withholding judgment on the Emprise AIDS project at this time. On one hand, we do not see how an unbiased database can come from an organization going into the project with so strongly held an agenda, viewpoint, and commitment as Emprise has in this case. Yet even a negative database could be valuable. For physicians and patients urgently need professional information about all treatments they are considering using. And negative information is often the hardest to find, partly because people are afraid of lawsuits, but even more because usually no one has much motive for researching and publishing the case *against* a treatment. As a result, the only information available often comes from promoters.

Yet not all treatments evolve on the same straight path starting with academic science, proceeding to peer-reviewed articles, and then to competent, rational development by a major pharmaceutical company able to afford the $120 million average development cost per new drug approved in the United States. Treatments which in fact have value can evolve from systems of traditional medicine, from popular culture, or from a scientific or even unscientific hunch. Any treatment which acquires a popular following before acquiring a professional one is at risk of being labeled illegitimate, and then being ignored by institutions and researchers who are fearful of damaging their reputations. Therefore the treatment remains "unproven."

We have long suspected that the AIDS movement might best stay away from what could be called "the old wars"—the unending battles between mainstream medicine and unorthodox treatments for cancer and other diseases. For the old wars have gone on for decades and therefore they are locked into a time scale of decades, while AIDS activists do not have that time. We are concerned that the old wars might now have come to us.

Perhaps the best outcome would be for Emprise to produce its database, but do so under a cloud of controversy (fortunately now provided by the open letter from ACT UP/New York). Then the public will know that the project represents not pure Science above the politics of competing views, but rather one view among the others. If the Emprise AIDS database is ever to obtain a reputation for fair and unbiased reporting, then it must earn that reputation. It cannot legitimately be born with it.

## Note

As we went to press, Ms. Monaco told us that because of the controversy Emprise is withdrawing the NIAID grant application, and is working with universities and others to determine how an untested-and-unproven-treatment database could be resubmitted under other auspices, so that the project can proceed with a more collegial relationship. She still feels there is a great need for expert, peer-reviewed critiques of the science alleged to support unproven treatments.

She also pointed out that the cancer monographs (on which the AIDS database can be modeled) include suggested future research to answer interesting questions about the proposed treatment—including the possibility of legitimate uses.

## For More Information

Emprise, Inc. may be able to provide their response to the ACT UP mailing, or other information about the database project. It can be reached at 1312 18th St. NW, Suite 200, Washington, DC 20036.

An article by Grace Powers Monaco, "Counseling Patients About Dubious and Rip-Off Remedies for AIDS and ARC," appears in *PAACNOTES*, May/June 1989, page 80.

For the case against the database project, contact ACT UP/New York, Attn. Alternative and Holistic Treatment Subcommittee, 496-A Hudson St., #6-A, New York, NY 10014, 212/989-1114.

## BURROUGHS WELLCOME SEEKS PROTOCOL-SECRECY LAW

*by John S. James*

A proposed Massachusetts law (bill number S. 464), initiated by Burroughs Wellcome Co., would make it difficult for the public to obtain protocols for clinical trials, including the informed-consent statements which volunteers entering trials are given to sign. While this particular law would only affect Massachusetts, it could be a precedent for similar legislation elsewhere.

The bill, which recently passed one legislative committee despite widespread opposition by AIDS organizations, arose from a dispute between Burroughs Wellcome and ACT UP/Boston over a test of AZT syrup in newborns with HIV-positive mothers. According to Steven Busby of the Community Research Initiative of New England, Burroughs Wellcome had required Boston City Hospital, which conducted the study, not to release any information about it. As a result, even the Massachusetts Department of Public Health (DPH) did not know that the trial was happening, and the study was not listed in the *Massachusetts Clinical Trials Registry*.

ACT UP learned about the study in April 1989. After it proved to the Department of Public Health that the study existed, the DPH requested a copy of the protocol, to which it was legally entitled. Current Massachusetts public-records law allows the release of the protocol to the public. Burroughs Wellcome claimed that the protocol contained trade secrets, and obtained a temporary injunction to prevent its release. But ACT UP then obtained a copy from the U.S. National Institutes of Health (NIH), which had determined that the protocol did not contain trade secrets, making the injunction moot. Burroughs Wellcome then went to the legislature to change the law for the future. Meanwhile, ACT UP found both ethical and scientific problems with the protocol, and significant changes were made in the study as a result.

(According to Busby, NIH policy strongly supports the public release of protocols of drug trials using human subjects if the trials receive public funds, and requires it for phase II studies and above. Opponents of S. 464 could find no other case in which a pharmaceutical company strongly objected to such release; certainly there is no other such case in Massachusetts.)

The proposed new law (S. 464) would allow a company required to file a protocol for a clinical trial to claim that the protocol contained trade secrets. If anyone asked for release of the information, a DPH staff person would examine the protocol to decide if there were trade secrets. Either party—the pharmaceutical company, or the member of the public—could appeal an unfavorable decision in the courts.

Burroughs Wellcome says that this change in the law would give it due-process protection against public release of its proprietary information. But the likely practical effect would be to make it much harder for the public to obtain in-depth information about clinical trials, even if there was in fact no real issue of trade secrets. Companies could routinely claim trade secrets, requiring court action before protocols are released. Litigation favors the richest party, and pharmaceutical companies are usually far better financed than public-interest groups. The result will be to further remove research from public scrutiny.

Burroughs Wellcome also says that its bill would make Massachusetts law consistent with Federal law, under which the FDA keeps proprietary drug-testing information confidential. But the proper comparison is with NIH, which routinely requires companies to agree to release protocols of clinical trials as a condition for receiving public funds for those trials. The FDA receives far more detailed and sensitive information from drug companies than ever appears in protocols.

Organizations supporting S. 464 include Burroughs Wellcome Co., Massachusetts Biotechnology Council, Inc., Massachusetts Hospital Association, Massachusetts Medical Society, and the Pharmaceutical Manufacturers Association. Legislators are being told that the biotechnology industry fears that competitors might work backward from a protocol to obtain proprietary information. Because of current economic problems, Massachusetts is especially concerned about being attractive to industry.

The following organizations are opposed to S. 464:

ACT UP/Boston
AIDS Action Committee
AIDS Watchdog Group
Boston AIDS Consortium
Children's Hospital AIDS Program
Community Research Initiative of New England

Dimock Community Health Center
Fenway Community Health Center
Gay and Lesbian Advocates and Defenders
Massachusetts Department of Public Health
Massachusetts Law Reform Institute
Massachusetts Lesbian and Gay Bar Association
Northern Lights Alternative
People With AIDS Coalition of Boston
Roxbury Comprehensive Health Clinic

Note: A December 21 memo from Burroughs Wellcome lists the Massachusetts Department of Public Health as supporting their legislation. In fact the Department opposes the bill, according to Sara Bachrach, it's Director of Government Relations, because it does not want to decrease access by persons with AIDS to information about protocols. A legislative committee ordered the Department to write compromise language for the legislation. The Department did so, but it opposes the bill even with the new language.


# AZT ASYMPTOMATIC STUDY PUBLISHED—NEW PUSH FOR EARLY DIAGNOSIS, TREATMENT

Results of the major U.S. trial of AZT for early intervention in asymptomatic HIV-positive patients (ACTG 019) were published April 5 in the *New England Journal of Medicine*. The major findings were already known, but physicians have needed more details to guide them in deciding when to recommend AZT.

ACTG 019 compared daily doses of 500 mg, 1500 mg, and placebo. AZT clearly reduced progression to AIDS, as well as showing benefit in other measurements, such as T-helper cell increases and p24 antigen reductions. The 500 mg dose not only had lower toxicity than 1500 mg, but also the low dose may have been more effective. For example, the rates of progression to AIDS per 100 person-years were 6.6 with placebo, 2.3 with 500 mg (low dose) of AZT, and 3.1 with 1500 mg.

Toxicity not only was less with the lower dose, it was also less for asymptomatic patients than for those more seriously ill. When used in low doses for early treatment, AZT seems not to deserve the reputation for toxicity which it had in the past. For example, there was no statistically significant difference in hematologic toxicity (anemia or neutropenia) or in elevated liver enzymes between the placebo and 500 mg group; nausea (reported by 3.3 percent of the low-dose group vs 0.2 percent on placebo) was the only severe side effect significantly more common with the low dose than with the placebo. (Anemia was found in 1.1 percent of the low-dose group, but was not severe enough in any patient to require a transfusion.)

This study re-emphasized the need for people to learn their HIV status and start treatment early. The message is getting out. On March 28 about 300 people had to be turned away from a San Francisco talk by Paul Volberding, M.D., the principal investigator of ACTG 019, on new information about AZT, due to unexpected turnout. The presentation will be repeated in a larger hall on Friday, April 13, at the UCSF Laurel Heights Auditorium, California St. at Presidio, 7:00 - 9:00 PM.

These AZT results also highlight the problems of getting treatment to those who cannot afford the price of AZT (currently about $2,200 per year *to wholesalers* at the 500 mg dose). And even if money is available, many persons with HIV have never had access to primary care; they seek medical treatment in hospital emergency rooms, only when they are very sick. An editorial in the April 5 *New England Journal of Medicine* ("Early Treatment for HIV: The Time Has Come") commented that "For these persons, the health care needed to provide the demonstrated benefit of early therapy is simply not available. Thus this major advance will result in a cruel and painful irony, and it highlights the urgent need to marshal resources and implement systems of care for all people with HIV infection."

# KS: INFORMATION NEEDED

A statement by Robert Gallo, M.D., of the U.S. National Cancer Institute, suggested that a much-improved potential treatment for KS may have been discovered (see *AIDS Treatment News* #99). But neither Gallo nor anyone else is saying more. We do not know what the drug is, nor what tests have been done.

Some rumors are *not* correct:

• The report that the drug is "MDS," from the Kowa company, is erroneous. This rumor started when a government press office, which itself did not know the name of the drug, asked a Japanese dermatology expert—who guessed that it might be "MDS," as he knew that American researchers had been interested in that. In fact, "MDS Kowa" is the name of the most popular brand of dextran sulfate, which is no longer in widespread use as an AIDS treatment.

• A report in a Japanese-language newspaper about 26 patients treated success-fully with a drug from Japan refers to Kemron—a low-dose oral interferon tested in Kenya. This research is interesting (see *The New York Times*, April 4; also see *AIDS Treatment News* #97), but almost certainly it is not what Gallo's lab is studying.

• In our last issue we published one physician's guess that the chemical Gallo referred to may be a form of beta cyclodextrin. We have since heard nothing to confirm that this is the drug.

If there has been an important advance against KS, why would it be kept secret? There could be many reasons, some more legitimate than others: serious danger of toxicity, supply problems, need to make business arrangements, desire to be published in a medical journal which wants a news splash, or simply business as usual. But even the better reasons do not justify secrecy if it leads to delays—for example, by putting all responsibility on a few key people, who are often busy with competing obligations or problems. If something important has been discovered, it should be shared with the public so that others can use their resources and influence to help overcoming obstacles (such as red tape, lack of money, or just being too busy). But people cannot help if they do not know that anything has happened.

*AIDS Treatment News* would like to hear, anonymously if necessary, from anybody with treatment information which is too important to be kept secret due to business as usual.

# Issue Number 101
# April 20, 1990

## ORAL INTERFERON: HOPE OR HYPE?

*by John S. James*

Startling claims, press reports, and rumors have turned a proposed AIDS treatment into the latest "miracle cure." Meanwhile, almost all AIDS experts who have looked into this matter are deeply skeptical, and often distressed, at how it has been handled. This article tells what is happening, and outlines some unanswered questions and reasons for skepticism.

## History and Background

On February 7 of this year, researchers in Kenya reported success in treating AIDS with "Kemron," their name for a treatment consisting of very low doses of a kind of alpha interferon, held in the mouth but not swallowed. *AIDS Treatment News* published a short article (issue #97); as far as we know, no other news outlet in the United States mentioned the development for the next month and a half. The silence was broken this month, after Dr. Koech spoke in Japan, with articles in the newsletter *Biotechnology Newswatch* ("Oral IFN vs. AIDS Scores in Kenya; U.S. Trials Next," April 2); in *The New York Times* ("New AIDS Experiments Stir Hope Mixed with Wariness," April 4); in *The Associated Press* ("Medical Experts Skeptical of Interferon Results in AIDS Patients," April 5); and in the *New York Native* ("The Cure?"—in two-inch-high letters on the cover—with the subtitle, "Is Oral Alpha Interferon Too Good To Be True?" April 16). (In Kenya, a magazine called *The Weekly Review* published a cover article February 9, titled "KEMRON: A Miracle Drug Against AIDS—At Last!")

Interferons, produced by the body during viral infections, have been studied for about 30 years. Alpha interferon has been available as a prescription drug in the United

States since 1986. In November of 1988 the U.S. Food and Drug Administration (FDA) also approved interferon as a treatment for Kaposi's sarcoma (KS); it had previously been used to treat hairy cell leukemia, and genital warts. The drug is normally given by injection, as it is believed that it would be digested in the stomach and destroyed if taken orally. Typical doses range from hundreds of thousands to millions of international units.

Most interferon used in the United States is produced by genetically engineered microorganisms (the two brands available are 'Roferon-a' and 'Intron a'). In November 1989 the FDA also approved a "natural" interferon (produced by cultured human cells deliberately infected with a virus) to treat genital warts. This product ('Alferon N Injection') contains at least 14 variations of the interferon molecule, whereas each of the recombinant (genetically engineered) products contains only one. This natural interferon is the variety approved in the United States that is closest to the interferon used in Kenya; the latter is produced by Hayashibara Biochemical Laboratories in Japan by a different cell line and contains at least nine variations of the interferon molecule. (Although approved for prescription use, Alferon N Injection is not yet generally available because it is new and supplies are still limited. At this time it has been made available to physicians who treat genital warts, to familiarize them with the product. The Japanese product is not available in the United States, apparently not even for a formal clinical trial intended to replicate the Kenya studies.)

Some experts doubt that it makes any difference whether interferon is "natural" or recombinant. This issue is an example of the broader fact that there is much confusion and disagreement among experts about interferons in general.

The treatment tested in Kenya consisted of extremely small doses of alpha interferon, about 100 to 150 international units, thousands of times less than the doses routinely given by injection. The greatly diluted drug was held in the mouth but not swallowed. Possibly the drug could be absorbed in the mouth (some conventional drugs are given under the tongue), but no one knows how so small a dose would have any effect. (Somewhat larger doses were found to cause nausea, and the experimenters suspect that the dose must be within a critical range, with too much of the drug being less effective than the correct amount.) Because the dose is so small, the cost of the drug is only pennies per dose, even though interferon is very expensive in its normal use.

Where did the idea come from to try using alpha interferon in such an unusual and seemingly implausible way—less than a thousandth of the usual dose, and held in the mouth, not injected? The idea came from veterinary experiments. Interferon has been tried for treating viral diseases of agricultural animals and also for feline leukemia in cats. Some veterinarians have tried administering interferon by squirting it into the mouth. Dr. Joseph M. Cummins, a veterinarian and president of Amarillo Cell Culture Co., Inc. in Amarillo, TX, is working with the Kenyan researchers and suggested the low-dose, oral route of administration based on this animal experience.

In Kenya, the leading spokesman for the treatment is Davy K. Koech, Ph.D., a well-respected medical researcher with dozens of published papers, mostly on tropical diseases such as malaria and schistosomiasis. The other principal investigator in Kenya is Arthur O. Obel, M.D.; he also has published dozens of papers. Very few of these articles concern AIDS.

## The Claims

Two claims have most caught the attention of the AIDS community:

• Every U.S. press report we have been able to find has quoted the claim that 99 out of 101 (some say 99 out of 100, or 99 out of 99) AIDS patients treated with Kemron had all their AIDS symptoms disappear within several weeks.

• Equally astounding is the claim that eight out of 40 patients "serodeconverted"—changed from HIV-positive to HIV-negative—during four to six weeks of treatment.

T-helper count increases were also reported, especially in those who had low counts to begin with (contrary to conventional experience with alpha interferon, which usually works best for those with higher counts).

Dr. Koech announced results of the 101 patients in late March at a conference in Okayama, Japan. A scientific paper about a more detailed study of the 40 patients mentioned above has been accepted for publication in June in *Molecular Biotherapy*, a journal published in the U.S. Some of the results of this 40-patient study appeared in *The New York Native*, April 16. According to Dr. Koech, the British journal *Lancet* rejected the paper because there was no control group (which in this case would probably have received a placebo).

## Questions and Doubts

• No one, including its advocates, knows how the treatment could work. The dose is tiny compared to what is used in other interferon treatment. The drug might be absorbed under the tongue, or there might be interferon receptors in the mouth; some kind of cascade of effects must be produced. But so far these are only speculations, not supported by evidence.

• The scientific study of 40 patients includes a table showing T-helper cell improvements. When we examined this table, we found that the *initial* T-helper counts, before treatment, had a median over 500; 33 of the 40 patients had T-helper counts over 270, with 18 being over 700. The mean T-helper count for these 18 patients— *almost half* the total patients in the study—*was over 1000 before treatment began*. Many if not most of the 40 patients would be expected to be asymptomatic.

But patients were accepted for the study if they were HIV-positive and had certain symptoms which might be AIDS-related. The symptoms were: appetite loss or weight loss; fatigue or weakness; mouth sores or ulcers or candidiasis; fever; diarrhea; respiratory tract infection; night sweats; lymphadenopathy; and skin rash. (The average patient had 5.2 of these symptoms. Two in this study were HIV-positive but asymptomatic; the others did have symptoms.)

It is possible that some of these symptomatic patients in fact had no AIDS-related symptoms, but instead had ordinary, minor infections which caused the fever, diarrhea, appetite loss, rash, night sweats, etc. Being HIV-positive and having symptoms which can be AIDS-related, they were included in the study and started on oral interferon treatment. Then they recovered—just as they would have if they had had no treatment at all—and were counted as having all their AIDS symptoms go away after the treatment.

We called Dr. Koech in Kenya and asked him about this possibility. He said that the molecular spectrum was not directly related to clinical symptoms, and that he was not trying to relate the U.S. and African diagnostic systems. He also noted that the disease itself and the results of testing are not directly comparable between Africa and the U.S. The scientific report of the 40 patients mentions that "Patients in Kenya were not staged by CDC or Walter Reed systems as might be expected in the USA." But the concern we raised above—that the symptoms observed in these patients may not have been AIDS related, and that in any case a group of patients selected only for being HIV-positive and having non-specific symptoms would, if followed for a few weeks, be expected to show many cases of recovery even without any treatment—has not been answered.

• A literature search conducted by *AIDS Treatment News* found no evidence that anyone associated with the Kemron studies, in Kenya or elsewhere, had much experience with AIDS. Lack of solid AIDS experience might have allowed errors to remain uncorrected.

We used Medline, a computer database maintained by the U.S. National Library of Medicine, to look for medical articles published during the last seven years (1983 through 1990) by any of the five authors of the scientific paper on the results of 40 patients in Kenya. Not all articles are included in the database, but it is usually complete enough to show the major fields in which a medical scientist has worked.

Davy K. Koech, Ph.D., of the Kenya Medical Research Institute in Nairobi, was listed as author or co-author of 52 articles or other scientific publications. Most concerned tropical diseases such as malaria and schistosomiasis. We found only two which mentioned AIDS, immunodeficiency, or HIV in the title, descriptors, or abstract. These concerned false positives in HIV testing in Kenya (published in 1988), and AIDS in Nairobi prostitutes (1986).

Arthur O. Obel, M.D., F.R.C.P., also of the Kenya Medical Research Institute, is the only other study author located in Kenya. He is author or co-author of 25 medical and scientific publications since 1983. But the only one we found on AIDS was a single case report published in 1984.

Jun Minowada, M.D., D.M.S., of Hayashibara Biochemical Laboratories, Inc. in Okayama, Japan, was listed as author or co-author of 126 publications since 1983. We only found two concerning AIDS; both of them are highly technical studies of blood cells.

Joseph M. Cummins, D.V.M., Ph.D., of Amarillo Cell Culture Company, Inc., Amarillo, Texas, was listed as author or co-author of 26 publications. Only one concerns AIDS, however: a 1987 letter on low-dose oral interferon in one patient.

The other U.S. author of the 40-patient study, Val A. Hutchinson, M.D., of Amarillo Virology Research, was co-author with Cummins of the low-dose interferon letter in 1987. Our search found one other published article, not involving AIDS.

The fact that AIDS was not a major field of anyone involved in the study does not mean that the results are wrong. But people are making decisions now on the basis of the Kenya results, which are completely different from what all other AIDS research would lead us to expect. The relative inexperience in AIDS of everybody involved might reasonably be considered in deciding how much practical weight to give these claims before they have been confirmed by at least one other research team.

• There was no control group. In other contexts this writer has argued that good science is possible without placebos. But in this case a randomized controlled trial would be very important (for example, to answer our questions above, about whether these patients would have improved anyway without treatment). And a placebo study could be ethical, since many patients had high T-helper counts and would not be endangered by going without treatment for six to eight weeks (the time required to see all symptoms vanish in 99 of 101 patients). Not everyone would have to risk getting a placebo—only a small number volunteers healthy enough to not face serious risk by remaining untreated for a few weeks. Most of the 40 patients had over 500 T-cells, and would not receive any AIDS-specific treatment anyway under standard medical care.

• What about the completely unprecedented claim that eight of the 40 patients went from HIV-positive to negative after a few weeks of oral interferon? The two obvious possibilities are (1) that what Koech has called "serodeconversion" did in fact take place, or (2) that there were errors in the tests. Dr. Koech has published several papers on immunologic tests; his expertise in the area gives greater weight to the test results. ELISA tests were confirmed by Western blot.

On the other hand, note that if any errors did occur—either false positives letting uninfected patients into the study, or false negatives when they left—all the errors would be cumulative, with no tendency to cancel each other out. Of the 80 tests (40 before treatment, and 40 after), a total of eight errors of either kind would be necessary to account for the reported result. It makes sense to wait for confirmation before accepting the unprecedented claim that this treatment can cause some patients to become seronegative.

• A great increase in T-cell counts—averaging over 500 for the 40 patients during six weeks of treatment—was also reported. Again we would like to see confirmation by another study. T-cell counts vary greatly, for many reasons. All but two of the 40 patients were selected and entered into the study at a time when they were ill (showing non-specific AIDS symptoms). Perhaps the (non AIDS related?) illness they had when they began the study temporarily depressed the counts, leading to a spontaneous rise as they recovered.

## Business Arrangements

According to its April 2 issue of *Biotechnology Newswatch*, Dr. Joseph Cummins holds four U.S. use patents on alpha interferon, giving Amarillo Cell Culture exclusive worldwide rights to oral use.

On April 4, 1990, Interferon Sciences (which makes Alferon N Injection) announced that it had licensed co-exclusive rights from Amarillo Cell Culture to human oral use of low doses of interferon. Interferon Sciences obtained worldwide rights except in Japan, where Hayashibara (which makes the drug used in Kenya) has exclusive rights. (According to the April 4 Interferon Sciences press release, Hayashibara owns 24 percent of the equity of Amarillo Cell Culture.) Under the new licencing agreement, Interferon Sciences aquired three percent of the equity of Amarillo Cell Culture.

Interferon Sciences is an 82-percent-controlled subsidiary of National Patent Development Corp.

Dr. Cummins is president of Amarillo Cell Culture. Dun & Bradstreet lists this company, incorporated in 1984, as having seven employees and a net worth of $309,351. Its current value would appear to depend heavily on how the world regards oral interferon.

## Plans for Trials

In the U.S., a small study is planned at Mount Sinai Medical Center in New York. Joseph M. Hassett, M.D., heard Dr. Koech in Japan; he told *Biotechnology Newswatch* that, "If even one-half of what Koesch reports in his uncontrolled study is correct, it's important to repeat the studies. If he is generally correct, we will know in a matter of weeks." This study plans to use the U.S. "natural" interferon product (Alferon N Injection). It would be better to replicate the Kenya trial with the same medication used there, but apparently there was some problem in obtaining it for this study. The Mount Sinai trial still needs Institutional Review Board and FDA approvals.

Another trial studied some patients in Amarillo and Lubbock, Texas, treated orally with Roferon, one of the recombinant interferons available in the United States. In a preliminary analysis, some blood improvements were seen. Now this study is being ended, and a new one will begin with a different dosing schedule and with the Alferon natural interferon, which was not previously available.

Internationally, a number of trials are being planned or at least discussed, some by the World Health Organization and some by Amarillo Cell Culture. On March 28, Tanzania announced that it was planning a trial, to prevent its citizens from going to Kenya in an attempt to obtain the drug.

## LABORATORY TEST SUGGESTS POSSIBLE DEMENTIA TREATMENT

*by John S. James*

A study published in *Science* (April 20) showed that in a laboratory test, rat brain cells were injured by very small amounts of gp120, a protein made by the AIDS virus. The cells could be protected by small concentrations (100 nM) of nimodipine, a prescription drug used to reduce neurological damage in certain cases of bleeding in the brain. The concentrations effective in the laboratory test can be attained in patients.

In the laboratory study, gp120 appeared to harm nerve cells by causing them to absorb too much calcium—over 30 times the normal level. That is why nimodipine, a calcium channel blocker, was tried in this test-tube study. The authors suggested more research to see if this drug might be useful in treating or preventing AIDS-related dementia or other neurological damage.

## What Happens Next?

Results from a laboratory study of rat brain cells cannot predict what will happen in patients. Even if the drug could work, no one knows the right dose. While nimodipine is fairly safe in its standard use (the most common side effect is decreased blood pressure), there is no information on its use by persons with AIDS, or on combining the drug with AZT or other treatments which would still be necessary, since nimodipine would have no effect on the HIV infection itself.

*AIDS Treatment News* called the senior researcher of this study, Stuart A. Lipton, M.D., a neurologist at Children's Hospital in Boston and at Harvard Medical School. He told us that he has a clinical trial ready to go; he is now talking with Miles Pharmaceutical, the company which owns the drug, seeking support for it. We mentioned that other funding might be found, but Dr. Lipton feels strongly that the company which owns the drug should pay for the study.

We called Miles Pharmaceutical and reached a spokesman in the public relations office. He said that while Miles was ready to support *pre-clinical* and *animal* studies (he emphasized those words in our conversation), they wanted more information before trying it in patients—for example, a test with another animal model. He mentioned that Miles had no experience with AIDS, but had been told that rats do not get the disease; scientific implications of that fact might be considered.

## Comment

It became clear that here was another example of the kind of misunderstanding that repeatedly derails practical AIDS research, due to the lack of national leadership ready to move in an emergency. It is understandable that a pharmaceutical company unfamiliar with AIDS would want more than a study of rat cells in a laboratory dish before sponsoring a trial. And yet the drug is believed safe, and ultimately—no matter how much animal work is done—the only way to see if it works will be for patients to try it. Dr. Lipton wants a trial now so that people will not start using the drug on the basis of one laboratory study, in the absence of any human trial for its use in treating AIDS-related neurological damage. We sensed that the parties had been talking to each other for some time before the article was published; they seemed to have reached an impasse.

Since no one knows if the drug will work at all for AIDS-related dementia or other neurological problems, no one knows if it would only be preventive, or if it could reverse symptoms already present. Fortunately AZT can often reverse dementia, showing that the damage is not irreparable. If nimodipine can clearly improve patients' condition, then a clinical trial would be relatively easy; it could be conducted by a community-based trials organization, or by an individual physician. But if the drug could only prevent the problem and had to be given in advance, a clinical trial would be difficult to administer, because it would require many patients and a long time to obtain the required evidence.

If no trial happens soon—we especially need the easy trial, for treatment as opposed to prevention—it is inevitable that people will start trying the drug without waiting for a scientific study.

## ACT UP CALLS FOR NIH DEMONSTRATION MAY 21

*by John S. James*

A national demonstration for more effective AIDS research will take place May 21 at the headquarters of the National Institutes of Health (NIH), located in Bethesda,

Maryland, near Washington, DC. NIH oversees most of the federal government's research into AIDS treatments through its AIDS Clinical Trials Group (ACTG). Other ACT UP chapters may hold simultaneous demonstrations at ACTG centers around the country.

Research problems (the quotes below are from an April 16 press release from ACT UP/New York) include:

• Lack of productivity. "After three years, not one single drug has been approved as a result of trials conducted by the ACTG."

• Poor priorities. "More than 80 percent of people in ACTG trials were given AZT," which was approved three years ago. AZT itself was developed outside the ACTG—as was aerosol pentamidine, after NIH refused to fund the critical trial.

• Conflict of interest issues. Almost all ACTG researchers have outside industrial consulting arrangements—and many of them opposed recent proposals to require disclosure. Have these secret arrangements had undue influence on the closed meetings which set ACTG priorities and thereby influence the spending of hundreds of millions of dollars of public funds?

• Lack of small, rapid phase I/II tests for new drugs.

*Note:* One new and interesting demand of this demonstration is for tests of 30 or more new AIDS drugs each year in small phase I/II trials. Dozens if not hundreds of appropriate candidate drugs are ready. Almost none are being tested. We believe that the basic problem is that money, personnel, and other resources are being diverted to extra testing of existing drugs, because the latter have more commercial momentum.

• Poorly designed trials, delays in releasing lifesaving information, too little research on treatment for children, lack of enrollment of women and people of color, and other problems.

Note: A *Critique of the AIDS Clinical Trials Group*, an in-depth background paper on what is wrong with the Federal program of AIDS clinical trials, will be published next week by ACT UP/New York. Authors are Mark Harrington, Jim Eigo, and Ken Fornataro, all of ACT UP's Treatment + Data Committee. For a copy, send a 9 by 12 or larger self-addressed envelope with $1.65 postage to: Mark Harrington, 611 E. 11th St., Apt. #7-A, New York, NY 10009. (A donation to ACT UP would be appreciated, but is not required.)

For an introduction to the basics of what is wrong with the trials and what needs to be improved, see Mark Harrington's "Anatomy of a Disaster," *Village Voice*, March 13, 1990.

## Comment

On November 11, 1988, a demonstration organized by ACT NOW, the national coordinating committee of ACT UP groups, brought at least 1,000 demonstrators to the headquarters of the U.S. Food and Drug Administration (FDA) and shut down the building for the entire day. Now activists are beginning to see problems associated with NIH as more serious impediments to effective AIDS treatment than problems at the FDA.

But moving the target to NIH involves much more than just a different subway stop and another government agency. The NIH demonstration presents new challenges which must be handled well:

•   The public does not understand the NIH issues (by contrast to the FDA, which it can easily picture as the "heavy" keeping promising treatments away from patients). NIH issues center around scientific judgments and priorities; it is hard for the public to judge whether or not criticisms have merit. And FDA battles focus on known, existing treatments; it is harder to organize people around deaths caused by drugs which do not exist and perhaps never will, but should. It is our impression that awareness of research issues is not well developed even in the AIDS community, except in New York City, where ACT UP has taken a leading role in understanding what is happening in research, and informing others.

•   Productivity of AIDS research has been slow to emerge as an issue because activists fear that too many people would just as well abandon treatment development and let people die. For those fighting for AIDS research budgets, there is seldom or never a right time to air criticism of the program. But now the glaring lack of new drugs out of the ACTG, and lack of hopeful signs for the future, are forcing the issue.

•   Most NIH-related problems have nothing to do with the employees who work at NIH headquarters, who have long had a well-deserved reputation for dedication and usually could make more money in industry. Clinical trials at NIH itself ("intramural" trials) have long been models of humane, courteous patient care, and they have been medically and scientifically productive; ddI, for example, was first tested there by the National Cancer Institute. The problems have been with the "extramural" research contracted out to academic institutions through the ACTG. NIH employees do not decide who gets the money; that is done by outside experts in peer-review committees. In theory, the peer review system is excellent. In fact, it is highly vulnerable to manipulation and abuse by industrial interests, old-boy networks, and empire build-ers—especially in AIDS, where outside scrutiny has been lacking due to the prevailing national unwillingness to deal with AIDS.

•   Tactically the demonstration must be organized with special care, because both inpatients and outpatients are being treated at NIH, and critical scientific experiments are being conducted; shutting down certain buildings, as was done at FDA, could endanger patients and be a public-relations disaster. ACT UP demonstrations often work through autonomous organizations and affinity groups. Organizers responsible for this demonstration must make sure that everyone involved—demonstrators, em-ployees, police, press, etc.—knows exactly what is legitimate and part of the ACT UP demonstration, and what is not.

Most of the problems associated with NIH do not really start at that agency. They arise instead from the national ambiguity about AIDS, and the resulting lack of high-level leadership and commitment. The ACTG program was set up several years ago, at a time when saving lives was not only unfashionable, but taboo even in the AIDS service community; virtually every organization assumed that its services would end only in death. This national lack of interest in practical saving of lives happened to mesh with the traditional value system of academic science, which most valued "pure" research, conducted without regard to the practical world. (Today's academic science is abandoning unworldliness in favor of money and deals—*not* an improvement.)

ACT UP's NIH demonstration conveys the message that glaring research deficiencies can no longer be kept out of sight. If it lets people know that medical research is *not* immune to national denial and lack of leadership, that these failures *do* kill, then the demonstration will have served its purpose.

# Issue Number 102
# May 4, 1990

## SAN FRANCISCO AIDS CONFERENCE, RELATED EVENTS: ISSUES AND UPDATE

*by John S. James*

The Sixth International Conference on AIDS, the largest scientific meeting on AIDS in 1990, will take place June 20-24 in San Francisco, at the Moscone Convention Center and at the Marriott Hotel one block away. A number of related events—some officially connected to the International Conference and some not—are also scheduled in or near that time. And two related international meetings originally planned for San Francisco—of the International Red Cross and of AIDS-related non-governmental organizations—have been rescheduled and moved elsewhere, because U.S. travel restrictions make it difficult and potentially dangerous for HIV-positive participants to enter the United States.

This article provides an overview and calendar of the Sixth International Conference, the international boycott by dozens of organizations because of the travel restrictions, and the many related conferences, educational meetings, marches and demonstrations, art events, video coverage plans, and other activities planned to coincide with the Conference. We also address the unmet needs for international communication on AIDS, needs requiring improvements in the annual International Conference in the future, and we propose a computerized system for peer-reviewed publication of scientific and medical findings.

### The Travel Ban and the Boycott

The law barring HIV-positive persons from entering the United States was passed by Congress in 1987. In April 1989 the ban gained international attention when Dutch AIDS educator Hans Verhoef was jailed in Minnesota, while attempting to change planes to attend an AIDS conference in San Francisco. (Months before that incident, however, Canadians had been prevented from entering the United States to seek medical treatment for AIDS. At least one earlier incident made front-page, headline news in Canada but was unknown in the United States as it was not reported in any news media here.)

In May 1989 the U.S. Immigration and Naturalization Service (INS) instituted a 30-day waiver to allow HIV-positive persons to enter the United States for certain purposes, including to attend conferences, obtain medical treatment, or visit family members. The waiver process was burdensome, however; a San Francisco law firm published a 62-page guide on how to apply. And there was no protection for confidentiality, as a code known to border agents throughout the world would be stamped in the visitor's passport, leading to risk of discrimination by other countries.

In September 1989 the UK Hemophilia Society wrote to all member organizations of the World Federation of Hemophilia that it could not participate in the August 1990 biannual hemophilia conference in Washington, D.C. because of the entry ban. A separate boycott of the Sixth International Conference on AIDS includes 79 organizations, as of May 4. The list is too long to reproduce here, but just the 'A' section of the alphabetical list gives a sense of the organizations involved: Action AIDS (UK), Action Health 2000 (Britain), AHRTAG (UK), AIDES Solidarite Plus (France), AIDS Action Council of New South Wales, AIDS Interfaith Network, AIDS Linean (Denmark), APARTS Solidarity Plus (France), Australian Federation of AIDS Organizations (AFAO), and Austrian AIDS Help. Other boycotting organizations include the International League of Red Cross and Red Crescent Societies, the British Medical Association, and the European Parliament.

Due mainly to the boycott and to pressure from the organizers of the Six International Conference, the U.S. Government twice made changes in the waiver procedure. First, it allowed the visa to be stamped on a separate piece of paper instead of the passport (only if applicants request that), a system modeled on that used by Israel for travelers who do not want to be barred from entering Arab countries. Later, the White House announced that instead of the 30-day HIV waiver, visitors could request a special 10-day waiver which would not require them to state that they are HIV-positive. These 10-day waivers are available only for the AIDS and hemophilia conferences, and for any future conferences which may be specifically approved as "in the public interest" by the U.S. Department of Health and Human Services. No "record of ineligibility" will be created by use of the 10-day waiver, and the U.S. State Department assured the Sixth International Conference that use of a ten-day visa will not affect later entry into the United States. (Either the 10-day or 30-day visa is required from HIV-positive visitors even if they would not otherwise need any visa.) The National Association of People With AIDS has maintained a list of boycotting organizations, and no group to its knowledge has withdrawn from the boycott because of the new 10-day visa option or other administrative changes.

A bill was introduced in Congress to give the U.S. Centers for Disease Control (CDC) the authority to repeal the travel ban—an authority it has for all diseases except HIV, which alone was added to the list by Congress—but the White House refused to support the bill, so it is not expected to pass in time for the Sixth International Conference. Lawyers disagree on whether the White House has the authority to allow the CDC to remove the ban without an act of Congress.

The Sixth International Conference has written a five-page letter to all Conference participants registered from outside the United States, to explain the current visa situation and requirements for HIV-positive persons planning to attend. For example, for the 30-day waiver applicants must show evidence that they can pay for emergency medical treatment if needed in the United States (so that there can be no cost to the government), while for the 10-day waiver applicants should be prepared to present proof of their intent to attend the Conference. Application for the 30-day waiver should be made at least 30 days in advance, whereas the 10-day waiver should be applied for two to four weeks before beginning travel. Obviously we cannot safely summarize the letter.

## Comment: Entry Restrictions and the Boycott

*AIDS Treatment News* is often asked if we are boycotting the Conference. As press, we must cover the news—the Conference, and the boycott, too.

We completely respect both positions, to attend or to boycott; people and organizations differ in how they can best serve in the common effort against AIDS. The boycott is not like a strike, intended to shut the Conference down; no one wants to do that. The boycott's main purpose, beyond bringing pressure to change U.S. policy, is to make the statement that the entry restrictions are unacceptable, and here it has succeeded. The worldwide revulsion against a policy based solely on bigotry and not at all on public health, a policy which damages international action against the epidemic for no benefit to anyone, has been critically important in preventing a stampede of retaliatory border restrictions which would have increased discrimination against persons with HIV and greatly impeded international action against the epidemic.

Note that of the two largest ACT UP groups in the world, one is attending the Conference (ACT UP/New York) and one is boycotting (ACT UP/San Francisco). Of the two largest AIDS service organizations in San Francisco, one is attending (San Francisco AIDS Foundation), and one is boycotting (Shanti). The American Red Cross will attend the Conference, although it has strongly opposed the HIV entry restrictions; the International League of Red Cross and Red Crescent Societies is boycotting. In either choice, one has good company. The question is not who is right, but how each can help in the overall effort.

## Scientific Program Published: Half of Abstracts Rejected

In a major departure from the earlier conferences in Montreal, Stockholm, and elsewhere, organizers of the San Francisco conference rejected half of the 4,900 abstracts submitted—about ten times as many as were rejected at Montreal—"to assure the highest quality presentation at the Conference." The Conference announced the rejection of over 2,000 submitted abstracts in a news release dated April 25. Because the rules allowed each person to be the presenting author of only a single abstract, it is clear that the work of over 2,000 different people was rejected (see "Comment" section, below). The rejected abstracts will not be made public, and most are expected to be permanently lost.

The accepted abstracts were divided into three basic categories: oral presentation, poster presentation, and publication-only. The most valued papers were usually given one of several kinds of oral presentations: a 20-minute slot in one of two concurrent plenary sessions from 8:00 to 10:30AM; a place in a poster-discussion panel during the poster-viewing session from 10:30 to 1:00 PM; or a 15- or 20- minute slot in one of eight concurrent oral sessions from 1:00 to 3:00 PM, or from 3:30 to 5:30 PM.

Each day the two concurrent morning plenary sessions focus on "State of the Art" and "Science to Policy." All the other presentations (oral or poster) are divided into four tracks: Basic Science (track A), Clinical Science and Trials (track B), Epidemiology and Prevention (track C), and Social Science and Policy (track D).

Some of the accepted abstracts not selected for an oral presentation will be shown as posters; hundreds of posters will be displayed each day. Authors are asked to be at their posters at certain times, so that anyone interested can meet them to discuss their work.

All abstracts considered for the Conference had to arrive by January 22, and their authors cannot change them before they are published in the book given to everyone attending; the published abstracts are therefore five months old when participants receive them. But the posters themselves can include whatever their authors want, so they can be changed right up to the day of presentation; information often appears on posters which is not available anywhere else. For the oral sessions, tapes can be purchased from the Conference; but to quickly gather new information from the posters, some people bring cameras, or tape recorders which they dictate into.

Many abstracts were accepted as "publication only," meaning that they only appear in the abstract book, but are not scheduled for oral or poster presentation.

Unfortunately the abstract books themselves will not be available in advance of the Conference. As with the previous international AIDS conferences, a major practical problem will be lack of time to read or scan the abstracts and select which posters to seek out. It is advisable to pick up registration material early, to leave more time to examine abstracts before the meetings start.

Titles of oral sessions, and of categories of posters (but not of the individual poster presentations themselves) are available in an advance program released to the press. We plan to summarize highlights in coming issues. But press cannot examine the accepted abstracts or their titles until the Conference begins—or the rejected abstracts ever.

## What Was Rejected?

Since the Conference will not say what abstracts were rejected, we can only report what we have heard from informal networking. As we go to press we have heard of five papers rejected:

• Also accepted for publication only was the hypericin observational study by the Community Research Alliance (also reported in *AIDS Treatment News* issue #96). This study followed 33 volunteers from baseline through four months' use of an herbal extract containing hypericin, one of the most important potential new antivirals, under a protocol providing the same blood tests and other data gathering used in most clinical trials. There was no control group. This research, organized by people with AIDS, reported human efficacy results at least a year ahead of those of any academic, government, or industry study of this treatment.

• A report on the effect of publication delays on AIDS research. The author investigates new treatments for a major AIDS research organization.

• Experience with providing research-nurse support to help physicians conduct AIDS treatment research in their practices. The author, a research nurse, does just that.

• Our own abstract on *AIDS Treatment News* and the unmet communication needs in the epidemic.

• An improved antibody test which shows unexpected fluctuations in antibody levels during the course of HIV disease, with possible clinical implications. This report was initially rejected; the author asked for reconsideration, and the abstract was finally accepted for publication only (no poster or oral presentation).

The Sixth International Conference organized international panels of hundreds of reviewers to rate the 4,900 abstracts submitted. But we have heard from two people involved later in the decision-making process that the work of the reviewers was often disregarded, with final decisions depending on politics and on who was known to those making the decisions.

It is harder to judge abstracts than to judge longer reports, because so little information is available. Reviewers are forced to base decisions on the credibility of the authors, to the disadvantage of authors not known to them.

The rejected abstracts are expected to be lost permanently. The Conference cannot publish them later or give them to anyone else to do so, because it only has permission from the authors to provide them to the Conference delegates. Members of a community task force set up by the Conference can view the rejected abstracts and write to selected authors to request permission to publish their work elsewhere, but there is little chance that this system will prove workable.

## Comment: Rejected Abstracts

We question whether anyone knows enough about AIDS today to justify taking half of the work submitted to the major scientific conference of 1990 and making it unavailable to the public. No one can be sure about what will be important later. The above examples of rejected work are not reassuring.

What could still be done would be to allow those attending the Conference to purchase the rejected abstracts—or at least to place an order there for later delivery. This plan would not exceed the authority of the Conference organizers to make submitted abstracts available to participants. It would be administratively possible, since the only action needed in the hectic final weeks before the June meeting would be to insert an order blank into the packets of materials to be given out. And there would be no additional expense, as costs would be paid by the purchasers.

But this or any other resolution to the vanishing-abstracts problem will require public pressure, as there is a conflict between the interests of the Conference organization and the interests of the public. The public interest is best served by having the over 2,000 abstracts somehow available. But keeping the rejected papers secret avoids possible criticism of the organization, by obliterating over 2,000 specific cases in which its decision might be questioned.

If the Conference organizers will not make the concealed abstracts available, then efforts will continue to contact as many of their authors as possible and offer to publish their work in a separate volume (suggested title: *AIDS Apocrypha*). In addition, those rejected abstracts which can be found could help to provide the nucleus of an international AIDS computer conference which could provide instant, peer-reviewed publication of scientific, medical, and other AIDS developments every day of the year, throughout the world. (See "Proposal: Computerized International Publication of AIDS Research Results," below.)

## PROPOSAL: COMPUTERIZED INTERNATIONAL PUBLICATION OF AIDS RESEARCH RESULTS

*by John S. James*

Despite the annual international conferences on AIDS, serious obstacles impede the rapid dissemination of research information. For example, the abstracts published at each Conference are due in January but not available to the public until five months later. Each Conference casts a shadow ahead during this five-month period; as the June meeting approaches, researchers become less and less willing to talk about their results. (Part of the problem here is the language on the abstract submission forms. Technically it does not require authors to avoid publishing their work during the five-month interval before the Conference, but the language does suggest such a requirement, and most researchers have interpreted it that way.) And aside from the Conference, the mechanics of journal publication usually delay information sharing for months, often for over a year.

Two years ago, organizers of the international AIDS conference in Stockholm had a "computer conference" system running at the meeting. Intended to provide international communication and publication for AIDS researchers, this system ran on a computer in Sweden but could be accessed internationally. However, we found that it was difficult for persons without academic affiliation to reach the Swedish system from a home computer in the United States. It may be less difficult today. (Note the International Global Teleconference now being organized in Sweden; it is listed above at the end of "Satellite Meetings and Conferences.")

How can we combine the need for selecting, editing, and peer review with the desire for an open system which avoids censorship by old-boy networks and narrow viewpoints? Here computerization can provide a unique advantage. Almost any abstract submitted could go onto the system; but also, expert referees, usually known to the system's users, would mark those abstracts which they considered interesting. These reviewers would usually be leading physicians and scientists, but they could also include representatives of grassroots organizations like ACT UP. Referees could make new recommendations, or cancel their previous ones, at any time. System users could choose the referees whose judgment they trusted, and then have the computer ignore all abstracts not recommended by any of them. (Users could also choose to ignore the referees entirely and look at any abstracts.)

How would the referees have time to look at all the abstracts, when thousands would eventually be submitted? They would not need to. Instead, the *authors* of new abstracts would be responsible for bringing them to the attention of those referees whose approval they wanted. Improvements could be negotiated, as is done with conventional peer-reviewed journals today. Authors could publish a rough draft immediately, then revise it later to obtain referee endorsements. This "instant peer review" provides the benefit of traditional refereed journals, while completely eliminating the publication delay which is their major disadvantage. It provides selectivity without censorship, by allowing readers to choose exactly whose selectivity they want.

Many medical and scientific journals which otherwise demand an exclusive from their authors will now allow publication of abstracts at scientific conferences, without ruling the work ineligible for formal publication. (Otherwise scientists would be reluctant to submit work to the International Conference on AIDS, for example.) This precedent should allow researchers to publish an abstract on a "computer conference," too.

For this system to work, it needs software which is easy to use. We frequently use online research databases, and we have found that two commands—FIND and PRINT—would be enough for all but advanced users. For example, a typical search might be

FIND AZT AND DDC

which would immediately print the titles of all abstracts which contained both those words, starting with the most recent. Beside each title would be a sequence number. Then

PRINT (followed by sequence numbers)

would print the full abstracts corresponding to the sequence numbers selected—or PRINT by itself, with no sequence numbers, would print them all. Anyone could learn this software in minutes. Yet these two commands would be powerful enough to provide convenient access to databases containing tens of thousands of abstracts.

Such a system would provide instant publication and communication, at all times and in all countries. The instant peer review with customized selection of referees *by the reader*, which we described above, would allow the same system to serve researchers, practicing physicians, AIDS activists, educators, legal experts, and others, giving each group its own view of the data, while allowing anyone to experiment with other views if they want. It would be like a permanent International Conference which anyone could attend at any time, without leaving their home or office.

Many components of such a system already exist; there is no need to re-invent them. The purpose of this article is to give one picture of how a useful computer publication system could work. If you can help with computer publication and communication, write to us at *AIDS Treatment News*, attn: computer conference.

# HEMOPHILIA AND HIV: A DOUBLE CHALLENGE

*by Denny Smith*

Before the current policies for screening HIV in blood supplies were instituted, many people were exposed to the virus through intravenous transfusions of blood or blood products. People with hemophilia routinely need certain blood-clotting components, and so for several years, primarily 1978 through 1985, many were inadvertently put at extremely high risk for acquiring HIV through the public blood supply. Hemophiliacs now represent one percent of all people with AIDS in the U.S., but that equals four percent of people with hemophilia. Another **50 percent**, about 10,000 people, are asymptomatic but HIV seropositive.

Hemophilia is a blood disorder involving deficiencies in one of two types of the body's coagulation proteins, factor VIII or factor IX. Deficiencies in factor VIII are more common and more serious. While both can be inherited, at least one third of all instances are new genetic mutations. Women who carry the hemophilia genes do not manifest the deficiency, but transmit hemophilia to approximately half of their male children and carrier genes to half of their female children. Men with hemophilia cannot transmit the deficiency to sons, but do transmit carrier status to all their daughters.

No matter which individuals in an affected family may carry genes for hemophilia, all members will eventually cope in varying degrees with the disorder. And the enormous prevalence of HIV infection in a community already coping with chronic health concerns has had severe medical and emotional consequences.

## Physicians Who Have Learned To Balance Both

Physicians who follow hemophiliac patients have historically nurtured a close relationship with them. Over a period of years the patient and doctor may meet many times, from controlling a hemorrhage crisis in the emergency room to working out a pain-relief program which avoids anti-coagulants. Obviously, these physicians were destined to become familiar with HIV diagnoses and therapies.

We spoke to Brad Lewis, M.D., who cares for hemophiliac and HIV+ patients at Alta Bates Hospital in Berkeley. He described to us ways in which health concerns related to hemophilia can be affected or unaffected by HIV infection. In at least one way, people with hemophilia were better prepared than most to cope with a health crisis—frequent hospitalizations and intermittent illness were familiar experiences. But for the same reasons, HIV at least doubles the emotional and economic stress on their lives. In terms of the physiological interaction of hemophilia and HIV, Dr. Lewis shared these observations:

- For reasons not fully understood, people with hemophilia and HIV are rarely troubled by Kaposi's sarcoma or active CMV infections.

- The hemorrhaging allowed by the clotting deficiency frequently causes serious joint pain. AZT appears to exacerbate this pain.

- HIV infection is often associated with decreased numbers of platelets, another of the body's clotting agents. This situation, called idiopathic thrombocytopenic purpura (ITP), is distinct from the mechanisms which cause hemophilia, but each can make bleeding caused by the other harder to manage.

- Hemophiliacs experience higher rates of liver-related problems, such as chronic hepatitis, resulting from repeated infusions of pooled blood products. Some of the drugs currently used in the treatment of HIV and AIDS are also taxing on liver functions, increasing the danger of toxicity for anyone already coping with liver dysfunction. However, Dr. Lewis notes that while liver enzymes are usually elevated in people with hemophilia, they are also usually stable and not necessarily indicative of progressive liver disease. He noted that monitoring a patient's levels of immune globulin may help predict if their liver abnormalities are stable or deteriorating.

(Chronic hepatitis is a serious problem for many hemophiliacs, and often for HIV+ gay men and I.V. drug users as well. Interferon has been studied as a treatment for hepatitis, and for HIV as well. Another substance called glycyrrhizin, currently used in Japan to treat liver disease, is being studied as a possible complementary therapy for a number of conditions involving hepatic dysfunction. *AIDS Treatment News* is now collecting information on glycyrrhizin, which we discussed over three years ago in issue #17; the treatment is attracting attention because of new research in Japan.)

To improve treatment development for the HIV+ hemophiliac population, Dr. Lewis suggested a few changes in the manner that clinical trials are designed. For one, entry criteria, particularly liver function parameters, could be relaxed for candidates with hemophilia. Additionally, the locations of HIV clinical trials should be expanded to established hemophilia treatment centers, in order to reach potential participants where they already receive healthcare, rather than expecting them to travel hundreds of miles to the nearest ACTG (AIDS Clinical Trials Group) site.

Dr. Lewis added that HIV and hemophilia each require specialized care, meaning that patients coping with both need access to medical care which is also familiar with both.

## Interview: Skip Harris

*AIDS Treatment News* interviewed Skip Harris, a Bay Area activist in the HIV community, and president of the local chapter of the Hemophilia Society from 1983 to 1985. He is familiar with each community's concerns, and with the general crisis in U.S. health care.

**DS:** How do you identify yourself in two different communities, Skip?

**SH:** I'm very public about my condition. When I was young, starting about eight years old, we ran blood drives every other year. I was always helping with the publicity for that—it was so nice asking people for help with something that didn't involve money!

**DS:** How is the hemophilia community dealing internally with HIV—is there a single consensus or strategy, or many different approaches?

**SH:** There are a variety of strategies; unfortunately the most pervasive that I've seen is one of denial. It results partially from our training. Around 1970 there was a dramatic development in the treatment of hemophilia, when the use of fresh-frozen plasma gave way to concentrates of the missing clotting factor. The concentrate was much more effective, and the medical community then tried to teach hemophiliacs that they could lead a relatively normal life. Well, HIV came along, and many of us found out we were infected. But most people weren't sick, so they went on living a "normal life". It was common then for doctors involved with HIV to say "don't do anything until you're sick," a sentiment easily and unfortunately echoed by doctors dealing with both HIV and hemophilia.

**DS:** Well, since early intervention has proven to be a more effective response to HIV, has that idea found acceptance among people with hemophilia?

**SH:** Yes, our Northern California chapter of the Hemophilia Society, and I believe the New Jersey chapter as well, are very aggressive about getting such information to their members through publications. I feel very fortunate having moved here by chance before the epidemic, and having access to HIV information developed by the San Francisco gay community. I think it's been a leader in the world. Even though it's smaller, it's been much more together, more politically active and involved than those in larger cities like New York or Los Angeles.

**DS:** Do hemophilia communities around the country look to the Bay Area as a model, like HIV communities do?

**SH:** Yes, and not just in HIV or hemophilia, but in health care generally, California is a leader. I'm fortunate to be part of an aggressive push in the local hemophilia community. For example, we reprinted several pages of text from Project Inform's compound Q study. Otherwise, there was no real source of news regarding Q for our members outside of the Bay Area. I know at least one person with hemophilia who has tried compound Q.

**DS:** In light of that, I wonder if the hemophilia community feels included or excluded in terms of HIV research or funding, or news in general.

**SH:** Well, the hemophilia community amazes me in terms of its diversity. People often think of it as a white, middle class disease. But it's an experience just as varied as the world at large in terms of race, color, creed and economic group.

**DS:** How did people respond to the recent "shortage" of clotting factor and the out-of-sight cost of medical care . . . particularly the combined costs of clotting factor and HIV treatments?

**SH:** Clotting factor's price makes HIV treatment look like pocket change. We were very angry when the price went up about 600 percent. People are enraged into numbness. The manufacturers tried to come up with all kinds of "pretty" reasons. But as far as I'm concerned, they just did what any drug pusher does to an unruly client—cut off their supply for awhile, let 'em squirm.

**DS:** It's a dynamic parallel to the profits wrought by Burroughs Wellcome, and Lyphomed, and all the pharmaceutical giants. It hardly seems to matter who their target patient population is; they just try to wring out as much as they possibly, possibly can. What do you think the breadth of HIV treatment knowledge is among people with hemophilia?

**SH:** Not good. Because of conditioning, the system, the doctors. Many hemophilia physicians weren't prepared to deal with HIV, and yet didn't want to give up control of the patients by referring them out.

**DS:** That's an interesting contrast to the many doctors who refer PWA's elsewhere precisely because they won't work with HIV patients.

**SH:** Yes, they've dumped responsibility on some "HIV specialist." But a number of the hemophilia specialists were actually too proprietary to consult an HIV specialist.

**DS:** Now, ten years into the epidemic, do you think the average physician caring for hemophiliac patients is familiar with AZT dosing, or the use of acyclovir, or the approval of EPO and aerosol pentamidine, etc.?

**SH:** Probably most are familiar with AZT and aerosol pentamidine, not necessarily with acyclovir and EPO.

**DS:** If you could make one or two things go in a different direction for people with hemophilia and HIV, what would you want?

**SH:** I'd want much more education disseminated through all the local chapters of the Hemophilia Society. . . just last year I spoke to a nurse in Chicago who works with hemophilia and who didn't know what aerosol pentamidine was, probably because Cook County wouldn't pay for it. Secondly, the government needs to fulfill a commitment to make treatment available. This year treatment was finally the recipient of some of the giant fundraising benefits. For a long time I found it very disturbing that AIDS prevention was the only idea addressed by those benefits, never AIDS treatment. The Reagan administration's policy toward AIDS very deliberately was to write off those who were already infected.

**DS:** Right, and that hasn't substantially changed.

**SH:** No—Bush has talked more about treatment but hasn't put his money where his mouth is. I really think the value of coalitions will grow in the future, coalitions of all the communities affected by HIV.

**DS:** When a couple of us from *AIDS Treatment News* attended the national "AIDS and Minorities" conference last August, we sensed very much a common realization that this is not a Black or Latino or gay or hemophiliac problem. If there is any silver lining to the epidemic, it's that people understand they deserve health care, no matter what. Why should someone have to struggle for either clotting factor **or** AZT? It's stupid.

**SH:** And what happens with health care will make or break this country.

# Issue Number 103
# May 18, 1990

## DDI EARLY RESULTS

Two separate reports of small trials of ddI appeared in the May 10 *New England Journal of Medicine*. These papers are unrelated to the current trials of ddI, and to the expanded access program under which several thousand people have been treated with the drug. Instead these papers describe earlier "phase I" studies: one at New York University, the University of Rochester, and the National Institutes of Health, the other at two medical centers in Boston (in order to distinguish, we will call them "the New York study" and "the Boston study" in this article).

The results of these studies have already been used (before they were formally published) in the design of the current phase II trials and the expanded access program; therefore there are no big surprises. But some of the information now published may be useful to persons taking or considering ddI.

In the same issue of the *Journal*, an editorial by Anthony Fauci, M.D., director of the National Institute of Allergy and Infectious Diseases (NIAID), compares and evaluates the studies. Both of them reported a number of different indications that the drug was working: T-helper increases, p24 antigen decreases, improved hematological measures, and substantial weight gain and energy level increases. In the Boston study, which used less ddI and gave the drug only once a day, 11 patients had had mild peripheral neuropathy before they started the ddI; this symptom resolved for eight of the 11 while they were using the drug. (Since peripheral neuropathy can be a side effect of ddI, it is interesting that peripheral neuropathy due to HIV infection would improve during treatment with the drug.) P24 and T-helper improvements were seen even at the lowest doses—adding to the increasing suspicion that the doses of ddI now generally used (in the clinical trials and in the expanded-access program) might be too high.

The most serious side effect of ddI is pancreatitis, which has caused several deaths among the several thousand patients who have used the drug. In the New York study, which gave the larger total doses of ddI, five of 37 patients developed pancreatitis. In the Boston study, only two of 34 developed pancreatitis. But the New York study had better p24 results. Dr. Fauci speculated that since the active form of ddI inside the cells has a half-life of 12 hours, the best regimen might be lower doses twice a day; but he noted that more trials are necessary to determine if this is true.

Both studies were short-term, giving ddI for a mean of 17 weeks in New York and 15.8 weeks in Boston—another reason why the ongoing trials are necessary.

## Symptoms of Toxicity

Some of the descriptions of the more common side effects published in the report of the New York study might help patients who are using ddI recognize them if they occur. It is very important to notify one's physician immediately in case of side effects, so that the dose can be reduced or the drug discontinued. In the latter case, it is often possible to restart later, at a lower dose.

The neuropathy "consisted of a tingling, burning, or aching in the lower extremities, particularly in the soles of the feet. The pain was particularly prominent at night but was also present throughout the day. Initially, the discomfort was noted in walking, but in more advanced cases pain interfered with sleep and routine daily activities... The onset of neuropathy occurred from 55 to 201 days after the initiation of therapy."

Pancreatitis was "manifested by abdominal pain and elevated amylase levels. The episodes began with vague abdominal pain, nausea, and vomiting and progressed to moderate or severe epigastric pain, which required narcotic analgesics in three of the five patients... The symptoms resolved within one to three weeks after the cessation of ddI therapy."

There have also been other side effects, such as seizures in a few patients. Physicians who are using ddI under the expanded-access program receive updates from the sponsor, Bristol-Myers Squibb Co., and from other doctors, as new information becomes available.

Some patients in the expanded-access program have decided to reduce their doses of ddI, often by taking only one of the two daily doses. There is some confusion on whether it is possible to do this with the knowledge of Bristol-Myers, or whether the drug would be cut off in such a case. We do not know the answer. In order to assure the accuracy of the safety information being collected from the expanded-access program, Bristol-Myers should make it clear that patients can reduce their doses and report that fact, without threatening access to the drug which some have found to be a lifeline.

## GLYCYRRHIZIN: RESEARCH STILL PROMISING, STILL LIMITED

*by Denny Smith*

An extract from the root of Glycyrrhiza, the licorice plant, has been studied for several years by Japanese researchers for anti-viral and immunomodulatory activity against HIV, and for therapeutic effects on liver disease.

The extracted substance, glycyrrhizin sulfate, has been observed in laboratory tests to inhibit HIV replication, interfere with virus-to-cell binding and cell-to-cell infection, suppress the clumping of infected cells and induce interferon activity. Of related interest, glycyrrhizin also inactivated herpes simplex virus and varicella zoster virus, both of which can become serious opportunistic infections. Among existing applications it is used in Europe and China to treat stomach ulcers and in Japan to treat hepatitis. Botanic and medical literature refer to two species of *Glycyrrhiza* as a source for the component: *G. radix* and *G. glabra*. Most of the articles discussing HIV refer to the first species.

Glycyrrhizin is one of several members of a chemical group called sulfated polysaccharides which have demonstrated varying degrees of anti-HIV activity. These include lentinan, Carrisyn, heparin and dextran sulfate. Glycyrrhizin's potential as an HIV therapy is not confirmed to be stronger or weaker than any of its chemical relatives, but anti-inflammatory characteristics and protective action against liver damage may make it useful for many people with HIV or hemophilia who must cope with chronic hepatitis or drug-related liver toxicity.

Over three years ago *AIDS Treatment News* reported at length on glycyrrhizin (issue #17). Since then, the other sulfated polysaccharides have captured more media and research attention. However work on glycyrrhizin continued, and within the last year several studies in Japan reported promising results with oral and intravenous formulations given to people with HIV or AIDS. At least two of the studies involved people who also have hemophilia.

One study of twenty asymptomatic seropositives at Osaka National Hospital was reported at the V International Conference on AIDS in Montreal last June. Of ten participants in this study who were given daily oral doses of glycyrrhizin, ranging from 150 to 225 mg, none progressed to symptoms over periods of one to two years. In the control group of ten who were not treated, one developed lymphadenopathy, and two others were diagnosed with AIDS and subsequently have died (Ikegami and others, 1989).

Another study was sponsored by Tohoku University, Fukushima Medical College, and Akita University. Nine patients with hemophilia who were HIV+ but asymptomatic were given 200-800 mg of intravenous glycyrrhizin daily for over eight weeks. Eight patients experienced an average 88.9% increase in T4-helper cells, and six experienced an average 66.7% improvement in their T4/T8 ratio. Liver dysfunction noted in four patients improved, and no serious side effects were observed (Mori and others, 1989).

A study conducted at Kumamoto University Medical School and Tokyo Medical College involved glycyrrhizin administered intravenously to three hemophiliac patients with AIDS. Six different courses of treatment were reported, using 400-1600 mg daily (adjusted by body weight) for at least one month. p24 antigenemia was detectable at the beginning of five of the six treatment episodes, but undetectable by the end of three of those five; for the other two, the levels decreased. The authors suggest that glycyrrhizin might inhibit HIV replication (Hattori and others, 1989).

Glycyrrhizin appears relatively nontoxic, but is capable of causing some side effects, including hypokalemia (low potassium levels), myopathy (muscle soreness or fatigue), high blood pressure, and sodium and fluid retention. Persons currently experiencing these symptoms are advised against using glycyrrhizin. Even in the absence of these conditions, we advocate supervision by an HIV-knowledgeable health provider for people considering a new treatment.

A friend of *AIDS Treatment News* has been using Glycyron 2, a Japanese pharmaceutical preparation of glycyrrhizin for oral use, since last October. He shared with us these impressions so far: For several years prior, his helper cells had remained very stable, in the 500 range. Then, last summer they began to decline rapidly in a trend apparent over consecutive tests. By October they registered 320, and he began taking glycyrrhizin in daily doses of 500 mg. After a month his helper cell count rose to 420, liver enzymes which had been slightly elevated were decreased, and he noticed an increase in energy.

Of course, helper cells fluctuate notoriously in many people, even without HIV involvement, and no one would claim that T-cell counts alone are predictive of illness or the efficacy of a given treatment. But together with symptom improvement, they are a first step toward more intensive monitoring of a trend. Our friend is always careful to have his bloodwork sent to the same lab. In November he began treatments with Compound Q, and has continued since then with both Q and glycyrrhizin, with good results in his bloodwork. His p24 antigen tests were negative before starting either treatment, but in January his p24 antibodies registered 400, compared to a pre-treatment count of 50. (Do not confuse p24 antibodies with p24 antigen. For the antibodies, a high value is desirable; for antigen, the reverse is true.) Attributing the improvements to one treatment or the other is not possible for certain; he feels that they complement each other.

Glycyrrhizin is available over the counter in Japan, where it costs about 10 cents per one 25 mg tablet. Depending on the desired dose, which varied widely in the above studies, glycyrrhizin could be an inexpensive complement in an HIV treatment program. Licorice root is the natural source and is widely available as a tea in health food stores in the U.S. Apparently, glycyrrhizin components comprise from 8 to 12% of licorice root, and they are available simply by drinking the tea. But obviously, this would be a haphazard and not a methodical way to obtain measured, standard amounts of glycyrrhizin. Chinese medicine often employs licorice root, but usually in small amounts combined with other therapeutic plants. We do not know of any U.S. source of the Japanese tablets at this time, but some buyers' clubs are considering carrying them.

## REFERENCES

Ikegami, N and others. Clinical Evaluation of Glycyrrhizin on HIV-Infected Asymptomatic Hemophiliac Patients in Japan. V International Conference on AIDS. Abstract W.B.P. 298, June, 1989.

Mori, K and others. Effects of Glycyrrhizin (SNMC: Stronger Neo-Minophagen C) in Hemophilia Patients with HIV Infection. *Tohoku Journal of Experimental Medicine*, volume 158, pages 25-35, 1989.

Hattori, T and others. Preliminary evidence for inhibitory effect of glycyrrhizin on HIV replication in patients with AIDS. *Antiviral Research*, volume 11, pages 255-262, 1989.

Tochikura, TS and others. Antiviral Agents with Activity Against Human Retroviruses. *Journal of Acquired Immune Deficiency Syndromes*, volume 2, number 5, pages 442-447, 1989.

Tochikura, TS and others. Human Immunodeficiency Virus (HIV)-Induced Cell Fusion: Quantification and Its Application for the Simple and Rapid Screening of Anti-HIV Substances *in Vitro*. *Virology*, volume 164, pages 542-546, June, 1988.

Ito, M and others. Mechanism of inhibitory effect of glycyrrhizin on replication of human immunodeficiency virus (HIV). *Antiviral Research*, volume 10, number 6, pages 289-298, December 1988.

# ACT UP, SENATOR HELMS, AND TOBACCO: A PROPOSAL

*by John S. James*

ACT UP groups and others have called for a boycott of Marlboro cigarettes, because Philip Morris is a major corporate contributor to the election campaigns of Senator Jesse Helms, Republican of North Carolina, who has consistently sabotaged U.S. AIDS policy and impeded Federal efforts against the epidemic. The boycott is now supported by ACT UP chapters in Washington DC, New York, Boston, Provincetown, Atlanta, Shreveport, Indianapolis, San Francisco, Seattle, Portland, and Paris, France. This article proposes another tactic which we believe could be effective against Helms, and also valuable in its own right in building national and international health coalitions.

Recently, public opinion and government policies in the United States have turned strongly against smoking. But as smoking declines here, it is increasing in the rest of the world. Export to other countries has become a life-or-death issue to the tobacco industry, since its future may rest on international sales.

So while U.S. health officials are strongly discouraging smoking at home, U.S trade officials are forcing other countries to accept U.S. tobacco, and to allow U.S.-based multinationals to aggressively promote smoking within their domestic populations, even to children—under threat of trade sanctions which can amount to sabotage of those countries' economies. South Korea, Taiwan, and Japan have already been forced to accept U.S. tobacco imports and advertising, and now the pressure is on Thailand. If Thailand refuses, all its imports to the United States could be stopped in retaliation, under the Trade Act of 1974, according to a *New York Times* article of May 18.

How do tobacco companies promote their products abroad, after the U.S. government has used its economic clout to prevent sovereign nations from implementing antismoking policies to protect their citizens? "In Kuwait the companies take photos of children next to Formula One race cars and hand out the photo, cigarettes, a lighter, and T-shirts to the children; in Thailand, where cigarette advertising is outlawed, Marlboro and Winston logos appear on schoolbook covers, kites, and T-shirts in anticipation of a favorable trade ruling; in Germany, citizens were handed packs of Camels as they came through the Berlin Wall," according to a recent issue of *Cancer News*, published by the American Cancer Society. After Taiwan and South Korea gave in to U.S. pressure, "cigarette promotion surged in these markets, and for the first time, advertising has been directly targeted to women who traditionally had very low smoking rates in these countries," according to the same source. If present trends continue, smoking will become a leading cause of death worldwide, especially in Third World countries; it is projected to kill 12 million people each year by 2050.

U.S. officials have argued that tobacco export is a trade issue, not a health issue—that under the law it does not matter that smoking is dangerous to health, all that matters is that tobacco is a product. Last week Congressman Henry A. Waxman (Democrat of California) and others were outraged when Dr. James O. Mason, Assistant Secretary for Health, cancelled a May 17 appearance before Waxman's subcommittee on the tobacco-export issue. Dr. Mason had strongly criticized tobacco export last month at the World Conference on Tobacco and Health, but later he was apparently silenced by the Bush Administration.

How can the United States continue to protect its own citizens while forbidding other countries from protecting theirs? The answer is that those who suffer from these unconscionable export policies have no voice in them because they are not citizens here. It has been much harder to raise U.S. grassroots opposition to the export policies than to issues which affect millions of Americans directly (like secondhand smoke in public buildings and vehicles).

This situation presents a special opportunity for AIDS activists and groups like ACT UP—and also for the arts community, which has its own problems with Senator Helms—to have a disproportionately large impact. Tobacco is widely grown in North Carolina, and tobacco companies are among Helms' leading supporters. Exports are the future of the tobacco industry, because of the strong turn against smoking by the U.S. public. No country wants future deaths and huge medical bills, so exports depend on U.S. policies which force other countries to take the product. These reprehensible policies, opposed by the countries affected, by international organizations, and by U.S. organizations like the American Cancer Society, continue because it is hard to personalize export policy as a grassroots issue.

But Senator Helms could be the key to personalizing this issue as it could never be personalized before. For example, actions by AIDS activists or by artists at the offices of the U.S. trade negotiators, or directed at members of Congress who support the unconscionable policies, could force the press to explain the issue, amplifying the testimony of anti-smoking experts and mobilizing public revulsion at the hypocrisy and national dishonor of discouraging cigarettes at home while forcing them abroad. Endless grassroots projects are possible. Groups like ACT UP, or arts activists, could contribute unique visibility to the campaign against tobacco exports, which otherwise consists largely of testimony by experts to august bodies.

Helms himself provides the motivation to bring a colorful, ongoing, and permanent grassroots presence into an issue of vital importance to his biggest supporters. Such a campaign could change him from an asset to the tobacco industry into a central threat to its future.

And the same campaign would also help to build coalitions between AIDS activists and those of other diseases, in the U.S. and internationally. Last week the American Cancer Society launched its "Trade for Life" plan against the tobacco-export policies. Developed earlier in the year at a consensus conference of international tobacco control experts from 16 countries, the Trade for Life Global Plan was overwhelmingly adopted by nearly 700 delegates representing 67 countries at the Seventh World Congress on Tobacco and Health last month in Australia. A key element in the plan is an international computer network of the American Cancer Society—ACS Globalink—to provide tobacco control information and expert assistance throughout the world.

Over 100 healthcare leaders, representing all major international health groups, have agreed to join this computer network.

# IN MEMORIAM: SKIP HARRIS

Hemophilia/HIV activist Skip Harris died on May 14. His death is a serious loss to both the AIDS and hemophilia communities in the San Francisco Bay Area. *AIDS Treatment News* had interviewed Mr. Harris and published his remarks in our last issue, in an article addressing the challenges faced by people with both hemophilia and HIV. When asked what he would like to see in the future for each community, Skip responded:

"I'd want much more education disseminated through all the local chapters of the Hemophilia Council . . . secondly, the government needs to fulfill a commitment to make treatment available. This year treatment was finally the recipient of some of the giant fundraising benefits. For a long time I found it very disturbing that AIDS prevention was the only idea addressed by those benefits, never AIDS treatment. The Reagan administration's policy toward AIDS very deliberately was to write off those who were already infected . . . Bush has talked more about treatment but hasn't put his money where his mouth is. I really think the value of coalitions will grow in the future, coalitions of all the communities affected by HIV . . . what happens with health care will make or break this country."

Skip also worked with us as a board member of the Community Research Alliance.

# IN MEMORIAM: DON GORMAN

Don Gorman's name has not appeared in *AIDS Treatment News*, but without him there would have been no newsletter. Over five years ago John James approached the newly formed Mobilization Against AIDS, and asked how he could help by researching and writing articles. Mobilization suggested calling the Documentation of AIDS Issues and Research Foundation, Inc. (DAIR)—a group which had evolved from a documentation and library committee within Mobilization. Don Gorman, the president of DAIR, suggested writing articles about experimental treatments—and provided the names of about a dozen treatments of interest. He published our first article in April 1986 in the newsletter *DAIR Update*, then introduced us to the *San Francisco Sentinel*, where our articles appeared every two weeks. *AIDS Treatment News* began several months later; the *DAIR Update* article, on AL 721, appears today as issue #1.

Don's DAIR Foundation also provided critical support for the early development of Project Inform.

As a registered nurse, Don approached AIDS information as a person with AIDS, an activist, and one trained in medical management. He published articles about medical management, especially about pneumocystis and the availability of aerosol pentamidine, early in the epidemic.

The DAIR Foundation, which maintains AIDS archives open to the public and prepares reports to support AIDS organizations, continues today in San Francisco; it can be reached at 415/552-1665. Anyone who could volunteer time to help continue Don's work is encouraged to get in touch.

# NEWS NOTES

## Senate Votes Overwhelmingly for AIDS Care

On May 15 the U.S. Senate voted 95 to 3 to override objections by Senator Jesse Helms, Republican of North Carolina, and vote on a bill to provide emergency disaster relief to cities and states with many AIDS cases. The next day, the Senate passed the bill by a vote of 95 to 4. The bill had been introduced by Senators Edward M. Kennedy, Democrat of Massachusetts, and Orrin Hatch, Republican of Utah; it has 65 other co-sponsors.

Much more is necessary before the bill becomes law—especially the separate appropriations process in Congress. But the degree of consensus signals a welcome change in Washington on dealing with AIDS.

Most observers see two reasons for the change. First, more members of Congress now know someone with AIDS, or someone who has died of it. The second factor is the excellent work of the AIDS Action Council and other lobbying groups. They drafted solid, practical legislation representing a consensus on AIDS by dozens of major, mainstream health and medical organizations.

## NIAID Recommends Fluconazole for Cryptococcal Meningitis Maintenance Therapy

On May 11 the U.S. Public Health Service announced preliminary results of a clinical trial of fluconazole vs. amphotericin B for preventing recurrence of cryptococcal meningitis. All 205 patients in the trial had first been treated successfully with amphotericin B for the acute phase of the disease. Then they were randomly assigned to either fluconazole or amphotericin B for continuing treatment to prevent relapses.

Of 106 patients who received fluconazole (200 mg by mouth daily), only two developed recurrent cryptococcal meningitis, in a median time of 212 days. But of the 77 who received intravenous amphotericin B, 13 had relapses. (These numbers do not add up to the 205 patients total, because some could not be evaluated in the analysis.) Because of these results, the trial was ended, and all participants were offered fluconazole, which has far less toxicity than amphotericin B.

As a result of this study, the National Institute of Allergy and Infectious Diseases now recommends that fluconazole replace amphotericin B for maintenance therapy of cryptococcal meningitis.

NOTE: *AIDS Treatment News* covered fluconazole treatment for cryptococcal meningitis in a five-page article almost three years ago, on September 25, 1987 (issue #41). At that time the drug had been used to treat over 2,000 people in Europe, mostly for less serious fungal infections; it had also worked well in the few cases in which it had been tried for cryptococcal meningitis. However, fluconazole was not approved in the United States until January 29 of this year. It is very expensive, and some people are using itraconazole instead. Itraconazole is not approved in the United States but is available in Mexico, and perhaps other countries, at a fraction of the U.S. fluconazole price. More information about itraconazole may be obtained from buyers' clubs; also see "Itraconazole: Affordable Fluconazole Substitute," *AIDS Treatment News* #80.

## AZT Early-Intervention Study Published

On May 15 the *Annals of Internal Medicine* published a formal report of ACTG 016, the major national study of persons with mildly symptomatic HIV and T-helper counts over 200. The results of this trial have already been incorporated into the recommendations concerning treatment of persons with T-helper counts between 200 and 500. While the conclusions are not new, the 11-page report includes many details which may be helpful to physicians in refining treatment strategies.

## REFERENCE

Fischl, M.D., Richman, D.D., Hansen, N. and others. The safety and efficacy of zidovudine (AZT) in the treatment of patients with mildly symptomatic human immunodeficiency virus type 1 (HIV) infection. A double-blind, placebo-controlled trial. *Annals of Internal Medicine* vol. 112, pages 727-737, May 15, 1990.

## WHO Names New AIDS Program Director

On May 14 the World Health Organization (WHO) appointed Michael Merson, M.D., as head of the Global Programme on AIDS. He had been temporary head since March 26, when Dr. Jonathan Mann was forced out (see *AIDS Treatment News* #99). Dr. Merson, a WHO employee for 12 years, directed its Control of Diarrheal Diseases Programme. He had also worked for the U.S. Centers for Disease Control (CDC).

WHO also appointed the deputy director of the CDC, Walter Dowdle, M.D., as consultant to Dr. Merson, when the latter assumed the interim position.

# Issue Number 104
# June 1, 1990

## HYPERTHERMIA REPORT: ONLY ONE PATIENT

*by John S. James*

In the last week of May, CNN television and other media reported a single case of a patient with AIDS and Kaposi's sarcoma (KS), who seemed to be much improved after hyperthermia, a treatment which consists of artificially raising the body temperature. Hyperthermia was previously used for treating certain infections, such as syphilis, and is still used in some advanced cases of cancer.

According to a brief written report by doctors Kenneth Alonso and William D. Logan Jr. of the Atlanta Heart and Lung Clinic at Atlanta Hospital, the patient had worsening KS and a T-helper count of 50 before beginning the treatment. AZT and alpha interferon had not prevented the symptoms from worsening. Since standard treatments had not worked, the hospital's Institutional Review Board gave permission to try hyperthermia.

Using tubes inserted in an artery and a vein in the thigh, blood was withdrawn, heated outside the body with a heat exchanger, and then put back into the circulation. With temperature carefully monitored by thermometers in the pulmonary artery and in the bladder, body temperature was gradually raised to 42 degrees C (between 107 and 108 degrees F) for two hours. The patient, who was under general anesthesia, was then cooled gradually.

Lesions started to improve within 48 hours, and by seven days some were less than half of their original size. Maximum improvement had occurred at six weeks; some but not all of the lesions had disappeared. The patient's T-helper count had increased from 50 to 330. HIV cultures were negative (which may mean little, however, because of the unreliability of most viral cultures), and reverse transcriptase in the blood (a measure of viral activity) had fallen by 70 percent.

The physicians submitted a report of this case for publication in a medical journal. When the story got into the press, they insisted that the treatment was not a cure. But some of the press reports suggested that despite the doctors' caution, the patient believed he was cured. Extensive coverage has led to hundreds of phone calls to the physicians and to AIDS service organizations.

## Comment

It is hard to evaluate this report without detailed peer review. Most AIDS experts reached by reporters have been reluctant to say much on the record until they know more. Most do seem to agree that the treatment *might* be useful, and that it must be investigated further.

Why would a report of a single case lead to national publicity? May is a "sweeps" month, when the audiences of TV stations are carefully measured in order to set advertising rates, and when, therefore, the stations do everything possible to boost their audiences. One media expert speculated that if the report had arrived a few days later, in June, it would not have been a story.

It is unfortunate when widespread reporting raises hopes prematurely. But in this case the publicity may also have made an important contribution. Despite the widespread agreement that the treatment might be useful and should be investigated, there is a serious risk that no followup trial will be organized. Hyperthermia has little commercial potential, since it generates only one sale of a relatively simple and inexpensive machine to each center which uses it; it does not lead to repeat sales, as pharmaceuticals do. Hyperthermia has no constituency in the government or in any part of the AIDS research establishment. Hopefully the widespread publicity will generate enough interest so that someone will follow up with a small trial.

Hyperthermia is dangerous if done improperly; it must be performed by knowledgeable physicians. Published articles on this technique describe extensive precautions which are taken for the patient's safety. If formal studies are not conducted, the treatment may instead come into use in the offices or clinics of physicians not trained to employ it properly. Fortunately, the procedure tried in one case with AIDS is exactly the same as that often used in treating cancer, meaning that the technology, staff training, precautions, risk estimates, etc. are already in place.

As far as we know, the patient in Atlanta is the only person with AIDS who has been treated with hyperthermia. The idea had previously been suggested; see References, below.

## REFERENCES

Brenner, S. HIV appears to have some susceptibility to heat [letter]. *AIDS Research and Human Retroviruses*, volume 5 number 1, pages 5-6, February 1989.

Bull, JM. A review of systemic hyperthermia. *Front. Radiat. Ther. Onc.*, volume 18, pages 171-176, 1984.

Weatherburn, H. Hyperthermia and AIDS treatment [letter]. *The British Journal of Radiology*, volume 61 number 729, pages 863-864, September 1988.

Yatvin, Milton B. An approach to AIDS therapy using hyperthermia and membrane modification. *Medical Hypotheses*, volume 27, pages 163-165, 1988.

# DDC: EXPANDED ACCESS ANNOUNCED FOR PATIENTS WITHOUT OTHER OPTIONS

On June 25 Hoffmann-LaRoche will begin an expanded access program to provide ddC (proprietary name HIVID) to patients who have failed or been intolerant to AZT and are intolerant to ddI. This program will proceed in parallel with the formal clinical trials of the drug (for more information about the trials, see the last issue of *AIDS Treatment News*). Those eligible for the new program could not participate in the trials, since they must be unable to use AZT in order to qualify for the expanded access; those in the formal trials of ddI must be able to use AZT, since they might be randomly assigned to it.

Because ddC has never been tested on this patient population, the new program will begin gradually. At first only 50 people will be accepted—and only from physicians who have prior experience with ddC. After 25 of them have been monitored for at least four weeks without serious problems, the program will be expanded to 200 people, and any physician with AIDS experience will be allowed to enter patients. After 100 people have been followed for 16 weeks without unexpected problems, there will be no numerical limit to how many may enter the program, if they meet the medical qualifications.

All patients will be randomized to one of two doses; the highest dose will be the same as that used in the formal trials. Random assignment of doses greatly increases the useful information a trial can provide, because it allows scientists to look for a dose-response relationship in both toxicity and efficacy. (In this program the main reason for varying the dose is to collect safety information for these patients.)

To be eligible for this program, patients must:

• Either be unable to tolerate AZT (under the criteria used in the ddI expanded-access program), or meet other criteria indicating that AZT was ineffective for them;

• Also be unable to tolerate ddI, for reasons *other than* peripheral neuropathy (which is a toxicity of ddC as well as of ddI);

• And also not have cancer (KS is OK, however, and so is basal cell carcinoma).

# PARALLEL TRACK PROPOSAL RELEASED: PUBLIC COMMENT ACCEPTED THROUGH JULY 20

The long-awaited proposal for a formal "parallel track" for early access to certain experimental drugs in phase II clinical trials, for people not eligible for those trials, has been published in the *Federal Register* (May 21, pages 20856-20860). The public-comment period ends July 20, and it is important to write to the address below to support this program.

How is the official "parallel track" different from the expanded-access program for ddI (and now for ddC also—see article in this issue of *AIDS Treatment News*)? The ddI program is like the parallel track, but it was started separately to avoid being delayed until the formal program could begin.

# The AIDS Research Advisory Committee (ARAC)

The parallel track proposal provides an official structure for deciding which drugs to recommend for early-access release. A major part of this structure, the AIDS Research Advisory Committee (ARAC), is "composed of outside scientists and physicians experienced with AIDS, persons with HIV-related diseases, and others." It will be administered by the U. S. National Institute for Allergy and Infectious Diseases (NIAID).

The ARAC is only advisory; the FDA makes the final decision of whether a drug will be released. And of course the pharmaceutical-company sponsor must be willing and able to make the drug available.

The parallel-track proposal allows sponsors to bypass the ARAC if they want, and submit their proposals directly to the FDA instead. (We consider this option a good idea, simply because nobody knows for sure how the ARAC will work in practice. Pharmaceutical companies will usually choose to go through the ARAC, because if they have a good program, that body will be an ally—and if they don't, they will be stopped at the FDA in any case. But if by mischance the ARAC becomes bogged down or otherwise fails to work properly, another option would be available.)

We consider the ARAC especially important because it creates a public body with official status to determine which drugs in clinical trials should become more available.

# Other Parts of the Parallel-Track Proposal

Besides ARAC, the parallel-track proposal also calls for:

• Creation of a national IRB (Institutional Review Board) for the parallel-track protocols. While local IRBs could still review any protocol, the national IRB could avoid delays and other problems which would result from relying only on the local groups. Until the national IRB is established, the ARAC will appoint a subcommittee to do its job temporarily.

• Emphasis on education of physicians and potential participants in parallel-track programs, to make sure that physicians are informed on how to use the drugs, and that the risks and benefits of participating are understood.

• Use of existing IND regulations to allow pharmaceutical companies to recover costs in some cases by charging for participation, but only " in the unusual circumstance in which the trial could not continue" (without charging fees), and only with the permission of the FDA.

• Criteria for terminating parallel-track access to a particular drug, for example if there is unreasonable risk to participants, if a better product becomes available, or if the parallel-track access interferes with clinical trials of any drug.

The parallel-track proposal as now published will apply only to HIV-related drugs at this time. It is, however, described as a pilot effort; if successful it could be expanded to include treatments for other diseases also.

# CONSENSUS STATEMENT: AIDS GROUPS SEEK BETTER RESEARCH PRIORITIES

Over 45 major AIDS and health organizations (see list below) have endorsed a consensus statement, "HIV/AIDS Biomedical Research Priorities: Recommendations to the National Institutes of Health." Some of the highlights:

• Three areas of HIV research—prevention, treatment, and health care—must all be strengthened.

• Of all the research proposals approved for funding by NIH peer review, only 24 percent are actually funded, due to lack of money. This proportion should be raised to 40–50 percent, as it was in the early 1970s.

• Three particular areas singled out for increased funding include community-based research, the National Cooperative Drug Discovery Groups for Opportunistic Infections, and NIH salary levels and training grants.

• Improved coordination of AIDS/HIV research is needed, through the Secretary of Health and Human Services.

• The ACTG (AIDS Clinical Trials Group) should focus on (small) technology-intensive phase I/II studies, with more new compounds than tested in the past. Larger, later trials should be sponsored by pharmaceutical companies, through community-based or other research groups.

Other recommendations concern focus on opportunistic infections, a national AIDS research database on disease progression, outreach to excluded groups, trials and other research concerning women and children, methodological research to improve trial designs, acceptance and implementation of the "parallel track" (see article above), community advisory panels at each ACTG site, publication of NIH guidelines for state-of-the-art medical care, NIH help to researchers in speedy dissemination of their results, full disclosure of all consulting or equity relationships between pharmaceutical companies and researchers involved in setting national AIDS research priorities, and reimbursement for the cost of standard medical care associated with trials by Medicare, Medicaid, or private insurance.

The organizations endorsing the consensus statement are:

AID Atlanta

AIDS Action Committee of Massachusetts

AIDS Action Council

AIDS Coalition to Unleash Power (ACT UP)/NY

AIDS Foundation of Chicago

AIDS National Interfaith Network

AIDS Project Los Angeles (APLA)

American Academy of Pediatrics

American Anthropological Association's Task Force on AIDS

American Association for Counseling and Development

American Association for Marriage and Family Therapy

American Federation of State, County and Municipal Employees

American Foundation for AIDS Research (AmFAR)

American Red Cross

Association of Schools of Public Health

Center for Women's Policy Studies

Child Welfare League of America

Chronic Fatigue Syndrome Information Institute, Inc.

Citizen's Commission on AIDS

Coalition for Compassion/Los Angeles

Community Research Initiative (CRI)/New York

Consortium of Social Science Associations

Dallas Gay Alliance/AIDS Resource Center

Federation of Parents and Friends of Lesbians and Gays

Gay Men's Health Crisis (GMHC)/New York

Human Rights Campaign Fund (HRCF)

International Association of Fire Fighters

Lambda Legal Defense & Education Fund

Minority Task Force on AIDS/New York

Mobilization Against AIDS/San Francisco

National AIDS Network (NAN)

National Assembly of State Arts Agencies

National Association of Community Health Centers, Inc.

National Association of People with AIDS (NAPWA)

National Association of Protection and Advocacy Systems

National Association of Social Workers

National Association of State Alcohol and Drug Abuse Directors

National Gay and Lesbian Task Force

National Hemophilia Foundation

National Minority AIDS Council

National Network of Runaway and Youth Services

Pediatric AIDS Foundation

People With AIDS (PWA) Health Group/New York

Planned Parenthood Federation of America

Project Inform/San Francisco

San Francisco AIDS Foundation

Synagogue Council of America

Women and AIDS Resource Network (WARN)/NY

Copies of the recommendations can be obtained from the AIDS Action Council (212/293-2886), or from the American Foundation for AIDS Research (212/719-0712, ask for Spencer Cox).

Note: We consider this consensus statement an excellent summary of improvements needed in AIDS research.

# TOXOPLASMOSIS UPDATE

*by Denny Smith*

Opportunistic infections of the protozoan *Toxoplasma gondii* are usually controlled by the standard therapies, pyrimethamine with sulfadiazine, or pyrimethamine with clindamycin for people who are allergic to sulfa drugs. (The toxicity of pyrimethamine can be countered with leucovorin). These drugs kill the mature parasites but unfortunately not the cysts from which more protozoa will emerge. So the treatments must be continued indefinitely on a "chronic suppressive" basis. Even during maintenance therapy, relapses are not uncommon.

Researchers at the University of Geneva reported last month that doxycycline, a commonly prescribed antibiotic, worked better than pyrimethamine for protecting mice infected with *T. gondii* (Chang and others, 1990). A combination of the two worked better than either drug alone. We could not find any physicians in this country who had tried doxycycline to treat patients with toxoplasmosis, even though an abstract of the Swiss work was presented last September in Houston at the Twenty-Ninth Interscience Conference on Antimicrobial Agents and Chemotherapy. Doxycycline may provide an option in future situations when the standard drugs fail.

Neither could we find anyone who had tried the other possibilities sometimes discussed for use against toxoplasmosis: arprinocid, azithromycin or trimetrexate. *AIDS Treatment News* #79 reported at length on these and other aspects of this infection, and although that was over a year ago, little has changed to improve significantly the survival rates for this diagnosis. We hope that the upcoming International Conference will report experience with new treatments.

Some success has been obtained with fresh applications of the drugs at hand. Using an idea presented at the last International Conference in Montreal, Larry Waites, M.D. of San Francisco has improved the outlook for his patients by pulse-dosing the treatments for toxoplasmosis, giving them two times a week instead of daily (see Pedrol, E and others, 1989).

Another source of optimism comes from trials now under consideration which would try low doses of pyrimethamine or clindamycin to prevent reactivation of latent infections in patients at risk. Fansidar has been tried as a prophylaxis, but this drug has been associated with fatal allergic reactions in some people. Fansidar was discussed at length in the January issue of *Treatment Issues*, published by the Gay Men's Health Crisis in New York, and again in the May issue of *BETA*, published by the San Francisco AIDS Foundation.

The notion of some prophylactic measure makes sense for people with HIV who have been exposed to *T. gondii*—if the risk of side effects from such therapy is outweighed by the benefit of preventing disease. Prophylaxis is already the norm for people at risk for *Pneumocystis* pneumonia (using septra, dapsone or aerosol pentamidine), and is gaining interest for suppressing latent infections of MAI (clofazimine or ansamycin) and *Cryptococcus* (fluconazole). Incidentally, although all of these microbes are widely present in the environment, *T. gondii* could be the easiest to avoid, since many people acquire the infection by eating undercooked meat. Also, cats are the natural hosts of the parasite's reproductive cycle. All HIV+ people should avoid contact with cat feces, whether or not they test positive for past exposure. Careful hand washing is critical after handling a pet cat and before eating or preparing food.

Toxoplasmosis usually presents itself as encephalitis, an inflammation of the brain from lesions caused by *T. gondii*. Robert Neger, M.D., reported in April to the Community Consortium in San Francisco the less frequent but real danger of retinal and optic nerve manifestations. This would be of obvious interest to other ophthalmologists who are consulted by HIV+ patients reporting vision problems which ordinarily would be approached as CMV retinitis. Dr. Neger noted that the most complete exam of the retina must use **indirect** ophthalmoscopy, after dilating the pupils.

A contrasting example of misdiagnosis was presented to the Community Consortium last January. Martin Mass, M.D., discussed the case of a patient who showed symptoms of neurological problems—memory loss and walking balance difficulty. An MRI scan showed multiple brain lesions, but this scan cannot distinguish toxoplasma infections from lesions caused by PML, herpes or lymphoma. The patient's bloodwork tested positive for antibodies to *T. gondii*, and in accordance with standard practice, he was started presumptively on drugs to treat toxoplasmosis. Unfortunately, his condition did not improve, and a subsequent brain biopsy identified the lesions conclusively as lymphoma. Dr. Mass suggested that if biopsies were performed earlier for patients with neurologic symptoms, the resulting diagnosis would be more accurate and treatment more timely. Other physicians discussing the case felt that the current three-week trial of presumptive toxo treatment is still appropriate.

We wonder why the development of new toxoplasmosis therapies and prophylaxes appears to be so snail-paced. Perhaps the existence of an already-approved treatment regimen translates into a disincentive for pharmaceutical companies which are primarily interested in first-line drugs targeted for large "hostage" markets. If this is true, patients who cannot tolerate the approved treatments, or who face drug-failure relapses are casualties of the ubiquitous "health for profits" motivating medical research today. This epidemic will be haunting the world for decades to come unless that motivating force of research is replaced by "health for people."

We plan to report developments, or the vacuum of developments, in treating toxoplasmosis and other opportunistic infections after the International Conference later this month.

## REFERENCES

Pedrol, E and others. Central nervous system toxoplasmosis in AIDS patients. Efficacy of an intermittent maintenance therapy. V International Conference on AIDS, abstract M.B.O. 37, Montreal, June 5, 1989.

Chang, HR and others. In vitro and In vivo effects of doxycycline on *Toxoplasma gondii*. *Antimicrobial Agents and Chemotherapy*, volume 34, number 5, pages 775-780, May, 1990.

# COMPOUND Q: CONTINUING GOOD NEWS

*by Denny Smith*

Anecdotal reports and at least one published article point to continued optimism around the use of trichosanthin, or compound Q, against HIV. *AIDS Treatment News* has heard from at least three people who have experienced significant improvement in blood values and HIV-related symptoms since trying compound Q. All three were given the drug under the supervision of a knowledgeable physician, and none of them experienced any serious side effects.

However, many instances of toxicity **have** been attributed to trichosanthin, and the physicians most familiar with the drug strongly advise against self-administration. Drs. Larry A. Waites, Vera S. Byers and Alan S. Levin have issued a public letter explaining this advice. Their clinic is willing to consult with other physicians interested in trichosanthin infusion information.

In addition to positive anecdotal reports, Project Inform has published an "interim update" of its "underground" trial of last year, as well as a description of a new trichosanthin protocol designed by the recently merged Project Inform Community Research Alliance (PICRA) and sanctioned by the FDA. Both reports appear in the May 1990 issue of *PI Perspective*. The first study organized by Project Inform used trichosanthin imported from China. Several buyers' clubs around the U.S. have since started to make the same product available. The PICRA study will use trichosanthin supplied by Genelabs, a California pharmaceutical manufacturer.

Meanwhile, four other sites in the San Francisco area continue other trichosanthin studies, also using drug provided by Genelabs. PICRA and San Francisco General Hospital are each expected to report on their trials at the International Conference later this month.

# Issue Number 105
# June 15, 1990

## CONFLICT OF INTEREST: CLOUD OVER AIDS RESEARCH?

*by John S. James*

In December 1989 the U.S. Department of Health and Human Services (HHS) rejected proposed guidelines intended to control conflict of interest in research supported by the U.S. National Institutes of Health (NIH). These guidelines would have greatly restricted Federally-supported biomedical researchers from having consulting arrangements with, or owning stock in, companies affected by their research. Many scientists strongly objected to the proposed restrictions, on the grounds that they would not allow the best scientists to work for both industry and government, and also because, they believed, the paperwork would be unduly burdensome.

Others are concerned that the present system means that anything is legal, as there are no rules or standards governing conflict of interest by academic biomedical researchers supported by public money. For example, nobody would allow Federal *employees* to have undisclosed consulting contracts with companies affected by their official decisions. But in biomedical research, the real funding decisions (and often regulatory decisions) are increasingly made by outside experts (not Federal employees), in peer-review or other advisory committees. These non-employees can legally have consulting arrangements with anyone; they might or might not disqualify themselves in cases of conflict. So just changing how the decision-makers are paid, from Federal *salaries* to Federal *contracts or grants*, summarily discards the entire structure of conflict-of-interest regulation which has developed over decades, potentially threatening the integrity of the public decision-making process.

In recent months there has been public suspicion of conflict-of-interest abuses, but few cited examples. The lack of confidence may result because the public has no way to know how serious a problem exists. This article outlines some of the prevalent fears and issues, not only in the financial arrangements normally considered "conflict of interest," but also in other cases in which the public pays for research but is ill served by decisions which place private over public interests. This article will include these broader issues, suggest questions to raise, and show why conflict of interest may be a critical obstacle to AIDS treatment development.

## Does Conflict of Interest Impede New Drugs?

In testimony against the NIH conflict-of-interest guidelines, it was revealed that almost all the principal investigators in the ACTG (AIDS Clinical Trials Group) system have industrial consulting arrangements—usually not disclosed to the public. Could these private arrangements result in bias against competing drugs when decisions are made on how to spend public money? The current issue of *Boston Magazine*, June 1990, has a long article on the background of Peptide T, and on the widespread suspicions that this potential treatment may have been dismissed unfairly because of fears that it could be a competitor to CD4 ("Peptide T and the Research Establishment," by Seth Rolbein).

Others are suspicious about exactly what pharmaceutical companies are buying through these consulting arrangements. Many view the ACTG system as unproductive, with little useful information to show for hundreds of millions of dollars and several years of time invested. Pharmaceutical companies have often been frustrated and unhappy in working with the ACTG. Why then are they paying money to almost all of its principal investigators? Are they buying scientific productivity—or influence over the flow of hundreds of millions of dollars of public money for AIDS clinical research?

Perhaps the worst suspicions concern the lack of promising new treatments in clinical trials. Dozens, probably hundreds of promising chemicals have emerged from laboratories, but then almost all of them are abandoned; they do not move on to human trials. The worst drug logjam occurs early in development, at the stage of finishing preclinical work (such as the manufacturing quality assurance and the animal toxicity testing required by the FDA), in order to obtain the "IND" (Investigational New Drug) approval which is required before human testing can begin. The public does not notice this early drugjam, because the potential drugs in question are not yet real treatment options for people; also, information about preclinical development is proprietary and usually secret—even the existence of a Federally-granted IND is not public information. Only years later does the public realize that the pipeline is largely empty, and few or no new treatments are becoming available.

Could conflict of interest be the major cause of this central problem? The possible scenario—not proven, only a suspicion at this time—is that products early in development do not have the commercial momentum to pay the consulting fees necessary to be taken seriously by the AIDS research establishment. Could new possibilities be abandoned in favor of still more research on products like AZT, which are already on the market and therefore have the cash flow necessary to buy their way into the professional community?

Many researchers, not surprisingly, have a very different view. They see their decisions as reflecting only the higher worlds of Science and Medicine, independent of such mundane matters as who pays the bill. Many are angry that anyone would think otherwise. They feel that such ideas challenge their integrity.

One middle-ground position acknowledges that the large majority of researchers do remain independent of undue financial influence. It sees the problem instead in the narrow outlook which develops when people interact constantly with small groups of others who have the same viewpoints they do. Activists as well as researchers face this problem.

But research costs much more than activism, so research cliques will seldom come into being except where there is money to support them. Money builds influence which brings in more money, leading to increasing concentrations of power in small and narrow groups, whose members quite correctly do not see themselves as being bought off, but as doing what they sincerely believe is right. Yet new treatments may be abandoned just the same, shut out as the groups which have coalesced around cash-rich commercial products compete for increasingly scarce Federal funds. The issue is not personal integrity, but the fact that the system does not work.

## Publication Embargos: A Different Conflict of Interest

An issue usually considered separately from conflict of interest, because it does not directly involve money, is the common requirement that scientists conceal their work for months or years, from the public and often from scientific colleagues as well, in order to enhance the news value of journals or conferences. (The common news embargos which last only a few days, and are intended to allow orderly release of information which does not depend on whose mail is delivered first, present much less serious problems.)

A recent article in *The New York Times* (May 22, 1990) reported one particularly serious example. The *Times* interviewed the former head of the U.S. National Cancer Institute concerning a large 1981 study which found that breast cancer in women could often be treated as well by removing a small lump as by removing the entire breast. "But the data were kept secret for 14 months while the paper was considered at *The New England Journal of Medicine*. During that time...some 100,000 American women were found to have breast cancer and were unaware that complete removal of the breast was unnecessary." The article did not estimate how many thousands of women had their breasts removed needlessly so that the researchers could publish in the most prestigious journal, and so that the *Journal* could have a scoop to further its business interests.

Recently *The New England Journal of Medicine* and some other major journals have allowed early release of information with urgent public-health importance; *The New York Times* article included several examples. But areas like AIDS, complex emergencies without a single solution, present a more fundamental problem. Scientists build on each other's work; long pre-publication secrecy, even when not immediately life-threatening, slows the entire research process and delays the ultimate development of better treatments, costing lives eventually although not immediately.

A recent book (*Covering the Plague: AIDS and the American Media*, by James Kinsella, Rutgers University Press, 1989) traces the history of pre-publication secrecy to the large increase in the number of scientists, beginning in the early 1970s, which allowed *The New England Journal of Medicine* to be very selective. "The surplus of manuscripts at the *Journal* allowed then-editor Dr. Franz Inglefinger to demand an 'exclusive' on every article that appeared in the *Journal*. The publication would run no manuscript that had been reported in detail anywhere else, including the popular press." Since there was a backlog of articles, scientific results were regularly withheld from the public, and from many scientific colleagues, for months. Hundreds of other journals followed and imposed the notorious "Inglefinger rule," but others (such as the *Lancet*, according to Kinsella) have not.

It might be hoped that the Sixth International Conference on AIDS would take the lead against this destructive system, but it has failed to do so. Authors had to certify that their abstract "has not been published elsewhere or submitted for presentation at another national or international meeting." Technically this wording does not require pre-publication secrecy—authors could present the material elsewhere *after* they signed the certification, which, with the abstracts themselves, was due in January. But in fact researchers have been tight-lipped about what they plan to present, maintaining the five-month "shadow" which each annual Conference casts before it—the time each year when researchers are most reluctant to talk about their latest results. (The Sixth International Conference also threatened journalists with loss of credentials, and therefore expulsion from the meeting, if they did not honor a press embargo on the Advance Program by withholding "all information related to program content...for release only after presentation at the Conference.")

Early public discussion of results to be presented would improve the Conference, by letting participants orient themselves before the whirlwind of events begins. The value of this meeting is not in the release of scoops—let us hope that nothing truly important was concealed for five months to be presented in San Francisco—but rather in status reports from leading researchers. Good business meetings provide information in advance, so that participants can have in-depth discussions instead of spending their time figuring out what is going on.

Unfortunately, next year's Seventh International Conference on AIDS, June 16-21, 1991, in Florence, Italy, already has similar restrictions on its form for submission of abstracts.

## What Can Be Done?

The initial attempt to control conflict of interest in NIH-funded research (mentioned above) has been rejected, after vehement opposition by many scientists. Efforts are now continuing to develop milder standards—perhaps not forbidding certain practices but only requiring disclosure. According to an assistant in the office of Congressman Ted Weiss, Democrat from New York, who has long pushed NIH to develop such standards, nothing will be in place for at least a year. (Congressman Weiss' subcommittee will soon publish recommendations on what it believes should be done. It has few specific examples of conflict of interest, however, and none concerning AIDS research. Anyone with a documented case—clear evidence of something, not just suspicion—should call or write to Weiss' office.)

Dr. Janet Newburgh, of the Institutional Liaison Office at NIH, told *AIDS Treatment News* that development of proposed conflict of interest rules is proceeding in two parts. The faster track concerns *commercial products*, or items close to being commercial products. The slower track concerns *invention development*, ideas farther from commercialization.

Unfortunately it seems clear that if we have a major problem, these NIH efforts will not solve it in the time frame needed. Nothing is likely to be done for over a year. And then if anything happens to restrain conflict of interest, and if it is successful, it will only gradually lead to improvement in government research priorities, which in turn will gradually lead to improvement in research and then to better treatments. This effort must be pursued, but we cannot hold our breath.

Another approach that we can take now is to investigate the problems around conflict of interest, understand the situation better ourselves, and increase awareness within the professional community and the public. Better awareness, and the resulting informal pressures and influences, may bring effective change faster than formal regulation can. Activists and investigative reporters can make a critical contribution, by informing the public about the dimensions of the problem.

Still another approach, suggested in the article below, is to continue to strengthen the ability of PWA, activist, and front-line physician organizations to work together to develop the community's own priorities for treatment research. Developing consensus on a few treatments which most deserve public help to shepherd them through the research system will also build the constituency to overcome the obstacles blocking their progress.

# CALL FOR ACTION: COMMUNITY CONSENSUS ON TREATMENTS NEEDING DEVELOPMENT

*by John S. James*

Recently a number of AIDS treatment stories have appeared in the press. Most of this news is good, although sometimes there is less to it than meets the eye. Yet critical problems remain. This article shows how community organizations can help to overcome the perennial problem of the lack of development of major new drugs.

The bad news is what *isn't* happening. Most policy problems in AIDS stem from lack of national coordination, lack of anyone responsible for developing, implementing, and monitoring coherent national strategy. In treatment development, there is no public office able to investigate any potential treatment (regardless of who owns it, or its stage of development), select those few which are most critical for the public interest and most urgently need attention, identify obstacles to their speedy development, and place those obstacles on the national agenda. As a result, the most important drugs today are failing to move into the clinical-trials pipeline. Unless we act now to invest in the future, little will come out over the next two to three years except ddI and ddC—important new options, yes, but not enough by themselves to prevent many deaths.

Ideally, some official body with well-respected medical and scientific leadership and staff would have done this job for the last ten years. It would take time, however, to bring any such group into being, and it would be difficult to assure its independence from the problems of the past. But there is an alternative which could be started immediately, and would in some ways be better than an official body.

By working with the organizations and the networking which already exist, we can develop community consensus—among PWA groups, advocacy groups, front-line physicians, research organizations, and others—on which potential treatments are most important, and what must be done to move them forward. While such an effort would not have the automatic authority of a government body, it could in practice have even more influence. Official reports often collect dust on library shelves, because they have no constituency. But the process of building a consensus also builds a constituency for carrying it out.

## Is Anyone Doing This Already?

Several existing or proposed bodies are concerned with setting AIDS treatment research priorities:

• **The ACDDC (AIDS Clinical Drug Development Committee).** This committee within the ACTG (AIDS Clinical Trials Group) meets four times a year to divide drugs into four priorities: high, medium low, and not recommended for clinical trials at this time. The meetings are closed, and we do not know the committee's operation in detail, but there have long been serious concerns about drug priorities within the ACTG.

About two years ago, a physician trying to get a drug into the ACTG system said that the drugs were taken up by the committee in no particular order. Usually at least one of the drugs proposed would provoke argument among the competitive scientists, and once the time for the meeting had elapsed, all the other proposals behind it in the queue were put off for the next meeting, months away. While we have never seen an ACDDC meeting, this scenario rings true, in that a committee charged with setting priorities could hardly pre-prioritize without raising questions about the need for the committee's existence.

We question whether a committee meeting four times a year, with busy members presumably supplied with stacks of paper to inform them about the decisions they are to make, is the best way to set priorities for treatment research. In almost every other aspect of human affairs, a new idea needs a "champion" to push it, or it will not progress. Without an ongoing relationship with the advocate, committees almost always reject important new ideas, because of political dynamics. It is easy to score points by criticizing a novel proposal, but dangerous to become identified with something unfamiliar.

For this article, we picked the three drugs that we would most recommend for urgent attention: hypericin, TIBO derivatives, and HPMPC (see below). The most recent list of ACDDC priorities which we have obtained—through the December 1989 meeting—included none of these three in any category, suggesting that none had been considered by that time; we have heard that one or more have been given high priority since. (For TIBO derivatives, the first paper was not published until February 1, 1990; however, study results usually circulate in the scientific community for months before publication.)

The ACTG is built on investigator-initiated research. Almost all of its principal investigators have consulting arrangements with pharmaceutical companies (usually not disclosed), in addition to their Federal grants or contracts. It seems unlikely that a drug would come to the ACTG (and therefore to the ACDDC within it), unless it has a sponsoring pharmaceutical company, and that company was ready to move the drug and had decided to seek Federal help in doing so.

The ACDDC, as an advisory body of the ACTG, presumably considers only drugs which the ACTG could test. It does not seek out new drugs (even if they are not yet ready for clinical trials, or are not commercially viable, and/or if their owner is busy elsewhere or does not want to bother with an AIDS drug) and then mobilize whatever resources are needed, including public pressure, to get them tested quickly. Yet this is what needs to be done.

• **The ARAC (AIDS Research Advisory Committee).** This group, to include people with AIDS, is part of the proposed "parallel track" system published last month in the *Federal Register* (see article on parallel track in *AIDS Treatment News* #104). If parallel track is accepted, after the 60-day period for public comments, then the ARAC will be a major advance; for the first time there will be an official body able to take an integrated approach in deciding which drugs are important. (Pharmaceutical companies cannot do so, because each will only promote its own products; and the FDA usually does not compare different drugs, but says "yes" or "no" to each drug separately, based on paperwork placed in front of it.)

But the ARAC has not yet met. And even if parallel track is accepted and the system works perfectly, it will focus primarily on drugs well along in clinical trials and ready for parallel-track access. Yet today the biggest bottleneck seems to be the business negotiations which occur as a promising compound finishes its pre-clinical development and moves into human trials for the first time. At that stage, an organization focused only on parallel track can do nothing.

• **HIV/AIDS Biomedical Research Priorities document.** Over 45 major AIDS and health organizations have endorsed 15 recommendations to the U.S. National Institutes of Health on AIDS/HIV biomedical research priorities (see article in *AIDS Treatment News* #104, June 1). This important effort embodies the kind of consensus building which is needed. We are suggesting a companion effort, to develop consensus on *specific treatments* which need public and professional attention to facilitate their progress through the research system. The May 17 document does not mention any treatments. Both kinds of efforts are needed.

• **New ACT UP list of potential treatments.** ACT UP/New York is preparing a list of drugs and treatment approaches which the ACTG has not researched. The pre-publication draft we have seen lists dozens of drugs and classes of drugs, mostly high-tech approaches to treatment, some of which we had not heard of.

The research to create this list is exactly the kind of effort needed to develop community consensus on a research agenda. The information comes from scientists, physicians, and others with specialized knowledge. The activists make sure that priorities reflect the interests of persons with AIDS or HIV, above those of companies with products to sell, or of professionals with careers to advance.

Even harder than preparing the initial list will be setting priorities. We believe that this effort should focus on finding a short list, perhaps five to ten treatments most needing public and research attention—not on trying to rate or categorize every treatment suggested.

## Treatment Examples Show Unmet Needs

Since U.S. media coverage of AIDS research usually consists of rewriting official press releases, most of the public believes that the slow pace of treatment development primarily reflects the scientific difficulty of the problem, and appropriate medical caution. In fact, business and administrative problems cause most of the delays in treatment development. Glaring past examples include aerosol pentamidine, used to prevent pneumocystis, and fluconazole, an important new antifungal. These cases are not unusual; most drugs suffer similar delays, only there is less publicity about what happened. (A few drugs *have* been developed rapidly—for example, the initial approval of AZT, and the progress of ddI since last summer.)

In the cases of aerosol pentamidine and fluconazole, the delays occurred after considerable human experience with the drugs in question was already available. But the biggest problem today seems to be the obstacles to taking a promising compound from pre-clinical laboratory and animal studies into the first human trials and then into early efficacy studies. The three drugs below were *not* picked as examples of delays— indeed they are progressing faster than most. They do show how much could be gained if there were a public voice to insist that the most critical potential treatments be expedited, not left to usual procedures.

• **Hypericin.** This chemical, in human use in Europe as an antidepressant and long used in herbal medicine, has been extensively covered in *AIDS Treatment News* starting August 26, 1988 (issue #63). It works very well against HIV in the test tube, and against other retroviruses in animals. A community-based study in San Francisco, using available herbal extracts, showed sustained T-helper improvements in those who started with high T-helper counts (the average baseline value was over 500); these patients were not using any other antiviral. But with the very small hypericin doses in the herbal extracts now available, most of those with low T-helper counts (mean under 200) continued to show T-helper declines. P-24 levels did decrease or become negative in four of six patients, but they were also using AZT, which might have caused the improvement. (For more information about this study, see *AIDS Treatment News* #96.) Another study of the herbal extract found no significant improvement in T-helper counts or p24 levels, whether or not the extract was combined with AZT (see *AIDS/ HIV Experimental Treatment Directory*—published by AmFAR—December 1989, page 35).

However, the herbal preparations contain very low concentrations of hypericin; animal studies suggest that larger amounts of the chemical are needed. Animals can tolerate large doses of pure hypericin, suggesting that people might be able to do so (long-term human tolerance of low doses is already established through the history of use of the herbal extracts). And hypericin works very differently than AZT; it is not a nucleoside analog (like AZT, ddI, and ddC). Therefore if it does work in people as an anti-HIV treatment, it could open a new world of therapeutic options, used either alone or in combination with AZT or other drugs.

All this, except for the community studies of the herbal extract, was known two years ago, and was published in a leading journal (*Proceedings of the National Academy of Sciences, USA*, July 1988). But because of the lack of effective national mobilization for AIDS treatment development, this very promising compound had to go through the usual procedures: finding investors, chemistry research to improve methods for synthesis, creation of a large enough batch so that the same supply could be tested in animals before being given to humans, and toxicity tests in animals.

According to the February 19 issue of *FDC Reports (The Pink Sheet)*, hypericin was being tested in monkeys at that time (February 1990), and if all went well, could begin human efficacy testing in late 1990, with filing for an NDA (permission from the FDA to market the drug) in early 1993, "if the drug shows 'dramatic' efficacy and lack of toxicity in humans." (And if no ordinary problems develop in business, administration, personnel turnover, etc.)

By the standards of business as usual, four and a half years from the first published laboratory report of antiviral activity to application for the NDA is fast. But if the nation would mobilize to save lives, it could have been done many times faster, without undue risk. Once the drug looked promising, enough could be extracted from plants, or synthesized by the already-known procedures, for animal tests for acute toxicity, then small, efficient human tests of safe doses for short-term evidence of efficacy (p24 decrease, T-helper improvement, weight gain, decline of AIDS-related symptoms, etc.) If the drug showed clear signs of working, then an all-out effort would be justified to solve any supply problems, get the treatment to those who had no other alternative, continue collecting data on long-term toxicity, begin combination trials with AZT, and begin trials to establish conclusive proof of efficacy. Note that despite its speed, this approach to developing key drugs would cost little until a drug was all but known to work, at which time money would be easy to raise.

What we are suggesting here is not very different from what in fact was done with AZT, ddC, and ddI. The early phase I trials, in theory designed to test for toxicity and determine maximum tolerated dose, in fact also provided the efficacy information which motivated larger trials. But the early human testing of all three of these drugs depended on a single individual—Samuel Broder, M.D., who has since been promoted to director of the National Cancer Institute (NCI). Since Broder now has other duties, new drugs are not following expeditiously from preclinical work into clinical trials. We suspect that the fundamental problem is that new drugs have not yet built (bought?) a constituency within the AIDS research establishment. The lucky chance of the right individual in a strategic position (the NCI has more power than pharmaceutical companies to overcome Federal obstacles in early stages of clinical trials) temporarily masked the major weakness and bottleneck in the whole U.S. drug-development process—the lack of movement of promising compounds through completion of preclinical development and into trials. With Broder no longer in position, this stage in the AIDS drug-development process has largely shut down. But the public has not noticed, because the problem is at the *beginning* of the clinical-trials pipeline, so its practical effects are delayed. Only a year or two later does the public become aware that the new drugs are not there.

When government experts say that there are no new antivirals ready to test, most people accept their statements on faith, because few have been prepared to challenge them. But the AIDS community can do its own investigation, by networking among organizations and individuals with many different talents and skills. With our own consensus about which treatments most urgently need public attention, we can discuss options like hypericin when experts say that no new drugs are ready. Sometimes the experts may be right. And sometimes they may be protecting themselves, as bureaucrats often do, by providing standard answers suggesting that whatever is already happening is all that could or should be done.

• **TIBO derivatives.** This class of drugs was developed in Belgium, by researchers using a process of intelligent trial and error to create new anti-HIV drugs. The first report, published in *Nature* on February 1 of this year, especially concerned one compound called R82150.

Laboratory tests showed that the drug was effective against HIV in extremely small concentrations—31,000 times less than the dose which harmed cells (compared to 6,200 for AZT). Then in another test, dogs were given in a single dose a thousand times the amount expected to be effective, with no harm. Finally, six healthy people volunteered to take the drug, and no toxicity was found.

On May 16 the U.S. National Institute of Allergy and Infections Diseases (NIAID) distributed a reply to ACT UP/New York, which had strongly criticized NIAID's ACTG research system. ACT UP had urged that TIBO derivatives be tested, but NIAID replied that they were not yet ready for clinical trials.

We find it hard to understand how a drug which appears to have a huge margin of safety, and which has already been given to humans, is not ready for clinical trials—especially when there is so urgent a need for new anti-HIV drugs. We suspect that this drug "is not yet ready for clinical trials" because the *business and administrative arrangements* are not ready.

A small clinical trial has in fact started in Europe. If the United States, with more AIDS cases and also more research resources than any other country, is behind in the development of some of the most important treatments, no one would be surprised.

By building a community consensus on the most important priorities for development, we can focus on the critical drugs and make sure that all necessary resources are available for their development. Without community input, it will take many years for drugs like R82150 to become available.

• **HPMPC.** This chemical, now being developed by Bristol-Myers, acts against CMV and herpes (not against HIV). HPMPC was discovered in Belgium by a team which included one of the researchers who discovered the TIBO derivatives. Technical articles about HPMPC have appeared in journals for several years.

Much of the research on HPMPC has tested it for herpes, but in AIDS the most important use may be for treating CMV (cytomegalovirus), which can cause blindness, or other serious infections. Two drugs, ganciclovir and foscarnet, are already used for CMV, but both have drawbacks.

In the laboratory HPMPC is active against human CMV in very small concentrations, .04 micrograms per milliliter. Yet a toxicity study found that mice could tolerate up to 200 milligrams per kilogram per day.

One animal study (abstract #751) was presented last September at ICAAC (Interscience Conference on Antimicrobial Agents and Chemotherapy), an annual conference on new antibiotics. Animals cannot be infected with human CMV, so a related virus, murine cytomegalovirus, was used in mice instead; experience with foscarnet had indicated that this animal model might help predict which drugs would be useful for human CMV infection. The study compared ganciclovir, the only CMV drug approved in the United States, with HPMPC. Ganciclovir reduced viral titers in blood and organs by 10 to 100 times, during the 21 days of the test. HPMPC reduced the titers by 100,000 to 1,000,000 times (to undetectable levels) in four to six days.

Another study presented at the same conference (abstract #739) reported that laboratory tests with cell cultures suggested that infrequent dosing might be effective.

In all the animal studies we have seen, the drug has been administered by injection (or applied topically to herpes lesions); one paper found some efficacy with oral administration of a related drug (HPMPA), but large doses were necessary, suggesting that oral availability might be poor.

Supply problems are unlikely for HPMPC, as at least three papers have published methods for making it.

We do not know the current status of HPMPC at Bristol-Myers; pharmaceutical companies seldom release details about their preclinical drug development. Apparently the next step is for Bristol-Myers to complete preclinical tests, obtain an IND (permission for human testing) from the FDA, and begin clinical trials.

We do not know whether or not development is moving rapidly. There does seem to be considerable enthusiasm for this drug among the few medical and research professionals who are familiar with it. On the other hand, there may be a limited market—for CMV because the infection does not need treatment except for persons with immune deficiencies, and for herpes because there is already a well-established treatment, acyclovir.

Under the U.S. system of drug development, companies which have exclusive rights to even vitally important drugs have no obligation to do anything with them; the public interest has no place in the decision. The FDA can bring pressure informally if it wants to, because companies must stay on its good side. But the law requires the FDA to keep much of its information secret, so usually the public does not know what is happening until there are clinical trials, which are hard to conceal. Often it is difficult to know whether a drug is being actively and effectively developed, or whether there are unnecessary obstacles. Fortunately, some companies have done much more than they had to in support of the public interest. Perhaps the remaining problems will be ameliorated by the growing belief that the lives of persons with AIDS are worth saving.

• **Other treatments.** While preparing this article we made a list of treatments which *might* deserve high-priority, expedited development. We made no attempt to be complete; for example, we omitted some important drugs like ddI and ddC, which are already in high-profile development. Also, we did not include non-drug treatments such as nutrition or exercise in this particular list. The treatments are in alphabetical order.

This list should show that there are many treatments which need to be investigated, and it may suggest leads that others will want to pursue:

AS101 (for HIV)
AzdU (HIV)
Azithromycin (MAI; toxoplasmosis)
ddC or ddI in combination with AZT (HIV)
Compound Q (HIV)
d4T (HIV)
Diclazuril (cryptosporidiosis)
G-CSF (a colony stimulating factor)
Glycyrrhizin (HIV)

HIVIG, or other passive immunotherapy (HIV)
HPMPC (CMV; herpes)
Hypericin (HIV)
Imuthiol (immune modulator)
Itraconazole (many fungal infections)
KS secret treatment
Levamisole (immune modulator)
Milk antibodies (cryptosporidiosis)
NAC (HIV, indirectly)
Oxophenarsine (HIV—see 1989 Montreal conference abstract #M.C.P.133)
Peptide T (treatment for neurological effects of HIV)
Sulfolipids (HIV)
TIBO Derivatives (HIV)
Vaccines: Salk, HGP-30, some others (HIV)

## The Next Step

The way to develop community consensus on which treatments need a public voice to assist and expedite their development is through expanding discussions among PWA, advocacy, physician, and other organizations. No one needs to play gatekeeper to designate who is or is not part of this process; treatment investigation is labor intensive, and it is clear who is doing the work. People usually start by investigating treatments which interest them, and bringing what they find to others. Leadership emerges spontaneously, without formal machinery.

Such discussions are already going on; for example, ACT UP groups in several cities (including New York, San Francisco, Boston, Providence, and Washington, DC) now have treatment committees. PWA coalitions have long been interested in treatments. Front-line physicians and community-based research organizations are primary sources of information—as well as friendly researchers in academia, government, or industry. This work is not new. More people need to become involved, however, and let each other know what they are doing. Also, we should discuss specific goals for this effort—for example, do we agree that we should reach consensus on a few high-priority treatments, and then focus on expediting their development?

Many people are ready to contribute money or other resources to research, but are stopped by the confusing jumble of so many voices advocating so many different approaches and directions. Potential investors or contributors cannot find information they can trust, because those close enough to the research to evaluate it usually have personal interests in the decisions or personal loyalties to those who do. A public process of dialog and consensus, centered in organizations interested in treatment of patients instead of commercial or professional promotion, could provide a clear context in treatment research and open the door for those ready to apply their talents and energies.

# SIXTH INTERNATIONAL CONFERENCE NEWS

## Boycott Update

• At this time over 130 AIDS and health organizations are boycotting or withdrawing from the Sixth International Conference on AIDS in protest of U.S. visa and immigration policies, according to a list released June 14 by the NAMES Project in San Francisco.

• The Bay Area Physicians for Human Rights, a San Francisco gay physicians' organization which will attend the Conference, has suggested wearing red armbands at the Conference in solidarity with those boycotting.

• The second International NGO (Non-Governmental Organization) AIDS conference, originally scheduled for San Francisco during the three days before the Sixth International Conference but called off because of the travel restrictions on persons who are HIV positive, has now been rescheduled for Paris, November 1-4. Its cosponsors are the National Minority AIDS Council in Washington, DC, and the Comite France SIDA in Paris. For more information, call Chris Castle, National Minority AIDS Council, 202/544-1076.

• Harvard University has announced that it will not co-sponsor the 1992 International AIDS Conference in Boston if U.S. policy continues to make it difficult for HIV-positive persons to attend. It is possible that the 1992 Conference could be cancelled, as two years may not be enough time to reserve space and make necessary arrangements elsewhere.

## Rejected Abstracts: Progress in Sight

On April 25 the Sixth International Conference announced that 50 percent of the 4,900 abstracts submitted to the conference had been rejected—compared to almost no abstracts rejected last year at Montreal. The high rate of rejection raised concern because: (1) no one can be sure what will turn out to be important in AIDS; (2) it is hard to judge short abstracts because so little information is available, leading to summary judgments based on who is known to the reviewer, or on superficial "gotcha" criteria; and (3) there was no way for the public to ever see the rejected abstracts.

Today progress is being made in addressing these concerns. About 800 more abstracts have been accepted, leaving 1,600 still rejected. While arrangements are not final, it is likely that the Conference will be willing to inform the authors of the rejected abstracts that another organization—probably Project Inform in San Francisco—is willing to publish them.

Publication will probably consist of delivering one 8.5 by 11 inch sheet (21.5 by 28 cm) for each abstract to a photocopy shop which will fulfill orders as received; a similar system was used two years ago to make copies of the Stockholm Conference abstracts available.

# NATIONAL AIDS BENEFITS HANDBOOK

*The AIDS Benefits Handbook*, subtitled "Everything You Need to Know to Get Social Security, Welfare, Medicaid, Medicare, Food Stamps, Housing, Drugs, and Other Benefits," by Thomas P. McCormack (Yale University Press, 1990), tells how to qualify for medical and disability benefits throughout the United States. The first half of the 257-page paperback provides an easy-to-read introduction to the different programs, including how procedures differ in different states. The second half consists of appendices with addresses, phone numbers, tables of benefit amounts, government regulations, and forms.

We asked a benefits expert at AIDS Benefits Counsellors in San Francisco to help us evaluate the book. She said that because they specialize in California, they could not judge the information for other states, but that everything they could evaluate was correct.

We believe that this book will be especially useful in providing introduction and background on different benefits programs and how to meet their requirements. Persons with AIDS or HIV may want to read it before seeking local advice about the programs in their areas.

# Issue Number 106
# July 6, 1990

## CONFERENCE REPORT, PART I

*by John S. James*

The headline story from the Sixth International Conference on AIDS is that (as expected) no "blockbuster" advances were announced. But behind the headline, this Conference produced much useful information—more than any previous meeting. Few reporters, scientists, or physicians can look through all the information presented; therefore many potentially useful developments may be lost, and never be reported in the general press or even in scientific journals.

During the Conference we focused mainly on examining and photographing poster presentations, and talking with people we met in the poster aisles. Many important oral sessions had scheduling conflicts with other meetings, so we bought audio tapes. The most convenient single information source remains the Conference abstracts, about three thousand of them published in a three-volume set. Although the abstracts could not be changed after January, the "bottom line" results reported seldom changed between then and June, so the abstracts remain useful. They are generally well organized into topics, easier to read than in previous years, and have subject and author indexes.

We plan to examine thoroughly two of the four tracks of the Conference—Basic Science (Track A), and Clinical Science and Trials (Track B)—seeking reports we believe could be useful to our readers. We will cover the other two tracks, Epidemiology and Prevention (Track C), and Social Science and Policy (Track D), only sporadically. We are now looking through the voluminous Tracks A and B information to pick out potentially useful items, and group them by specific opportunistic infection, particular HIV treatment, or under other practical headings. We expect our next few issues to be largely devoted to this Conference, but we cannot be sure, since issues of *AIDS Treatment News* are not planned in advance but cover whatever seems most important at the time.

We are also following political developments concerning the Conference. Some of them raise issues about the fundamental contract between government and the governed. We have chosen to wait to see what develops on these matters, and to focus on scientific and medical information for now.

For this issue we are lucky to have the report from Dr. Marcus Conant, below, on some of the major Conference developments as seen by one of the country's leading HIV physicians.

## SIXTH INTERNATIONAL CONFERENCE OVERVIEW FROM MARCUS CONANT, M.D.

Marcus Conant, M.D., is in private practice in San Francisco, where he has one of the largest HIV practices in the United States. He has treated AIDS since it was first discovered, and has conducted clinical trials of experimental treatments and published over 30 papers on AIDS and HIV since 1983. Immediately after the Sixth International Conference on AIDS in San Francisco (June 20-24), Dr. Conant met informally with other leading physicians to review the information reported, and to seek consensus on how it should affect their practices.

On July 2 Dr. Conant called a two-hour public meeting in San Francisco to tell his patients and others about results of the Conference and the physicians' review session afterwards. The following is from our notes of the July 2 meeting. We thank Dr. Conant for permission to use this material, and for reviewing it for accuracy.

### History of the Annual International Conference on AIDS

Each year's International Conference has had its own theme.

"The first Conference in Atlanta, in 1985, was clearly a meeting with a lot of hope; everybody went there saying, finally it's coming together, finally after five years of the epidemic we're going to see some movement. The next year in Paris was clearly the meeting of despair. People were expecting some real breakthroughs, and there weren't any; everyone came away depressed.

"The third year in Washington (June 1987) AIDS came of age scientifically; that was the first international meeting where the heavy hitters moved into the field— people from immunology and virology, specialists in other viral diseases, people who had made vaccines. With those heavy hitters came their young turks who want to get Nobel prizes, because if you're really bright in science you hang around with somebody who's really bright. AIDS also came of age politically, as the White House recognized AIDS as important enough to send George Bush, then Vice-President, to address the meeting; Bush's speech was booed by the audience.

"The next year in Stockholm (1988) was a period of confirmation. The studies on AZT were being done, and everybody was finding the same result, in Africa, Europe, or the United States. Last year in Montreal, one of the major themes was women and children and AIDS.

"Before this year's Conference in San Francisco, some of us had despaired of having more international meetings. There was so much concern about turmoil that many were saying that there may be no place for an international AIDS meeting, each specialty will have its own. To the great credit of Paul Volberding and John Ziegler, they organized a meeting that did bring it together for everybody. They assured that for the next few years we will continue to have international AIDS meetings. I think unfortunately that the behavior of the United States government will assure that those meetings will not occur in this country."

## AZT

No big surprizes about AZT came from the Conference, but Dr. Conant mentioned some significant results:

- We did not hear of any new toxicities.

- We are seeing much less myopathy, probably because of the lower dose. "More people are seeing what we had observed, that if you are on high-dose AZT, 1200 mg per day, and are exercising a lot, that may trigger the myopathy, and if you stop working out for a while and reduce your AZT, you may then go back to work out moderately and see your CPK (creatine phosphokinase level) stay down and not rise."

- We are seeing no liver toxicity on the lower dose. "So if you are on AZT and your liver enzymes start going up, and your doctor thinks it is due to the AZT, tell him or her that we need to look further. Could there be something else that's causing liver toxicity?"

A questioner asked how long people have been followed on the lower dose (500 or 600 mg per day). Dr. Conant answered that people have been on this dose and followed for a little over two years. Some people have been on the high dose for about five years.

- Only about one percent of patients with over 250 T-helper cells need to stop AZT because of toxicity, when using the low dose. That compares with up to 40 percent in the early trials, for people who had had pneumocystis and took the high 1200 mg dose.

- The lower the CD4 (T-helper cell) count when patients start AZT, the less likely they will be to lower p24 levels (a measure of viral activity in some patients). "Clinicians need to hear this. If you start AZT at 200, you have less chance to lower the p24 than if you start at 400 or 500."

- AZT is working about the same in children as in adults, and the same in women as in men.

- A very small study has shown AZT to be effective at 300 mg per day. "I would keep that figure in the back of my mind. If you have to do dose reductions, and you want to know how low to go, I would try not to go below 300 mg per day; that's for a 150 lb man or woman."

- European data has shown that AZT does not need to be given every four hours. "So (at the physicians' meeting after the Conference) we largely agreed that we would be recommending 200 mg three times a day."

- What about viral resistance? "We spent three hours talking about that, and the bottom line is we don't know at this time. The consensus was that resistance is a concern, but at this point there is more compelling data that people with below 500 T-helper cells do better with AZT than without it.

"Also, we don't know if people who develop resistant virus are therefore going to get sick; does that really constitute drug failure? For example, if ddI became available tomorrow by prescription, and you had been on AZT for two years, and I found you had resistant virus, and you tolerated the AZT well, would I stop the AZT and put you on ddI, or would I reduce the AZT to 300 to 500 a day and put you on ddI in addition to the AZT? Does resistance mean that the drug has totally failed, or only that we might want to add another antiviral? We are far from any definitive answer.

"Will resistant virus be transmitted? If so, treating persons who caught the virus could be a more difficult problem."

## ddl

Question from the audience about the risks and benefits of ddI: "Some two percent of patients on the drug for seven months have experienced pancreatitis. The high dose is associated with pancreatitis; low doses do not appear to be. Pancreatitis is much more common in persons with a prior history of pancreatitis, or of liver disease. If someone has chronic active hepatitis, or elevated liver enzymes, the physician will probably want to watch even more closely.

"Hemorrhagic pancreatitis with death has been seen. There have also been deaths, probably due to arrhythmias (heart-rhythym abnormalities), in people simultaneously taking rifabutin, clofazimine, and ddI.

"Triglycerides may be elevated prior to elevated pancreatic enzymes (amylase).

"On the positive side, T-helper cells rose about 30 percent in a group of people on ddI. Physicians are seeing p24 reduction, and viral culture going negative, but nothing more dramatic than with either AZT or ddC.

"ddI appears to be working in children.

"The ddI dose they're using is around 250 mg twice a day for a 70-kilo man, 375 for heavier people. (Note: we reported in the May 18 issue of *AIDS Treatment News* that some patients in the open-label study—the expanded-access program—have reduced their dose by taking only one of the two daily doses—preferably with the knowledge of their physician and Bristol-Myers.)

"Concerning the rise of T-helper cells, there has been a statistical problem in some studies. To take an illustrative example, suppose everyone in a study stays the same, except for some of the people with the lowest T-helper counts, who have big declines in the count and therefore decide to drop out of the study. Then the overall average would go up—even though not a single patient went up—just because those at the lower end dropped out. Studies can be adjusted for this particular bias by taking each patient's baseline T-helper count as that person's starting point, and averaging the changes, plus or minus. But simply reporting the average or median T-helper cells in the group before treatment, and in the group after treatment when some patients have dropped out, can be misleading.

"One of the criticisms of the ddI open-label study is that those for whom the drug doesn't work drop out."

## ddC

"ddC looks more promising than it did last year. T-helper counts are up. A lower dose of ddC has lower toxicity, and the toxicity is predictable. There have been no fatalities from ddC.

"ddC is probably safer than ddI. I think if you polled half a dozen experts now and asked if you had to go off AZT, what would be the next drug you would choose, ddC would be the choice. Unfortunately, access will be limited for a time.

"The best ddC data yet is in the paper Gottlieb presented to the Montreal AIDS conference last year."

## Antiviral Combinations

A member of the audience asked whether to add ddI to AZT, if ddI were available. "I don't have an answer. But if I had been on AZT for a year and a half, and had evidence of disease progression, and I could take both drugs, I would consider doing so. There's a place for combination therapy.

"I liked having the AIDS activists in the Conference; sometimes they raised the most cutting questions. On combinations, the traditional way is to test drug A, get to know everything about it, then test drug B, and only later try combining the two. But since everybody seems to agree that combinations is the way to go—they've been talking about it for years now—activists asked why not go ahead and do it? The answer was, 'That's not the way we do it.' The question was useful, because if you watched the speaker who was answering it, you could see written all over his face the thought, 'Isn't this stupid?' That may be the first time the thought occurred to him—having to say it publicly—that maybe we ought to move on."

Question: is there any data based on previous experience with other diseases as to how the drugs should be combined? "The answer unfortunately is no. These are synthetic nucleoside analogs, and except for acyclovir to treat herpes, there is not yet another model; it is not the same as chemotherapy.

"It's not as bleak as it sounds. We think that much of this data now will come from animal models, and that we won't have to wait to do the whole thing.

"There are some experiments on combining drugs, for example the ddC study at Stanford which is testing alternations of this drug with AZT."

## Surrogate Markers

"What about p24 or virus in the blood as a surrogate marker? The answer at this time seems to be that they are not reliable enough to use for clinical management. About 20 percent of patients who have negative p24 still die of AIDS.

"Even the Ho quantitative viral assay is not sensitive enough that we can say that you should stop AZT at this point and go to ddI.

"We're hearing that p24 and viral-culture tests are useful markers, and can be used by the clinician from time to time, but you would not stop a study based on those. I asked at the meeting—with Volberding, Fischl, Schooley, and others—is there a surrogate marker other than disease progression or death that you would choose to use to stop a study? Their answer is still no. That is the science at this time, unfortunately."

## Soluble CD4

"Bad news. It has no toxicity, but it does not cross the blood-brain barrier. But the worst news was reported by David Ho. He tested soluble CD4 with virus grown in the test tube, and it was very effective in removing virus. He then took native virus from patients, and the CD4 didn't work. Smart people are still researching CD4; they are not giving up. But these results are not what we wanted to hear."

## Compound Q

"If you ask, 'Does compound Q work?' I don't know. 'Should I do it?' That would depend on many other variables. There's not enough data to say. There has been frightening toxicity with coma in some cases.

"Some of the compound Q results which have been discussed were not presented at the Conference. We need to ask the hard questions. If the researchers say the T-helper counts are going up, we need to ask how they figured that." (See note on statistical problems with T-cell group means, above.)

"Clearly we need a lot more information."

## Peptide T

"There is little good data with peptide T alone. But in one study, with AZT and peptide T given nasally, it improved cognitive function compared to AZT alone. If confirmed, that's very promising. Unfortunately, Dr. Candace Pert is having trouble now finding funding for her peptide T studies, so whether we see more peptide T research soon will depend on funding."

## Isoprinosine

"A recent article in the *New England Journal of Medicine* (June 21) showed that 17 patients on placebo progressed as opposed to two on isoprinosine. I think you will see more isoprinosine studies. Clearly this data looks very good; it looks like hard data. There is a question that it may be blocking the pneumocystis, not treating the HIV.

"Mark Illeman and I did some of the early isoprinosine studies back in 1983. One study, which we never could get the company to fund again, was fascinating. We had 20 men taking isoprinosine or placebo, and then we would measure how much CMV (cytomegalovirus) there was in the semen. There was a large drop in CMV in the people on isoprinosine.

"The trouble was that when the data was analyzed, we had ten patients on placebo, and their baseline CMV concentrations ranged from low to high; we had four on drug, and all of them started low. The company had all the data, and they just told us that this is all they had to analyze. We didn't know why the other six had not been included. Without being able to break the code myself and be sure that we had a good comparison, I was unwilling to publish the results until we could repeat the study to be sure. We never could get the funding to do it again."

(Note: Isoprinosine is approved in dozens of countries but not in the U.S., and is used for treating herpes simplex and some other viral diseases. A literature search found no published report of any test of isoprinosine and CMV—meaning that if the drug is useful in suppressing or treating this infection, we would not know it.)

## Oral Interferon

"Sublingual alpha interferon? Nobody knows. The consensus of our small meeting was that if it does work, it's without rationale; we don't understand how it could work. People are waiting for more data."

## Hyperthermia

"Dr. Alonso was here, and presented some of his data. I met later with an internationally recognized immunologist who had met with Dr. Alonso. We all want that to work; it's easy to do. But the immunologist was concerned that Alonso's team had not brought with them all the data they were claiming. For example, they claimed that scans had shown that KS in the lung had improved—but they didn't bring the scans to San Francisco. The immunologist offered at his own expense to fly to Georgia and look at the data; we don't know what will happen with that.

"It's so sad, because something like that comes and you've got lots of desperate people who want answers, including the doctors . . .

"The claim is that they're heating the blood higher than 107-108 degrees outside the body. We've seen lots of patients with a temperature of 107 for a few hours, and it didn't cure their AIDS.

"I'm also concerned that Dr. Alonso is already saying that he can determine who will get better after this therapy and who will not."

## GM-CSF

"The data looks very promising; access to the drug is still limited."

## AZT/Interferon Combination

"There is much enthusiasm for using very low doses of alpha interferon, such as a million units a day, or three million units three times a week, for people with high T-helper counts, 300 to 500, to see if this can prevent disease progression."

## Acyclovir

"I had thought we had seen the end of the AZT combined with high-dose acyclovir treatment. But Dr. David Cooper from Australia, a leading AIDS expert, is still reporting better survival in 60 patients, with CD4 counts around 30, if they are on very high dose of acyclovir, 800 mg four times a day. It does not seem to be CMV-related, but does appear to stop progression of other OIs."

Question about Conant's use of acyclovir:

"Everybody who had herpes, I'll give 400 mg twice a day—that's easy and safe, and won't bankrupt you. Earlier, based on Dr. Cooper's previous reports of less CMV, we were putting people on high-dose acyclovir, but we didn't see that much difference.

"About four years ago there was a laboratory study suggesting that acyclovir potentiated AZT. The hope was that low-dose acyclovir would make the AZT work better. But later laboratory studies showed that not to be true. So we have been less enthusiastic about recommending the high doses to people with less than 100 T-helper cells.

"But at the Conference, the data was from a good investigator, with good controls, and 60 patients; the ones on acyclovir are surviving better than the ones not."

Question about long-term side effects of acyclovir:

"We are not seeing any. The biggest concern on the high dose would be kidney toxicity, and as long as you remain hydrated, that's not a major concern. You would not want to take that much acyclovir and hike out of Grand Canyon, however. We didn't see any toxicity when we were giving the high-dose acyclovir."

## Passive Immunotherapy

"Keep in touch; hopefully a study will be starting soon."

## Pneumocystis Prophylaxis

"Out of this Conference came almost irrefutable data that trimethoprim sulfamethoxazole (brand names Septra, or Bactrim) is as effective as aerosolized pentamidine in preventing pneumocystis. It was given as one double-strength tablet per day—or given three times a week. Cooper in Australia gives it on two days each week, one twice on Monday and one twice on Thursday, and has never had a pneumocystis breakthrough. We will probably recommend that patients with more than 100 T-helper cells consider going on one double-strength Septra a day as your basic prophylaxis for pneumocystis. Then if you get below 100 T-helper cells and want to do aerosol pentamidine in addition to that, you're welcome to do it, although we're not sure it's going to help that much more. But the good news is you can trade a pill that costs about $30 a month for the cost of over $300 a month for aerosolized pentamidine.

"There were no dissenting votes in the small group of people we assembled, from here and Australia and Europe. The developing consensus is that somewhere below 500 T-helper cells you go on AZT, somewhere below 250 T-helper cells you go on one Septra a day, and if it continues to fall down below 100 T-helper cells a day you may want to go on aerosolized pentamidine also.

"There are other advantages of Septra over aerosolized pentamidine, besides the cost. Pneumocystis is not just a lung disease, it can be a systemic disease as well. With Septra, you are prophylaxing systemically, not just in the lung.

"Also, there is emerging evidence that with Septra you are also prophylaxing against toxoplasmosis, and shigella (a kind of food poisoning, which also occurs from handling reptiles).

"The bad news is that 20 percent of the people are going to get a drug eruption (a rash caused by the drug). You may be able to treat through the drug eruption, by lowering the dose greatly and coming back up, or you may have to stop the Septra and go to aerosolized pentamidine."

(Dr. Conant said that if he had to guess, once a day might be less likely to cause side effects than twice a week, because it would be easier to build tolerance with the drug every day.)

Question about dapsone for pneumocystis prophylaxis:

"We don't know, there isn't enough data yet. If you are on dapsone, it's probably reasonable to stay there."

Question: if on pneumocystis prophylaxis and T-helper cells went over 300, OK to stop?

"Yes, but you might wait for the next T-cell test in four months to make sure the result was not an aberration."

Question: is there a problem of losing the use of Septra if a reaction develops (in case one gets pneumocystis in the future)?

"Yes, this is a concern. We are trying to design a study to attempt to desensitize people to Septra, the same way as you can desensitize people to penicillin."

Question: if someone has a T-helper count of about 25 and cannot stop aerosol pentamidine because he's in a study, should he consider Septra also? He cannot take dapsone because of the rules of the study.

"Aside from the issue of damaging the study, we have been telling people for about a year that if they have under 100 T-helper cells they should consider dapsone in addition to aerosol pentamidine, to protect against systemic pneumocystis. But if a study does not allow dapsone, it is unlikely to allow Septra, either.

"When the standard of care changes, the studies have to change. They cannot do things to you that are below the standard of care. So next time you're in, mention hearing experts from the Conference saying that the standard of care may be changing to include Septra for people at risk for pneumocystis; ask what's their reaction to this."

Question: any information about long-term side effects of aerosol pentamidine?

"Yes. Diabetes has been seen in some cases with long-term use. The drug may contribute to pancreatitis in patients on ddI. However, there have been no drug eruptions (rashes). Also, no loss of elasticity of the lung has been reported."

In response to a question about dapsone vs. Septra for prophylaxis, Dr. Conant said he guessed they would prove about equally effective. (The reason the physicians' meeting chose Septra is that there is more data on it than on dapsone at this time.) Some dapsone data was presented last year at the International AIDS Conference in Montreal. Side effects about the same; Dr. Conant thinks the number of drug eruptions will probably be less with dapsone.

## Treatment of Pneumocystis

"There is now a growing consensus that corticosteroids do play a role. It looks like cortisone is safe if done properly and judiciously—high-dose cortisone, then tapered gradually."

Dr. Poscher, on Conant's staff, explained that "This is used in severe pneumocystis—not mild cases—when patients present to the hospital requiring oxygen or ventilators. They should be started on steroids early, within the first 24 to 36 hours of their hospital admission. In the past the tendency was to salvage them with steroids three or four days after they did not respond to treatment. That's been shown not to work at all. It is the early use of steroids that causes 50 percent reduction in mortality from pneumocystis."

## Toxoplasmosis

Dr. Conant reported that toxoplasmosis is much more common in Europe than in the United States; the best guess for the reason why is raw meat in European diets.

Some physicians are trying prophylaxis with dapsone, or Septra. Dr. Conant said that if he had less than 100 T-helper cells, he would be on one of these.

There is some enthusiasm for clindamycin for therapy instead of sulfadiazine.

## Tuberculosis

"Tuberculosis is frightening. We are seeing a lot of it among HIV-positive people in some areas: for example in Miami, among Asians here in San Francisco, and in Africa. Up to a third of those cases disseminate, instead of only infecting the lung."

Dr. Conant heard that Dr. Margaret Fischl has 51 cases in the Miami area, some in gay men, that are resistant to the standard four-drug combination. This is worrisome, especially because tuberculosis can spread easily.

Question: if a friend has TB, is on medication for it, is it not safe to assume he is not infectious?

"Correct. If you have a friend who's just coughing—I wouldn't kiss people with coughs, until we learn more about this.

"Every HIV-positive person should have a TB skin test; the earlier the better. It tells you whether your body has ever seen TB before; it doesn't mean you're infectious. But the TB you had (and controlled) could become reactivated, so your doctor would watch your chest film more carefully. If the test was negative, you should probably repeat it every year. It's another reason for having a routine chest X-ray.

"If your immune system is already suppressed, the skin test might read negative even if it should be positive. The way to find out is to do a skin test with other antigens; if you react to them, then you probably would react to TB if you had been exposed to it"—meaning that the TB test would be accurate.

(Note: previous reports of TB treatment, before the occurrence of the drug-resistant strain, had shown that standard treatment worked about as well for HIV-positive persons as for anyone else.)

"AIDS presents very differently in different geographic areas. For example, TB has not been a problem in the gay community in San Francisco—but there has been a lot of it in Miami, and there is no reason it could not spread to immune-suppressed people elsewhere."

Another geographic example: "In an AIDS ward in Memphis, many patients have histoplasmosis. But in our practice in San Francisco we have seen only one case."

## Mycobacterium Avium Complex (MAC; also called MAI)

"Dr. Harold Kessler and others presented some beautiful work (see poster #Th.B.517) showing that 5-drug therapy with Amikacin gives the best response in the treatment of MAI. Clearly the position some were taking two years ago that it is not useful to treat MAI is wrong; patients live longer and their quality of life is better if you aggressively treat MAI. The consensus is becoming that if the disease is diagnosed, treat it aggressively.

"What about using the PCR test to diagnose MAI in two hours—instead of six weeks for culture? The problem so far is that this test may be too sensitive, and diagnose MAI in everybody."

Question about clarithromycin for treating MAI. Dr. Conant is aware of work in France, but no paper was presented at the Conference.

## Cryptococcal Meningitis

"Fluconazole does not seem as effective as amphotericin (AmB) for initial treatment. Don't use both, because the drugs compete. After initial treatment, fluconazole is clearly best for maintenance.

"The jury is still out on whether to prophylax with fluconazole—using one fluconazole a day for persons with very low T-helper cells—to avoid the possibility of getting the disease. There is no data to show whether this is beneficial. It could possibly be harmful, because there could be unknown interactions with other drugs the patient was using."

## Cryptosporidiosis

"Cryptosporidiosis is becoming less frequent; we do not know why. Data was presented on diclazuril (poster #Th.B.520 and talk by Dr. Rosemary Soave) as a possible treatment."

## Syphilis

"Standard blood tests do seem to be effective to detect syphilis, despite immune deficiency. There are only a few cases where the tests have been known to fail."

## CMV: Oral Ganciclovir

"Oral ganciclovir is not as promising as had been hoped, as it has poor bioavailability. No benefit was found for CMV colitis."

## Lymphoma

"We are seeing much more lymphoma. A third of those cases are apparently caused by Epstein-Barr virus. The lymphomas seem to be coming from chronic infection with some agent—maybe Epstein-Barr, or other viruses which have not been identified—which immortalize the B-cells (making them cancerous) or T-cells. One speculation—could it be that Dr. Cooper's patients in Australia are doing better with high-dose acyclovir because it is suppressing viruses which cause lymphoma? There is no data for this yet, it is just a possible hypothesis.

"People who have had KS and survived for many years have very high levels of IL6. The concern is that large amounts of IL6 might trigger B-cell lymphomas. So people who have had KS for several years, who develop a new node that's not been there before, should talk to their doctor about whether it could be a lymphoma. We don't know for sure yet about the risk factors, but this is one to consider."

## Other Cancer

"Basal-cell carcinomas are becoming more common—especially body basal cells as opposed to facial basal cells. Basal cells very seldom metastasize, so these cancers are usually not very serious.

"But there has also been much squamous-cell carcinoma in the anal-genital area, especially in people who had perianal warts. If you had warts in the anal area and get a bump there that's growing, get your doctor to make sure it's not a malignancy. If early diagnosed, it can be excised and is no problem. If you ignore it for several months, this cancer may metastasize and be serious.

"We may see more liver cancer in HIV-positive men—especially with chronic active hepatitis and alcohol."

## Vaccines

"There is much optimism now about vaccines, both for treatment for those already infected, and for the uninfected. Much new information is becoming available.

"Dr. Jay Levy reported one case of a chimpanzee which has now cleared an HIV infection and is antibody negative.

"Other researchers found that women with antibodies to the V3 loop of the virus do not infect their babies. These antibodies must therefore be protective. If so, they could be made either in humans or synthetically and given to patients.

"Salk has been testing his vaccine in persons with HIV for three years now. Passive immunotherapy is another approach to providing protective antibodies.

"Murray Gardner presented a magnificent paper on SIV in primates. Jay Berzofsky showed how you can take the part of the virus you want to make antibody to, put augmenters on it, and make even higher antibody levels. But some epitopes of the virus can facilitate viral replication. So you must design a vaccine that has the parts you want, with augmenters that make it multiply, and eliminate the parts that facilitate viral replication.

"Phil Berman a week before the Conference announced that he had protected two out of two chimps with a genetically engineered vaccine."

Dr. Conant attended a Genentech cocktail party and found the leading vaccine experts there, and much enthusiasm for making a vaccine.

## Epidemiology, Partner Notification, Health-Care Workers

"Belgium has started a partner notification program, and is finding it very useful in picking up asymptomatic infected individuals. I think you'll see more discussion of partner notification in this country in the next year or two. One of the problems that plagues the government is that, with the gay community, they can treat the entire community as a cohort, and say that if you've ever had sex with another man, you are at risk. But with the heterosexual community, do you test every heterosexual in America, or do you try to target those heterosexuals who are at risk? Clearly the latter is the most cost effective. It may not be the best way to do it, but if you were managing a government program, you would ask how to target the people at highest risk. One way to do that would be by partner notification. That has not been widely done, for civil liberties reasons. I think you will be seeing it discussed more.

"There is much concern about occupational risks to health-care workers. At least two have become HIV positive after a serious needlestick injury, despite high dose AZT given immediately. We had hoped that AZT would be something workers could do to protect themselves."

Question: how accurate have been projections from five years ago?

"From most reasonable people, projections have been sometimes inflammatory, but they have been accurate at least in pointing to where the epidemic is going. If you look at people like Dr. Donald Francis, he has been quite accurate the whole time. The conservative right, and some of the stories hyped in the media, have often been wrong.

"Clearly we are seeing different diseases emerging as people live longer. One reason is that antivirals may change the natural course of HIV disease. We are prophylaxing against pneumocystis, so people who were dying of it live to get something else. And KS is going away by itself, for reasons we do not understand.

"We're seeing more toxoplasmosis, more cryptococcosis, and a lot more lymphoma.

"As in cancer, each person with AIDS is their own individual case. Some people will do very well over time, but others with the same laboratory tests will do poorly. The challenge continues to be to find out what that difference is, so that you can do for the ones doing poorly what the others are doing for themselves.

# Issue Number 107
# July 20, 1990

## CONFERENCE REPORT, PART II
*by John S. James*

Our previous issue included an overview of the most important practical treatment information from the Sixth International Conference on AIDS, from a public talk by Marcus Conant, M.D. This issue continues our Conference coverage:

• New discoveries of potential drugs outside of the dominant preconceptions may offer the most promising possibilities for future development—because with them, the easy research has not already been done. But these new developments risk being ignored. Newspapers seldom acknowledge their existence, and few scientists, physicians, or reporters have time to read or listen to all the Conference presentations. Our article on experimental antivirals examines two scientific papers which deserve attention.

• Many Conference presentations concerned AZT dosage, combination therapy, and antiviral resistance. The article by Michelle Roland on AZT outlines these developments.

• Opportunistic infections are potentially easier to treat than HIV, and yet they have often been neglected in the research conducted up to now. As a result, advances against opportunistic infections have been among the most practical of new developments, and at the same time among the most disappointing. In this issue, Denny Smith reviews cryptosporidiosis reports presented at the Conference.

## EXPERIMENTAL ANTIVIRALS
*by John S. James*

Dozens of different potential antivirals were mentioned in presentations at the Sixth International Conference on AIDS. But usually the results were too sketchy to be useful, or otherwise relevant to only a handful of specialists.

If we were asked to name one "sleeper" at the Conference—one project which we believe may have great importance but which received little attention—it would be the work on melanins, described below. It is too early to know if this treatment will be useful—but it would be easy to find out.

By contrast, the paper on Chinese medicines with anti-HIV activity in laboratory tests (below) did attract attention—partly because virologist David Ho, known for his work on plasma viremia, assisted in the project. As with melanins, we highlighted this work because it offers practical advantages. A medicine already in routine human use can clearly be developed faster as an AIDS/HIV treatment than a new chemical never used before. But Chinese medicines may be unpatentable, and they fit poorly into the Western medical-industrial complex, so the research needed is hard to fund. Community-based organizations should pay special attention to treatments which could be developed rapidly, but may not be developed at all without community pressure.

Readers should note that this article is based mainly on information presented at the Conference, as we have not had time to contact the researchers or do other followup.

# Melanins

This work, by researchers at Vanderbilt University Medical School, could easily be missed, because the interesting information appeared for only one day on the poster presentation itself (poster #Th.A.228), not in the published abstract or in an article published by the investigators. To anyone not at the poster that day, melanins would look like just another of the dozens of potential treatments which appear promising in laboratory tests and ought to be investigated further for possible human use for treating AIDS.

Melanins are pigments which are already found in the body in hair, skin, and eyes. Although recognized for at least 60 years, their chemical structure is not known, and no therapeutic use for these chemicals has been found. The melanins which occur naturally in the body are insoluble in water, but the synthetic forms studied as an anti-HIV treatment are soluble. Melanins are easy to make, can be given orally, and are inexpensive.

The published abstract (reference above) reported that small concentrations of melanins (0.3 to 10 ug/ml) blocked infection of human T-helper cells with HIV in laboratory tests; three different cell lines and three different viruses (including HIV-2) were used. A more detailed report of the same work was published in April of this year. (Montefiori, D.C. and others. Inhibition of human immunodeficiency virus type 1 replication and cytopathicity by synthetic soluble catecholamine melanins in vitro. *Biochemical and Biophysical Research Communications*, volume 168, number 1, pages 200-205, April 16, 1990.) The mechanism of action is not known, but melanins did *not* inhibit reverse transcriptase, so clearly they work entirely differently than AZT. (One test suggested that they probably did not get inside the cells.)

Another report, apparently of research too recent for inclusion in the published abstract or the journal article, appeared only on the poster itself. Synthetic melanins were given to mice in their drinking water, and their urine had anti-HIV activity even when diluted up to 200 times; control urine of mice given plain water had no effect.

The mice showed no toxicity from the chemical, and they ate and drank as much as the control mice during the five-day test. (Much larger doses of melanin given by injection did kill mice, however, and the researchers estimated the lethal dose for the animals at between one and ten grams per kilogram of body weight.)

**Comment:** Although this research is preliminary and much uncertainty remains, we find it especially significant that urine concentration 200 times that needed to show anti-HIV activity could be achieved with no apparent harm to the animals (blood concentrations were not reported). Other reasons why this work deserves high-priority followup is that melanins are considered relatively innocuous, can be given orally (at least in the animal tests), are very easy to produce (the synthesis could be carried out in a high school chemistry lab), and are inexpensive. Also, since melanins work very differently than the available antivirals like AZT, combinations might be especially effective.

Many questions can be raised. Melanins worked with laboratory cell lines and viruses; would they work with fresh cells and viruses from patients? What is the toxicity of these chemicals in humans? And melanins may interact with certain antibiotics or other drugs; how might this complicate their use?

Yet the existing information suggests a strong possibility that melanins might have an important impact on AIDS/HIV treatment worldwide. We are concerned that this opportunity may not be realized, since under the commercial and regulatory structure of drug development in the United States it will take years before any standard drug could become available from this early research—due to delays with patents, business negotiations, corporate restructuring, etc., as well as Federal requirements such as excessive animal tests which should not be allowed to impede progress in an emergency. Scattered reforms have been made, but no one has studied the practical operation of drug development from beginning to end, or has the authority necessary to make the changes needed to meet the AIDS emergency effectively.

We suggest that community-based and other research organizations—including institutions outside of the United States—investigate melanins further, and proceed if justified to develop this information into a practical AIDS/HIV treatment.

## Chinese Medicines

At the UCLA School of Medicine and Cedars-Sinai Medical Center in Los Angeles, 57 injectable Chinese medicines were screened against HIV in laboratory-cell cultures; 10 showed activity (poster #Th.A.237). These ten were then screened against primary HIV-1 isolates (and also against HIV-2). Using primary isolates is important because recently it has been found that tests with cells and viruses which have lived for years in laboratories—the ones most convenient for scientists to use—can show very different results than the same tests with cells and viruses taken recently from patients.

In the first phase of testing (using cultured cells and viruses), the therapeutic index (ratio between the concentration which was effective and that which was harmful to the cells) ranged from 22 to 333. Of the ten drugs which passed the first test, the two with the greatest therapeutic index were Injection Yin Huang (333), and Injection Co. Dan Shen (174). We do not have the result of the second-phase tests.

**Comment:** Treatments based on Chinese medicine are usually ignored in the U.S. drug-development system. The cultural bias of Western science and medicine is to isolate one or more pure chemicals which are effective, and then hopefully synthesize them—adding years of research time when an adequate herbal treatment may already be available.

Community-based research organizations could make a major and cost-effective contribution by organizing professional investigation of and advocacy for treatments which, due to cultural or commercial biases, are unlikely to get a prompt hearing otherwise. Then small phase I/II trials could obtain initial information about effectiveness in patients, using standard measurements such as T-helper counts, and p24 antigen and antibody levels. These trials could be conducted easily when the treatments being tested are already in widespread human use.

# AZT, ANTIVIRAL COMBINATIONS, AND RESISTANCE

*by Michelle Roland*

Most of the clinically useful information from the Sixth International Conference on AIDS concerned either fine-tuning of the use of drugs that are already approved and in standard use (e.g., AZT, alpha-interferon, and various prophylaxes for pneumocystis), or preliminary suggestions on how to use drugs that are not yet FDA-approved but are likely to become more broadly available in the coming months and years (e.g., the anti-HIV drugs ddC and ddI, and the anti-CMV drug foscarnet). Much of the remaining information was more useful to researchers, doctors who are also involved in designing clinical trials, and policy makers and activists who are trying to implement increasingly efficient and attractive ways to test potential treatments.

The major focus of this article will be on information which people can use today in making treatment choices. We will also discuss some of the important information on the use of treatments and combinations of treatments which may be available in the foreseeable future.

## AZT: When and How Much?

Much discussion concerned data already thoroughly critiqued in the past several months about when to start AZT and how much to use. The latest official recommendations suggest 600 mg per day for persons with fewer than 500 T-helper cells. Most physicians now use either 500 or 600 mg.

What about AZT for people with more than 500 T-helper cells? Margaret Fischl, M.D., a leading researcher on AZT, reported that the large government-sponsored study with asymptomatic patients has not at this time found a statistically significant difference in disease progression between patients with more than 500 T-helper cells who took AZT and those who took a placebo. However she also noted that this data is inconclusive, and does not show whether or not AZT would be helpful for these people.

At this time very few early studies are designed to test the effects of drugs in asymptomatic patients. Pharmaceutical companies may avoid studies in groups of people where the effect may not be big enough to earn FDA approval of their drug. But answers for these patients will become increasingly important to those who are wondering when they should start using an anti-retroviral, or prophylaxis for specific opportunistic infections.

One very small study suggested that 300 mg of AZT per day may be effective. This study was designed to test the effect of combining high dose acyclovir with AZT. Only 22 patients were enrolled; approximately half took 600 mg of AZT and the others took 300 mg. Although the addition of acyclovir in half of the patients on each dose did not produce differences in tests used to assess viral activity (p24 antigen and plasma viremia), the 300 mg dose appeared as effective in lowering these measures, and perhaps even more effective in sustaining an increase in T-helper cell counts, as the 600 mg dose.

This small study is far from conclusive, but it does suggest that people who have to lower their AZT dosage because of side effects or the use of other drugs which depress blood cell counts may still benefit. It also supports the growing suspicion that we have not yet found the minimum effective dose of AZT.

This confusion about dosage has implications for how early tests of anti-viral drugs in humans are designed and interpreted. Currently, the standard approach is to look for what is called the "maximum tolerated dose." As we have seen with the example of AZT, this dose was quite toxic. Yet early studies continue to look for the maximum dose, and then later studies use that dose, because it is the best studied. Treatment activists have long pointed out this flaw in drug development, and have suggested using the infectious-disease approach of seeking the minimum effective dose, instead of the cancer-chemotherapy approach of maximum dose. But pharmaceutical companies have an incentive to use larger doses, because if their drug fails to show efficacy in a controlled trial, they may not get another chance to test it, and their drug will be dead; yet they can reduce the dose later if necessary to manage toxicity.

## AZT in Combination with Approved Drugs

• Acyclovir: It has long been believed that high doses of acyclovir may increase the effectiveness of AZT. One small study reported on AZT plus high dose acyclovir; it did not show any increased anti-viral benefit from the addition of acyclovir. It is important to remember that acyclovir is still useful in treating herpes infections and often in preventing their recurrence.

• Alpha Interferon: Alpha interferon is currently approved for the treatment of Kaposi's sarcoma in some people with AIDS. Some scientists and doctors believe that it might increase the effectiveness of AZT. Preliminary data from an ongoing study on the use of alpha interferon with AZT (600 mg) in patients with more than 500 T-helper cells does not yet answer this question. Unfortunately, more subjective and laboratory toxicities have occurred in the combination group than in patients on either drug alone. These side effects included fatigue, loss of appetite, nausea, elevated liver enzymes, and decreased red and white blood cell counts. However, so far the numbers of people who have withdrawn from the three parts of the study are the same (suggesting that there was no great difference in side effects severe enough to require stopping treatment), and dose modifications were required in all three parts to reach safe and comfortable doses. Therefore, if this combination is found to be effective, it may be possible to tailor doses to individual patients to manage side effects.

After one year there were no significant differences in changes in T-helper cell counts between the group taking 600 mg AZT with alpha interferon, and the group taking 1200 mg of AZT alone. About 10 percent of the patients were p24 antigen positive when they entered the study and all experienced a decrease in this lab value, which may be a marker of disease progression. Although the numbers are very small (a total of only 10 patients), there appeared to be a more sustained decrease in p24 antigen levels in the combination group than in the AZT-only group. It has been difficult to complete enrollment in the study; therefore the data is incomplete and not entirely useful.

[Note: readers should be careful in interpreting statements that "no statistically significant difference" has been found in an incomplete study; this does *not* mean no difference has been found. There may be a big difference—but just not enough patients yet to provide statistical proof. Also, the criteria for claiming statistical significance for an incomplete study—and terminating the study as a result—are extremely conservative, often several times as severe as the criteria for claiming statistical significance at the end of the study; for background on this statistical quirk, see *AIDS Treatment News* #81. In addition, researchers may be reluctant to give out any early information about a trial which is continuing (unless those results are so extreme that they force the trial to be stopped), because early information could cause patients to drop out of the arms which seem less effective, which could bias or otherwise damage the study.]

## AZT in Combination with Experimental Drugs

The only information on the combination of AZT with an experimental drug that was presented at the Conference was on ddC, which works in the same way as AZT as an inhibitor of the enzyme reverse transcriptase, but is different enough that it has different side effects. The idea of combining antiretroviral treatments has three main attractions. First, combining or alternating treatments may make it possible to manage the toxic side effects of each treatment better than with a single treatment. Second, the problem of drug-resistant strains of HIV may be reduced by using more than one drug with a similar mechanism, like the nucleoside analogs AZT, ddC and ddI (more on resistance below). Third, by combining drugs that block different parts of the viral life cycle, it should be possible to limit HIV replication more completely than we have been able to accomplish with a single anti-viral drug alone.

The consensus at the Conference was that drug combination (either using the drugs at the same time, or in alternation) is the wave of the future. As more antivirals become available to patients through expanded access programs and eventually through FDA approval, the questions which need to be answered today are how to use these drugs together safely and effectively.

The ddC plus AZT studies presented at the Conference show us more about how complex the problem of interpreting and comparing studies has become than about how best to use these drugs together. None of the three studies used the same dose combinations, thus the different ways of combining these drugs cannot be compared across the studies. Two of the studies tested alternating the two drugs every week or month, or using each one intermittently (with a period of no treatment), one in patients who were intolerant to AZT and one in patients who were not intolerant to AZT when they entered the study. The third tested combinations of the drug used concurrently. Each study compared various dose combinations.

The worst side effect of ddC is peripheral neuropathy, while the primary side effects of AZT are on the bone marrow, leading to depressed blood cell counts. So the challenge of studying combinations or alternations of these drugs is to minimize peripheral neuropathy and red and white blood cell count depression while maximizing increases in T-helper cell counts and other markers of anti-viral activity.

Unfortunately, the major study showed that the most effective dose of ddC (high) was also the most toxic. This toxicity seems to be decreased by alternating AZT and ddC on a monthly rather than weekly schedule. Thus, the conclusion of the researchers who presented this data is that the optimum dosing schedule is monthly alternating high dose ddC with AZT. Although that is one conclusion which could be reached, some people may prefer to continue to look for more desirable combinations of these two drugs. It is important to note that this study used 1200 mg of AZT.

In patients who were intolerant of AZT, there was more depression of blood cell counts in the monthly than weekly alternating dose group; the least blood-count toxicity was in the group that used ddC on an intermittent basis without AZT at all. The researchers who conducted this study concluded that monthly alternating low dose ddC with AZT may be an acceptable "salvage therapy" for patients who have failed AZT. Again, some people would probably rather try other combinations, including longer periods on ddC than AZT, and lower doses of AZT, before reaching a conclusion about optimum dosing of these drugs in people who are intolerant of AZT.

Finally, the study which tested the use of AZT and ddC at the same time found no statistically significant differences in either safety or effectiveness between the various combinations tested—at least in the partial data available at this time. It used lower dosages of both AZT and ddC than did the two studies discussed above. Because this study is not completed, the data did not yet provide much useful information. It will be impossible to compare this study directly with the other two because of differences in the dosages used.

How can drug combinations be tested better in the future? One approach, called response-surface methodology, was developed in chemical engineering, where it is often necessary to vary the concentrations of two or more chemicals to find the specific combination which works best. In this kind of trial, a matrix of many different dosage combinations of two drugs is tested simultaneously, but very few patients are needed for each "cell"—each specific dose combination—perhaps only three or four patients, far too few for an arm of a standard drug trial. The reason so few are needed is that the overall pattern which emerges shows the best combination, although each individual cell may be too small to provide statistical information by itself. As far as we know, response-surface methodology has not yet been used in AIDS research, although it is being discussed. It offers the advantage of testing all reasonable dosage combinations at the same time and for about the same expense and number of patients as a standard trial which only compares a few dosage combinations.

## HIV Resistance to Anti-Viral Treatments

Antiviral drug resistance was a significant topic at the Conference. Because one of the key enzymes involved in the replication of HIV, reverse transcriptase, is quite error prone, HIV mutates frequently. Some of the strains that are formed as a result of the mutations are resistant to antiviral drugs like AZT. AZT-resistant strains of the virus can be found in patients who have never taken AZT, but are most frequently isolated from patients who have been taking AZT for more than 6 months. AZT resistance appears to increase with the amount of time one has taken the drug, although some scientists believe that resistance may develop more slowly when antiretrovirals are started earlier in HIV infection. Fortunately, cross resistance does not seem to be a problem with the nucleoside analogs that are being tested today (AZT, ddC, ddI). Therefore, even if AZT has stopped working because viral resistance has developed, ddI or ddC should still work.

The clinical importance of AZT resistance has not been proven. But some scientists believe that all future clinical trials of antiretroviral drugs should include laboratory tests of resistance. Managing the ability of HIV to mutate into resistant forms is one of the reasons that many researchers believe that combination anti-retroviral therapies will be so important.

Other viruses that affect people with HIV infection also form drug resistant strains. For example, herpes viruses can become resistant to acyclovir; the good news is that they often still respond to the experimental anti-viral drug, foscarnet. Also, CMV (cytomegalovirus), which often affects the retina of the eye but can also cause problems in the colon, spleen and other organs, has been shown to develop resistance to ganciclovir, the only approved therapy for its treatment. The resistance issue is one of the crucial reasons that test tube and human trials of new antivirals for virally induced opportunistic infections are in great need of research attention and money.

## For More Information

More information is available in the following Conference audio tapes. Note that each of these sessions is recorded on two cassettes.

Talk by Margaret Fischl, Thursday plenary session. Tapes #90ICA-10 and 90ICA-11.

New Concepts Regarding the Use of Zidovudine (AZT). Tapes #90ICA-46 and 90ICA-47.

Clinical Trials with New Antiretrovirals. Tapes #90ICA-50 and 90ICA-51.

CMV and Other Viral Opportunistic Infections. Tapes #90ICA-60 and 90ICA-61.

Resistance to Antiretrovirals. Tapes #90ICA-66 and 90ICA-67.

In addition, information from the following abstracts was used in this article:

On viral resistance: S.B.81 through S.B.88.

Foscarnet for acyclovir-resistant herpes: Th.B.446 and Th.B.447

Ganciclovir resistance in CMV retinitis: F.B.93.

AZT plus alpha interferon: Th.B.22.

ddC studies: Th.B.23, S.B.425, S.B.426.

AZT plus acyclovir: Th.B.24.

# CRYPTOSPORIDIOSIS: SCATTERED SUCCESS, RESEARCH DELAYS

*by Denny Smith*

Several antibiotics and antidiarrheals were among the treatments discussed at the International AIDS Conference last month for use against AIDS-related infections of *Cryptosporidium parvum*. Rosemary Soave, M.D., has been investigating new therapies for cryptosporidiosis at Cornell University. She presented results of her studies of diclazuril and spiramycin, as well as data on other agents under investigation.

The results regarding diclazuril were approximately the same as those reported in our last update on treatment for cryptosporidiosis (see *AIDS Treatment News* #95). Various responses of symptom improvement and decreases in counts of the parasite's oocysts were seen using doses ranging from 200 mg to 600 mg a day, with stronger responses at the higher doses.

Dr. Soave noted that serum (blood) levels of diclazuril were measurably higher in participants who had the strongest response. The drug used in these studies was hastily prepared for human consumption after a veterinary version for treating parasites in poultry, under the trade name Clinicox, was also discovered recently to be useful in some people. Ironically, the original compound formulated for chickens was apparently better absorbed than the newer "human" version. We have not heard of any ill effects in people who tried the veterinary product.

Dr. Soave is eager to continue studies of diclazuril, but the manufacturer claims there are limited supplies of the drug for humans. We spoke to Mr. Bob Lagendre, spokesperson for Janssen Pharmaceutica in the U.S., who said that they are now revising the formulation to improve absorption and that within a few months the manufacturing headquarters in Belgium hopes to make available two new analogs, dubbed "clazuril" and "letrazuril." These will be studied in six new trials around the U.S.

In the past, oral spiramycin did not appear to affect cryptosporidiosis significantly. But administered intravenously, spiramycin is now obtaining some good results. Of fifteen patients who completed a regimen of IV spiramycin, four experienced a complete response in symptom improvements and a decrease in cyst counts. Two of the four exhibited a complete absence of parasites in stool specimens after the treatment.

Other therapies presented at the Conference included hyperimmune bovine colostrum, transfer factor, paromomycin, loperamide oxide, and two analogs of the drug somatostatin, SMS 201-995 and Vapreotide.

Hyperimmune colostrum has been discussed now for several years as a potential therapy for cryptosporidiosis. The particular study presented at the Conference was authored by several Danish institutions and offered mildly positive results. Another study of colostrum was recently reported in *AIDS* (volume 4, number 6) by researchers at St. Vincent's Hospital in New York. A very small study of five patients produced results which warrant larger, more carefully-designed trials of colostrum.

The transfer factor discussed by Dr. Soave was an extract of lymphocytes derived from infected cows. Fourteen people who received this transfer factor demonstrated both improved symptoms and decreased cyst counts. Neither hyperimmune colostrum nor transfer factor are widely accessible now to people diagnosed with cryptosporidiosis.

Paromomycin, a prescription drug available under the brand name Humatin, is used for treating intestinal parasites. Park Plaza Hospital in Houston presented a 24-month chart review of 23 episodes of gastrointestinal cryptosporidiosis in 12 patients who were treated with paromomycin. All the patients showed some degree of symptom improvement after receiving the antibiotic, and in seven patients' stools the organism became undetectable. Minimal toxicity was reported. The dosing ranged from 1500 to 2000 mg daily, for a median duration of two weeks.

Loperamide, marketed as an antidiarrheal under the trade name Imodium, and the investigational somatostatin analogs were discussed as attempts to control AIDS-related diarrhea, and not as a cryptosporidia treatment *per se*. Managing the debilitating symptoms of diarrhea and weight loss of cryptosporidiosis is a critical measure, though only a stop-gap one.

Meanwhile, a truly effective treatment for eradicating this infection is urgently needed.

## REFERENCES

The Conference tape of Dr. Soave's presentation is tape #90ICA-63. (For information on ordering Conference tapes or abstracts, see "Obtaining Conference Information," below.)

The following references are to the three-volume set of abstracts of the Sixth International Conference on AIDS:

Gathe, J and others. Treatment of gastrointestinal cryptosporidiosis with paromomycin. Park Plaza Hospital, Houston, Texas. Abstract #2121.

Girard, PM and others. Preliminary results of Vapreotide (a new somatostatin analog) in AIDS related diarrhea. Hopitaux Bichat-C Bernard, Necker, St Antoine, Paris, France. Abstract #Th.B365.

Hojlyng, N and others. Cryptosporidium diarrhoea in AIDS patients treated with hyperimmune bovine colostrum. Statens Seruminstitut, Copenhagen, Denmark. Abstract #Th.B.521.

Mallolas, J and others. Efficacy and tolerance of SMS 201-995 (a somatostatin analog) in HIV infected patients with diarrhea. Hospital Clinic, Barcelona, Spain. Abstract #Th.B.364.

Mukololo, P and others. Efficacy of loperamide oxide in HIV-related diarrhoea. University Teaching Hospital, Lusaka, Zambia. Abstract #2025.

Soave, R and others. Oral diclazuril therapy for cryptosporidiosis. Cornell Medical Center, New York University and St. Luke's/Roosevelt, New York. Abstract #Th.B.520.

# Issue Number 108
# August 3, 1990

## MYCOPLASMA: CRI PLANS DOXYCYCLINE TREATMENT STUDY

*by John S. James*

New York's Community Research Initiative (CRI), one of the pioneers of community-based AIDS research, is developing a trial to see whether the antibiotic doxycycline can help certain patients with an ARC diagnosis—and whether a blood test for mycoplasma infection can predict who might benefit. This trial will test the hypothesis of Luc Montagnier, M.D.—one of the discoverers of the AIDS virus—that mycoplasma infection might be an important cofactor in the development of AIDS.

### Background

Mycoplasmas are organisms between viruses and bacteria in complexity. They are known to cause some human diseases, and they can be controlled with certain antibiotics. During the last several years, Shyh-Ching Lo, M.D., and other researchers at the U.S. Armed Forces Institute of Pathology found a mycoplasma which appeared to be a previously unknown species in organs of 22 of 34 persons who had died of AIDS, and reported evidence that this mycoplasma may be causing organ failures. (For more information on this work, see *AIDS Treatment News* #95.) In laboratory tests, the antibiotics most active against this mycoplasma appear to be doxycycline and ciprofloxicin (see Lo, SC and others, Sixth International Conference, abstract #Th.B.536).

At a special meeting organized at the Sixth International Conference on AIDS last month in San Francisco, Dr. Montagnier reported laboratory studies supporting a hypothesis that mycoplasma might be a major cofactor in the development of AIDS—not just an opportunistic infection. His team found mycoplasma in the blood of about one third of AIDS patients; the organisms are hard to detect, so they may be present in others, too.

Also, the researchers found that antibiotics which inhibited the mycoplasma prevented HIV from killing cells in the laboratory, although the drugs did not affect HIV directly. Dr. Montagnier speculated that HIV might become more destructive later in the disease than early after infection, because of later mycoplasma infection. An abstract by Dr. Montagnier and others (#1072, accepted for publication-only at the Conference, without a talk or a poster presentation) reported that doxycycline protected cells against destruction by HIV, even though the virus continued to multiply within the already-infected cells. HIV cultures treated with tetracycline lost their ability to kill cells even after the tetracycline was removed, suggesting that a tetracycline-susceptible contaminant in the culture (probably a mycoplasma) enabled the HIV to kill the cells.

Dr. Montagnier has given high priority to further investigation of the possible role of mycoplasma in AIDS, and has assigned 15 people, half of his unit, to work on it.

For more information on this research, see the interview with Dr. Montagnier by Martin Delaney of Project Inform, published in *The Advocate*, July 3, 1990.

## The CRI Study

The treatment study now being planned by the Community Research Initiative will randomize 150 patients with an ARC diagnosis to one of three daily doses of doxycycline: 50, 100, or 200 mg twice a day. Researchers will monitor patients' clinical status and do the usual blood work; in addition, a special laboratory will test blood samples for mycoplasma, at baseline and at three-month intervals. Because clinical evaluations can be subjective, the mycoplasma test results will be blinded; a Data Safety Monitoring Board will examine the unblinded data after six months, in order to halt the study if the results are dramatic enough to justify that step.

The CRI has raised about half of the $300,000 required for this study; it wants to have at least two thirds of the funding before beginning, to assure that the trial can be completed. Doxycycline is a generic drug, as its patent has expired; therefore pharmaceutical companies have no incentive to fund research. Federal agencies are not yet ready to conduct a treatment trial for mycoplasma, although they may do a prevalence study by analyzing blood and tissue samples.

This CRI study is important for several reasons:

• Even before mycoplasma became an issue, some physicians have prescribed doxycycline empirically for people with HIV who had unknown illnesses. The rationale is that many people with AIDS have opportunistic infections which have not been diagnosed (as has been shown by autopsy studies); doxycycline is fairly safe, and effective against many disease-causing organisms, so it could be worth trying when attempts to diagnose a problem have failed. The doxycycline trial will provide the best available data to guide empirical use of the antibiotic by persons with HIV—whether or not mycoplasma is important.

• The study will test Dr. Montagnier's hypothesis that mycoplasma infection may be a major cofactor in AIDS. It will show whether the available mycoplasma blood test is helpful in guiding the use of doxycycline, and whether testing for mycoplasma has prognostic value.

- Doxycycline is readily available, very well known in human use, and inexpensive. Therefore if the study does find a positive result, it could have rapid impact on AIDS treatment in the United States and elsewhere.

If you can help in the fundraising or otherwise in the development of this study, call Bernard Bihari, M.D., Executive Director, Community Research Initiative, 212/481-1050.

# NEW LAW WOULD ALLOW PROPERTY SEIZURE FOR "HEALTH FRAUD"; HEARING AUGUST 7

*by John S. James*

A bill to expand "war on drugs" property seizure to cases involving unapproved medical treatments has passed the California State Senate, and could soon become law. The last chance for public input may be early next week. While this law would only affect California, it has national importance because other state legislatures often follow California's example, and because of the extensive medical research conducted here.

The proposed law, SB 2872, would allow seizure and forfeiture proceedings against property—including entire companies—in some cases even before conviction of a crime. After expenses were paid, proceeds would be split 50-50 between State and local prosecutors—financing more health-fraud investigations, and creating an organizational incentive for prosecution against unapproved medical treatment, apart from any public-policy objective.

## Arguments For and Against

SB 2872 was introduced by Senator Marian Bergeson at the request of the California Department of Health Services. The initiative did not come from industry, the professions, or the public; in fact, as late as April 17, when the bill was considered by a Senate committee, not one person or organization had contacted the legislature to support it.

By July 27, there were three supporters: the American Cancer Society, the American Council on Science and Health, and the Cancer Advisory Council of the State Department of Health Services. The American Cancer Society could only give us its 91-word letter to the legislature. This letter does not address the merits of this particular bill, and shows no evidence that anyone in the organization examined the bill's specifics.

The American Council on Science and Health could give us even less. Its president was on vacation, and no one in the office knew that the organization had taken any such position.

The short letter from the Cancer Advisory Council said that the bill had been discussed briefly at its last meeting, and it did give an argument in support. It praised California's existing laws against unorthodox cancer treatment, but said that "funding is not readily available for enforcement activities, and thus some of our very effective laws tend to have a hollow ring to them. The Bergeson Bill will help to rectify this."

As of July 27, two organizations were listed as opposing the bill: the pharmaceutical company Genentech, Inc., and the California Attorneys for Criminal Justice. The two and a half page letter from Genentech's lawyers did provide a detailed critique:

"Under the provisions of SB 2872, a pharmaceutical company such as Genentech could have its entire manufacturing and research facility seized and made subject to forfeiture proceedings, even if a conviction has not yet been won. In addition, the bill allows for the entire forfeiture of a company's facility if intent is proven in even minor violations of the instances enumerated in Division 21."

Division 21 (of the Health and Safety Code) covers "no fewer than thirty activities which may be violated," Genentech's letter explained. "The following list is just a sampling of those activities which, if violated, would cause a pharmaceutical company operating in California to become subject to forfeiture proceedings," if there was a second violation, or any violation "with intent to defraud or mislead." The list of 14 items summarized in the letter mostly concerned drug labeling deficiencies, prescribing or administering an experimental drug in violation of State requirements, claiming that a new drug is effective, or failing to maintain adequate records. A company could also be seized if a product label failed to carry a warning message required by California's Proposition 65. Inadequate filing of paperwork with the State could also lead to a company's seizure.

Another problem mentioned by the letter is that it is common practice for a pharmaceutical company to make claims for a drug which may later be contested by the FDA, based on a different interpretation of the data. In such a case, SB 2872 would allow the State to "arrest an appropriate company employee and thus cease the operations of the company until the FDA matter is settled."

The other letter opposed to SB 2872, from the California Attorneys for Criminal Justice, said that the current forfeiture law, in effect now for about one year, was "the result of careful and lengthy negotiations by all parties and interests concerned. It was generally agreed that the new law would be in effect for a period of five years, at which time it could be closely evaluated *before* it was expanded to other areas or eliminated."

An April 17 legislative analysis by the Senate Committee on Judiciary pointed to other possible problems:

• Bounties could cause district attorneys to unduly emphasize crimes which provide financing to their offices, to the neglect of other serious crimes, such as rape, which do not.

• Increased prosecutions due to bounties could strain courts, jails, or other parts of the criminal-justice system.

• Expenses could be recovered from persons not convicted of or even charged with any crime. And the debt for such expenses, unlike other debts, could not be discharged in bankruptcy.

## Comment

Our concern is that funding law-enforcement agencies through seizure of property could lead to enforcement actions conducted primarily for generation of revenue, reducing patients' treatment options and slowing the pace of research. People may believe it is impossible that a major company like Genentech, capitalized at four billion dollars, could be seized and sold as a result of minor or technical law violations. But SB 2872 creates strong incentives for prosecutors to build their budgets by seizing assets. This kind of bounty hunting happens routinely in the "war against drugs"; under SB

2872, it could happen in pharmaceuticals, too, threatening California's industry and its leadership in research.

Options for medical care not explicitly approved by the FDA would be at even greater risk. California's existing laws against unorthodox treatment acknowledge no right of patients to make their own choices. Advertising that any kind of non-approved treatment has any effect on AIDS or ARC is illegal; the fact that the claim is true, and the person making it can prove it, is legally irrelevant. Other laws allow astronomical fines for even minor violations. SB 2872 would provide incentives for prosecutions which could reduce accepted treatment for AIDS to little more than giving patients AZT until they die.

Until recently, U.S. law has minimized seizure of property as a way to fund prosecution. Historical examples show the danger of creating such monetary incentives for prosecution which otherwise would not need to occur. In the Middle Ages, witchcraft trials became prevalent only in countries which allowed seizure of property, which could be shared by religious authorities, civil authorities, and accusers. Generation of revenue—not popular hysteria, as commonly assumed—was the real engine of the witch-hunts. So much property was transferred in this way that after a century of the trials, one inquisitor lamented that there were "no more rich heretics," and therefore the future of his office was in doubt.

No one can guarantee a monopoly on truth. Law enforcement should compete for funding with other public priorities, not fund itself through seizures to expand prosecution without regard to real needs.


# SIXTH INTERNATIONAL CONFERENCE, PART III: TOXOPLASMOSIS

*by Denny Smith*

The Conference news on *Toxoplasma gondii* infections largely consisted of refinements in diagnosis and a growing acknowledgement of the value of prophylaxis for people at risk for toxoplasmosis. Although the Conference published abstracts of more than twenty studies of this infection, no truly new therapies available for use were among them.

Jack S. Remington, M.D. of Stanford University presented the Conference's oral session on toxoplasmosis management, and opened his discussion by commenting on the low priority assigned thus far to combatting this major problem. Following is a survey of his remarks and selected studies from the Conference abstracts.

Toxoplasmosis usually, but not exclusively, presents as symptoms of encephalitis or neurologic difficulties. Computerized tomography (CT) scans are often used to screen possible causes of neurologic symptoms, but they are not always reliable for distinguishing the lesions of *Toxoplasma* from those of lymphoma, Kaposi's sarcoma, PML, CMV or herpes. Magnetic resonance imaging (MRI) is more useful, and brain biopsy or aspiration the most conclusive.

To avoid losing critical time until a diagnosis is absolutely certain, treatment for cerebral masses is often initiated under the presumption of toxoplasmosis; a good response to the treatment becomes a marker for an accurate diagnosis. But not every case responds, and meanwhile some other cause of the symptoms may have progressed untreated. An example of lymphoma misdiagnosed as toxoplasmosis was mentioned in *AIDS Treatment News* #104. A Conference abstract from Rio de Janeiro described how an increase in the number of presumptive toxoplasmosis diagnoses for cerebral masses was accompanied by an increase in deaths of patients who did not respond to toxoplasmosis treatment. The authors cite the need for better criteria for presumptive diagnosis of this infection (abstract #2115, Sohler, MP and others).

Dr. Remington pointed out that the retina, GI tract, pancreas, heart and lungs have been reported as sites of infection as well, so toxoplasmosis must be approached as a possibly disseminated infection. He added that he and American and French colleagues have developed better methods (differential agglutination) of testing *Toxoplasma* titers, but they can only wait for private industry to make these widely available.

A study from the University of Miami and New York University reported four instances of congenital *Toxoplasma* infections in infants born to mothers who were seropositive for both HIV and toxoplasmosis (abstract #F.B.476, Mastrucci, M and others). This information could be helpful for pediatricians trying to diagnose encephalitis in newborns, since two of the mothers in the study had no history of active toxoplasmosis. The infants were born with HIV as well.

The treatments discussed in the oral session included the standard regimen combining pyrimethamine with sulfadiazine, as well as agents under study: clindamycin, dapsone, doxycycline, 566C80, gamma interferon and a class of drugs called macrolide antibiotics, which include roxithromycin, azithromycin, spiramycin and clarithromycin. (An important note for researchers regarded the importance of different strains of *Toxoplasma*. Since this variable often determines the agents to which the protozoa will be susceptible, a number of strains should be subjected to a given compound, in research studies.)

When sulfa drugs cannot be tolerated, recent clinical practice has been to replace sulfadiazine with clindamycin. Dr. Remington said that the combination of clindamycin with pyrimethamine is generally considered effective, but no evidence yet proves it equal or superior to pyrimethamine with a sulfonamide. IV clindamycin offers more data so far than oral clindamycin.

Doxycycline, which has shown positive results against *Toxoplasma* in animal data, did not control toxoplasmic encephalitis in humans, according to doctors at Elmhurst Hospital Center in New York. Their abstract was a chart review of six patients who had shown intolerance to treatment with sulfadiazine and pyrimethamine, and who were then given doxycycline for at least one month. Five of the six experienced a return of lesions during therapy. Three of those five responded to retreatment with the standard drugs (abstract #TH.B.479, Turett, G and others). We were hoping for more success with doxycycline, perhaps in some combination therapy if not by itself, for people who cannot continue with sulfadiazine. A related study from Sidney described the successful desensitization to sulfadiazine in some people known to have sulfa allergies by giving gradually increasing increments of the drug over several days. Of sixteen patients with toxoplasmosis, ten were reported to be desensitized (abstract #TH.B.480, Tenant-Flowers, M and others).

Of the macrolide antibiotics, azithromycin looks the best in mice studies. To control *Toxoplasma*, a drug must reach significant concentrations in body tissues and not just blood. Azithromycin is exceptionally effective in this regard. Dr. Remington pointed out that azithromycin's strong potential as a toxoplasmosis therapy has been common knowledge for over two years, and not a single controlled human trial of the drug has yet been conducted.

566C80 is a new agent from Burroughs-Wellcome with strong activity against *Toxoplasma*, perhaps including the capacity to kill the parasite's cysts. This compound is also under study to treat *Pneumocystis* infections. Clinical studies of this drug are planned by the NIH.

Gamma interferon, which is probably the body's prime natural defense against *Toxoplasma*, has been shown to have additive or synergistic effect with some antibiotics—namely clindamycin, roxithromycin and pyrimethamine. (On the other hand, AZT may block the activity of pyrimethamine in mice, underscoring the need for access to more than one anti-HIV drug for people requiring treatments for opportunistic infections.) ACTG trials of gamma interferon to treat toxoplasmosis are being developed.

An abstract from the University of Genoa described Septra as an effective alternative to pyrimethamine and sulfadiazine for treating toxoplasmosis (abstract Th.B.477, Canessa, A and others).

Trimetrexate, under investigation to treat *Pneumocystis* infections, also has strong *in vitro* activity against *Toxoplasma*.

Authors of a Belgian abstract emphasized the importance of environmental precautions for people who are HIV+ but who test negative for toxoplasmosis. They advise their patients to avoid gardening, exposure to cat feces, and eating raw meat or uncooked vegetables (abstract F.B.426, Liesnard, C and others). People whose blood tests show evidence of a latent *Toxoplasma* infection could of course also benefit from those precautions, as well as the use of some preventive therapy to thwart a reactivation. Dr. Remington mentioned that there are no data solidly supporting a particular toxoplasmosis prophylaxis.

But recently, Septra, clindamycin and pyrimethamine have been suggested as candidates for clinical prophylaxis trials. A study from Spain described success with Fansidar in lowering the incidence of toxoplasmosis (abstract #2116, Iribarren, JA and others). Fansidar may have unacceptable risks, however, since it has been linked to some fatal allergic reactions. Another chart review at Elmhurst Hospital found that patients who were taking a double-strength tablet of trimethoprim-sulfamethoxazole (Septra or Bactrim) twice a day to prevent *Pneumocystis* pneumonia experienced a lower incidence of toxoplasmosis than patients on aerosol pentamidine (abstract Th.B.482, Nicholas, P and others).

After an episode of toxoplasmosis is treated, some suppressive therapy must be continued since no drug tested in humans has been able to kill the oocysts (resting forms of the organism) which can produce live parasites again in people with compromised immunity. Researchers in Barcelona have found that pulse-dosing, or intermittent maintenance treatment, of pyrimethamine and sulfadiazine twice a week effectively prevented relapses of active infections in fifteen patients. (A similar finding was presented last year at the Montreal conference). This could help many people who cannot tolerate the toxicity of daily dosing. However, other experts have cautioned that the half-life of pyrimethamine can vary from person to person, so pulse-dosing may be reliable for persons whose bodies retain such a drug long enough, and not for others.

Incidentally, in the comparison groups of the study's participants who could be followed, fifteen patients decided, against medical advice, to not continue with any maintenance therapy. Eight of those developed a relapse of toxoplasmosis between two to fifteen months after their first episode. Ten other participants tried intermittent treatments of pyrimethamine with clindamycin, instead of sulfadiazine. Unfortunately, four of them experienced a relapse after two to nine months (abstract TH.B.483, Gonzalez-Clemente, JM and others).

In spite of the good efforts and intentions evident in all of these studies, people are still dying of toxoplasmosis. Survival is better with early diagnosis and concurrent anti-HIV therapy, but even given these advantages something less toxic and more effective than pyrimethamine with sulfadiazine is needed. Dr. Remington spoke for many when he expressed frustration with the static situation of treatment research for this infection. For example, more than a year ago an update on toxoplasmosis in *AIDS Treatment News* (#79) included a report on arprinocid, at that time considered one of the most promising compounds to be laboratory tested against *Toxoplasma*. We could find no mention of arprinocid at this Conference, nor of trimetrexate, nor of any human experience with azithromycin, as Dr. Remington noted.

If arprinocid, azithromycin, 566C80, gamma interferon, or trimetrexate are not safe or useful in humans, we need to know. And if they **are** safe and effective, we need to know that too, as soon as possible.

# SIXTH INTERNATIONAL CONFERENCE: TREATMENT OF CMV INFECTIONS

*by Michelle Roland*

CMV (cytomegalovirus) is responsible for several serious opportunistic infections in people with AIDS. It most commonly infects the retina of the eye (CMV retinitis), resulting in blindness if untreated. CMV can also cause colitis and pneumonia and can infect other organs, including the spleen. The one approved treatment for CMV retinitis in the U.S. is intravenous ganciclovir (also called DHPG). Because of its limited long-term effectiveness, often serious side effects, and the inconvenience of the intravenous formulation, alternative treatments for CMV infections are urgently needed. In addition, very little is known about the safety and effectiveness of ganciclovir or any experimental treatment for other manifestations of CMV infection, e.g. colitis and pneumonia; increased research attention in this area is also crucial.

This article will cover the information presented at the Conference on the use of ganciclovir by itself and in combination with the experimental drugs ddI and GM-CSF. In addition, we will discuss the unapproved drugs foscarnet (which is furthest along the U.S. regulatory pipeline), oral ganciclovir, and TI-23 (anti-CMV monoclonal antibodies). Preliminary results of a study on high dose intravenous acyclovir, which is FDA approved for herpes infections, will also be summarized. Finally, we will suggest some research directions which should be pursued immediately to maximize the effectiveness and minimize the toxicity of currently and soon to be available treatments for CMV retinitis. (Note: for our last CMV update, see *AIDS Treatment News* #96.)

## Intravenous Ganciclovir

Patients and health care workers familiar with ganciclovir know that, although ganciclovir is quite effective in initially stopping the progression of CMV retinitis, its long term effectiveness is often limited, either by time, or by its serious side effects. Data presented at the Conference shows that CMV cultured from some patients develops resistance to ganciclovir after three months of treatment, offering at least a partial explanation for the time-limited effectiveness of this treatment in many people with CMV infections. The amount of time for which this drug is effective varies among patients. In a large study of over 700 patients, almost half had experienced progression of their retinitis in a mean of approximately 97 days (with a range of 4 to 220 days); the other 56% had not experienced any progression at the time the data was presented. (References to this and other studies are listed at the end of this article.)

Although ganciclovir's effectiveness is often time-limited, it is the only drug currently available in the United States for use by people with CMV infections; it is important to learn how to use it as safely, effectively and conveniently as possible until better treatments are available, either by combining it with other drugs and/or by altering the frequency of its administration.

## Ganciclovir with GM-CSF

Ganciclovir's most serious side effect is its depression of the development of a type of white blood cells called neutrophils. These cells are important in fighting off bacterial infections. Many scientists and activists have believed that a drug called GM-CSF (granulocyte macrophage colony stimulating factor), which stimulates the growth of some types of white blood cells in the bone marrow, might counter the neutropenia (depressed neutrophil count) experienced by many people using ganciclovir.

Preliminary results from a small study comparing patients treated with GM-CSF with others who received only ganciclovir suggest that neutropenia severe enough to require discontinuation of ganciclovir may be reduced with the use of GM-CSF, although the differences between the two groups were not outstanding.

What is the clinical significance of the small decreased incidence of severe neutropenia? It is believed by many that temporary or permanent discontinuation of ganciclovir contributes to progression of CMV retinitis. Although the difference in percentage of patients in the two groups who experienced progression of their retinitis was not statistically significant, the mean time to progression was 102 vs 156 days. There were also fewer bacterial infections in those patients who received GM-CSF (47%) than in those who did not (62%).

The preliminary results of this study appear to many to be encouraging. There were some side effects, including more muscle aches in the GM-CSF group, and an increase in the number of another type of white blood cell called eosinophils. However, the overall trend seemed to indicate that GM-CSF may help reduce some of the adverse effects of ganciclovir and should be available to patients who wish to use it. GM-CSF has long been one of the drugs that treatment activists have advocated for immediate expanded access before FDA approval.

## Ganciclovir with ddI

Because ganciclovir and AZT have similar toxicities with respect to bone marrow suppression and a decrease in the white blood cell count, it was believed until recently by most doctors and researchers that the two drugs should not be used together. As the standard dose of AZT is lowered, more physicians are recommending that patients may continue to take low doses of AZT with ganciclovir, as long as their blood counts are monitored frequently. With the widened availability of ddI, and the knowledge that ddI does not depress white blood cell counts when used alone, there is much hope that ganciclovir and ddI can be used together safely. This combination would provide patients with anti-retroviral therapy in addition to their anti-CMV treatment.

Preliminary results from an extremely small ongoing study (five people) support the hope that ddI and ganciclovir can be taken together without any additional toxicities. All of these patients had taken AZT previously and four of them had had to discontinue the AZT because of neutropenia. No one developed decreased blood cell counts in the short time of the study (2-7 weeks). The initial findings are far from conclusive, but do support the belief that ddI may well be a better anti-retroviral than AZT for people who need to use ganciclovir.

## Ganciclovir Three Times Per Week?

Ganciclovir is currently administered twice a day for 14 days (induction phase), followed by once a day, five days a week administration as maintenance therapy. An Australian study tested the use of ganciclovir three times per week in the maintenance phase, at approximately twice the dose used in the five days per week schedule. Although this study did not have a control group with which to compare its results, it did find rates of progression of CMV retinitis similar to those reported in many other studies. 40% of the patients had experienced progression of their retinitis at a mean of 4.1 months; 38% continued to have inactive retinitis on maintenance therapy at a mean of 6.1 months in the study. (As mentioned above, the large ganciclovir study presented at the Conference reported 44% progression at a mean of 97 days.)

Again, this study is not conclusive, but it does suggest that ganciclovir may be used effectively less frequently than it is being used now. Given the inconvenience of the intravenous therapy, if this data were to be confirmed, it would be very good news. We believe that this type of information is of critical importance to people with AIDS and CMV infections and should be seriously pursued by other researchers.

## Ganciclovir for CMV Colitis

Very few studies have been conducted with treatments for CMV infections other than retinitis. A single placebo-controlled study of ganciclovir in colitis showed some improvement in weight loss and significant improvement in progression to CMV retinitis and laboratory assessment of infection as compared to the placebo group. Unfortunately, although the incidence of diarrhea and abdominal pain decreased in the ganciclovir group, the group receiving placebo experienced the same degree of improvement in these symptoms, suggesting that the drug was not responsible for the improvements.

Ganciclovir appears to be useful in at least some aspects of the treatment of CMV colitis; however no studies have been done to answer such questions as whether treatment should be continued indefinitely or just until symptoms resolve. Different doctors and researchers have different opinions about ganciclovir maintenance therapy in CMV colitis. Further investigation in this area is certainly warranted.

## Foscarnet

Given the limits of ganciclovir, the development of other treatments for CMV infections is essential. Furthest along the developmental and regulatory pipeline is foscarnet. Although this drug also has serious limitations (can be toxic to the kidneys; also requires daily intravenous infusion), it is essential that more than one drug be available to treat this viral infection. Data from the Conference continues to suggest that foscarnet is effective in stopping CMV retinitis for a limited time and delaying its future progression. The relapse rates appear to be similar to those found with ganciclovir. In addition, one study found a consistent decrease in p24 antigen levels (in those who were initially p24 antigen positive); these researchers concluded that due to it's potent anti-HIV and anti-CMV activities, foscarnet may prove to be the treatment of choice in CMV retinitis.

Foscarnet is not without its problems, however, and not all scientists believe that it will prove to be superior to ganciclovir. In addition to the already identified side effect of reversible kidney toxicity, reversible penile lesions have also been identified in a number of people taking foscarnet. These lesions often require cessation of therapy to heal. Also, one study found dose limiting neurotoxicity in 2 of 16 patients at a seemingly more effective but higher dose of foscarnet. Finally, another study demonstrated that, although calcium levels in the blood were not altered, the two hormones involved in keeping calcium levels steady in the body were elevated in people taking foscarnet. The clinical implication of this observation is not known at this time.

## Comment

A note about the design of clinical trials for CMV retinitis: Researchers do not like to design clinical trials without a control group which receives either a placebo, no treatment, a different treatment, or a different dosage of the same treatment. In designing clinical trials for CMV, some researchers have invented a new category which they call "non-sight-threatening CMV retinitis" based on the location of the CMV lesions on the retina. They created this category of patients so they could justify withholding treatment from one group to compare against a treatment group. In their abstract, these researchers write, "Data previously presented demonstrated that [immediate treatment] was more effective than delay in postponing progression of CMV retinitis." Any clinician treating patients with CMV retinitis could have told them that. It is essential that this dangerous distinction between non-sight-threatening and sight-threatening retinitis not be used in any future clinical trials of agents against CMV retinitis.

## Ganciclovir vs Foscarnet . . . or Better Yet, Together?

It is believed by many researchers that foscarnet and ganciclovir are approximately equally effective. A comparison study of the two drugs under way in England has found that the initial response of CMV retinitis may be a bit slower with foscarnet than with ganciclovir. Although the mean time to reactivation of the retinitis was about 4 months in both groups, the British researcher stated that there may be a trend to later and fewer reactivations with ganciclovir than with foscarnet. Importantly, regardless of small differences in efficacy, most patients on both treatments required an interruption or change in their medication at some point during treatment; many of those who did switch therapies responded to the second drug.

As expected, both drugs have their limitations. However, because of their different toxicities, they may be more effective if used concurrently or in alternation than when used alone. Clinicians and researchers familiar with the two drugs find that people respond differently to each, but that what is most important is having an alternative treatment available if the first one does not work.

## Comment

What should be the next step in testing ganciclovir and foscarnet? Researchers associated with the AIDS Clinical Trials Group (ACTG), the government sponsored research group, are currently designing a comparative study of ganciclovir and foscarnet, to determine which one is a better treatment. But as we already know (and the English study supports), neither of these treatments is ultimately satisfactory on its own. People often either experience a relapse of their retinitis or have to discontinue treatment due to serious side effects. What seems clear is that, given the reality at this time of two imperfect drugs, the most important information we need now is how best to use them together. This is the same question that is starting to be asked about the use of the anti-retroviral drugs AZT, ddC and ddI.

Instead of asking which one works better, we need to ask if it would be more efficacious and less toxic to use the two drugs concurrently or in alternation. (We have heard a report that one or more doctors may be using them concurrently now.) If used concurrently, how much of each drug should be combined? If used in alternation, when should they be switched? Business as usual in this case would be to compare the two drugs alone; business as usual is a luxury that people with AIDS cannot afford, particularly in this case. We believe that the next step should be to design a trial which intelligently examines options for using these two drugs together.

Note that activists have been pressuring foscarnet's manufacturer, Astra Pharmaceuticals, to release the drug broadly on compassionate use for about two years. In the United States, foscarnet is still only available to those patients who qualify for, and have access to, a clinical trial.

## Other Treatment Possibilities

### High Dose Intravenous Acyclovir

A very small study suggested that high dose intravenous acyclovir, taken with AZT, may be an acceptable alternative treatment for people who are intolerant of or have failed ganciclovir or for those patients who cannot tolerate both AZT and ganciclovir together but wish to continue taking AZT.

Patients were initially treated with ganciclovir and switched to intravenous acyclovir plus AZT for maintenance. The published abstract of this study states that 2 of the initial eight patients treated experienced progression of retinitis at weeks seven and eight after the completion of the ganciclovir induction. This study is ongoing and is too small at this time to allow us to draw any reliable conclusions.

## TI-23 (CMV Monoclonal Antibody)

Results from a small, dose-ranging study of intravenous TI-23, a monoclonal antibody against CMV, suggested that this approach may be a safe alternative to other anti-CMV drugs currently available or being studied. Since this drug is a foreign protein, it was important to make sure that the body would not create antibodies against the drug as a normal immune response. No such antibodies were detected and there were no objective side effects observed in the CMV positive, asymptomatic patients who were studied.

This study was not designed to determine if the drug is effective; the second phase of the study, which is currently ongoing in symptomatic patients with CMV infection, was reported to be showing encouraging early results.

## Oral Ganciclovir

Alternatives to intravenous treatment for CMV infections are greatly desirable; preliminary data was presented at the Conference on an oral form of ganciclovir. Although this study was designed to determine safety rather than effectiveness, some preliminary observations can be made. At the doses studied so far in this initial dose-ranging study (designed to find the maximum tolerated dose), all 11 of the patients had experienced a relapse of their CMV retinitis in a median time of 62 days (range of 3 to 131 days). There were no problems observed with toxicity, although resistant strains of CMV were isolated in two of the patients.

With the formulation of the drug which was tested, only 6-8% of the drug was found to be active in the blood stream. It is possible that if better formulations of the drug can be developed, effectiveness will be improved.

## Other Possibilities

Other oral drugs, such as FIAC and HPMPC, are also in development, but no data was presented on them at the Conference (See ATN 94 for information about FIAC and ATN 76 and 96 for information on HPMPC.)

## REFERENCES

Ganciclovir and GM-CSF: F.B.92
Ganciclovir and ddI S.B.474
Ganciclovir 3 times per week: Th.B.433
Ganciclovir in colitis: F.B.94

Foscarnet: Th.B.434, Th.B.435, Th.B.436,
Th.B.437, Th.B.438*, Th.B.439, Th.B.440,
F.B.96   *non-sight-threatening
Foscarnet vs Ganciclovir: F.B.95
Intravenous Acyclovir: Th.B.441
TI-23: Th.B.442
Oral Ganciclovir: F.B.9

# CPFs: RESEARCHERS DESIGN NEW ANTI-HIV COMPOUNDS

On July 20 researchers at the Dana-Farber Cancer Institute at Harvard Medical School, and at the Harvard University Department of Chemistry, reported the development of a new class of anti-HIV chemicals, in an article in *Science* magazine (Prevention of HIV-1 Infection and Preservation of CD4 Function by the Binding of CPFs to gp120. Finberg RW and others, *Science*, vol. 249, pages 287-291, July 20, 1990.) A brief flurry of news reports followed. While these chemicals are not yet ready for human tests, their development is important.

The new substances, called CPFs, are chemical variants of small peptides—short fragments of amino acids, the building blocks of proteins. CPFs contain only two amino acids. They work like soluble CD4, binding to the gp120 molecules on the AIDS virus—the molecules which attach to T-helper cells and allow the virus to enter. They may also protect the T-cells from being damaged by free gp120 in the blood.

In laboratory tests, the chemicals already developed required relatively high concentrations to protect cells against infection—40 micrograms/ml or more. A good antibiotic would usually work at lower concentrations—suggesting that the CPFs already studied might not become useful drugs themselves. But the researchers have found that small changes in the molecule can make big differences in effectiveness, suggesting that better versions might be created in the future.

At this time, no one knows if humans can tolerate CPFs—or if they will be stable in the body. But mice given 20 to 50 times the dose expected to be effective showed no toxicity, according to a UPI report based on a recent interview with one of the researchers.

CPFs may be important because:

• They were rationally designed to block a specific part of gp 120 which is essential for viral binding to T-helper cells (and other cells with the CD4 marker, which HIV apparently uses to gain entry into uninfected cells). Test after test has shown that CPFs behaved as expected in laboratory cultures. The existence of a clear rationale helps chemists design new versions of the chemical which may work better.

• HIV binding to uninfected cells seems to depend on a critical arrangement of molecules in the virus. Therefore, scientists expect that HIV may not be able to develop resistance to CPFs, as it appears to do with AZT-type drugs. If the virus mutates so that its gp 120 cannot bind to CPFs, then it may also be unable to bind to CD4 receptors and infect cells.

- Unlike soluble CD4, CPFs are easy and inexpensive to manufacture. And they could probably be given orally.

# Issue Number 109
# August 17, 1990

## ASPIRIN AND AIDS

*by John S. James*

Since early in the AIDS epidemic, some research has suggested that ordinary aspirin (or certain aspirin substitutes) might have a role in treating the disease, other than the relief of minor symptoms. Aspirin could not be the whole answer, of course. But laboratory studies have suggested that reducing certain inflammatory reactions, as aspirin does, may affect the pathogenesis of the disease, improving some immune functions, and possibly slowing the replication of HIV by reducing the levels of certain chemical messengers which may trigger the growth of the virus. Some anecdotal reports which have come to our attention also support the possibility that aspirin may have a role in the treatment of AIDS or HIV.

For several years a number of physicians have used aspirin or other anti-inflammatory drugs to help patients with AIDS feel better—especially to relieve fever or diarrhea when these symptoms are unexplained, and in some other cases such as fevers caused by MAI. While aspirin works for these purposes, until recently the treatment of choice was usually indomethacin, a nonsteroidal anti-inflammatory drug (NSAID); the reason for preferring indomethacin is that published information was available, since most of the early research was done with that drug. But new research is now suggesting that aspirin might be better than indomethacin or other NSAIDs. Both provide symptomatic relief from fever and diarrhea, and both reduce synthesis of a certain prostaglandin (see explanation below), which appears to be excessive in persons with AIDS and may make the disease worse. But aspirin might also have an anti-HIV effect which indomethacin does not.

Aside from a small study recruiting now, we know of no clinical trials to find out whether aspirin or similar drugs might have use in AIDS treatment. Without trials, the possibility remains theoretical; it is not known what dose, if any, might be useful.

It may seem impossible that if something as simple as aspirin might have value in treating AIDS, it could have been overlooked. But in fact, that outcome would be most likely. Aspirin is a generic drug, so there is no commercial incentive to run trials. Governments would have incentive to learn about an inexpensive treatment, but Federal research is based on letting scientists decide what they want to study. Usually this is a good policy, but in AIDS it has led to control of most funds by small groups of scientists, whose research interests have been narrowly focused and have been influenced by the availability of funding from pharmaceutical companies. Few private physicians conduct their own research without funding, or use treatments not already accepted as standard of practice and not proven in clinical trials. The essence of the problem here is that no person or office has, or ever has had, overall responsibility for managing government or public-policy response to the epidemic. Therefore when there are hints that a safe and readily available treatment may be useful, it is nobody's job to make sure that those hints are followed up.

## Background and Literature Review

Aspirin is considered the prototype of the nonsteroidal anti-inflammatory drugs. These agents work by reducing the synthesis of certain prostaglandins (especially prostaglandin E2), which are part of the inflammatory response. Other drugs which may be similar to aspirin as potential HIV treatments are indomethacin (a prescription drug) and ibuprofen (e.g., Advil), but *not* acetaminophen (e.g., Tylenol), which is not believed to have the same effect.

Early in the AIDS epidemic, before the discovery of HIV, a number of scientists interested in the pathogenesis (origin and development) of AIDS saw certain inflammatory reactions as part of the disease process. This approach led to a number of laboratory studies, which were later published. Most of these early studies used indomethacin instead of aspirin, probably because the former was a proprietary drug until 1984 (when it became generic). After the announcement of HIV, also in 1984, most research interest focused on it and on nucleoside analogs like AZT; pathogenesis was neglected. Some indomethacin studies were published after 1984, mostly in 1985 or 1986—probably reflecting the time required to complete and publish work which was conceived in the earlier era. (But one study published in 1985[1] was funded by the Gay Men's Health Crisis, which would be open to funding research on non-proprietary drugs.)

We have only found one abstract on anti-inflammatory drugs and AIDS or HIV published since 1987. Recent research seems to be preferring aspirin to indomethacin. A small clinical trial of a proprietary aspirin derivative, now recruiting at St. Luke's/ Roosevelt Hospital in New York, may provide the first scientific test in humans of whether or not aspirin can reduce HIV activity. (See additional information, below, on this trial.)

A literature search using the Medline computer database found only nine articles or letters about acetylsalicylic acid (aspirin) or indomethacin, that were also about AIDS. The earliest article, in 1984, reported that indomethacin enhanced the proliferation of lymphocytes from gay men with lymphadenopathy[2]. (Research on immunological effects of indomethacin, especially in the context of cancer, goes back to the 1970s.) A 1985 article[1] found that the enhanced proliferation of lymphocytes applied only to cells from persons with AIDS or ARC, not to those of normal volunteers; the article suggested that indomethacin might have therapeutic use in treating these diseases. A 1986 paper[3] found two separate immunological impairments in cells of patients with KS and AIDS; both were improved with indomethacin. But a 1987 laboratory study[4] found no difference between the cells of persons with AIDS or ARC vs. controls, in the effect of indomethacin; however, this study only measured production of IL2, a T-cell growth factor, in the indomethacin test.

Letters from two different groups in Spain concerned indomethacin for relief of AIDS symptoms. The first, published in 1986[5], reported experience with six patients with HIV. The first patient had been treated with indomethacin in 1983, due to a wrong diagnosis. This patient had generalized lymphadenopathy, malaise, fever, and severely reduced lymphocyte count; when treated with 150 mg of indomethacin daily, all symptoms disappeared, and they had not returned after three years, during which the treatment was continued. Because of that case, the physicians tried indomethacin in five persons with AIDS; they found no toxicity, and four of the five showed "considerable clinical improvement" after four weeks of indomethacin (the other patient died of pneumocystis). Two of the four successful patients needed doses raised to 75 mg every eight hours for the best results.

The other letter[6] was published in Barcelona in Spanish in 1988. It reported on three patients with AIDS or HIV who were treated with indomethacin. While all three seemed to be helped by the drug, two of them had died, one from a recurrence of pneumocystis, and the other from a recurrence of an unspecified infection.

Also from Spain, a different research group reported to the III International Conference on AIDS in Washington, D.C. in 1987[7] that they found increased levels of prostaglandin E2 (PGE2, believed to inhibit immunological functions and possibly stimulate replication of HIV) in persons with HIV. In HIV positive patients with depressed cell-mediated immunity, the level of PGE2 was ten times higher than normal; high levels of PGE2 correlated significantly with low lymphocyte count, low T-helper count, and impaired response to mitogens; it was also observed to correlate with clinical deterioration. (These observations are significant because both aspirin and indomethacin are known to reduce PGE2 levels in patients.)

In a computer search of tens of thousands of newspaper and wire-service stories, we found only one story mentioning a possible use of aspirin in treating AIDS. An Associated Press report in 1986[8] quoted researchers from the George Washington University Medical Center as suggesting that aspirin might be useful in AIDS and other immunological disorders. Preliminary trials had found that "one to two aspirin tablets daily can triple interferon production and double interleukin output." None of these volunteers were HIV positive, however. (See "Current Research," below, for more information about this work.)

Two earlier studies, in the 1970s, had found antiviral effects of aspirin in tests in animals and in plants[9,10].

## Current Research

A laboratory study published this May reported a difference between aspirin and indomethacin in their effect on HIV[11]. The same research group had already reported that intestinal mucosal cells from persons with AIDS or HIV, taken by rectal biopsy, would produce p24, a protein of the AIDS virus, during incubation for 48 hours in the laboratory. The new report found that indomethacin failed to change the p24 level, while an aspirin derivative reduced it by half. The researchers speculated that this effect of aspirin might be related to inhibition of the enzyme lipoxygenase.

Based on this result, a small clinical trial now recruiting in New York is testing the aspirin derivative (aminosalicylic acid, brand name Asacol, an experimental drug now in phase III trials) as a treatment for non-specific colonic inflammation in persons with HIV. This aspirin derivative is designed to be poorly absorbed, and formulated to pass through the stomach unchanged, so that it can deliver a very large aspirin dose directly to the intestines. This special form of aspirin is being used in the research in order to allow a clean study design, but it is suspected that ordinary aspirin would work, too.

Perhaps the most interesting result of this study will come later, when the p24 tests are run on the frozen samples. (These tests are usually run together as one batch, to reduce random variation caused by laboratory errors.) This data may provide the first scientific hint on whether aspirin can reduce HIV activity in patients. Later in this article we suggest other trials which could be carried out by community-based research organizations, to answer the question directly, using ordinary aspirin.

For information about a completely different project, we spoke with Dr. Judith Hsia at George Washington University to follow up on the 1986 report on aspirin research, mentioned above. She told us that researchers there are still actively looking at aspirin as an immune modulator; however, none of the volunteers so far have been HIV positive. (One of the scientists in this study, Dr. Allan Goldstein, is also the developer of the HGP-30 AIDS vaccine.)

A 1989 publication from the George Washington group[12] documented large increases in levels of gamma interferon and IL2 in normal volunteers after aspirin treatment. The dose was surprisingly small; 325 mg (one ordinary aspirin tablet) every *other* day worked much better than one tablet every day, during the one week of the study. Later, volunteers were deliberately infected with a common-cold virus; not surprisingly, the small aspirin dose did not protect them.

In a current study by the same research team, aspirin is being given to elderly mice (elderly so that they would be immune deficient) in order to see if it would make flu vaccine work better. No results are available yet.

## Practical Experience: Interviews with Physicians

Joseph Sonnabend, M.D., is a well-known AIDS physician in New York and one of the founders of the Community Research Initiative (CRI), a leading organization in community-based research. Dr. Sonnabend has long been critical of the overemphasis on HIV as the cause of AIDS to the virtual exclusion of other promising research areas such as pathogenesis. He has used anti-inflammatory drugs for years in treating AIDS and related conditions.

In our recent interview, Dr. Sonnabend made the following points:

• He had used indomethacin, because of the experience with it reflected in published literature (reviewed above). Now he uses aspirin instead.

• He has used anti-inflammatory drugs when patients are seriously ill, with recurring fevers not due to opportunistic infections. (Dr. Sonnabend is notably aggressive about prompt diagnosis and treatment of opportunistic diseases; anti-inflammatory drugs must not be used instead of such medical care.) These patients usually take one gram of aspirin (two 500 mg tablets) four times a day.

Continuous use of this high dose is likely to cause stomach ulcers, unless another drug is used to protect the stomach. Dr. Sonnabend uses misoprostol (brand name Cytotec). Another physician we spoke with preferred sucralfate (brand name Carafate) to protect the stomach; he was concerned that misoprostol would reduce stomach acidity so much that the antifungal Nizoral (used by some AIDS patients) would not work. Also, Cytotec is expensive. And it is an abortifaciant, so it cannot be used during pregnancy.

• While there is no scientific proof that aspirin can or cannot slow the progression of AIDS, it is clear that many patients feel much better while on the treatment.

• Enteric-coated aspirin—and also aspirin suppositories—are available, and they might be better than the tablets because they avoid direct irritation of the stomach. (They would not eliminate the need for a drug to protect the stomach, however, because high-dose aspirin can cause ulcers through systemic effects, even without direct contact with the stomach.)

For another view, we called James Campbell, M.D., in San Francisco. He was aware of the research interest in anti-inflammatory drugs as immune modulators, but added that they have been used most extensively to help patients feel better: to suppress fevers caused by MAI, for example, or to reduce diarrhea when it is unexplained. With large doses there can be toxicity to the kidney and to the stomach.

## Anecdotal Reports

We have heard four anecdotal reports relevant to aspirin as a component of AIDS or HIV treatment.

One person with AIDS had fever most of the time, and noticed that he felt dramatically better when using aspirin. His physician warned that he should stop, because of the danger of stomach ulcers. We lost touch with this person over a year ago, and do not know what treatment he used, or with what result.

Two other people had taken aspirin daily for years, for reasons unrelated to AIDS, and both had done unexpectedly well in remaining alive and healthy. One takes two aspirin tablets every night; we do not know what dose the other uses.

One physician with AIDS told us he tried anti-inflammatory drugs, without apparent value. He had used both NSAIDs and aspirin.

## Precautions

Continuous use of large doses of aspirin can be dangerous, and it is important to discuss the risks of this treatment possibility with one's physician.

Here is a partial list of some of the concerns which have come to our attention:

• Precautions against stomach ulcers were discussed above. In addition, aspirin should be taken with "food, milk, antacid, or large glass of water"[13] to reduce stomach irritation. Effervescent preparations may be helpful. Alcohol makes the stomach problems worse, and should be avoided by persons using long-term aspirin therapy.

• Aspirin delays blood clotting. Persons with hemophilia or other blood-clotting disorders, or who are taking medications which affect clotting, must get medical advice before using aspirin.

• One case of Reye's syndrome in an adult with AIDS who was using aspirin was recently reported[14]. This rare but serious disease is usually found in children, and aspirin is believed to increase the risk. The authors had not heard of any other case in an adult with AIDS.

• Large doses of vitamin C can cause aspirin to be excreted more slowly, increasing its concentration in the body.

• Aspirin can interact with other drugs.

For these and other reasons, persons should consult their physician before using large doses of aspirin.

## Suggestions for Trials

Community-based research organizations could easily conduct trials of aspirin in the treatment of AIDS or HIV, and could make an important contribution by doing so. Here are some of the trials that we think most need to be done. The goal is to obtain objective evidence relevant to the usefulness of aspirin in AIDS treatment.

• Can aspirin reduce HIV replication or activity? One way to find out would be a randomized trial with p24-positive volunteers assigned to take aspirin or not to take it. Volunteers could continue AZT and other medications they were using.

How long would this trial have to run, and how many patients would be necessary? To find out, an initial pilot study would watch changes in p24 levels in several patients treated with aspirin. This pilot data may already be available in existing medical records.

• Could aspirin have a role in early HIV treatment? Here most patients would be p24 negative, so p24 could not be used as a marker of viral activity.

One physician suggested that a good time to try aspirin might be at around 300 T-helper cells, when the first symptoms of HIV, such as inflammation in the mouth, were beginning to develop. He thought that large doses, such as used by persons with arthritis, would be necessary.

To test this theory, a study could look at T-helper counts, in patients with starting counts in a range of about 200 to 500. In this range, the T-cell count appears to be a sensitive indicator of whether a treatment is working. Different doses should be tried, to obtain information about dose-response. If a low dose can be helpful, it would be important to know that.

A pilot study could suggest how much of an effect to expect, and how long to wait for it. Again, this pilot data may already be available.

• What is the long-term effect of aspirin on health and survival? The problem here is to design a study which is feasible to carry out.

Nobody knows for sure that p24 and T-cell improvements necessarily predict improved long-range outcome. But to get statistical proof that a treatment affects "hard" clinical endpoints like death or disease progression requires a huge study with hundreds of patients, some randomly assigned to a control group. For aspirin, no such study will happen.

The alternative of "historical controls"—comparing treated patients with others who were not treated in the past—presents problems because of the changes in the epidemic. Treatments have changed, and the virus has changed. Patients are different, too; for example, those now becoming ill were often infected in the early 1980s, before safe-sex campaigns, so they are patients in whom the disease has progressed relatively slowly. But those who became ill in the early 1980s clearly had a more rapid progression, since the virus had not been prevalent until shortly before that time; perhaps they were more susceptible to it. With historical controls, such changes in the patient population might make a treatment look like it is working even if it is not.

One approach to this problem might be called a computer-model control; we believe it was first suggested by San Francisco AIDS activist Michelle Roland, who occasionally writes for *AIDS Treatment News*. A computer model would be prepared based on the best statistical data available about predictors of disease progression—the relative importance of T-helper count, other blood tests, clinical symptoms, use of treatments such as AZT and OI prophylaxis, information such as age, sex, and race, etc. Whenever epidemiologists, clinicians, or other experts find errors in the model, they could correct them, building cumulative improvements. When they found trends in how the epidemic was changing over time, they could have the computer mathematically project the known trends to the present time. Eventually the model would contain information from thousands of patients, organized with the ideas of dozens of leading experts.

Then when a clinical trial is designed, the model could substitute for a placebo control group. All the study volunteers could be treated; and from their baseline blood work and other information, the model could predict how many deaths, infections, or other outcomes would statistically be expected at any given time in the future, in the absence of any new treatment. (The methods for making such calculations are well known, as they are routinely used for actuarial purposes in the insurance industry.) The group receiving the new drug could then be compared with the prediction, to see if the drug was working. These trials would be much easier to organize than those which require a no-treatment comparison, since patients who would want the treatment anyway would enroll in the trial to receive consistent followup. This approach to trial design might be called "smart" (computerized) historical controls.

Ms. Roland is preparing a proposal for initial development of such a computer model. Anyone interested can write to her c/o *AIDS Treatment News*, P.O. Box 411256, San Francisco, CA 94141.

## Comment

Until more trials are conducted, it is not possible to be sure that aspirin can be helpful in treating AIDS or HIV. We are concerned that as a result of this article, many people will start taking aspirin. But we are also concerned that a promising treatment lead is being dropped by default, because of lack of commercial incentive.

People should be cautious, and tell their physicians about this or any treatment they plan to use. We also hope that community-based or other research organizations will organize trials to obtain definitive information on whether or not aspirin can help to slow the progression of AIDS or HIV. This treatment possibility, until now almost unknown in the AIDS community, deserves serious attention.

## Please Send Us Information

If you have any experience with aspirin and AIDS or HIV, either as a physician or as a patient, please let us know. Contact John S. James, *AIDS Treatment News*, P.O. Box 411256, San Francisco, CA 94141, 415/255-0588. We are especially interested in experience with long-term use, and/or with high doses.

## REFERENCES

1.  Reddy MM, Manvar D, Ahuja KK, Moriarty ML, Grieco MH. Augmentation of mitogen-induced proliferative responses by *in vitro* indomethacin in patients with acquired immune deficiency syndrome and AIDS-related complex. *International Journal of Immunopharmacology*. June 1985; volume 7 number 6, pages 917-921.

2.  Valone FH, Payan DG, Abrams DI, Dohlman JG, Goetzl EJ. Indomethacin enhances the proliferation of mitogen-stimulated T lymphocytes of homosexual males with persistent generalized lymphadenopathy. *Journal of Clinical Immunology*. September 1984; volume 4 number 5, pages 383-387.

3.  Braun DP, Harris JE. Abnormal monocyte function in patients with Kaposi's sarcoma. *Cancer*. April 15, 1986; volume 57 number 8, pages 1501-1506.

4.  Hofmann B, Fugger L, Ryder LP, and others. Immunological studies in acquired immunodeficiency syndrome: effects of TCGF and indomethacin on the *in vitro* lymphocyte response. *Cancer Detection and Prevention Supplement*. 1987; number 1, pages 619-626.

5.  Ramirez J, Alcami J, Arnaiz-Villena A, and others. Indomethacin in the relief of AIDS symptoms [letter]. *Lancet*. September 6, 1986; 2 (8506), page 570.

6.  Salinas Argenta R, Sans-Sabrafen J, Martin E, Zaragoza J. Indomethacin as symptomatic medication in patients with advanced HIV infection [letter]. (English translation of title.) *Med. Clin.* (Barcelona). April 2, 1988; volume 90 number 13, pages 556-557.

7.  Fernando-Cruz E, Fernandez A, Gutierrez C, Garcia Montes M, Rodriguez M, Zabay JM. Increased levels in plasma of Prostaglandin E2 (PGE2) could account for the abnormalities of cellular immune function in drug addicts with HIV infection [abstract]. III International Conference on AIDS, abstract number WP.120.

8.  Associated Press. Aspirin may be useful in battling cancer, AIDS, pregnancy problems. December 3, 1986.

9.  Seifter E, Rettura G, Levenson SM, Appleman M, Seifter J. Aspirin inhibits a murine viral infection. *Life Sci.* 1975; 16, page 629.

10. White RF. Acetylsalicylic acid (aspirin) induces resistance to tobacco mosaic virus in tobacco. *Virology*. 1979; 99, page 410.

11. Kotler DP, Reka S. Modulation of HIV production by rectal mucosa *in vitro* [abstract]. *Gastroenterology*. May 1990; volume 98 number 5 part 2, page A-457.

12. Hsia J, Simon GL, Higgins N, Goldstein AL, Hayden FG. Immune modulation by aspirin during experimental rhinovirus colds. *Bulletin of the New York Academy of Medicine*. January 1989; volume 65 number 1, pages 45-56.

13. *Nursing89 Drug Handbook*. Springhouse Corporation, Springhouse, Pennsylvania.

14. Jolliet P, Widmann JJ. Reye's syndrome in adult with AIDS [letter]. *Lancet*. June 16, 1990; volume 335 number 8703, page 1457.

# MAI, TOXOPLASMOSIS PROGRESS REPORTS

*by Denny Smith*

Infection with *Mycobacterium avium intracellulare* (MAI), also known as *M. avium* complex (MAC), is a frequent AIDS-defining diagnosis, and often these infections are disseminated throughout the body. Several interesting developments have recently been set in motion for improving the treatment of MAI. They are surveyed below, followed by highlights of MAI research presented at the Sixth International Conference on AIDS in June, and an announcement of a study of a new drug to treat infections of *Toxoplasma gondii*. (The last issue of *AIDS Treatment News*, #108, included a more complete report of treatment news for toxoplasmosis.)

Azithromycin, an antimicrobial drug which has been discussed for over two years as a potential treatment for toxoplasmosis, is now in a pilot study at Pacific Presbyterian Medical Center in San Francisco to treat MAI. Since this is a pilot study looking essentially for drug safety, only fifteen persons will be followed. Participants will receive 500 mg of an oral formulation daily. When safety is established, trials will begin at other sites around the U.S.

We spoke to the principle investigator of the study, Lowell Young, M.D., who is Chief of Infectious Disease at Pacific Presbyterian Medical Center and Director of the Center's Kuzell Institute, which will oversee the azithromycin trial. Dr. Lowell shared several thoughts with us about the future of research for MAI therapies.

Azithromycin has appeared promising for some time in laboratory studies for activity against MAI, *Toxoplasma*, and *Pneumocystis*. There may soon be a decision to begin human trials of the drug for toxoplasmosis. Another new compound, called clarithromycin, which was disappointing when applied to *Toxoplasma*, was shown to be as promising as azithromycin against MAI in French and German pilot studies. Dr. Young said that the main distinction so far is that azithromycin remains in the body longer than clarithromycin. He is eager for trials of both drugs to progress, but acknowledges the unlikelihood that either of them alone will be effective against MAI, since the history of mycobacterial therapies points to a reliance on combinations of treatments. Both of these drugs are available in some countries outside the U.S.

The Food and Drug Administration recently granted orphan drug status to TLC G-65, or Gentamicin Liposome Injection, manufactured by the Liposome Company. Gentamicin sulfate is already approved to treat certain bacterial infections, but like many antibiotics, it does not adequately reach the interior of human cells, where MAI resides. Liposomes naturally penetrate cell walls and so are sometimes used to encapsulate and deliver a given drug to intracellular targets. The use of liposomal preparations represents a welcome expansion of options to treat MAI and possibly other opportunistic infections as well. TLC-65 is nearing clinical trials, and interested physicians can call the manufacturer at 609/452-7060, and speak to Mr. Ed Silverman.

The Houston Clinical Research Network and St. Francis Hospital in San Francisco are among 16 trial sites nationwide now recruiting for studies of rifabutin (Ansamycin), an experimental drug, as a prophylactic measure for controlling latent MAI infections. (Clofazimine, an approved medication, is another agent under study for this purpose, given 50 mg daily.) The rifabutin trials are placebo-controlled. Interested persons in the Houston area can call 713/528-5554, and in San Francisco 415/775-4321, ext. 2512.

Other rifabutin trial sites are located in Arizona, the District of Columbia, California, Florida, Georgia, Maryland, Missouri, New Jersey, New York, Ohio, Pennsylvania, Texas, Virginia, and Wisconsin. Information on local trials can be obtained by calling the manufacturer, Adria Laboratories, at 614/764-8382.

The Treatment + Data Committee of ACT UP/New York has designed a survey for collecting data or opinions from physicians who have had experience treating MAI. Their successes or failures with various drugs could provide valuable information when the results are compiled and studied for trends. To obtain a copy of the survey, interested persons can call Garance France-Ruta at 212/532-0363, or mail a request to Garance, c/o the PWA Health Group, 31 W. 26th St., Fourth Floor, New York, NY, 10010. The analyzed results will be available to participating physicians.

*AIDS Treatment News* has received anecdotal reports from or about several people who experienced serious hearing loss due to inner ear nerve damage during treatment with amikacin, one of the drugs frequently used in MAI treatment regimens. "Ototoxicity," including balance difficulties as well as hearing loss, is already known to be a possible side effect of drugs called aminoglycosides, which include amikacin as well as gentamicin, mentioned above. We urge people diagnosed with MAI and their physicians to be cautious and aware of this potentially irreversible problem. (Dr. Young told us that the toxicity of amikacin should be well-known and that it is not usually a worry when using the drug for less than a month; he noted that the danger is heightened in older people. The question of whether the liposomal gentamicin will carry the same risks as the standard formulation has not yet been answered).

Note: AIDS-related hearing loss is not always caused by drugs. We have received two other reports of hearing loss, one caused by lymphoma and the other by candidiasis.

The abstracts published at the recent International Conference included a study from Chicago which reviewed the response to treatment in 20 patients diagnosed with disseminated MAI infections. The treatment used was a common combination of four oral drugs, administered indefinitely—clofazimine, rifampin, ethambutol, and ciprofloxacin— with an initial limited course of intravenous amikacin. The authors discerned a "favorable clinical/microbiological response" to this therapy in 19 of the 20 patients. Bacteremia in four was either controlled with the addition of amikacin or persisted in its absence. But three patients experienced severe ototoxicity after 60 days of amikacin (abstract Th.B.517).

Another of the abstracts presented at the Conference discussed the incidence of MAI from a review of the medical records of eleven pediatric patients at Children's Hospital of New Jersey. The authors concluded that diagnosis of atypical mycobacterial infections in children may be delayed for as much as a year and a half, and that symptoms to watch for are abdominal distress, persistent fever or failure to thrive (abstract #2060, Hoyt L and others).

The above items of information may be undramatic by themselves, but represent a net optimism for controlling MAI. Only a year ago, many doctors declined to treat this infection at all, on the assumption that no single drug was convincingly effective against it. Now AIDS-knowledgeable physicians are experimenting with various combinations of agents, and we expect that the ACT UP survey will be of real assistance to them.

566C80 is a new treatment possibility for toxoplasmic encephalitis, which is entering a pilot study for people who have already tried the standard therapy, pyrimethamine with sulfadiazine, but failed to respond or could not tolerate the side effects. Interested persons should contact Barbara Baird, R.N., at the National Institute of Allergy and Infectious Disease, 301/402-0980.

The progress of 566C80, azithromycin, and liposomal drugs into clinical trials is welcome and long-awaited. If these agents continue to look useful, we hope the journey from pilot studies to expanded access is timed to save lives in the very near future.

# Issue Number 110
# September 7, 1990

## GOOD NEWS ON DDI

A new report on the longest-running study of human use of ddI, at the U.S. National Cancer Institute, shows a very good survival rate in patients using doses of the drug which were well tolerated. A total of 58 patients were involved in the study, 22 with AIDS and 36 with related conditions; their median T-helper count when they started ddI was 47 (range 4 to 267). The survival rate after 21 months was 80 percent for patients with AIDS and 93 percent for those with symptomatic HIV infection who did not meet the definition of AIDS. (Many patients were on the study for less than 21 months, but survival to that time was estimated by the Kaplan-Meier statistical method, which is well accepted for this purpose.) The paper was published in *The Lancet*, September 1, 1990[1]; additional information from interviews with scientists involved in the study appeared in *The Wall Street Journal*, August 31, and in other newspapers through a United Press International story.

How does this survival compare with that of AZT or no treatment? The *Lancet* article cautions that this data may not be comparable with past experience because most patients were stable when they began the study, many received pneumocystis prophylaxis, and 10 were treated with AZT while their ddI was temporarily stopped. News stories reported that earlier studies with similar patients had found about a 50 percent survival at 21 months among those treated with AZT, and 25 percent survival with no treatment; but we do not know if those figures reflect pneumocystis prophylaxis.

Other highlights of the *Lancet* paper:

• Of the 13 patients who received long-term (median 17 months) treatment with well-tolerated doses of ddI (no more than 9.6 mg/kg per day), mean T-helper count started at 157 and increased by 50 percent (at the time of maximum increase, after nine months of treatment). T-helper cell and p24 antigen improvements continued for some

372

patients for up to 15 months, after which there were too few patients to draw firm conclusions.

- Patients with little or no prior treatment with AZT (no more than four months) showed much better T-helper improvements than those who had used AZT for much longer. But p24 antigen, a measure of viral activity, decreased substantially in both groups during ddI treatment. The article does not speculate on why the T-helper count increased less in patients who had had long-term use of AZT, but lead investigator Dr. Robert Yarchoan, interviewed in *The Wall Street Journal*, suggested that the reason may have been the effect of AZT on the bone marrow, which produces T-helper as well as other blood cells. (The AZT doses of these patients were not reported, but presumably they would have taken the "high" dose, 1200 mg, which was standard at that time, and which causes much more toxicity than the lower doses now in use.)

- Of five patients in the study who had dementia or other cognitive dysfunction, all had improved cognitive measurements after six to 12 weeks of ddI.

- Toxicities were severe at high doses of ddI, with most patients developing neuropathy, pancreatitis, or hepatitis within six months; no one died of drug effects in this study. But at doses of 3.2 to 9.6 mg/kg per day, only three of 35 patients developed any of these serious toxicities. Many patients had less severe side effects, such as insomnia, irritability, abdominal pains, and headache; we do not know what doses these patients used. To reduce pancreatitis, the most serious toxicity of ddI, the researchers now "measure serum amylase and triglyceride and temporarily stop ddI when the amylase rises to 1.5-2 times the upper limit of normal or when the triglyceride concentration rises above 7 g/l; ddI is then re-instituted when the levels approach normal."

## Comment

This small study does not prove that ddI is better than AZT, although the good survival rate for patients with AIDS or serious symptoms, and low T-helper counts when they began the study, suggests that it might be. The important question, however, is not whether ddI is better on the average, but whether it is better for some patients. It seems clear that the answer is yes, and that the drug should be approved as a treatment option.

## REFERENCES

1. Yarchoan R, Pluda JM, Thomas RV, and others. Long-term toxicity/activity profile of 2',3'-dideoxyinosine in AIDS or AIDS-related complex. *The Lancet*. September 1, 1990; volume 336, pages 526-529.

# TOWARD FASTER ANTIVIRAL DEVELOPMENT: "RAPID SCREENING" TRIALS PROPOSED

*by John S. James*

Last year AIDS treatment activists joined with government and academic statisticians in an ongoing working group for improving the design of clinical trials. This Statistical

Working Group, operating within the AIDS Clinical Trials Group of the U.S. National Institute of Allergy and Infectious Diseases, is developing a new kind of eight- to 15-week clinical trial to compare and prioritize new drugs which successfully complete phase I (early dosage and toxicity studies). The winners from the rapid screening process would then go immediately into larger trials designed to lead to drug approval.

Dozens of potential AIDS antivirals are now coming out of laboratories, and there is no way that all could get the full-scale clinical trials required to convince the FDA that the drugs are good enough for general use. Even if more money were available, there are not enough experienced scientists, research nurses, or patients meeting entry criteria, to run so many large trials. The proposed new system could quickly screen all the promising drugs, so that the truly important ones could quickly be moved into larger, definitive trials.

The importance of the Statistical Working Group is that the people needed to make the proposal work are part of the process, so most issues could be resolved immediately. At a key meeting on July 10, 1990, statistical experts from NIAID (the U.S. National Institute of Allergy and Infectious Diseases), made sure that ideas were scientifically acceptable. Sometimes they did not know what the FDA would think, but then they could ask Ellen Cooper, M.D., head of the antiviral division of the FDA, who was at the same meeting. And the AIDS activists there knew what was or was not likely to be acceptable to patients. Also at the meeting were statisticians from the U.S. National Cancer Institute, NIAID's statistical contractors from Harvard and the University of Minnesota, and at least two pharmaceutical companies involved in AIDS trials, Bristol-Myers Squibb and Hoffmann-La Roche.

Pharmaceutical companies seldom run clinical trials to compare drugs, because each company only develops its own, and at any given time seldom has more than one drug at the same stage of development for the same disease. The screening trials must be sponsored by a neutral party, for example a government agency or a community-based or academic research organization. Pharmaceutical companies must be consulted early, however, because they will be involved when their drugs are tested. There is concern that some companies may be reluctant to put their drugs to an early test.

The Statistical Working Group would not have succeeded without good ideas going in. The basic elements of the screening trials were already familiar to the scientific community, as a similar system has been used successfully in cancer research.

## How the Trials Will Work

### (1)  Outcome Measurements

For over a year, scientists have debated the use of viral or immunological "markers" to tell if a drug is working against HIV. At this time the scientific mainstream has not been willing to accept improvement in available markers, like T-cells or p24 antigen or antibody, as good enough proof of efficacy to lead to drug approval. As a result, trials take years instead of weeks, because in order to prove a treatment works, enough people must die or suffer disease progression to generate statistically significant numbers in favor of the treatment. (Note that even a perfect drug which cured instantly would also take a long time in this system, since the delay depends on what happens to the volunteers who are **not** treated.) Also recruitment is difficult when patients need to enter a long (e.g., two year) trial in which their treatment must be controlled by a protocol written in advance. Such trials can require long-term sacrifice of medical options which otherwise would have been chosen.

However, the anti-HIV drugs which have been tested and are believed to benefit patients—AZT, ddI, and ddC—all cause average T-helper cells to rise within a short time, usually eight weeks of starting the treatment. There is no reason to believe that these drugs themselves raise T-cells directly; instead they appear to be inhibiting HIV, allowing the immune system to recover. Therefore other drugs which inhibit HIV at least as well would also probably cause the T-cells to rise, within the same time frame. By using T-helper count not as definitive proof of efficacy but only as a preliminary indication, the Statistical Working Group sidestepped the currently-deadlocked debate on whether such markers are good enough for final, definitive trials.

## (2) Placebos

Brainstorming among clinical-trials experts at the July 10 meeting led to an idea for avoiding placebos in the screening trials without sacrificing their scientific power. The first suggestion was to test many drugs at the same time. Most proposed drugs will not work, so they will in effect be the placebo. As one scientist put it, if five drugs are being tested, then if there are one or two winners, these should stand out from the others (in T-helper improvement). And if by luck one of the drugs was a superwinner, that would be obvious, too.

The trials would be kept short, probably two or three months, to avoid exposing participants to ineffective drugs for long.

Alternatively, in some cases a placebo or no-treatment arm might be acceptable in these trials. Since many drugs would be tested, patients would have only a small chance, probably less than one in five, of receiving no treatment. And the trial would not last long. Persons who were not critically ill might be willing to risk entering a no-treatment arm for two or three months.

## (3) Blinding

An administrative problem with a trial comparing many drugs is the difficulty of making all the pills look the same, to maintain "blinding"—not let patients, physicians, or staff know who is getting what drug. But recent thinking among clinical-trials experts is de-emphasizing the importance of blinding for studies with objective outcome measures like T-helper counts.

What **is** important is randomization—assigning patients randomly among different arms in the trial. If volunteers choose which drug they will get instead of being randomly assigned, it would be impossible to be sure there were no hidden biases caused by certain groups of patients, with better or worse prognosis, choosing certain drugs. Without randomization it would be impossible to fully trust the result.

If trial designers can avoid blinding the rapid-screening trials—no decision has yet been made—it would greatly simplify trial administration, especially since these trials will be testing many drugs.

## (4)  How Many Patients?

Statisticians are still working out the details, but preliminary discussions suggested that trial size might be about 30 to 50 patients for each drug being tested.

## (5)  Efficiency: Rapid Screening Trial and Master Protocol

This system would not need to be limited to comparing any particular group of drugs. New drugs could be added at any time, provided there were enough volunteers. Drugs would be finishing at different times, as their respective study arms were filled and the volunteers completed the two- or three-month test.

Administration could be greatly streamlined by use of a master protocol—a concept which has been used in cancer research. The protocol for the trial is developed in advance, even before all the drugs to be tested are known. With each new study arm, only the drug and method of administration must change. Everything else—entry criteria, blood work, data collection forms, data analysis, etc.—stays the same.

Of course each new drug would have to be approved by the FDA, and by all IRBs (institutional review boards) involved. But it's much easier and faster to approve just one drug, under the master protocol, than an entire study design.

Another advantage of using a master protocol is that all the different drugs can be compared, because entry criteria, measurements made, etc. are the same. Because the epidemic changes over time, exact comparisons can only be made between two or more treatments when patients have been randomized among them at the same time. But even when some drugs become available later and are tested months or even a year or more after others, comparisons between them will be much better than comparisons between drugs tested in different, unrelated studies. To a large extent, each new drug tested could be compared with all previous ones in the same master protocol.

## Overall Picture

This drug-screening system would be testing several different drugs at any one time. Any volunteer who met the entry criteria would be randomized to one of the currently available drugs, and take it for a short time, probably about 12 weeks. About 30 to 50 patients would be given each drug.

Improved T-helper count would be the primary measure of efficacy, although other data would of course be collected and analyzed. The drugs would be compared to pick those few which stood out from the others. These would quickly go into larger, more conventional trials designed for fast-track drug approval. They might also be made available for early access, through a system like parallel track.

## Interviews with the Developers

We attended the July 10 meeting, but this article is based mainly on phone interviews with some of the people who have developed the screening-trial concept. There are different versions of the idea, however, and to simplify this presentation we combined them into the unified picture above.

**September 7, 1990**

So far only one article has been published on this rapid-trial idea—"New Screening Proposal Could Speed AIDS Drug Trials," by Sari Staver, *American Medical News* (published by the American Medical Association), August 10, 1990. Ms. Staver interviewed Daniel Hoth, M.D., director of the AIDS program at the National Institute of Allergy and Infectious Diseases, and Ellen Cooper, M.D., from the FDA, who was at the meeting. Both endorsed the idea. Dr. Hoth said it might be implemented in 12 to 18 months.

We spoke with Susan Ellenberg, Ph.D., Chief of the Biostatistics Research Branch of the Division of AIDS at NIAID. She is one of the organizers of the Statistical Working Group, and clarified several points about the rapid screening trial idea:

• It is still in the discussion phase, primarily among statisticians. Physicians and pharmaceutical companies still need to be convinced of its value.

• Testing four or five drugs at at time, in a short trial looking at virological or immunological markers for a preliminary screen, seems "a very sensible idea; clearly many people were interested." While some concerns were raised at the meeting, the general consensus was positive; no one said the idea could not work.

• The main concern is that some drugs may be valuable but not show benefits early. Pharmaceutical companies may be afraid that their products could be rejected too early. But any drug showing potential would be followed up; the screening trials are to help set priorities, not to kill drugs which have other evidence in their favor.

Another key person in the development of this rapid screening proposal is David Schoenfeld, Ph.D., a statistician at Harvard Medical School and Harvard School of Public Health, who has worked with a similar system in cancer research for several years. The cancer trials tested many drugs for melanoma, brain tumors, and other cancers. They used tumor size as the outcome measure, but Dr. Schoenfeld thinks that the T-helper count may be a more useful measure, potentially making the rapid screening trials even more successful in AIDS than they have been in cancer.

We asked Dr. Schoenfeld about the contributions of AIDS activists in the development of the screening-trials concept. He said that the activists had been "very important and helpful in the AIDS Clinical Trials Group. They have been in a sense the initiative" for ideas like the screening trials. And they bring to the statisticians knowledge of what patients are thinking, what their concerns are. Usually the statisticians who design trials do not have contact with patients; and yet if trials are not acceptable to potential volunteers, they will not be able to recruit, and cannot be run. The activists "keep things moving in the ACTG, reminding us this is a crisis. They are very knowledgeable about clinical trials, and have good ideas."

Dr. Schoenfeld explained that a key advantage of the rapid screening trials is to speed the development of really new therapies—that now there is no good vehicle for quickly testing them.

Another member of the Statistical Working Group saw in the rapid screening trials a rapprochement between the short-term needs of patients and the long-term needs of research. "They are short enough to ask questions without putting people in a bad situation. For example, in a 12-week trial patients could risk a sub-active dose. Trials using means such as response-surface methodology could show optimum doses for combination therapies." She noted that the United States is not doing well at this time in trial design, and that the "pre-trial trial" of the screening system will help us minimize the consequences. (Note: response-surface methodology, a technique developed in chemical engineering, is a way of designing studies to find the best doses of two drugs used in combination.)

Memos written by Bob Huff of the Treatment and Data Committee of ACT UP/New York, and other activists in the Statistical Working Group list some advantages and problems of the concept. "A screening trial could identify early activity in a high-quality study before phase II trials begin." It would "provide information to support prioritization decisions for phase II trials," "give the earlier definition of a drug's efficacy profile," and "provide much useful information to phase II trial designers." The system would also allow combination therapies to be tested as easily as single drugs. The single study would cost less than multiple small trials. The trials could easily find volunteers, both because of the short time commitment required, and because it would be easier to publicize one trial than many separate ones.

Limitations and problems include lack of long-term data, the possibility that entry and safety criteria unique to one drug might have to be applied to others to allow randomization, and the fact that "the trial only identifies 'winners' according to the criteria of the 'AZT model,' i.e., early T-cell count increases," meaning that a better drug that takes longer to be effective might be missed. There is also the question of whether drug companies will be willing "to go head to head with competitive drugs" and support the program.

Another issue (not mentioned in the above document) is whether there are enough promising new drugs that a screening system is even needed. Today some researchers are even saying that they do not know what drugs to test. There are many scientifically promising compounds; the problem is the great bottleneck in getting them through (or even into) the pre-clinical development required for the all-important IND (Investigational New Drug approval, the FDA's permission to test the drug in humans) and then through the early phase I human test. The new proposal for screening trials will not solve this problem, which must be handled separately (for example, by improving incentives for pharmaceutical companies by facilitating earlier marketing approval for critically important drugs). Screening trials cannot overcome all the bottlenecks in medical research, but they do address one of the major points of delay.

## What Happens Next?

Dr. Schoenfeld is now developing technical details of the proposal, and is preparing a paper for presentation to the next ACTG meeting in November. Notes from the July 10 meeting will also be available. Activists are circulating concept sheets among members of the Statistical Working Group for their comments.

Community-based research organizations and others should work with the rapid screening trial proposal; with more support, it may not take the predicted year or two to implement. Also, research groups which are too small to run the full system and test many drugs at once might still be able to borrow parts of it—for example, by testing one particularly important treatment against a no-treatment arm, using the same study design which the full screening proposal will use. Few people have known about the concept until now; we hope this article helps get the word out.

To contact the Statistical Working Group, which is developing the proposal, call Bob Huff, ACT UP/New York, 212/674-8381.

# FEDERAL PANEL SEEKS DRUG-APPROVAL REFORMS

Two years ago, then Vice-President George Bush asked the President's Cancer Panel to study the Federal role in new-drug development and approval of treatments for cancer and AIDS, and to suggest changes to speed research, improve patient access to new therapies, and facilitate their transfer to standard medical practice. The President's Cancer Panel appointed the National Committee to Review Current Procedures for Approval of Drugs for Cancer and AIDS—usually called the Lasagna Committee, after its chair, Louis Lasagna, M.D. The Lasagna Committee held ten hearings between January 1989 and April 1990; on August 15 it issued its final report, a 25-page document with 20 recommendations for improving the drug-approval process. Recommendations include:

• **Adopting "a national policy...to foster the development of new drugs for AIDS and cancer."** A permanent oversight committee, appointed by and reporting to the Secretary of Health and Human Services, would monitor the needs and performance of the FDA in drug regulation. (Note: the importance of this recommendation is that today there is no such national policy, and no one responsible when the system as a whole is not working. Each office just does its own job, even when it is clear that disaster will result.)

• **Severe staff and equipment shortage at the FDA** can be addressed not only by providing more resources, but also by allowing institutional review boards, and outside contractors approved by the FDA, to do some of the reviews now done by staff. The Committee recommended that phase I trials could optionally be approved by a qualified institutional review board (IRB) instead of by the FDA. Also, pharmaceutical companies could optionally pay the FDA to rapidly review an NDA (marketing) application by contracting the work to outside experts. These changes are necessary because "Congress has placed many new responsibilities on the FDA in the last decade, while the number of employees in the agency has decreased . . . In the short term no quick solution is apparent to these inadequate resources."

• **FDA advisory committees** should have a much larger role, with their own staffs, and responsibility for their own agendas.

• **Medicare, Medicaid, and private insurance should pay** for experimental drugs and unlabeled uses of approved drugs, and all associated medical care, "if the use has been approved by expert government agencies, in authoritative medical compendia, or by a committee established by the Secretary of Health and Human Services." Coverage should be the same under Medicare, Medicaid, and all private insurance, and should not vary between geographic areas. Individual insurance companies "should have no discretion with respect to such matters."

• **Earlier marketing approval for AIDS and cancer drugs** should occur as soon as there is credible evidence of efficacy, with other research being completed after approval. The Committee noted that the large phase III trials, which commonly take years, have little practical impact on approval, since 90 percent of drugs which pass phase II also pass phase III.

In addition, "It is only after initial NDA approval of the drug as a single entity that its full potential is realized, because physicians are then free to use it in combination with other drugs in accordance with their best clinical judgment. While still under investigation, such combination uses occur only infrequently and with little opportunity for full clinical exploration. For all of these reasons, large phase III studies have been, and should continue to be, conducted in the post-approval setting."

• Other recommendations include support for **community-based trials**, for **parallel track** if it does not delay trials, and for the FDA's responsiveness to **patient advocacy groups**. It urged improved relationships between **FDA and pharmaceutical-company personnel**, with more open communication.

To obtain a copy of the report, contact the Committee's executive secretary: Dr. Elliott H. Stonehill, National Cancer Institute, Bethesda, MD 20892, 301/496-1148.

## AZT AND LYMPHOMA

*by John S. James*

Non-Hodgkin's lymphoma, a cancer of certain blood cells, has been associated with AIDS since early in the epidemic; published reports go back to 1982, and one article reported 90 cases, in 1984[1]. More recently physicians have seen a major increase in the number of patients with AIDS and lymphoma (which has also increased in the general population, for unknown reasons). There is concern that as treatment for pneumocystis and other opportunistic infections improves, non-Hodgkin's lymphoma could become one of the major opportunistic diseases. Most physicians suspect that the main cause of the increase in AIDS-related lymphoma is that patients are living longer today, and therefore there is more time for the disease to develop. But there are also suspicions that AZT might be contributing to the increase.

In the August 15 issue of the *Annals of Internal Medicine*, researchers from the U.S. National Cancer Institute, and other branches of the National Institutes of Health, published a report on AZT therapy and incidence of non-Hodgkin's lymphoma[2]. While the figures on lymphoma are indeed alarming, we believe that a close look at the paper shows less reason to worry about AZT than first impressions might suggest.

## Results

To obtain long-term data on AZT, the researchers analyzed all patient records from three early trials of the drug at the National Cancer Institute; the patients are among the first to use AZT. A total of 55 patients were included. Eight of them (14.5 percent) had developed a high-grade non-Hodgkin's B-cell (or in one case, null-cell) lymphoma, after a median of two years of AZT treatment. However, statistical projections were that 28.6 percent (*of patients equally ill to begin with*) would develop lymphoma by 30 months of AZT treatment, and 46.4 percent by three years. These figures do not apply to people who start AZT earlier, and at lower doses, today.

Clearly these results imply that lymphoma will become an increasingly serious problem. But in evaluating the risk of lymphoma, and especially the question of whether AZT has any role in causing it, other facts also presented in the paper must be considered:

• These eight patients had advanced illness before they began treatment with AZT. All had AIDS or symptomatic HIV infection, and their median T-helper count when they started treatment was 26 (range 8-135). Their median T-helper count when they developed lymphoma was six. All eight had less than 50 T-helper cells for at least five months (median time 15.3 months with a count under 50) before they developed lymphoma.

The median T-helper count for all 55 patients when they started treatment was 74 (range 0-973), compared to the median of 26 for the eight who developed lymphoma— suggesting that those with higher T-helper counts did not develop lymphoma, although they also were taking AZT.

• These results must be considered in view of the fact that even before AIDS, and certainly before the use of AZT, it was well known that immune suppression due to other causes increased the risk of lymphoma. As of 1987, over 200 cases of non-Hodgkin's lymphoma were known among persons with hereditary immune deficiencies. In addition, patients using immune-suppressing drugs to control rejection after organ transplants have a high incidence of cancers, and 36 percent of those cancers were found to be non-Hodgkin's lymphomas. Immune suppression is known to cause lymphomas, without AIDS or AZT being involved.

• The lymphomas found in this study were the same kind as those generally found in AIDS, whether or not patients are taking AZT. This suggests that immune deficiency, not AZT, is more likely the cause of the lymphoma.

• If AZT did contribute to causing lymphoma, large doses would probably be more dangerous than smaller ones. All the patients in this study started AZT early, when the recommended dose was 1200 mg per day. Today most patients are using half that much or less.

At this time there seems to be a consensus among most physicians and scientists that while AZT cannot be ruled out as a cause of lymphoma, it is much more likely that the increase in this cancer is because patients with serious immune deficiency are living longer. The possibility that AZT could help cause the disease must be investigated. But meanwhile, experts are not recommending changes in treatment as a result of this study, and we have not heard of any physicians changing their practices because of it.

Note: for an overview of treatments for lymphoma, see "Lymphoma Treatments Update," below.

## REFERENCES

1. Ziegler JL, Beckstead JA, Volberding PA, and others. Non-Hodgkin's lymphoma in 90 homosexual men. Relation to generalized lymphadenopathy and the acquired immunodeficiency syndrome. *New England Journal of Medicine.* 1984; volume 311, pages 567-570.
2. Pluda JM, Yarchoan R, Jaffe ES, and others. Development of non-Hodgkin's lymphoma in a cohort of patients with severe human immunodeficiency virus (HIV) infection on long-term antiretroviral therapy. *Annals of Internal Medicine.* August 15, 1990; volume 113, number 4, pages 276-282.

# LYMPHOMA TREATMENTS UPDATE

*by Denny Smith*

Options for treating lymphoma have not increased much in number but have, like other AIDS-related therapies, grown in refinement. For background information on lymphoma, see *AIDS Treatment News* #93.

## Radiation and Chemotherapy

Radiation was one standard approach to lymphoma discussed at the Sixth International Conference on AIDS in June. A three-year chart review of 25 cases of non-Hodgkin's lymphoma of the central nervous system was described by researchers from New York's Montefiore Medical Center/Albert Einstein College of Medicine[1]. All patients received total cranial irradiation; few side effects were noted and twelve patients showed symptom improvement. Subsequently, opportunistic infections claimed more lives than the lymphomas.

Clinicians at the same institutions presented another chart review of 20 patients discussing various aspects of chemotherapy for lymphoma[2]. Although radiation or chemotherapy are often the most appropriate treatment choice and can achieve a complete tumor response in many people, they have a tendency to further impair the immune system by damaging the bone marrow's capacity to generate new blood cells. The authors of this abstract elaborated on the danger, suggesting that bone marrow toxicity from more than two cycles of chemotherapy may increase the chance of developing an opportunistic infection.

The authors also note that the risk for lymphomas appearing in the central nervous system, which is largely impervious to intravenous chemotherapy, warrants a chemotherapy prophylaxis, which is administered intrathecally (injected into the cerebrospinal fluid), to people under treatment for AIDS-related lymphoma.

We spoke to Lawrence Kaplan, M.D., and James Kahn, M.D., who supervise the lymphoma protocols at San Francisco General Hospital, and who discussed with us the current results from several lymphoma studies there.

Dr. Kahn described good responses from a chemotherapy regimen treating Hodgkin's disease: tumor regression, and little toxicity, was obtained from a combination of four chemotherapeutic agents—bleomycin, vincristine, streptozocin, and etoposide. Hodgkin's disease is much less common among AIDS-related cancers, however, than non-Hodgkin's lymphoma.

Another study at San Francisco General involved a new drug called chlorodeoxyadenosine (CDA), which was given to nine people who had failed standard chemotherapy for non-Hodgkin's lymphoma. Two partial responses were obtained from this agent; Dr. Kaplan surmised that CDA could be more useful in combination with other drugs.

## Controlling Toxicity: GM-CSF

Granulocyte Macrophage Colony Stimulating Factor (GM-CSF) is perhaps the best-known of many human growth factors now under investigation. GM-CSF is already widely considered to be useful for controlling the bone-marrow toxicity of such treatments as AZT, ganciclovir, and interferon. A trial at San Francisco General comparing lymphoma chemotherapy regimens with and without GM-CSF found that neutropenia, a common side-effect of chemotherapy, was reduced for those participants receiving GM-CSF[3]. This abstract reported an initial drop in p24 antigen levels for both groups in the study, probably because of cell killing by the chemotherapy drugs.

We interviewed Dr. Kaplan, who gave us later information not included in the abstract. The group receiving GM-CSF required fewer hospitalizations, due to the reduction in neutropenia. However, after falling in both groups, the p24 level later rose above baseline in the group receiving GM-CSF with chemotherapy, but not in the group treated with chemotherapy alone. Neither group was receiving AZT or other anti-HIV drugs. Dr. Kaplan cautioned that this is a laboratory observation, not a finding in a clinical care setting.

## Other Approaches

San Francisco General was also the site of a trial examining anti-idiotype antibody therapy, a relatively new technique to enhance a natural anti-tumor mechanism of the immune system. Dr. Kaplan said that because of the difficulty identifying tumors with shared idiotypes, this approach was largely unsuccessful. Other "immune-based" therapies are likely to be developed in the future for treating lymphoma. But for now, the practical question is whether chemotherapy is more effective and less toxic when given in low doses, or in large doses with GM-CSF used to control side-effects.

An important consideration during treatment for lymphoma, as with treatment for opportunistic infections, is the continuation of some anti-HIV therapy. But the combined toxicities of chemotherapeutic drugs and AZT or ddI can make this goal difficult to maintain. Dr. Kaplan suggests designing a treatment combination which avoids parallel toxicities, such as from vincristine and ddI.

## REFERENCES

1.  Goldstein J, Dickson D, Valentine E, Davis L. Radiation therapy of the central nervous system in AIDS related non-Hodgkin's Lymphoma. Sixth International Conference on AIDS, June 1990, abstract #2102.

2.  Sparano J, Goldstein J, Gucalp R, Davis L, Wiernik P. Patterns of failure and toxicity of chemotherapy in AIDS related non-Hodgkin's Lymphoma. Sixth International Conference on AIDS, June 1990, abstract #2092.

3.  Kaplan L, Kahn J, Crowe S, Volberding P, Grossberg H, McManus N, Mills J. A randomized trials of chemotherapy with or without recombinant granulocyte monocyte colony stimulating factor in HIV-associated non-Hodgkin's lymphoma. Sixth International Conference on AIDS, June 1990, abstract #S.B.510.

# FOSCARNET EXPANDED ACCESS ANNOUNCEMENT
*by Michelle Roland*

Astra Pharmaceuticals, the manufacturers of the anti-viral drug foscarnet (Foscavir), has instituted an "expanded access" program for specified patients with acyclovir resistant herpes and CMV infections including retinitis, colitis, hepatitis, encephalitis, and pneumonia. Physicians of patients who meet the criteria described in this announcement should call 1-800-388-4148 to discuss enrolling individual patients in this program. Astra requests that physicians have the patient's chart with them when they make the call.

Astra's expanded access program is basically an individual compassionate use protocol which requires that each patient's request for the drug be approved by both Astra and the FDA. According to Astra spokesperson Pat Williams, the application process should take one to three days to complete, at which time the drug will be Federal Expressed to the physician. It does require the physician's willingness to order lab tests, monitor the patient clinically, and complete necessary initial and on-going paperwork. It also requires three days of hospitalization to monitor allergic or other adverse reactions.

Like Bristol-Meyers' ddI expanded access program, Astra's program requires that patients requesting foscarnet not be eligible for any clinical trial with the drug, whether that trial is sponsored by Astra, the government ACTG (AIDS Clinical Trial Group) program, or any other sponsor. Patients and physicians should call 1-800-TRIALSA to determine if there are clinical trials for which the patient would be eligible within a reasonable geographical area.

## Eligibility Criteria for People with CMV

Three categories of patients with CMV retinitis may qualify for foscarnet through expanded access: 1) Patients who have been diagnosed with CMV retinitis who are ineligible for ganciclovir (also known as DHPG) therapy because of current and on-going myelosuppression (neutrophil count <500 cells/ml or platelet count <50,000/ml) or hypersensitivity to ganciclovir. Note that Ms. Williams indicated that there would be some flexibility in the required neutrophil count if the physician felt that failure could be documented with more than 500 cells/ml (up to 750 cells/ml) and that continued treatment with ganciclovir would be dangerous to the patient.

2) Patients on ganciclovir who are experiencing ganciclovir toxicity (neutrophil count <500 cells/ml or platelet count <50,000/ml or other dose-limiting toxicities considered on an individual basis) during either the induction or maintenance phase of treatment. Again, there will be some flexibility with the neutrophil count as described above.

3) Patients on ganciclovir therapy who are experiencing progression of their retinitis during induction or the first two weeks of maintenance therapy. Astra will require re-induction with ganciclovir in patients who are failing maintenance more than two weeks after their last induction phase. Ms. Williams stated that they want to ensure that ganciclovir failure has occurred before providing foscarnet to this group of patients.

Studies for which patients with CMV retinitis may be eligible include an Astra sponsored study in Houston for ganciclovir failure. All other studies with foscarnet at this time are comparative studies using ganciclovir in some patients and so should not interfere with eligibility for expanded access. (For more information call 1-800-TRIALSA about ACTG 129, and about a Phase I study at the National Eye Institute using laser therapy and ddI with foscarnet or ganciclovir.)

Patients with other manifestations of CMV infection, including colitis, pneumonia, hepatitis and encephalitis, who are not responding to or cannot tolerate ganciclovir may also qualify for this program. Ms. Williams encouraged the doctors of such patients to call Astra.

## Eligibility Criteria for Acyclovir Resistant Herpes

Patients must have experienced no improvement in their herpes lesions after at least ten days of intravenous acyclovir therapy at a dose of 10 mg/kg every eight hours. Alternatively, acyclovir resistance can be demonstrated by an *in vitro* resistance test.

Patients must not be eligible for (or able to get to) Astra's studies in Los Angeles or Houston on acyclovir resistant herpes.

## Additional Requirements for Women

All women must have a negative pregnancy test and agree to use contraception during treatment and for three months following treatment. The supply of foscarnet will be stopped if a female patient becomes pregnant. When asked about evidence of teratogenicity (harm to the fetus) with foscarnet, Ms. Williams stated that there is no evidence of danger in animal studies but that no human data exist about effects on the fetus. Note that this is the usual process in the U.S. with respect to testing drugs in women; i.e., the drug gets approved with either very little or no experience in women and the specific effects on women and fetuses are discovered in post-marketing studies or during clinical experience.

## Physician Responsibility

The physician must be willing to complete a case report form and regulatory paperwork. Ms. Williams estimated that the total time required for paperwork would be about 1 hour in the first week and 20 minutes weekly for the duration of the treatment. The physician must have hospital privileges; hospital review board approval is also required. The people at Astra are concerned about physicians lying about kidney problems in their patients in order to get them foscarnet since foscarnet's major side effect is on renal function. Ms. Williams suggested that if a physician is found to be lying about significant clinical or lab history, future applications by that physician may be denied.

## Costs

The drug is supplied at no cost and any "special studies" required by Astra will be paid for by them. However, the first three days of treatment must be administered in the hospital in order to monitor acute toxic or allergic reactions. All hospital associated costs must be paid for by insurance or the patient. In addition, routine lab work, also required by Astra, must be paid for by the insurance company or the patient. During the induction phase of treatment, this lab work is required approximately three times per week. It is required approximately every two weeks during maintenance therapy. In the case of CMV retinitis, routine monitoring includes eye exams. Photography is not required, but is requested by Astra for both retinitis and herpes.

# Issue Number 111
# September 21, 1990

## VITAMIN C: LABORATORY TESTS INDICATE ANTIVIRAL EFFECT

*by John S. James*

A series of laboratory tests at the Linus Pauling Institute of Science and Medicine in Palo Alto, California found that ascorbate (vitamin C) reduced the growth of HIV in cultured human lymphocytes, in concentrations not harmful to the cells. The experimental study, conducted by Steve Harakeh, Ph.D., and Raxit J. Jariwalla, Ph.D., appears in the September issue of the *Proceedings of the National Academy of Sciences, USA*; results were also presented September 11 at "Ascorbic Acid: Biological Functions and Relation to Cancer," an international symposium sponsored by the U.S. National Cancer Institute, and National Institute of Diabetes and Digestive and Kidney Diseases, in Bethesda, Maryland. The study is extensive and hard to summarize, but it showed a substantial reduction in measures of viral activity (p24, reverse transcriptase, and syncytia formation) without toxicity to cells at concentrations of 25 to 150 mcg/ml, with the higher concentrations working better.

How much vitamin C would be needed to reach these levels in blood serum? This study did not measure blood levels, but the published paper cited measurements by others. One researcher found an average blood level of 28.91 mcg/ml after oral use of 10 grams of vitamin C. Another found that intravenous infusion of 50 grams a day led to a peak plasma level of 796 mcg/ml.

## Comment

This research appears to have been carefully done; many measurements were made and the results all point in the same direction. We raised several questions, however, and gave Dr. Jariwalla a chance to respond.

One potential limitation is that this study used cultured cells and viruses, which have been bred in laboratories; recently scientists have learned that viruses and cells freshly obtained from patients can give different, and presumably more reliable, results in drug screening. In our interview, Dr. Jariwalla noted that at this time there is no evidence that strains differ in resistance to ascorbate—but that different strains have not yet been tested.

One question about the usefulness of vitamin C concerns the relatively narrow range between effective and toxic doses found in this study. Effectiveness began to be seen at 25 mcg/ml, but toxicity was found at 400 and above; half or more of the cells were killed by exposure to 400 mcg/ml or greater for four days. The therapeutic range is therefore fairly narrow; for some drugs, the corresponding ratio between effective and toxic doses is a thousand or more, compared to 16 (400 divided by 25) in this laboratory test of vitamin C.

Dr. Jariwalla said that "although this may be so, there is no evidence of ascorbate toxicity found in human beings when large doses have been taken. The only side effect of high doses of ascorbate is a mild laxative effect. There are no reliable reports of severe ascorbate toxicity, such as acidosis or kidney stones."

Several years ago there was much interest in high-dose vitamin C as an AIDS treatment. By the end of 1987 this interest had greatly diminished, although some people continue to use the treatment today. One reason we have been skeptical of vitamin C is that if the treatment had worked well, it seems unlikely that the community would have stopped using it.

Dr. Jariwalla said that interest in vitamin C as a potential AIDS treatment had diminished for several reasons. First, the emphasis shifted to AZT and other nucleoside analogs as antivirals. Second, no clinical trials of vitamin C and AIDS got off the ground. And third, no hard scientific evidence of the effect of ascorbate on the AIDS virus was available until now.

At least two clinical trials were proposed years ago by leading AIDS researchers, but no funding was available. The Linus Pauling Institute, which has long been interested in vitamin C, has heard "a number of reports . . . from AIDS patients who had taken high doses of vitamin C and had experienced a marked improvement in their condition" (quote from a press release accompanying the recently published article). It is possible that results today could be better than those of several years ago, when treatment was only used late in the illness. Today, treatments are started earlier; and AZT and other antivirals make possible combination therapies, which were not available during the time of great interest in vitamin C. The article suggests a rationale for such combinations.

We asked Dr. Jariwalla what the study suggested about an appropriate dose of vitamin C. He said other results indicate that at least 10 grams orally would be needed to obtain the minimum blood levels for antiviral effect. Higher doses can be obtained through intravenous infusion, to reach plasma levels in the range found most effective in the laboratory tests. He cautioned, however, that further clinical studies are required to establish the optimum method of administration for maintaining high levels of ascorbate in the blood.

(Note: large doses of vitamin C are usually taken as a powder, not as pills. We asked about the different forms of the vitamin which are available. The Linus Pauling Institute sent us an information sheet which said that "Vitamin C, from Bronson

Pharmaceuticals, La Canada, CA, is available in the form of ascorbic acid, sodium ascorbate, calcium ascorbate, or sodium ascorbate and ascorbic acid combination." The sodium or calcium ascorbate salts are used to reduce slight acidity in the urine due to ascorbic acid. Dr. Jariwalla said that for oral use of high doses, the mixture of sodium ascorbate and ascorbic acid should be used—or calcium ascorbate for persons on a sodium-restricted diet.)

We suggest that patients discuss vitamin C, or any treatment they are considering, with their physician. A nutritionist told us that some patients have sought treatment for diarrhea, not realizing that it was caused by taking too much vitamin C; until they told their physician that they were using the vitamin, the actual cause of the diarrhea was not suspected. Persons should also realize that suddenly stopping high doses of vitamin C can cause deficiency symptoms, as the body is used to the large amounts and temporarily unable to use the small amounts in the normal diet efficiently.

We also called Bonnie Broderick, R.D., M.P.H., who is HIV nutritionist for the early intervention project of the Santa Clara (California) Department of Public Health. She was concerned that large doses of vitamin C could interact with other nutrients, especially vitamin B12 and copper, possibly causing deficiency symptoms of those nutrients. She also referred us to a chart in *Nutrition Action Healthletter*, October 1987, which listed possible adverse effects of high doses of vitamin C; the chart is based on a book, *The Right Dose: How to Take Vitamins and Minerals Safely*, by Patricia Hausman, M.S., published by Rodale Press, Emmaus, Pennsylvania, 1987. Because of the possibility of adverse effects, she is not recommending high-dose vitamin C until clinical trials have shown an antiviral effect or other benefit in people.

We asked Dr. Jariwalla what he thought would be the next step in organizing studies. (Financing, of course, is a major requirement; the Linus Pauling Institute study was funded by private donations, and by the Japan Shipbuilding Industry Foundation; research grants will be sought for further studies.) Dr. Jariwalla replied that two main avenues are being explored. First, the Linus Pauling Institute is inviting researchers at hospitals, clinics, community-based organizations, etc., to start clinical studies. The Institute itself does not do clinical trials, but can collaborate with others who initiate them. And second, the Linus Pauling Institute has urged the National Institute of Allergy and Infectious Diseases to undertake clinical studies. Dr. Jariwalla said that "the new evidence provides a strong scientific basis to conduct clinical trials of vitamin C in AIDS."

## REFERENCES

1.　Harakeh S, Jariwalla RJ, and Pauling L. Suppression of human immunodeficiency virus replication by ascorbate in chronically and acutely infected cells. *Proceedings of the National Academy of Sciences, USA*. September 1990; volume 87, pages 7245-7249.

# CRYPTOSPORIDIOSIS: GUARDED PROGRESS
*by Denny Smith*

Some quiet developments may be breaking the miasma of research to find an effective treatment for *Cryptosporidium parvum* infection, which causes severe diarrhea. For background reports on various antibiotics and other approaches, see *AIDS Treatment News* #95 and #107. Following is additional information on some of the drugs discussed in those articles.

## Diclazuril, Related Developments

Diclazuril is a veterinary drug used to treat parasites in chickens, and over a year ago was found to help some some people with cryptosporidiosis. Contrary to what we implied in our previous articles, diclazuril is not marketed to U.S. veterinarians, although a number of people have acquired personal supplies from other countries.

A version redesigned by the manufacturer, Janssen Pharmaceutica, for human use was tested in recent clinical trials in New York. Rosemary Soave, M.D., reported the results thus far at the Sixth International Conference on AIDS in June. She tested daily doses from 200 mg to 600 mg, and saw the best responses at the higher doses.

Even though this infection is usually not a problem outside the gastrointestinal tract, Dr. Soave said that those people who experienced the best response to diclazuril also showed higher levels of the drug in their bloodstream. So Janssen is again reformulating diclazuril to improve absorbability. Trials of the improved compounds are planned, but details have not been released. Meanwhile, Janssen has applied to the Food and Drug Administration for permission to provide compassionate use access to diclazuril.

On a speculative note, a pharmacist told us that a close chemical relative of diclazuril, called toltrazuril, is also used for treating parasites in animals. Toltrazuril, a product of Bayer (under the trade name Baycox), is a broad-spectrum anti-protozoal used to treat sheep, poultry, and fish. Like diclazuril (trade name Clinicox), it is marketed in some Latin American countries for veterinary use. We were told that in animal studies, toltrazuril was as safe as diclazuril, and that it is formulated in a liquid more concentrated than the diclazuril powder mixed with poultry feed. However, we know of no human experience with toltrazuril nor of any laboratory data testing it against *Cryptosporidium*. A veterinarian friend of ours is looking further into toltrazuril, as well as other veterinary drugs which might be able to treat infections in humans.

## Humatin Success?

One of the studies of cryptosporidiosis presented at the Sixth International Conference was a hospital chart review of patients treated with the common anti-parasite drug paromomycin (brand name Humatin); the study found good results (see *AIDS Treatment News* #107). Surprised that an ordinary, available medicine was found useful after years of research into numerous possibilities, we contacted the author of the abstract, Joseph Gathe, M.D., at Park Plaza Hospital in Houston. Dr. Gathe said that he continues to see very good responses to paromomycin in about 90% of his patients with cryptosporidiosis. The improvements include a substantial decrease in the quantity and frequency of diarrhea, and often a decrease in stool counts of the parasite's cysts.

This drug is an intraluminal agent, which means it passes through the gastrointestinal tract with little absorption into the bloodstream. Dr. Gathe explained that this characteristic is an advantage for controlling toxicity (none was seen in his patients), but would make the drug useless for treating infections which have disseminated to other body systems. However, drug handbooks caution that if this drug should reach the bloodstream, such as through intestinal ulcers or blockage, it could lead to hearing loss or kidney toxicity or other side effects attributed to large or extended doses of aminoglycoside antibiotics.

We consulted three other physicians who have tried paromomycin in the past to treat cryptosporidiosis: two of them had not seen any response. One of the two pointed out that chart reviews can be unreliable methods of drawing conclusions about a treatment because they analyze data retrospectively, without control over variables which a prospective clinical study would eliminate or at least manage.

The third was Paula Sparti, M.D., a respected HIV physician in Miami. She has tried paromomycin with her patients diagnosed with cryptosporidiosis, sometimes without any results. But one of her patients responded dramatically within 36 hours after starting paromomycin, at 500 mg given four times daily. His profuse diarrhea completely cleared, and related abdominal pain subsided. Shortly after, a patient treated by an associate of Dr. Sparti's responded similarly to the drug.

Dr. Sparti's assessment is that some people, not all, may benefit from paromomycin. She feels that since it is available and safe, people with cryptosporidiosis should be offered a trial. If there is no improvement within 7 to 10 days, the drug can be discontinued.

It is possible that some of the differences in response to the drug may result from the difficulty in diagnosing intestinal infections. In the search for a cause of diarrhea or malabsorption, several organisms capable of causing illness might be identified in stool specimens. Other microbes may not be readily found in the specimens yet be present and causing problems in the intestinal tract. Given these uncertainties, the treatment for diarrhea and resulting weight loss can be hit and miss. If symptoms begin to clear up during the administration of a given drug, such as paromomycin, it might not always be possible to know which organism the drug acted upon, if any.

## Macrolide Antibiotics?

Two other drugs tried so far to treat this infection are spiramycin and clindamycin; there have been positive, but limited, results. Clindamycin is already approved to treat certain infections; spiramycin is an investigational macrolide antibiotic, available through compassionate use. A related drug called azithromycin, approved in Yugoslavia, has strong laboratory activity against another protozoal infection, toxoplasmosis. Human trials to test azithromycin against toxoplasmosis are long overdue. A pilot study testing the drug in MAI infections is already in progress. The manufacturer, Pfizer, Inc., is now working toward FDA approval as a treatment for certain respiratory infections and chlamydia. We have heard that some buyer's clubs are investigating how to increase access to azithromycin in this country.

Given azithromycin's broad potential, we wondered about trying it for cryptosporidial infections. We spoke to Shelley Gordon, M.D., an infectious disease specialist in San Francisco who usually tries clindamycin with primaquine to treat cryptosporidiosis, with some success. She noted that her patients with higher helper cells tend to have the best results. We asked her about the logic of trying azithromycin, and she agreed that it is worth considering. A spokesperson for Pfizer told us that they were not aware of any studies suggesting that azithromycin has activity against *Cryptosporidium.*

The safety and availability of paromomycin suggest that it is worth trying for cryptosporidiosis. Diclazuril and its future analogs appear promising, and speedy development could spare many people from resorting to veterinary versions. Azithromycin is a speculative possibility, but it warrants research attention. These drugs, like clindamycin, spiramycin and hyperimmune milk, may work for some people some of the time. Until one is proven consistently effective, we support aggressive experiments with the reasonable choices at hand.

# MANAGING YOUR DOCTOR

*by Michelle Roland*

## Introduction

Many patients find themselves dissatisfied with one or more aspects of their relationships with their health care providers. For some, the problem is the amount of time and attention they receive during office appointments or in-patient hospital visits; for other, philosophical differences in treatment approaches leave them feeling misunderstood or unsupported in their decision-making process. Still others find their symptoms undiagnosed and/or untreated for long periods of time.

In this article, we will present some suggestions about how to develop a constructive working relationship between patients and their physicians. In order to do this, we will attempt to explain how doctors are trained to think and how you, as a patient, can assist them in their thought process while having your questions answered to your satisfaction.

## What Kind of Patient Are You?

The first step in developing a good relationship with your doctor is to identify the role you wish to play in this relationship. The next step is to find a doctor who feels comfortable working with patients in this way. In order to find such a doctor, you must know what you are looking for.

Many people with HIV infection want to work as full partners with their doctors in managing their health. For such people, frank discussions of diagnostic and treatment possibilities are very important. Others would rather have the doctor do most of the thinking about what could be causing the symptoms and how to treat them without being included in this thought process. They would rather play a more passive role and accept the doctor's suggestions without a great deal of interaction.

This distinction is most often not quite as clear cut as it may sound. Many people fall somewhere in the middle, wanting to be included in the decision-making process, but not really wanting to know all of the details along the way. For these patients, brief explanations about what the doctor is looking for will suffice, followed with a more in-depth discussion of treatment options once a diagnosis has been made.

Determining which role you want to play does not mean that you need to be bound to that role irreversibly. There will be times when you want to know more or less than usual; the challenge will be in identifying those times and being able to communicate your needs to your doctor as they change. Most people, no matter how large a part they want to play in managing their health care, will at times find this role, and the information that comes with it, very scary and threatening. The emotional impact of such information should never be minimized, no matter how active you are in your health care.

## Finding the Right Doctor for You

In addition to determining how active you want to be in your health care relationship, you need to decide the general philosophical approach you think you will want to take in terms of treatments. Some people feel most comfortable following the standard of care in the medical community. At this time, that would include such suggestions as starting AZT when your T-helper cell count has fallen below 500 and prophylaxis for pneumocystis pneumonia if the count falls below 200. Most often, the standard of care includes FDA approved drugs or treatments for which there is much data supporting their safety and effectiveness.

Other people want to try new treatment approaches which have not yet been proven to be effective. Some recent examples of drugs which fall into this category include compound Q and oral alpha interferon. Some patients want to try new drugs in the context of a clinical trial; others prefer to use them with only their physicians' monitoring and advice. Finding a doctor who is already participating in clinical trials or who is willing to refer you to local trials will be important for patients who want to access potentially effective new treatments in this way. Finding a doctor who is willing to either provide you with largely untested compounds, or monitor you if you get them through another source, will be important if you want to try this approach. Not all doctors feel comfortable participating in the use of unproven drugs with their patients. It is a good idea to determine your doctor's willingness to monitor and support you in this area if you think you may want to try such a drug now or in the future.

Many people may want to add non-traditional (in the Western medical model) approaches like acupuncture, Chinese herbs, homeopathy, relaxation/visualization, vitamin therapy, etc. to their health care program. Finding a doctor who is supportive of your total health care approach is important in this case. If you want to use both unproven drugs and adjunctive therapies, you should find out how your doctor feels about each of these concepts.

Once you have determined the elements you are looking for in a doctor, you will have to talk about these issues with your current doctor or any new doctor you may be considering. You do have a right to have these conversations with your doctor. Realize, however, that your doctor may not be used to having this kind of discussion with his or her patients. Before launching into the details of the discussion, your doctor might be more open if you tell him or her that you want to talk about philosophy and style and arrange a time to have this discussion; this approach will allow the doctor to schedule the necessary time and prepare to switch gears from the purely medical issues with which she or he may be more comfortable to a frank discussion of partnership.

[Note that this article assumes that the patient has a high degree of privilege and accessibility to a variety of doctors from which to choose. The unfortunate reality is that in many of the public health and HMO systems, and in many geographical locations, the patient's ability to choose doctors is very limited. In such cases some of the later suggestions in this article may still be useful, although more difficult to implement.]

## Time

There almost never seems to be enough time in any health care setting, whether private, clinic, HMO (Health Maintenance Organization), or public hospital, although some of these settings are certainly worse than others. This problem will probably never be solved, but it may be helpful to think about a few of the reasons that time always seems unnecessarily limited.

In some settings, for example, many HMOs, the doctor essentially has no control over the length of each appointment. You will often find yourself waiting for long periods of time, and feeling very frustrated. Keep in mind, however, that you are most likely waiting because the doctor spent more than the allotted time with other patients. The doctor in this situation is constantly battling conflicting needs: the need to stay on schedule so you don't have to wait too long and the need to spend "extra" time with patients who need medical or emotional attention.

A simple solution may seem to be to schedule fewer patients each day. While it is certainly true that some physicians have large practices for financial reasons, more often the physician is again confronted with conflicting needs: to take patients who need a doctor (good HIV doctors are in high demand), to see patients on short notice (how often do you feel frustrated by having to wait days or weeks for an appointment?), and to schedule sufficient time with each patient. In this difficult equation, appointment time is often the loser.

In spite of this pessimistic assessment of time, some physicians and offices are better than others about staying on schedule and spending sufficient time with each patient for the patient to feel that his or her needs are being met. When possible, talking to other patients who see a particular doctor is probably the best way to determine how much of a problem scheduling will be.

A final comment on time: Often, a fair amount of time is spent thinking about each patient when the patient is not there. A responsible doctor reviews the chart before going in to see the patient, to refresh his or her memory about that patient's history, and then spends some time thinking about what the symptoms mean and how to approach them when they write the chart note after the patient leaves. This fact may not make you feel any better cared for when the doctor seems to be rushed and not giving you the attention you want and need, but it's good to keep it in mind when you are assessing the care you are receiving. Is the care good, even if you don't feel like you are getting enough time? If so, the doctor is probably doing a good job "behind your back." If not, you may need to talk to your doctor about the time issue and other reasons you may not be getting the care you need.

## How Do Doctors Think?

Doctors are trained to think in four main steps. Understanding this thought process can help you learn how to ask questions in a way that will help your doctor think better and provide you with answers to your questions. First, the doctor takes a *history*, or asks questions about your current complaint and pertinent aspects of your past medical history. At this time, the doctor tends not to examine you, but rather just to talk. This may seem a little awkward, as you may want to show the doctor what it is you are describing. He or she will probably ask you to show where your discomfort is, but will not focus on the physical exam until after asking you as many questions as he or she can think of. This may be an area where people feel cut short or ignored. The doctor is again working with conflicting needs: the need to listen to you and let you talk and the need to keep on schedule. You can help by trying to answer the doctor's questions completely but to the point, and the doctor can help by being attentive to you. Doctors are told all throughout their training that the majority of information they need to make a diagnosis will come from the history, so they should listen well.

You can also help in this area by reminding the doctor of important facts of which they may have lost track, like weight loss over an extended period of time, recent and past medication changes, adverse reactions to medications, visits to other doctors, recent lab tests or x-rays that have been ordered, etc.

Next, the doctor does a *physical exam* based on the information from the history. Again, this may seem awkward, because the doctor's thought process has shifted; he or she may not want to talk much while examining you. Some doctors will be able to put you more at ease during the physical by keeping up the conversation. Others may concentrate intently on the exam.

Once the doctor has collected the data from the history and physical, he or she makes an *assessment*, which should take the form of a *differential diagnosis*. This is the stage where he or she considers all the possible causes for your symptoms and physical signs found during the physical exam.

Finally, the doctor decides on a *plan* to determine which of the possible diagnoses is the correct one and how you should be treated.

You can play a crucial role in the last two stages: trying to figure out what is causing the problem and deciding how to treat the problem. This is the thinking that the doctor usually does in his or her own head, or while writing in your chart. If you want to be involved in the process, these are the kinds of questions you can ask: What are the possible diagnoses you are considering to explain my symptoms and physical findings? What makes you consider each of these possibilities? Is there anything else we should be considering? How will we figure out which of these possible diagnoses is the correct one? What tests should we run? How invasive is each test? How expensive? How accurate? Are there some tests we should run more than once (stool samples for ova and parasites, for example)? What are the risks and benefits of each test? In what order should we do these tests? What treatments should I consider at each stage: before we have a diagnosis and after we have it figured out?

The most important thing you can do to help your doctor think through the problem and to help you feel assured that you are getting the best possible care is to map out a plan with the doctor. What will you do first? If you cannot make a diagnosis after doing that, then what will you do? Then what? Then what? You can go through the same process with treatment possibilities once a diagnosis has been made. What are my treatment options? If I try this and it doesn't work, or the side effects are too bad, then what could I try? Then what? Are there any other medications I can take with the treatment that might make the side effects more tolerable? What side effects should I expect?

## Following Up

Chances are that you will still have questions when you leave the doctor's office or later as you think about all the information you have received. Write your questions and concerns down and bring them with you to your next appointment.

Working with an assertive patient can be threatening to even the most enlightened doctor. To soften the "threat," try to validate your doctor and to take his or her needs into consideration. Find something you like about what the doctor is doing before you jump into all your questions and concerns. Tell him or her that you'd like to talk about several issues and that you are aware there may not be time to cover all of them during this appointment. Ask how much time you do have, and if you can schedule another appointment soon to discuss the issues which are not highest priority. Make sure you know what your priorities are so you can have as many of your needs met as possible during each appointment.

Finally, ask yourself what questions you always seem to have after an appointment. What consistently frustrates you? Try to take those questions and frustrations and figure out how to talk to your doctor about them so that you can decide together how best to take care of all the parts of you.

## CARE ACT FUNDING THREATENED; LOBBYING HELP NEEDED

The Comprehensive AIDS Resource Emergency Act of 1990, passed by large majorities in Congress and recently signed into law by President Bush, provides $780 million in emergency impact aid to cities and states heavily affected by the epidemic. But while this bill *authorizes* the expenditure, the money must also be *appropriated* in a separate legislative process. On September 12, the Senate Appropriations Subcommittee of Labor, HHS and Education approved a budget plan funding only $110 million of the $780 million authorized—essentially continuing funding for AZT, but starting no new programs. Part of the remaining funds could be added next year.

The original bill, introduced by Senators Edward Kennedy (Democrat—Massachusetts) and Orrin Hatch (Republican—Utah), had included $275 million as disaster relief to 16 U.S. cities which have been especially hurt by the decade-long epidemic. In a statement addressing the cut, San Francisco Mayor Art Agnos said, "I understand that we are responding to the invasion of Kuwait by Iraq, but America is also facing its own invasion by a killer virus that is wiping out tens of thousands of lives. . . Today, nine years into the AIDS epidemic, we are still waiting for a meaningful response from Washington."

In addition to San Francisco, the cities slated for help were Atlanta, Boston, Chicago, Dallas, Ft. Lauderdale, Houston, Jersey City, Los Angeles, Miami, Newark, New York, Philadelphia, San Diego, San Juan, and Washington, D.C. As chair of the AIDS Task Force of the U.S. Conference of Mayors, Agnos sent telegrams to fellow mayors facing the loss, urging them to lobby for support of an amendment by Senator Brock Adams (Democrat—Washington) to restore full funding of the bill. An editorial in *The New York Times*, September 14, also called on the Senate Committee on Appropriations to reverse the decision.

Senator Adams likened the epidemic to other natural disasters, noting that tornadoes and earthquakes would never have to wait "another year" for a national response.

The funding could be restored by the full Committee on Appropriations, by the full Senate, or by the House/Senate conference which will occur later. No one knows when these votes will occur, because the schedule will depend on the the the current "budget summit" meeting between Congress and the White House.

The most important Senators are those on the Committee on Appropriations: Adams, Bumpers, Burdick, Byrd, Cochran, D'Amato, DeConcini, Domenici, Fowler, Garn, Gramm, Grassley, Harkin, Hatfield, Hollings, Inouye, Johnston, Kasten, Kerrey, Lautenberg, Leahy, McClure, Mikulski, Nickles, Reid, Rudman, Sasser, Specter, and Stevens. If you are a resident of any state represented by one of the above Senators, then your call to his or her office will be especially important.

Because the legislative picture keeps changing, you might want to call an expert AIDS organization to get current information. Any of the following could help: AIDS Action Council, 202/293-2886; Human Rights Campaign Fund, 202/628-4160; Mobilization Against AIDS, 415/863-4676; or National Minority AIDS Council, 202/544-1076.

## WOMEN DENIED AIDS BENEFITS: WASHINGTON, DC, PROTEST OCTOBER 2

The Women's Caucus of ACT UP/DC is planning a demonstration to be held on Tuesday, October 2, 1990 at the headquarters of the Social Security Administration in Washington, DC. The Social Security Administration is being targeted because of their reliance on the Centers for Disease Control's definition of AIDS, which prevents many women with HIV/AIDS from qualifying for Social Security Insurance. Because of the CDC's exclusive definition, 65% of women with HIV/AIDS are unable to qualify for benefits they need to help pay for food, shelter, transportation, or childcare.

The CDC's definition of "AIDS" is primarily based on the symptoms and infections seen in white gay men, and ignores the symptoms most often seen in women. Individuals who do not show CDC-defined symptoms are denied access to Medicaid, Medicare, and SSA benefits, since those are necessary to establish disability and qualify for federal money. Consequently, women with HIV/AIDS die before they receive any benefits. AIDS is a leading cause of death for women in New Jersey and New York City, and infection rates are rapidly increasing.

ACT UP plans to take action that will dramatize the government's ineffectual response to the needs of women with HIV/AIDS. The demonstration will take place at the Health & Human Services building at the corner of Independence and 3rd Streets SW at 12 noon on October 2, 1990. For more information, call ACT UP/DC at 202/728-7530.

## NATIONAL HEALTH CARE DAY, OCTOBER 3

*by John S. James*

At least 87 million people in the United States have either inadequate health insurance or none at all. Those people who can qualify for insurance have watched their premiums skyrocket during recent years, and many are frequently denied reimbursement for experimental, potentially life-saving treatments. Many others can neither qualify for nor afford private insurance, and their numbers have long outgrown the Reagan/Bush allotment for public resources.

To exacerbate this situation, millions of dollars a day are now drifting toward a war buildup and away from essential domestic needs, particularly health care programs. On September 12 a $780 million AIDS emergency spending act was slashed to $110 million by a Senate subcommittee, critically jeopardizing an already tardy federal response to AIDS (see announcement above, on CARE bill funding).

AIDS has become the rawest example of a larger, chronic disaster in U.S. health care. Millions of Americans must routinely wait "another year" to receive proper treatment. Jobs with Justice, a national coalition of labor unions and community organizations, is organizing a day of actions for Wednesday, October 3, to spotlight the general crisis of quality, access, and cost of the U.S. health care system, and to demand an equitable, comprehensive, national system of health care for all.

Sponsors of "Health Care Action Day" include the Communications Workers of America (CWA), Service Employees International Union (SEIU), and the International Association of Machinists (IAM). So far the cities planning for activities include Atlanta, Birmingham, Boston, Chicago, Columbus, Denver, Los Angeles, Miami, Nashville, Canterbury (New Hampshire), New York, Oklahoma City, Philadelphia, Pittsburgh, Providence, San Diego, San Francisco and Seattle. Unions will also hold noontime informational picket lines at their worksites. To contact Jobs With Justice, call 202/728-2395, or 800/4242-USA.

ACT UP/Boston has issued a call for ACT UP chapters around the country to participate in this effort with local actions: "ACT UP/Boston urges all groups to seize this opportunity to work with other groups that will be active on this day, and fight back against those who are responsible for the state of our healthcare system." They can be reached at 617/49-ACTUP.

# Issue Number 112
# October 5, 1990

## DDI AND DDC: THE CALL FOR EARLY APPROVAL

### by John S. James

On August 16, Martin Delaney of Project Inform wrote to physicians at the Antiviral Drugs Division of the U.S. Food and Drug Administration, to let the Agency know that in the coming months, many activists would be asking that two experimental AIDS treatments, ddI and ddC, be approved soon based on the data now available, without waiting two years or more for long-term trials currently under way to be completed. Interest in rapid approval of these drugs has developed surprisingly quickly; in San Francisco, for example, ACT UP/Golden Gate is planning a major demonstration for October 9 (see announcement, below).

The idea of approving ddI and ddC now did not begin with activists, however, but among leading physicians and researchers familiar with the drugs. For months, a consensus has been building among the researchers that both drugs would ultimately be approved anyway; why not, then, consider approving them now? What is new is that activists are taking this idea, which might otherwise have remained as conversation at scientific meetings, and placing it on the national agenda.

The issue of ddI and ddC is vitally important because there are tens of thousands of people unable to use AZT, or no longer able to benefit from it. In addition, among gay men, most HIV infections occurred between 1979 and 1985[1], before the cause of AIDS and ways to prevent transmission were widely known; since the median time from infection to AIDS is about 10 years, many people will become ill over the next several years. More treatment options, including early treatment, are essential.

How good are ddI and ddC? The important data generated by the ongoing large-scale controlled trials has not yet been compiled and analyzed, let alone published; therefore, the physicians, scientists, and other professionals involved in the trials are reluctant to make public statements. But informal conversations with those involved suggest a widespread consensus that both drugs will be approved because they do have

**398**

a role in AIDS/HIV treatment, especially in combination with AZT and/or for patients who cannot successfully use AZT alone. (For results of earlier human studies of ddI, see recent article by Yarchoan and others[2]; also see papers published by *Reviews of Infectious Diseases*, July-August 1990[3,4,5,6,7]; for background on human trials of ddC, see papers from a February 3, 1990 San Francisco symposium, published in May by *The American Journal of Medicine*[8,9,10,11,12,13,14,15,16]). The available evidence is not conclusive, but it is consistently positive.

Neither drug is risk free. Both can cause peripheral neuropathy, and must be administered carefully to avoid or control this side effect. In addition, ddI can cause pancreatitis, which in a few cases has been fatal; blood tests are necessary so that if this condition starts to develop, the drug can be stopped or have its dose reduced before it causes illness. ddC does not cause pancreatitis.

The new data, currently being accumulated in formal trials and in the large ddI expanded-access program, seems unlikely to change the current belief that these drugs can be beneficial to many patients, and that side effects are manageable. The new data will be analyzed before drug approval is given. Activists are not seeking instant approval of ddI and ddC, but rather approval in the near future, hopefully before the end of 1990. In the three months until then, the data could be analyzed, if an adequate effort is made.

No one wants unconditional approval regardless of the data—and presumably no one would deny approval regardless of the data, either. Therefore, the real issue is not whether these drugs should be approved, yes or no. The real issue is how to make the decision—how to evaluate all existing information to best respond to a public-health emergency.

## The Traditional Way to Decide

Protocols for the major ddI and ddC studies, like most clinical trials today, have provision for early termination of the trial if early results show definitively that one treatment arm is worse than others. A "data safety monitoring board" (DSMB) meets privately at pre-set intervals and unblinds the study, so that patients will not be continued on a treatment which is clearly worse. Usually, of course, the DSMB decides to continue the study. And in that case it seldom says anything publicly about what results were found, so as not to bias the trial, for example by causing patients on a treatment arm which seemed inferior to drop out. Because of this secrecy, the public cannot monitor what is happening within the DSMB, and must accept its work on faith.

We do not know what criteria the DSMB will use to decide whether or not to terminate the ongoing ddI and ddC studies. But there are several reasons to be seriously concerned that the business-as-usual approach, which is to make this decision according to criteria spelled out long ago, when the protocols were first designed, could lead to the wrong decision. And the decision will be vitally important, because if the trials are not terminated early, they could last for two years or more *after* enrollment problems are overcome—meaning that neither drug will be approved for a long time.

The first potential problem is that when these trials were designed, immunological and virological markers (T-helper counts, p24 antigen) were less accepted by researchers than they are today. Therefore the trials were designed statistically to compare two or more arms based on rates of death or major disease progression. That is why these studies require hundreds of volunteers and are likely to last two years. AIDS progresses slowly, so it takes a long time to accumulate enough deaths and major opportunistic infections for statistically definitive comparisons to be made—no matter how good the drug being tested may be. If the DSMB for each trial evaluates the interim data based on the original protocol, instead of today's knowledge, it is likely that neither study will be stopped, and we will have to wait out the two years for these drugs.

Another concern is that, for statistical reasons, the criteria for early termination for clinical trials are extremely conservative. The statistical methods in common use require that if you take an early look at a study's data, and *might* have stopped the trial but in fact do nothing, then at the end of the study, your claims for the drug must be weaker than they otherwise could have been. Although this is difficult even for researchers to understand, the unbelievable result is that just looking at the data could cause a drug which otherwise would have been declared effective to be declared unproven instead. (The reason for this is that the overall procedure of the trial must be designed to control the probability of erroneously accepting a worthless drug, and the early look does add to the probability of such an error. Therefore, the final criterion for ruling the drug effective at the end of the study must be tightened, in order to keep the overall probability of error within the limit claimed by the trial's designers.)

The problem is that to minimize this effect, to minimize the possibility of having to reject a drug which otherwise would have been accepted, trial designers require extremely severe standards for early termination of a trial, making such termination unlikely. A drug must do much better to cause a trial to end early, than to be considered proven effective if the trial had been scheduled to end at that point.

Another fundamental problem is that the largest trials being conducted now are testing ddI and ddC individually. But today it is becoming increasingly clear that the best way to use these drugs is in combination, such as ddC with AZT. Large studies can take so long to get into operation that they become obsolete even before they begin.

## Another Approach: Lasagna Committee Standards

On August 15, the National Committee To Review Current Procedures For Approval Of New Drugs For Cancer And AIDS (commonly known as the Lasagna Committee, after its chairman, Louis Lasagna, M.D.) issued its final report (see "Federal Panel Seeks Drug-Approval Reforms," *AIDS Treatment News* #110). The Lasagna Committee had been asked by then Vice-President George Bush to recommend better ways to study and approve drugs for life-threatening conditions, to make them available more rapidly to patients who need them. The Committee's recommendations are based on ten hearings held between January 1989 and April 1990.

Of the Committee's 20 recommendations, the one most relevant to ddI and ddC approval is number four, "The FDA Standard for Effectiveness of New Drugs." Because of its importance, we reproduce the entire recommendation here:

"Because of its special relevance to issues faced today in developing new drugs for cancer and AIDS, the FDA needs to pay particular attention to the congressional intent in requiring substantial evidence of effectiveness prior to approval of a new drug application (NDA), as described in the Senate Report on the Drug Amendments of 1962:

> " 'The term "substantial evidence" is used to require that therapeutic claims for new drugs be supported by reliable pharmacological and clinical studies. When a drug has been adequately tested by qualified experts and has been found to have the effect claimed for it, this claim should be permitted even though there may be preponderant evidence to the contrary based upon equally reliable studies. There may also be a situation in which a new drug has been studied and its effectiveness established only to the satisfaction of a few investigators qualified to use it. There may be many physicians who would deny the effectiveness simply on the basis of a disbelief growing out of their past experience with other drugs or with the diseases involved. Again, the studies may show that the drug will help a substantial percentage of the patients in a given disease condition but will not be effective in other cases. What the committee intends is to permit the claim for this new drug to be made to the medical profession with a proper explanation of the basis on which it rests. In such a delicate area of medicine, the committee wants to make sure that safe new drugs become available for use by the medical profession so long as they are supported as to effectiveness by a responsible body of opinion and scientific fact.'

"By applying these principles, patients suffering from AIDS and cancer will have available to them new drugs for the treatment of their disease at the earliest stage at which there is responsible scientific evidence to justify marketing.

"The committee recognizes that, by making new drugs available for marketing at this early stage, when there is substantial evidence but not yet definitive evidence of effectiveness, there is an attendant greater risk of serious adverse reactions that have not yet been discovered. Cancer and AIDS patients have made it clear to the committee, however, that in light of the seriousness of the diseases involved, they are willing to accept this greater risk. Earlier approval of new drugs will mean that the patient will bear greater responsibility, along with the physician, for understanding and accepting the risks involved."

It may seem unreasonable to urge that new drugs for life-threatening conditions like cancer and AIDS be approved when "reliable pharmacological and clinical studies" conclude that they work, but "preponderant evidence to the contrary based upon equally reliable studies" concludes that they do not. Why should it be national policy to approve a drug when there is such uncertainty?

Other parts of the Lasagna Report provide background for this recommendation. For example, from a section discussing cancer drugs but which also applied to AIDS, "It is only after initial NDA approval of the drug as a single entity that its full potential is realized, because physicians are then free to use it in combination with other drugs in accordance with their best clinical judgment. While still under investigation, such combination uses occur only infrequently and with little opportunity for full clinical exploration."

Before the current law on drug approval was passed in 1962 (the law to which the long quote above applied), drugs only had to be proven safe before they could be sold in the United States; they did not have to be proven effective. Although some analysts have estimated that we would be better off with that system than with the present one (claiming that earlier and less costly access to good drugs would more than balance the harm caused by the useless ones), very few people want to go back to the old system of not requiring efficacy proof, and politically there is no chance of that happening.

But in recent years, proof of efficacy may have been taken too far—to the extreme of requiring academically satisfying proof, unrelated to real-world concerns such as balancing cost vs. benefit, or the feasibility of actually carrying out some of the trials which are called for. The result is a price tag of over $200,000,000 for each new drug approved—money the public pays one way or another in drug prices. The more serious price is paid in lives of patients denied new drugs when no satisfactory alternative treatments are available.

The Lasagna Committee has issued an authoritative call for a more balanced and workable approach to developing treatments for life-threatening conditions. "When there is substantial evidence but not yet definitive evidence of effectiveness," critically important drugs should be approved for prescription use, with physicians properly informed of the state of the evidence.

The academic elegance theoretically available from rigidly controlled trials has led to an assumption that all new knowledge about drugs comes from formal trials, and that physicians merely apply that knowledge to patients. In fact, medical progress rests on two legs—scientific studies and also clinical experience—and they must work together for best results.

(Note: the Congressional intent and Lasagna Committee recommendation that a drug can be approved even when there is "preponderant evidence" against it does not describe ddI or ddC. The data on both of these drugs, while not conclusive, is overwhelmingly favorable; see references, below.)

## Early Approval and Clinical Trials

One argument *against* early approval of ddI and ddC—we think it is the strongest argument—is that early approval would probably result in the ending of the ongoing large-scale controlled trials. As a condition for approval, the manufacturers would, of course, be required to continue doing studies; the FDA is already moving in the direction recommended by the Lasagna Committee of approving critically important drugs at the earliest possible time, with more of the efficacy research being moved into the period after the drug is available by prescription. But usually such early approval is granted after phase II studies have finished—either at the end of their scheduled time, often about two years, or in extreme cases by early termination according to the very conservative pre-defined criteria applied by the DSMB, as discussed above. For ddI and ddC, however, activists want the existing data to be evaluated now, without waiting for the ongoing phase II trials to finish; the drugs would be approved if there is substantial evidence of their value.

Theoretically it would be possible to continue the existing large-scale phase II trials of both drugs, even after approval. But in practice, with ddI and ddC approved and with the growing belief that combination therapy with AZT is usually best, many patients, especially those not doing well in the trials, would leave them to choose other treatment options. Therefore, the existing large-scale controlled trials probably could not be completed.

A similar issue arose when AZT was approved; the long-term phase II trial was terminated early by the DSMB. At that time, there were 17 deaths in the placebo group compared to only one in the AZT group, a difference so great that it did meet the very conservative statistical criteria for ending the study early. But today, in retrospect, it seems clear that AZT is not that good; the extreme difference in the death rates must have resulted partly by chance. No one knows why so many patients in the placebo group had died at that time. Some researchers have since argued that they wished the study had been continued longer, so that we could have had more conclusive proof of efficacy, especially regarding long-term use. It has even been suggested that the early end of the AZT trial was a tragedy, since we will never have the data which it could have provided.

But the benefits of early approval of AZT far outweighed the costs. The benefits included not only getting AZT to the study volunteers in the placebo group, but also making the drug available to thousands of others not in the trials. The approval also opened up the field of combination studies, as the FDA almost never approves trials using more than one experimental drug at the same time. And the success of AZT greatly advanced all of AIDS research, by ending the earlier fatalism: the idea that no drug could possibly work to treat AIDS.

And today much more is known about ddI and ddC, especially about dose, side effects, and long-term human use, than was known about AZT when that drug was approved. But perhaps the most significant difference between the current situation and that of AZT is that if the analysis of all existing data (which activists are now calling for) confirms that combination therapies such as AZT and ddC are often better than any of the drugs alone—and we believe it is almost certain that this result will be confirmed—then it will mean that the ongoing large-scale controlled trials studying these drugs alone are fundamentally obsolete, since the treatment they are testing would be known to be less than the best. If the benefits of combination treatment are confirmed, then will it be worth sacrificing the interests not only of hundreds of volunteers in the ongoing trials, but of tens of thousands of others for whom existing treatments are unsatisfactory, to get more data on ddI and ddC as single-drug therapies which will never be widely used?

## Early Approval and Industry Incentives

Another argument against early approval of ddI and ddC is that approval is not necessary to provide access, which can be done through the proposed "parallel track" system, or a similar expanded access mechanism, to allow drugs to be used while the controlled clinical trials proceed. Parallel track and comparable approaches certainly need to be explored. Some people suspect, however, that early approval of drugs for prescription use, while research continues in post-marketing studies, may work better than expanded access systems such as parallel track, for the following reasons:

• We are in an emergency, and expanded-access systems will take time to work out, including the all-important physician education component. Consider how long it is taking to develop parallel track, since that concept was first proposed. But when drugs are approved for prescription use, the necessary systems are already in place.

• Expanded-access systems may not have the flexibility that physicians and patients want—for example, to allow use of drugs in combination.

• Paperwork and other difficulties often limit such programs to private physicians, raising equity issues because the treatments are not available to those who receive their medical care in public clinics.

• Expanded-access programs like parallel track will not happen unless the pharmaceutical companies which own the drugs are willing to participate. But the companies may not have enough incentive to put their products on parallel track. They cannot be allowed to earn money on a program to distribute drugs before marketing approval (since if they could, the program would become tantamount to marketing approval, and would have no reason for separate existence). Even recovering their costs from parallel-track distribution is not feasible, as pharmaceutical companies are unwilling to reveal what their costs are. And if companies are pressured to participate, then they have incentives to create restrictions which keep the programs small. Parallel track might turn out to be a good idea, except for one problem—that it seldom gets used in practice.

What *does* provide incentive to pharmaceutical companies? One expert on clinical trials described the companies' approach toward the FDA as, "Tell us what we must do, and that if we do it we will get the NDA," (New Drug Application approval, meaning permission to market the drug). The only incentive that counts for pharmaceutical companies is getting their drug approved. (And incidentally, bureaucratic dynamics may favor approval of unimportant drugs which break no new ground over major innovations.)

Therefore, a policy of the earliest possible approval of critically important drugs for life-threatening conditions such as AIDS and cancer—the policy recommended by the Lasagna Committee—has a hidden future benefit, in addition to the present benefit of making existing drugs available earlier to patients. It creates incentive which extends throughout the drug development process, all the way back to the earliest theoretical and laboratory studies, for companies to bring their most important drugs forward, to focus their research resources on critical, life-saving drugs, instead of pursuing the me-too products for existing markets, which consume so much effort today.

## REFERENCES

1. Hessol NA, O'Malley P, Lifson A, and others. Incidence and prevalence of HIV infection among homosexual and bisexual men, 1978-1988 [abstract #M.A.O.27]. Fifth International Conference on AIDS, Montreal, June 4-9, 1989.

2. Yarchoan R, Pluda JM, Thomas RV, and others. Long-term toxicity/activity profile of 2',3'-dideoxyinosine in AIDS or AIDS-related complex. *The Lancet*. September 1, 1990; volume 336, pages 526-529.

3. Rosencweig M, McLaren C, Beltangady M, and others. Overview of phase I trials of 2',3'-dideoxyinosine (ddI) conducted on adult patients. *Reviews of Infectious Diseases*. July-August 1990; volume 12, supplement 5, pages S570-S575.

4.  Cooley TP, Kunches LM, Sanders CA, and others. Treatment of AIDS and AIDS-related complex with 2',3'-dideoxyinosine given once daily. *Reviews of Infectious Diseases*. July-August 1990; volume 12, supplement 5, pages S552-S560.

5.  Dolin R, Lambert JS, Morse GD, and others. 2',3'-Dideoxyinosine in patients with AIDS or AIDS-related complex. *Reviews of Infectious Diseases*. July-August 1990; volume 12, supplement 5, pages S540-S551.

6.  Valentine FT, Seidlin M, Hochster H, and Laverty M. Phase I study of 2',3'-dideoxyinosine: Experience with 19 patients at New York University Medical Center. *Reviews of Infectious Diseases*. July-August 1990; volume 12, supplement 5, pages S534-S539.

7.  Richman DD. Zidovudine resistance of human immunodeficiency virus. *Reviews of Infectious Diseases*. July-August 1990; volume 12, supplement 5, pages S507-S510.

8.  Broder S and Yarchoan R. Dideoxycytidine: current clinical experience and future prospects—A summary. *The American Journal of Medicine*. May 21, 1990; volume 88, supplement 5B, pages 5B-31S to 5B-33S.

9.  Meng TC, Fischl MA, and Richman DD. AIDS Clinical Trials Group: Phase I/II study of combination 2'-3'-dideoxycytidine and zidovudine in patients with acquired immunodeficiency syndrome (AIDS) and advanced AIDS-related complex. *The American Journal of Medicine*. May 21, 1990; volume 88, supplement 5B, pages 5B-27S to 5B-30S.

10. Bozzette SA and Richman DD. Salvage therapy for zidovudine-intolerant HIV-infected patients with alternating and intermittent regimens of zidovudine and dideoxycytidine. *The American Journal of Medicine*. May 21, 1990; volume 88, supplement 5B, pages 5B-24S to 5B-26S.

11. Skowron G and Merigan TC. Alternating and intermittent regimens of zidovudine (3'-azido-3'-deoxythymidine) and dideoxycytidine (2',3'-dideoxycytidine) in the treatment of patients with acquired immunodeficiency syndrome (AIDS) and AIDS-related complex. *The American Journal of Medicine*. May 21, 1990; volume 88, supplement 5B, pages 5B-20S to 5B-23S.

12. Pizzo PA. Treatment of human immunodeficiency virus-infected infants and young children with dideoxynucleosides. *The American Journal of Medicine*. May 21, 1990; volume 88, supplement 5B, pages 5B-16S to 5B-19S.

13. Merigan TC and Skowron G. Safety and tolerance of dideoxycytidine as a single agent. *The American Journal of Medicine*. May 21, 1990; volume 88, supplement 5B, pages 5B-11S to 5B-15S.

14. Richman DD. Susceptibility of nucleoside analogues of zidovudine-resistant isolates of human immunodeficiency virus. *The American Journal of Medicine*. May 21, 1990; volume 88, supplement 5B, pages 5B-8S to 5B-10S.

15. Broder S. Pharmacodynamics of 2',3'-dideoxycytidine: An inhibitor of human immunodeficiency virus. *The American Journal of Medicine*. May 21, 1990; volume 88, supplement 5B, pages 5B-2S to 5B-7S.

16. Broder S. Dideoxycytidine (ddC): A Potent antiretroviral agent for human immunodeficiency virus infection—An introduction. *The American Journal of Medicine*. May 21, 1990; volume 88, supplement 5B, page 5B-1S.

# WOMEN AND HIV: NEW CONSCIOUSNESS, WORLD AIDS DAY

*by Denny Smith*

December 1 will mark the third annual "World AIDS Day," sponsored by the World Health Organization (WHO). The focus this year is on women and AIDS. In August,

WHO estimated that of the eight to ten million people with HIV infection around the world, at least two million are women. Although women have played a major role throughout the pandemic caring for others with AIDS, their own HIV status and concerns have been trivialized or ignored. A number of studies presented at the Sixth International Conference on AIDS in June examined situations faced by women, including unrecognized signs of HIV progression and social barriers keeping women from early treatment. Several of these studies and related upcoming events are discussed in this article.

## Examples of Inferior Diagnosis and Treatment

Within WHO's estimate of two million women with HIV, 80 percent are cases reported from sub-Saharan Africa. Most of the remainder are reports from Latin America and North America. Eastern Europe and Asia document the lowest incidence, although these are areas of the world least familiar with AIDS epidemiology, so many cases may be missed. Women have become the fastest-growing segment of reported HIV infections, but a consequence of their marginalization in the epidemic is the widespread incidence of undiagnosed or unreported infections. Even where reporting is meticulous, biased assumptions discount many people, such as lesbians and older women.

In the United States, a disproportionate number of women with HIV are from communities of color, where AIDS is a leading cause of death. In this country with the world's most reported HIV diagnoses, health care is an elitist commodity, largely available according to one's level of income. People with HIV who are unable to afford private insurance have a difficult time finding dependable care, and this inequity is worsened by economic barriers of race and sex. A study presented at the Conference by the Perinatal AIDS Center at San Francisco General Hospital revealed that pregnant, HIV+ women experience social and economic problems which pre-date their HIV infection and which interfere with their compliance in clinical protocols and care plans.[1]

The discrepancy between what women give to the health of the community and what they get is not unique to the AIDS crisis. Cultures everywhere rely on women to attend to the sick and to details of daily health. A Conference report from Rutgers University described results of interviews with care-givers of people with AIDS that resembled social patterns of care for the elderly and chronically ill: women provided the bulk of daily care. More pointedly, people with AIDS in every transmission and ethnic category received most of their unpaid care from women.[2]

This environment contributes to women putting their own health second, with resulting delays in medical care and increased susceptibility to opportunistic infections. An AIDS information center in Mexico City, seeking ways to improve psychological support for women with HIV, reported that women with children always gave priority to the child, and second place to themselves.[3] A demographic review of a cohort of urban women by Georgetown University Hospital found that women tended to discover their serostatus late in HIV progression. Thirty nine percent of this cohort already had T-cell counts below 200, and another 36 percent had a count under 500.[4] In other words, many had missed the opportunity to intervene early, and probably more effectively, in their infection.

The criteria for diagnosing AIDS have been defined largely from studies of HIV progression in gay men, providing guidelines for physicians who may apply them to all their patients and underrate symptoms like chronic vaginitis and pelvic inflammatory disease specific to women. Gynecologic problems can be the first signs of compromised immunity in women, and gynecologists may be less likely than internists to be familiar with manifestations of HIV. The Centers For Disease Control has been under pressure to revise the definitions of AIDS to account for women's symptoms.

One concern receiving attention now is the frequency of cervical and vaginal cell abnormalities which could develop into tumors. A number of studies from the Conference, from different countries, revealed a higher incidence of these in women with HIV, especially those with past infections of the human papilloma virus (HPV), which causes genital warts and is a sexually transmitted disease. To monitor the risk of cervical cancers in HIV+ women, some physicians now recommend pap smears every six months.

A Conference abstract submitted by three German universities described how alpha interferon production in women declined as HIV infection progressed, and this was accompanied by an increase in cervical and vaginal atypias and inflammation. They concluded that the drop in alpha interferon production could give predictive information for gynecological diseases.[5]

A number of factors may lead to lower survival rates in women. An evaluation of people with Kaposi's sarcoma who attended the Uganda Cancer Institute found that the incidence of KS was increasing in general, and that women with KS tended to have a more aggressive disease, involving lymph nodes, and died sooner than male patients. The evaluators suggest that hormonal factors be investigated for their role in the development of KS.[6] (In other countries, KS is diagnosed less frequently in women than in men.)

Pregnancy raises a variety of questions for HIV+ women, such as the potential for transmitting the virus to the baby, the effect of various drugs on the mother and the fetus, and the effect of pregnancy on the mother's HIV infection.

The chances for infants to acquire HIV from seropositive mothers has been reported recently to be 25 percent and lower, a drop from older estimates. The modes for mother to infant transmission are becoming better understood. Transmission is thought to be possible through the placenta (perhaps at any time of the pregnancy), during birth (contact with maternal blood), or, least likely, after birth through breast feeding. Scientists at the National Institute of Allergy and Infectious Diseases (NIAID) discovered that several types of cells in the placenta, like helper cells in the blood, exhibit a CD4 receptor to which HIV readily binds. NIAID is conducting a clinical trial to determine if AZT given during pregnancy can limit HIV transmission to the fetus, although the protocol deals only with the third trimester.

A French study at the Conference found that the incidence of perinatal transmission is increased in mothers with low helper cell counts and positive p24 antigenemia.[7] This would imply that early monitoring and antiviral intervention for women to halt the decline of immune markers could also lower the incidence of perinatal transmission.

A retrospective review of 403 women in Masaka, Uganda, compared the progress after childbirth between HIV+ and HIV- mothers. The seropositive mothers had longer hospitalizations, lower mean hemoglobin levels, and an increased incidence of thrush, herpes zoster, headaches and gastrointestinal upsets.[8]

However, among women who are seropositive, there is no evidence that pregnancy speeds the progression of HIV infection.

## Signs of Change

A new critical awareness of women's HIV health has generated a sequence of events this year.

•   At the International Conference on AIDS in San Francisco last June, ACT UP staged effective demonstrations to highlight issues pertinent to women with HIV, using civil disobedience to block downtown city traffic and capture the eye of the news media. More than 80 studies relating to women and HIV were published in the Conference abstracts, a sign that these issues have been receiving some private, if not public, attention. Unfortunately, AIDS research has been so obsessed with women's relationship to childbearing and transmission of the virus, that data from studies of women's health for the sake of women are still empty pages. We need news of options and experience for treating women's HIV infections.

•   In July, women and AIDS organizations around the San Francisco Bay Area held a public forum addressing the deficits in the design of clinical trials. Speakers included women living with HIV, physicians treating AIDS, and community service providers. The issues included clinical trials entry criteria, which can arbitrarily exclude women based on the theoretical risk of a new drug taken during pregnancy. Although the risk should be considered, the choice is illogically removed from those with the greatest interest—potential women participants. Another aspect of traditional trial design which can systematically exclude women consists of protocols which try to minimize variables in the data by recruiting from a homogeneous population, such as gay men.

The head of the AIDS Activities Office of San Francisco's Department of Health, Sandra Hernandez, M.D., who was one of the forum's speakers, called for a reassessment of inclusion/exclusion criteria for clinical trials, and a realignment of their purpose and scope to account for everyone coping with HIV.

•   At a recent meeting of the AIDS Clinical Trials Group in Bethesda, Maryland, Daniel M. Hoth, M.D., announced a future public conference to address women and HIV, in collaboration with the Centers for Disease Control. The announcement came after months of pressure from AIDS activist women. Researchers from NIAID then met with representatives from the AIDS community the week of September 24 to plan the details of the conference. We spoke with Lisa Auer, who was there representing the Project Inform Community Research Alliance in San Francisco.

Ms. Auer told us that the meeting was productive, and relayed some decisions about the conference: it will be held in Washington, D.C. on December 13 and 14; four separate focus tracks were named: epidemiology, clinical manifestations and therapeutics, psychosocial aspects of HIV, and education and prevention. Only 1000 participants will be registered, with 100 spaces reserved specifically for women with HIV. Attendance is free, and for information interested persons can call Carol Gordon or Debra Stewart at 301/770-0610. The next issue of Project Inform's *PI Perspectives* will contain an article by Ms. Auer on woman and HIV.

• New community models could facilitate women's access to consistent health care. One example is a living cooperative for women with AIDS or related conditions and their children now organizing in Oakland, California. The project is named Hale Laulima, a Hawaiian expression meaning "house of many hands"; it should be active by December. The goal is for residents to meet their individual needs, such as doctor visits, by pooling resources and sharing meal preparation and childcare. This could substantially improve access to medical care for women ordinarily not able to take time for their own needs. The residence also plans to foster discussions of treatment information, which frequently doesn't reach isolated women in a community. (Hale Laulima can use financial donations—the mailing address is 3871 Piedmont Avenue, Oakland, California, 94611.)

Another new community model was described in a Conference abstract from the New Jersey Medical School and Medical Hospital, where a full-service outpatient clinic for women with HIV was established. When the course of women followed by the clinic was compared to women seen only as hospital patients, the data suggested that those cared for in the clinic had better survival rates. The clinic provided psychological support and social work services as well as medical attention.[9]

The New Jersey Women and AIDS Network has printed a very useful brochure surveying the problems and answers pertinent to HIV+ women, and a similar booklet written for health providers. Requests for copies can be sent with a self-addressed stamped envelope to the New Jersey Women and AIDS Network, 5 Elm Row, Suite 112, New Brunswick, NJ, 08901. Their phone number is 201/846-4462. For bulk orders the brochure is 20 cents each, and the booklet is 30 cents.

The Women's AIDS Network, based in San Francisco, compiles topical information packets for women and for organizations dealing with HIV and AIDS. It can be reached at 415/864-4376, extension 2007.

The AIDS activist community, women with HIV, and many AIDS service-providers are calling for future AIDS research to address women directly. HIV progresses in women, even if no one notices until a serious crisis brings them to an emergency room, and even while they are depended on to maintain the health of others. Symptoms of HIV in women are late in gaining recognition, with an according lag in effective treatments.

1990 is more than past the time to acknowledge the pivotal position of women in the AIDS crisis, and begin to correct the pervasive, institutionalized neglect of their health. Information concerning World AIDS Day can be requested from WHO, 1211 Geneva 27, Switzerland. In the U.S., activities will be coordinated by the American Association for World Health, which can be reached at 202/265-0286.

## REFERENCES

1.  Hauer LB and others. Client compliance with perinatal AIDS research: the Bay Area Perinatal AIDS Center (BAPAC) experience [abstract Th.D.805]. Sixth International Conference on AIDS, San Francisco, June 20-24, 1990.
2.  Schiller NG and others. The role of kin in care giving for persons with AIDS in New Jersey [abstract Th.D.822]. Sixth International Conference on AIDS, San Francisco, June 20-24, 1990.

3.    Tovar P and others. Psychological aspects and particular problems in HIV infected women [abstract S.B.374]. Sixth International Conference on AIDS, San Francisco, June 20-24, 1990.

4.    Young MA and others. Natural history of HIV disease in an urban cohort of women [abstract F.B.432]. Sixth International Conference on AIDS, San Francisco, June 20-24, 1990.

5.    Friese K and others. Interferon alpha as a predictive parameter in the development of gynecological diseases in HIV-infected women [abstract F.B.461]. Sixth International Conference on AIDS, San Francisco, June 20-24, 1990.

6.    Mbidde EK and others. The epidemiology and clinical features of Kaposi's sarcoma (KS) in African women with HIV infection [abstract S.B. 508]. Sixth International Conference on AIDS, San Francisco, June 20-24, 1990.

7.    Boue F and others. Risk for HIV-1 perinatal transmission vary with the mother's stage of HIV infection [abstract Th.C.44]. Sixth International Conference on AIDS, San Francisco, June 20-24, 1990.

8.    Kalibala S and others. The relationship between HIV infection and maternal morbidity in Masaka, Uganda [abstract F.B.458]. Sixth International Conference on AIDS, San Francisco, June 20-24, 1990.

9.    Pinto RC and others. Women's clinic: a full service clinic for women with HIV disease [abstract S.D. 816]. Sixth International Conference on AIDS, San Francisco, June 20-24, 1990.

# ACT UP/SAN FRANCISCO SPLITS; NEW GOLDEN GATE CHAPTER

*by John S. James*

On September 13, about a third of the 200 members of ACT UP/San Francisco left the group and formed a new organization, ACT UP/Golden Gate. The split was covered remarkably well in the three major San Francisco gay newspapers (the *Bay Area Reporter,* the *Bay Times,* and the *San Francisco Sentinel),* in the general-interest *SF Weekly,* and later in one of the major daily newspapers, the *San Francisco Examiner* (October 1). We will not repeat their detailed information; but since we will be reporting on both groups in the future, we included this sketch of what is happening and why.

The split came after months of increasing tension, and many people think the division will be beneficial. Both organizations are now working well, and they have begun their relationship on good terms. Some individuals will be active in both, and weekly meeting nights have been arranged to accommodate. One committee, the Youth Action Caucus of ACT UP/San Francisco, applied to also be a committee of ACT UP/Golden Gate, and was accepted. The groups are expected to work together; for example, both unanimously endorsed a call for approval of ddI and ddC before the end of the year.

Why, then, the split? The immediate issue was whether to maintain consensus, or allow decisions by an 80 percent vote. The decision to adopt voting would have had to be made by consensus, and when several people blocked that decision, the group split. (ACT UP/Golden Gate now makes decisions by a two-thirds vote, although in practice many, if not most, are unanimous.)

For both groups, demonstrations and street theater are primary tools. But ACT UP/ Golden Gate also emphasizes working "within the system," as well as on the street, to get research done and make treatments available, and those who work with government agencies, pharmaceutical companies, and other mainstream organizations, want group support. ACT UP/San Francisco emphasizes the need for larger social change to end the epidemic, as well as the need for treatments. Consensus was a key issue, because giving anyone the power to block group action assured that minority voices would be heard and considered. But with 200 members with very diverse points of view (ACT UP/San Francisco had tripled in size since the June, 1990 Sixth International Conference on AIDS), it had become very difficult to get any significant action approved. Energy was increasingly devoted to process issues and infighting, instead of useful work.

Separation has freed both groups, ending paralysis, allowing productive competition, and opening the way for members who had previously left the group to now return to one or the other. Both groups will hold demonstrations in the next week (see announcement below).

The general meeting of ACT UP/San Francisco continues to be every Thursday at 7:30 PM at the Women's Building, 3543 18th St. (near Valencia). ACT UP/Golden Gate meets every Tuesday at 7:00 at 539 Hayes St.

# Issue Number 113
# October 19, 1990

## AZITHROMYCIN, CLARITHROMYCIN: BROAD POTENTIAL RECEIVING SERIOUS ATTENTION

*by Denny Smith*

For some time, laboratory studies of two relatively new drugs related to the antibiotic erythromycin suggest they might be very useful for treating a number of major and minor infections, including toxoplasmosis, MAI (also known as MAC), and cryptosporidiosis. A few reports of clinical experience which seem to support the animal or test tube results have come to us recently, and there are calls for wider access to both drugs.

They are azithromycin and clarithromycin, and the tantalizing potential to treat three opportunistic infections would logically give them the highest priority in AIDS research. Until now that has not been the case, and the plodding momentum of human trials of the drugs threatened to squander their value for thousands of people. Following is the clearest picture we could assemble of their current status, based on conversations with the commercial developers of the drugs, with members of the community, and with the Treatment and Data Committee of ACT UP/New York, which has posed a number of well-formulated questions to the manufacturers regarding the pace and efficiency of their investigations.

These two agents appear to be the strongest candidates for treating AIDS-related infections yet to emerge from a growing class of compounds called macrolide antibiotics. Other macrolides under study in AIDS research are roxithromycin and spiramycin. An article in *AIDS Treatment News* #75 reported with optimism the potential of azithromycin and roxithromycin to treat toxoplasmosis and cryptosporidiosis. But the following June 16, 1989, issue #81 reported the failure of roxithromycin to treat advanced toxoplasmosis in humans. Spiramycin has been tested as a treatment for cryptosporidiosis, with mixed results; an oral formulation was not useful, but intravenously the drug has helped some people. Spiramycin has also been tried to prevent transmission of *Toxoplasma* from mothers to fetuses.[1]

None of these drugs was listed by study title in the abstracts published for the Sixth International Conference on AIDS last June, although we heard them discussed in some contexts with other treatments or infections. They will be discussed in various studies to be presented this month at the 30th Interscience Conference on Antimicrobial Agents and Chemotherapy, October 21-24 in Atlanta. Some of the abstracts from these studies and a few other previously published reports are referenced at the end of this article.

We contacted the manufacturers of azithromycin and clarithromycin to ask about their plans for clinical trials and any other avenues of access until their products are proven and licensed.

Both drugs are well into phase III trials in the U.S.; both manufacturers have already applied for the NDA (New Drug Application, meaning permission to market the drug for prescription use). But the companies are pursuing Food and Drug Administration (FDA) approval for label indications *not* specifically related to treating AIDS. A newly approved drug, however, would be available to physicians treating AIDS infections, because an M.D. can administer a licensed treatment at his or her discretion for any diagnosis, whether named or not in the product labeling. In recent years, however, some health insurance carriers have been refusing to pay for many "off-label" uses of drugs, no matter how convincing the situation. So in spite of a physician's judgment, the exact labeling may ultimately determine who will or will not get the drug.

Both drugs also have Investigational New Drug (IND) status, for use in trials against MAI and toxoplasmosis.

Azithromycin has been studied in European trials, and is in Phase III trials in the U.S. to treat chlamydia, gonorrhea, and certain other infections not strictly associated with AIDS. It is marketed in Yugoslavia and Czechoslovakia under the brand name Sumamed, manufactured by Pliva. The pharmaceutical firm of Pfizer, Inc., holds the rights to develop azithromycin elsewhere, using the trade name Zithromax. In the U.S., the FDA is due to consider the NDA for azithromycin early next year.

An advantage of macrolides is their fat solubility, which increases concentrations of the drugs in body tissues. Azithromycin in particular surpasses the other macrolides in its "targeted delivery." Of great therapeutic value in some infections, this describes the capacity to penetrate the walls of some immune cells and remain inside for several hours; as the cells naturally migrate to sites of infections, so does their passenger, spilling out in the attack and enhancing the cell's fight against the infection.[2,3] Azithromycin is considered the prototype for developing a macrolide subclass called azalides.

Our recent report on MAI therapies in issue #109 referred to a San Francisco pilot study of azithromycin for treating MAI infections. Lowell Young, M.D., is the principal investigator of the study, conducted at Pacific Presbyterian Hospital in San Francisco; he has authored some of the past reports of *in vitro* macrolide studies.[4] He told us that the drug has been well tolerated in patients so far. This small, open-label study is still open to recruits because the entry criteria are strict. Interested persons can call 415/923-3262.

Pfizer researcher Scott J. Hopkins, M.D., explained to us the current status of other azithromycin studies for AIDS opportunistic infections. Pilot efforts to try azithromycin for cryptosporidiosis are being developed in the U.S. and the U.K., and for toxoplasmosis in France. The most welcome event now is the release of azithromycin through a compassionate use protocol for treating toxoplasmic brain infections in people who have failed the standard therapies, or are known to have a history of intolerance to those drugs. The protocol involves 600 mg of azithromycin daily for one month, then decreased to 600 mg weekly.

The physician requesting azithromycin must obtain at least verbal approval from an Institutional Review Board (IRB) for initial doses of the drug, and written approval for continuing access. Case report forms must be returned to Pfizer, so useful information can be compiled through this experience. Effective October 21, physicians can call Michael DeBruin, M.D., at 203/441-5701, or FAX 203/441-5702, to seek enrollment in this protocol for their patients.

Clarithromycin is a product of Abbott Laboratories, and has been approved for use in Ireland and Italy, under the trade names Klacid and Claricid. Abbott has submitted an NDA to the FDA for clarithromycin as a treatment for some skin and respiratory infections. Based on results of past studies, Abbott has plans to test clarithromycin in the treatment of toxoplasmosis and MAI, as well as for prophylaxis to suppress latent infections of the same.[5,6,7] These plans are apparently less developed than are Pfizer's for azithromycin, described above.

A recent trial with 14 patients found a 99.98 percent reduction in MAI blood levels after six weeks' treatment with clarithromycin, compared to an increase in levels in patients receiving a placebo[5]; a second phase of the trial found a 99.65 percent decrease with the drug. At the dosage used, toxicities required discontinuation of the drug by three patients.. We have heard anecdotal reports of several people who found some improvement in MAI symtptoms after trying a combination of clarithromycin and clofazimine, one of the standard MAI drugs.

## Azithromycin Anecdotal Experience

In response to articles in recent issues of *AIDS Treatment News* which raised the question of azithromycin's untapped potential, two readers called us to share first-hand experience with this drug.

The first report was offered by someone who began experiencing neurologic symptoms several months ago, and was diagnosed with toxoplasmic encephalitis after a computerized tomography (CT) scan revealed a brain lesion. These scans are not reliable for distinguishing lesions caused by *Toxoplasma* from those of cerebral lymphoma, and in fact this person had been diagnosed with lymphoma once before. His response to lymphoma treatment was complete, and the new lesion was not judged to be lymphoma by his physician or the consulting neurologist. So they initiated the standard treatment for toxoplasmosis—pyrimethamine with leucovorin and a sulfon-amide. When our friend developed a serious rash, the sulfa component was replaced by clindamycin, a frequent "next" choice. Unfortunately, this was followed by severe diarrhea, one of the side effects associated with clindamycin, and the treatment was discontinued.

By the time our friend could no longer tolerate either combination therapy, he had received about one month of treatment. Pyrimethamine alone is not considered adequate against active toxoplasmosis, and another CT scan showed the lesion persisting, although reduced in size by the treatments.

Our friend's doctor then offered to treat the infection with azithromycin. Upon signing an informed consent for using an investigational drug, our friend was given a loading dose of oral capsules totalling one gram of azithromycin, and then a maintenance dosage of 500 mg daily. After one week of treatment, a new CT scan showed no evidence of the lesion; another scan was performed at a different institution and verified the response.

We considered the question of whether the entire effort was applied to an incorrect diagnosis. But if the lesion had been lymphoma, it would not have been affected by any of the drugs tried, and symptoms would have lingered or worsened.

There is also the dilemma of understanding anecdotal successes—how to know which drugs in a multiple-drug regimen obtained the response. In this case, was azithromycin effective enough to replace the established treatment, or did it only play a complementary role after those drugs brought the infection under control? It is very improbable that the lesion would regress independently after the drug combinations were stopped, given the usual course of AIDS-related toxoplasmosis. Both our friend and his physician are convinced that azithromycin controlled the infection. They saw no obvious toxicities, and in line with the established treatment regimen, a suppressive maintenance dose will be continued indefinitely.

The other report came from Larry Bruni, M.D., who treats HIV in his Washington, D.C., practice, and who has advocated for investigations of both drugs for some time. He decided to offer azithromycin to two of his patients whose bloodwork revealed past exposure to *Toxoplasma*, and in whom high titers pointed to an increased risk for a reactivated infection. The titers were decreased in both patients on the drug, and Dr. Bruni feels it has been effective so far in preventing active toxoplasmosis.

He also tried azithromycin with three patients diagnosed with cryptosporidiosis. One of the patients said that he doubted the drug was helping, and he was lost to follow-up early in the experiment. The other two reported good responses to the drug, and they continue to use it.

## Comment Regarding Access

Unfortunately, the differences in healthcare systems and drug licensing among various countries have led to uneven access to many important drugs. In our reports of investigational treatments, we try not to take for granted the approval status of experimental drugs in countries outside the U.S., or the economic limits imposed on countless people who need AIDS treatments urgently. Where drugs are not licensed, or affordable, clinical trials may provide access to a treatment for some people. If participation in a trial is not feasible, physicians can sometimes secure an experimental drug by petitioning the manufacturer on behalf of patients in need, especially those who have failed standard treatments, or who have no other options.

We have not heard of any access to azithromycin outside of Yugoslavia, Czechoslovakia, or release by Pfizer. Dr. Bruni speculated that since they are quite close in structure, clarithromycin might be used to treat infections which are reported to have responded to azithromycin.

Clarithromycin is available in the U.S. through the PWA Health Group in New York City; the drug is expensive, and two to four weeks are required to obtain it from abroad. Requests must include a doctor's prescription; interested people can call 212/532-0280 to ask for a mail-order form.

Clarithromycin may be available immediately from a new buyers club in Los Angeles, called LABC/Staying Alive; their number is 213/748-1295. Both of these groups are non-profit organizations, run by people well known in the community.

One aspect of the clarithromycin research plans challenged by ACT UP/New York's Treatment and Data Committee is the decision of Abbott Laboratories to test clarithromycin alone against MAI, since clinical experience with treating mycobacterial infections generally has concluded that a multiple drug approach is necessary.

Proprietary interests could explain the single-agent focus, and yet if an effective drug fails to win results because of an ineffective application, no one's interests will be served. Trials implementing different approaches could be conducted at the same time, and should be soon, given the critical passage of time for people now ill.

On the other hand, high marks were given to Abbott's plans to design a trial of clarithromycin as a possible prophylaxis against several infections at once. The compassionate release of azithromycin for toxoplasmosis is a welcome gesture from Pfizer. Both Abbott and Pfizer have in their possession substances which at the moment may be the best, or only, options for treating many people. Whether these drugs are approved for lesser infections or continue on to larger studies, the only appropriate pace is one of urgency.

# REFERENCES

1.  McCabe RE and Oster S. Current recommendations and future prospects in the treatment of toxoplasmosis. *Drugs*, volume 38, number 6, pages 973-987, December 1989.

2.  Girard AE, Cimochowski CR, and Faiella JA. Correlation of increased azithromycin levels with phagocyte infiltration into sites of infection [abstract 762]. 30th Interscience Conference on Antimicrobial Agents and Chemotherapy, October 21-24, 1990, Atlanta.

3.  Wildfeur A, Laufen H, Muller-Wening D, and Haferkamp O. Interaction of azithromycin and human phagocytic cells. Uptake of the antibiotic and the effect on the survival of ingested bacteria in phagocytes. *Arzneimittelfurschung*, volume 39, number 7, pages 755-758, July 1989.

4.  Bermudez LE, Young LS. Activities of amikacin, roxithromycin, and azithromycin alone or in combination with tumor necrosis factor against Mycobacterium avium complex. *Antimicrobial Agents and Chemotherapy*, volume 32, number 8, pages 1149-1153, August, 1988.

5.  Dautzenberg B, Legris S, Truffot C, and others. Clarithromycin clears Mycobacterium Avium Intracellulare (MAIC) from blood of AIDS patients. A randomized trial [abstract 1264]. 30th Interscience Conference on Antimicrobial Agents and Chemotherapy, October 21-24, 1990, Atlanta.

6.  Prokocimer P, Dellerson M, Craft C, Pernet A, Ruff B, and Grosset J. Effect of clarithromycin on blood cultures positive for Mycobacterium Avium Complex in HIV+ patients [abstract 634]. 30th Interscience Conference on Antimicrobial Agents and Chemotherapy, October 21-24, 1990, Atlanta.

7.  Pichotta P, Gupta S, Prokocimer P, and Pernet A. The overall safety of oral clarithromycin in comparative clinical studies [abstract 1332]. 30th Interscience Conference on Antimicrobial Agents and Chemotherapy, October 21-24, 1990, Atlanta.

# AZT: 300 MG DOSE MAY BE EQUALLY EFFECTIVE

A study published October 11, 1990, in *The New England Journal of Medicine* compared three different doses of AZT (also called zidovudine, or Retrovir) and found all three equally effective, according to several different measures.[1] The doses were 300, 600, or 1500 mg per day; as expected, the low doses had less toxicity.

This phase II, unblinded, "pilot" study enrolled a total of 67 volunteers, all of whom had symptomatic HIV infection, but not AIDS. All had T-helper counts of 200 to 500, and were either p24 positive or had plasma viremia, when they began the trial. (For the viremia measure, this study used a quantitative test for the amount of virus present, not the older viral cultures which were only positive or negative but did not indicate an amount.)

Those randomly assigned to the 300-mg dose had the greatest T-helper improvement, from an average of 321 to 412 during the first 12 weeks of treatment. Several other measurements—the proportion who became p24 negative, the decrease in p24 levels in the others, and the reduction in plasma viremia—were the same in all dosage groups. Clinical improvement, measured by weight gain, Karnofsky performance scores, and reduced fatigue, was better in the low and medium doses (300 and 600 mg) than in the 1500-mg dose.

After the 12th week, patients continued in a second phase of the trial for a median of 28 additional weeks. None of the 22 who were p24 positive at the 12th week became p24 negative later—suggesting the limited effectiveness of AZT. In fact, the p24 levels increased 14 percent during this second phase (the median of 28 weeks after the 12th week of treatment). This increase was comparable in all three dosage groups.

As an additional test to see whether the different doses worked equally well, some patients were crossed over from 300 or 600 mg to 1500, or from 1500 to 300. This change in the dose of AZT had no effect on p24 levels.

This study also tested acyclovir (Zovirax) in combination with AZT, by randomly assigning some of the patients in each of the AZT dosage groups to 4.8 grams of acyclovir per day. There was no evidence that the combination had any more antiretroviral effect than AZT alone. But the authors pointed out that their study could not rule out the possibility that acyclovir might increase survival, as one study[2] suggested. Only additional trials could determine if suppressing certain herpes viruses with acyclovir would have clinical benefit. No toxicity was seen from the acyclovir, when combined with any dose of AZT.

The researchers concluded, "The consistency of the clinical and laboratory data . . . suggests that 300 mg of zidovudine a day has antiviral and CD4-lymphocyte-enhancing effects similar to those of a 600-mg dose, with less toxicity than higher doses." However, "Our findings must be corroborated before this dosage is routinely adopted." They also conclude that "The minimal effective dose of zidovudine for the treatment of HIV infection has yet to be determined, and further studies of very low daily doses are warranted."

This study was supported by grants from the National Institutes of Health and the AIDS Clinical Trials Group (ACTG) of the National Institute of Allergy and Infectious Diseases. The principal investigator was Lawrence Corey, M.D., of the University of Washington in Seattle.

## Comment

The fact that a small study was finding that 300 mg of AZT seemed to work as well as 600 mg had become widely known in the AIDS community. But formal publication provides the details which make the result more useful.

At this time the usual dose of AZT is 500 or 600 mg per day. It is unlikely that this standard will change just because of one relatively small study. But the new results should make physicians and patients more confident about lowering the dose when necessary, or when they are already inclined to do so.

This trial was well designed, in several ways. It used relatively few patients, and therefore could be conducted quickly, cleanly, and economically. It made good use of laboratory endpoints, including quantitative plasma viremia, and also used clinical endpoints such as weight gain and fatigue scores. While none of these measurements is by itself definitive, the consistency between them is convincing. The researchers tabulated results at 12 weeks (known to be long enough for AZT to show benefits), but then continued the study to obtain longer-term data. These aspects of this trial illustrate current developments in clinical-trial design.

## REFERENCES

1.  Collier AC, Bozzette S, Coombs RW, and others. A pilot study of low-dose zidovudine in human immunodeficiency virus infection. *The New England Journal of Medicine*, October 11, 1990, volume 323, number 15, pages 1015-1021.
2.  Fiddian AP. [Wellcome Research Laboratories, Beckenhham, Kent, U.K.] Preliminary report of a multicentre study of zidovudine plus or minus acyclovir in patients with acquired immune deficiency syndrome or acquired immune deficiency syndrome-related complex. *J. Infect.*, January 1989, volume 18 [supplement 1], pages 79-80.

# DDC: EXPANDED ACCESS ELIGIBILITY CRITERIA

On September 10 Hoffmann-La Roche announced that it planned to make ddC available through a compassionate access program for persons with AIDS or related conditions who could not effectively use other treatments. A number of patients are already on the program. This article summarizes the entry criteria now in use; the intent is to let patients and physicians know who is likely to qualify.

• To obtain ddC under this program, patients can qualify by AZT treatment failure, or AZT intolerance, or AZT ineligibility.

• To qualify under *AZT treatment failure*, patients must have received at least 500 mg/day of AZT for at least six months, and not been off of the drug for more than 30 days during that six-month period. They must have had at least one of the following:

— Three opportunistic infections or cancers in the last six months; or
— Drop of 50 T-helper cells, *and* a T-helper count of less than 50 on two occasions one month apart; or
— Sustained or increasing p24; or
— Involuntary weight loss of 2-2.5 pounds per week for at least four weeks; or

— Significant neurologic deterioration; or
— Karnofsky score less than or equal to 40 for at least one month, as a result of AIDS.

• To qualify under *AZT intolerance*, patients must have remained intolerant to AZT although the dose was reduced to 500 mg per day or less. Intolerance is defined as one or more of the following:

— Decrease in hemoglobin by 2 gm/month; or
— ANC less than 750; or
— Severe vomiting or intractable nausea due to AZT; or
— Severe headaches not treatable by analgesics; or
— Acute psychosis; or
— Severe agitation; or
— Declining muscle strength, such as inability to climb stairs, with CPK greater than 1000.

These toxicities must have required discontinuation of AZT, and must resolve to Grade 2 or better within 45 days after discontinuing AZT, and before entry into this ddC protocol.

• To qualify under *AZT ineligibility*, patients must:
— Be taking necessary treatment with drugs which cannot safely be given with AZT and could be given with ddC (e.g., ganciclovir for life-threatening or sight-threatening CMV infections); or
— Have baseline ANC less than 1000, and no prior use of AZT; or
— Have baseline hemoglobin less than 8.5.

• The protocol also defines ddI intolerance and ineligibility. Originally, patients could receive ddC only if they had failed *both* AZT and ddI. After protests by activists, who objected to patients being required to fail other than standard therapies, this "ddI loop" was eliminated. ddI intolerance or ineligibility are no longer required for access to ddC, but the information is still being collected, for research purposes.

• The AZT toxicities described above "would be considered 'probably' drug related if three of the following four criteria are met:

— Logical time course following drug administration;
— A known toxicity of the drug;
— Improvement after discontinuation of the drug;
— Recurrence with rechallenge with the drug."

(Note that these criteria do not necessarily require rechallenge, which would be dangerous in some circumstances.)

• Patients must also meet all of the following conditions:
— Hemoglobin at least 8.0 and not transfusion dependent;
— ANC at least 750;
— Platelet count at least 80,000;
— Estimated creatinine clearance greater than 50 ml/minute (a formula is given for making the estimate);
— SGOT and SGPT less then five times upper limit of normal (in some cases, a hepatitis B surface antigen test should be done);

— Both men and women must practice birth control, and women must have a negative serum beta HCG pregnancy test within seven days of entry into the protocol;

— Patients must be at least 12 years old, with consent of parent or guardian for those under 18.

- Exclusion criteria. Patients must not have any of the following:

— A history of peripheral neuropathy due to any cause—or any finding suggestive of peripheral neuropathy found at baseline neurological exam (An isolated finding of absent Achilles reflex may be allowed.); or

— Cancer other than KS or basal cell carcinoma; or

— Concomitant treatment with any other nucleoside analog (e.g., AZT); or

— Concomitant treatment with excluded medications. ("Excluded medications include other experimental drugs, immune modulators, systemic corticosteroids, drugs with known nephrotoxic or hepatotoxic potential, and drugs likely to cause peripheral neuropathy."); or

— Pregnancy or breast feeding; or

— Being unwilling or deemed unable to sign an informed consent.

- Concomitant medications. Most non-experimental medications are permitted when necessary. But any that could cause peripheral neuropathy should be avoided. And other precautions are recommended or required; for example, ddC must be stopped temporarily if certain drugs need to be administered.

## Disclaimer

This article summarizes the eligibility criteria of the ddC expanded-access program; it is not complete. In addition, the criteria will probably change over time. The above summary is for background only.

## PRIMAQUINE SUPPLY PROBLEM: HOW TO GET THE DRUG

Primaquine, a drug which is vitally important for a few people with AIDS, has been unavailable at pharmacies in the United States for about three months, and could remain unavailable for months longer. Affected patients and their physicians must be informed that it is possible to get the drug.

Primaquine is usually used to treat or prevent certain kinds of malaria. In AIDS it is used in combination with clindamycin to treat or prevent pneumocystis—but only for patients who cannot tolerate or do not benefit from all three of the preferred treatment regimens—Bactrim (Septra), pentamidine, and dapsone.

The supply was cut off because the sole U.S. manufacturer of primaquine, Winthrop Pharmaceuticals, has been unable to obtain a chemical precursor needed to make the drug. The U.S. Centers for Disease Control obtained an emergency supply, which it will provide free to physicians for treatment of certain kinds of malaria (but not for malaria prophylaxis, because the supply is limited). Apparently no provision was made for persons with AIDS, for whom use of the drug is "off label," as primaquine has not been officially approved specifically for pneumocystis.

What is not widely known is that this shortage exists only in the United States. Elsewhere, primaquine is cheap and plentiful. Apparently the foreign manufacturers are unwilling to invest the money required to obtain generic approval for their preparations, since there is little malaria here, few other patients need the drug, and the profit margin is low because primaquine is generic.

In response to this emergency, the PWA Health Group in New York has obtained primaquine from England. (Individuals can legally import small quantities of foreign pharmaceuticals for personal use.) A bottle of 1,000 tablets (7.5 mg) costs $34; a prescription is required. For more information, call the PWA Health Group at 212/532-0280.

Note: An article on the primaquine supply problem appears in the excellent September, 1990, issue of *Notes from the Underground*, the newsletter of the PWA Health Group. For a copy, call them at the number above. An article in the July 20, 1990, *Morbidity and Mortality Weekly Report,* published by the U.S. Centers for Disease Control, alerted the medical community to the supply problem, and explained the arrangements made for patients with malaria.

California note: The California legislature recently passed a law to add clindamycin (the drug used with primaquine) to the Medi-Cal (Medicaid) formulary, allowing it to be prescribed to Medi-Cal patients. State authorities had previously refused to pay for the drug.

## IMMUNE-BASED THERAPIES
## MEETING: CHICAGO, NOV. 8

A one-day meeting on "The Status of Immune-Based Therapies in HIV Infection and AIDS" will take place on November 8 in Chicago, in association with the 5th Annual Conference on Clinical Immunology, which is November 9-11.

Topics include interleukin-2, alpha interferon, other cytokines, DTC (Imuthiol), isoprinosine, levamisole, immune serum, anti-gp 160 monoclonal antibodies, CD4 blocking, CD4 adhesin, vaccines for HIV-infected individuals (gp 160 vaccine and others), and laboratory evaluation of immune-based therapies.

## *BETA*: FOOD PRECAUTIONS, ORAL PROBLEMS OF HIV

The sixth and current issue of the *Bulletin of Experimental Treatments for AIDS (BETA)*, published by the San Francisco AIDS Foundation, contains an excellent survey of food-preparation precautions which could prevent certain infections for people with HIV. The article is authored by Irene Baucom and traces the origin of various infections associated with compromised immunity, as well as reasons and measures for minimizing exposure to food-borne microbes.

In the same issue Caroline L. Dodd, B.D.S., and Deborah Greenspan, B.D.S., report on a spectrum of oral infections and lesions associated with HIV disease. Treatments as well as diagnoses are discussed. To ask for this edition, or to subscribe to *BETA*, call 800/327-9893 or 415/863-2437.

## *GOOD INTENTIONS:* NEW BOOK ATTACKS CONFLICT OF INTEREST IN MEDICAL RESEARCH

*by John S. James*

*Good Intentions*—subtitled *How Big Business and the Medical Establishment are Corrupting the Fight Against AIDS,* a sure-to-be-controversial book by Bruce Nussbaum, a senior writer at *Business Week*, appeared in bookstores this month. It is published by Atlantic Monthly Press.

*Good Intentions* is based on over 100 interviews between 1988 and 1990 with key figures in AIDS research, mostly in the Washington, DC, New York City, and Raleigh, North Carolina, areas; only one scientist refused to be interviewed. The author approached the subject without preconceptions: "I didn't begin the book angry but I did finish it that way." A quote from the introduction gives a better sense of the message than our description could:

"Despite my twenty years as a journalist, much of it covering business and finance for *Business Week*, I was not prepared for the behind-the-scenes realities of big-time medical research. Even after the wild and woolly eighties, where greed became a Wall Street theology, the corruption was startling.

"On Wall Street, the financial crooks, the insider traders, knew for the most part that they were cheating, breaking the law. The games they played were new—the LBOs, the hostile takeovers, the greenmail. But the corruption itself was as old-fashioned as embezzlement.

"Nothing of the sort exists in medical science. In that arena, people have good intentions. They believe they are doing good works for the general health of the nation. Indeed, personal corruption is still rare, although faking experimental data appears to be on the rise.

"The corruption in medical science goes much deeper. It derives from the very way the Food and Drug Administration, the National Institutes of Health, and the dozens or so elite academic biomedical research centers work with private drug companies.

"An old-boy network of powerful medical researchers dominates in every disease field, from AIDS to Alzheimer's. They control the major committees, they run the most important trials, they determine what gets published and who gets promoted. They are accountable to no one. Despite the billions of taxpayer dollars that go to them every year, there is no public oversight. Medical scientists have convinced society that only they can police themselves.

"Yet behind the closed doors of 'peer review,' conflicts of interest abound. These are not perceived as conflicts of interest by the scientists themselves. The researchers are convinced that they have only good intentions. This book will show that medical science is the graveyard of good intentions. It will indicate how medical science, in its own unique way, may turn out to be the Wall Street of the nineties.

"*Good Intentions* is about AIDS. It could be about cancer or heart disease or any other major disease. The social, political, and financial structure of the biomedical research behind each one is similar. Acquired Immune Deficiency Syndrome is relatively new. The deals, the arrangements, the conflicts of interest are therefore more open to the observer. They are only just now being constructed.

"AIDS is also a killer. It strikes young people in the prime of their lives. The AIDS virus is infectious. Anything that gets in the way of quickly developing safe and effective treatments is monstrous. Against this background, the behavior of medical science is thrown into stark relief. A long history of cancer would illustrate the same issues and problems."

(Copyright 1990 by Bruce Nussbaum, reproduced by permission.)

# Comment

*Good Intentions* seldom attacks individual researchers. Some emerge as heros, and most did the jobs they were supposed to do. The problems arise more from the system than from the people.

This is not the first book to allege that medical/scientific monopolies or conflicts of interest have grossly harmed research in AIDS and other diseases. But it may be the first to make the message accessible and credible to non-specialists—media people, politicians and their staffs, business and foundation leaders, and anybody else interested in current affairs.

Why is this book important? You can see for yourself by visiting any book or magazine store with a good public-affairs section. Shelves are loaded with general-interest books and articles on science and government, and on almost every national problem. But AIDS is strangely absent from this world of discourse—not mentioned at all, for example, in books on the Federal government during the Reagan years, or getting at best a few sentences of the most superficial comment. Many books have been published on AIDS, but few include anything about treatment research, and fewer still are ever seen by the general public.

Why has AIDS research suffered this neglect in the intellectual life of the nation? We believe the major reason is that non-specialists were afraid of the difficulty and complexity of the issue. They do not want to say anything about AIDS research, because they fear getting it wrong.

Until now, any non-specialists who wanted to know what really was happening in AIDS treatment development would have needed to undertake an extensive personal research project, finding information in newsletters, in Congressional hearings, through interviews with experts, etc., and then deciding what is relevant and what is credible. No wonder it was easier to accept the "mantram" that everything possible was being done, we're moving as fast as we can, good science takes time.

*Good Intentions* is far from the last word on AIDS research; no single book could tell the whole story. Many legitimate questions and criticisms will be raised. Some of those who appear in the book may have good reason to question how they are portrayed. But while not the last word, it is in a sense a first word, opening research issues for the first time to the normal process of public discussion and debate.

Some may say this book appears at the wrong time. For AIDS activists and researchers are now working together better than ever before; the spirit of cooperation calls for defending rather than attacking each other. Many believe there are too many personal attacks already. We should remember that the book is not accusing individuals of wrongdoing; instead it shows problems in the system, problems no one could have foretold and which few have imagined until now. It provides a first glimpse of the enormous inefficiencies and lost opportunities everywhere in medical research. We can only guess what progress could be made if these problems can be corrected.

Some may fear that the book is ill-timed because of the growing dangers to Congressional funding due to Federal financial problems. But a recent nationwide survey found that one American in five personally knows someone who has AIDS or is HIV positive (*Boston Globe*, July 17, 1990, page 1). Congress cannot walk away forever. We can and must address alleged problems openly, and correct them to make research more efficient and productive.

*Good Intentions* suggests that the fundamental problem in medical research, not just in AIDS, is that the real decisions are made for the benefit of powerful interests, not for the benefit of current and future patients, on whose behalf the whole enterprise is ostensibly being run. The best corrective may be the development of patient advocacy movements (like ACT UP and Project Inform), which do their homework on research, learn what really happens there, and represent the public interest in a way it has not been represented before. These movements are not always adversarial; they increasingly work together with professional, industrial, and regulatory interests. They provide a voice at the table for those who have had no voice until now.

In many areas of U.S. public life, most real power rests with what is called the "iron triangle," consisting of an industry, the Federal regulators of that industry, and the Congressional committees and staffs which oversee the regulators. In medical research the traditional structure might be called an iron quadrangle, including not only the usual three, but also the relevant professions (medicine and science), which have rules, independence, and interests of their own. The AIDS activist movement is adding a fifth group, as patients demand and win a place at the bargaining table, too.

A potential problem for this patient movement is that most of the public-affairs constituency has had no understanding of its issues. Groups in the liberal, public-interest, good-government, consumer-protection spirit should be allies of patient advocates, not opponents. It is easy for well-intended reformers, intimidated by the complexity of science, to uncritically accept the opinions of authorities, without realizing that these authorities have interests and agendas of their own. *Good Intentions* sheds light here; for the first time, it brings the hidden realities of drug development into general public view.

# Issue Number 114
# November 2, 1990

## PNEUMOCYSTIS PROPHYLAXIS OVERVIEW
*by Michelle Roland*

### Introduction

In spite of recent improvements in treatment, pneumocystis pneumonia remains the most frequent cause of death in people with HIV infection. In addition, all currently available treatments have potentially serious toxicities associated with them. Therefore, the best approach to dealing with pneumocystis is to avoid getting it by properly using an effective prophylaxis (preventive treatment) in all persons at risk of developing the infection.

This article provides an overview of current information and controversies about approved and experimental prophylaxis for pneumocystis. Because no currently available option is ideal, we discuss the potential advantages and disadvantages of each approach.

### When to Use Pneumocystis Prophylaxis

The official recommendation of the U.S. Public Health Service is that adults should use a prophylaxis against pneumocystis if they have: (1) a T-helper count of 200 or less, or (2) a T-helper cell percent of less than 20, or (3) a previous episode of pneumocystis.[1] (The T-helper cell percent is a laboratory marker of disease severity that doctors often take into account when recommending various treatments or prophylaxis. It measures the percent of all the white blood cells known as lymphocytes that are T-helper cells.)

There are additional situations in which prophylaxis may be helpful, although there is no consensus among physicians in this area. A recent survey of over 80 physicians and other health-care providers practicing in the San Francisco Bay Area demonstrated the following trends in pneumocystis prophylaxis:[2]

• Seventy-seven percent of the responding health-care providers would offer prophylaxis to patients with any AIDS-defining opportunistic infection, even if they did not meet the criteria outlined in the official recommendations described above.

• Fifty-eight percent would offer prophylaxis to patients with any AIDS-related malignancy irrespective of whether or not they met the official criteria.

• While approximately 80-90 percent would offer prophylaxis to patients with under 200 T-helper cells, whether symptomatic or not, less than half of those responding would do so for patients with less than 20 percent T-helper cells and no other reason for prophylaxis.

• Approximately half would offer prophylaxis to symptomatic patients with more than 200 but less than 300 T-helper cells; only about 30 percent would offer prophylaxis to asymptomatic patients in that range. Few would recommend prophylaxis for patients with more than 300 T-helper cells.

## A Note About Infants

Current recommendations suggest that all infants and children should receive pneumocystis prophylaxis when their T-helper cell count falls below 500. However, an important study presented at the Sixth International Conference on AIDS suggests that some infants (those who were infected with HIV perinatally as opposed to those infected by transfusion) may be at high risk of developing pneumocystis with well over 500 T-helper cells.[3]

A chart review of 38 infants in Los Angeles showed that 41 percent of the infants who acquired their HIV infection perinatally were diagnosed with pneumocystis with a T-helper cell count greater than 500. Of those who acquired their infection perinatally and developed pneumocystis when they were less than one year old, all had greater than 500 T-helper cells; in fact, many had more than 1000 T-helper cells.

Although 93 percent of the infants who acquired their HIV infection via transfusion and were diagnosed with pneumocystis did have less than 500 T-helper cells, the official recommendation for prophylaxis in some categories of infants, it seems, should be reassessed.

## Which Prophylaxis?

There are currently two different drugs for pneumocystis prophylaxis in widespread use in the U.S: aerosolized pentamidine, and Bactrim (also known as Septra, trimethoprim-sulfamethoxazole, TMP-SMX, or cotrimoxazole). Both have been officially recommended by the U.S. Department of Health and Human Services in the Center for Disease Control's *Morbidity and Mortality Weekly Report*, although neither was suggested to be the better choice in this document.[1] In addition to aerosolized pentamidine and Bactrim, dapsone and dapsone plus pyrimethamine are currently being used or considered by clinicians and patients and are being tested in clinical trials. These drugs may have the additional advantage of preventing toxoplasmosis.

Bactrim was the first successful pneumocystis prophylaxis used in adults and children with cancer or organ transplants. It was routinely used for this purpose in the late 1970s,[4,5] before AIDS was recognized. It was also the first drug used to prevent pneumocystis in people with HIV infection, before the development of aerosolized pentamidine. Even though it was shown to be very effective in preventing pneumocystis,[6] its toxicities (severe rash, anemia, neutropenia, nausea, etc.) encouraged doctors, researchers, and patients to search for alternative approaches.

By the late 1980s, the apparent effectiveness of aerosolized pentamidine, and the relatively fewer and milder side effects associated with it, made it the drug of choice among many patients and clinicians. Aerosolized pentamidine was preferable to some from a theoretical standpoint because delivering a toxic drug directly to the site of action seemed safer than delivering it to the whole body. This theory assumed, however, that pneumocystis only causes disease in the lungs, which we now know is not true.

Recently the following questions have been raised in an attempt to understand which of these two regimens, aerosolized pentamidine or Bactrim, may be best as a first choice for prophylaxis: (1) Is one drug more effective than the other? (2) Is there an increased incidence of pneumocystis infections in organs other than the lung (extrapulmonary pneumocystis) in patients using aerosolized pentamidine compared to those using the systemic drug Bactrim? (3) Is there an increased incidence in collapsed lungs (spontaneous pneumothorax) associated with the use of aerosolized pentamidine? (4) Can Bactrim be used more safely but just as effectively by using it less often? (5) Does the use of aerosolized pentamidine make diagnosis of break-through pneumocystis by chest x-ray, sputum, and bronchoalveolar lavage (fluid collected during a bronchoscopy) more difficult than does a systemic prophylaxis? (6) How do the issues of cost and convenience fit into the risk/benefit equation? While aerosolized pentamidine costs an average of $1,200 per year for the drug alone, not including the significant costs associated with administering the treatment, Bactrim (or generic equivalents) may cost as little as $12 per year.

## Aerosolized Pentamidine vs. Bactrim: Relative Safety and Efficacy

The ideal way to determine which prophylaxis works best is to compare the two directly in a large, controlled, prospective clinical trial. Unfortunately, no such data is yet available. An ongoing government-sponsored trial comparing these two drugs is completing enrollment of patients at this time (ACTG 021). According to David Hardy, M.D., one of the principal investigators overseeing the study, the results are not expected to be available in the next several months. The data will be looked at periodically by a panel of experts (called a Data and Safety Monitoring Board), however, and significant results will be publicized if they are found before completion of the study.

Many physicians suspect that dapsone is comparably effective to aerosolized pentamidine or Bactrim. Enrollment of a large government-sponsored trial comparing these three drugs has been completed (ACTG 081). This trial is scheduled to run until June of 1992. The principal investigator, Sam Bozette, M.D., of the University of California at San Diego, does not expect the trial to be completed early because he does not expect to see a large difference in the incidence of pneumocystis or adverse reactions among the three groups.

Results of these two clinical trials should provide important information about the relative efficacy of these three approaches. In addition to the relative incidence of both pulmonary and extrapulmonary pneumocystis, the incidence of toxoplasmosis and bacterial infections among the different groups will also be analyzed, with the expectation that the systemic drugs may decrease the incidence of those infections as well. Finally, the incidence of anemia will be compared among the groups to see if the systemic drugs cause a significantly greater incidence of anemia than does aerosolized pentamidine.

The only controlled trial of Bactrim for prophylaxis of AIDS-related pneumocystis published in a peer-reviewed journal to date is a Bactrim vs. no-treatment trial in patients with Kaposi's sarcoma which was published in 1988.[6] The treated group (2 tablets a day plus 5 mg of leucovorin calcium) experienced no pneumocystis, whereas 53 percent in the no-treatment group were diagnosed with pneumocystis. Although effective, 50 percent of those receiving Bactrim experienced toxicities (rash, nausea), and 17 percent had to discontinue the prophylaxis.

Several uncontrolled studies were presented in San Francisco at the Sixth International Conference on AIDS in June. Results from a Danish trial of 122 people who had previously had at least one episode of pneumocystis showed relapse in 8 of the 122 patients, who were using one double-strength tablet of Bactrim daily, in a mean time of 13.1 months.[7] In another study, a retrospective chart review found no pneumocystis in patients taking Bactrim once per day for 3, 6, 9, and 12 months.[8] The authors concluded that Bactrim was effective in preventing pneumocystis when compared to an expected rate of 13 percent at 6 months and 24 percent at 12 months in patients not using a prophylaxis. This study was small (21 patients at 12 months and 45 patients at 6 months) and uncontrolled, but strongly suggestive of Bactrim's efficacy.

A recently published controlled, randomized, dose-comparison study of aerosolized pentamidine initiated by the San Francisco County Community Consortium (now the Community Consortium) in 1987 showed a significant decrease in the incidence of pneumocystis in patients receiving 300 mg of aerosolized pentamidine once a month as compared to those receiving 30 mg every two weeks.[9] According to the principal investigator of this study, Gifford Leoung, M.D., of San Francisco General Hospital, the use of 300 mg of aerosolized pentamidine once a month reduced the incidence of pneumocystis to approximately 12 to 15 percent of that previously seen in patients who used no prophylaxis. This study, which was completed in December, 1988, was instrumental in obtaining official FDA approval of aerosolized pentamidine, making prophylaxis widely available to many people with AIDS for the first time.

Clearly, both Bactrim and aerosolized pentamidine are effective in decreasing the incidence of pneumocystis. But neither is 100 percent safe and effective. Although aerosolized pentamidine has become the most common prophylactic choice in many areas of the U.S., researchers and clinicians have raised a number of concerns about its use. We spoke with Sam Bozette, M.D., the principal investigator on the U.S. government-sponsored study of aerosolized pentamidine vs. Bactrim vs. Dapsone, discussed above. Although data from that study is not yet available, and Dr. Bozette has not seen any of it, he shared the following thoughts with us based on clinical experience and his understanding of the biology of the disease and the mechanisms of the drugs available:

- He believes Bactrim should be the first line prophylaxis. In his opinion, a systemic approach makes more sense than a local approach. While acknowledging that aerosolized pentamidine is effective, Dr. Bozette doubts the ability to deliver the drug to all the areas in the lung where it is needed. He pointed out the increased incidence of pneumocystis in the top portions of the lungs in patients on aerosolized pentamidine prophylaxis.

- Dr. Bozette also pointed out the increased incidence of extrapulmonary pneumocystis associated with the use of aerosolized pentamidine, which he believes would be prevented with the use of a systemic drug like Bactrim. Although several small studies presented at the Sixth International Conference on AIDS addressed the issue of extrapulmonary pneumocystis in patients using aerosolized pentamidine, none compared the incidence in those using aerosolized pentamidine with those using a systemic drug like Bactrim or Dapsone.[10] Therefore, while it may seem likely that delivering the prophylactic treatment to the whole body (as with Bactrim or dapsone) instead of only to the lung (as with aerosolized pentamidine) would reduce the incidence of extrapulmonary pneumocystis, we cannot be sure that this is, in fact, the case.

- Dr. Bozette also noted, with the same reservation about a lack of comparative data, the potential increased incidence of spontaneous pneumothorax (collapsed lung) in patients on aerosolized pentamidine. Clinicians and researchers disagree on whether aerosolized pentamidine directly causes this problem. A recent study found 12 pneumothoraces in 327 patients on aerosolized pentamidine; of these, 83 percent required a chest tube, and 6 of the 12 patients died. Seventy-five percent of those with pneumothorax had evidence of active pneumocystis. The researchers concluded that the pneumothorax was not directly caused by use of aerosolized pentamidine, but rather "represents a prophylaxis failure with a high mortality rate...[Their] pathologic and clinical observations in patients receiving aerosolized pentamidine with spontaneous pneumothorax indicate that there are areas of the lung with inadequately controlled infection with *P. carinii*."[11] The problem remains that there is no data to compare the rate of pneumothorax in patients treated with systemic drugs like Bactrim or dapsone to that in patients using aerosolized pentamidine.

- Dr. Bozette also addressed the concern that the use of aerosolized pentamidine might make diagnosis, and thus management, of pneumocystis more difficult, as the number of organisms would be decreased by the aerosolized pentamidine even if they are not eliminated completely. At the Sixth International Conference on AIDS in June, researcher Henry Masur, M.D., reported that both sputum yield and the ability to diagnose pneumocystis using bronchoalveolar lavage fluid are decreased with the use of aerosolized pentamidine. However, a study presented at the recent Thirtieth Interscience Conference on Antimicrobial Agents and Chemotherapy (ICAAC, October 21–24, 1990, in Atlanta) found no difference in the ability to detect the organism in sputum samples or bronchoalveolar lavage fluid of patients using or not using aerosolized pentamidine.[12] The question remains open.

When asked which prophylactic treatment he would recommend if a patient failed Bactrim, Dr. Bozette said that the following factors should be taken into account: 1) if the patient does not want to take more pills or is anemic or otherwise intolerant of antiretroviral therapy, he would recommend aerosolized pentamidine; 2) if, however, the patient were allergic to Bactrim, and did not have any of the other problems, he would recommend dapsone as the second choice. Dr. Bozette emphasized that the patient's preference is a very important variable in this decision-making process.

Dr. Leoung, principal investigator for the San Francisco aerosolized pentamidine study referred to above, suggested several circumstances in which aerosolized pentamidine may be a better first choice than one of the systemic drugs. Because aerosolized pentamidine does not get into the circulation, it may be a better choice in pregnant women, as there is some risk to the fetus associated with the use of the systemic drugs. Also, the government only pays for aerosolized pentamidine, because Bactrim is not FDA-approved for pneumocystis prophylaxis. Although Bactrim is much less expensive than aerosolized pentamidine, this bit of bureaucratic logic may pose a problem for some patients. Also, some patients may be taking other medication which should not be combined with Bactrim. And for some, the convenience of a monthly treatment is an important factor.

## If Bactrim, How Much? How Often?

Official US recommendations suggest that Bactrim should be used twice a day, together with daily leucovorin. Most physicians do not prescribe leucovorin, and many use Bactrim less often than every day. The data on Bactrim use in pediatric cancer patients demonstrated that there was no difference in its effectiveness when used daily as opposed to three times a week.[4,13] In *AIDS Treatment News* issue #106, Dr. Marcus Conant reported on the successful use of Bactrim two times a day, twice a week by Cooper, from Australia. A study published but not presented at the Sixth International Conference on AIDS reported a decrease in the incidence of moderate and severe side effects (rash, nausea) with one tablet per day as opposed to two tablets every day or two tablets three times a week; this study included almost 200 participants.[14]

Four studies presented at the recent ICAAC conference suggest that one tablet taken three times a week is safe and effective in preventing pneumocystis. Two of these studies were retrospective chart reviews which looked at the incidence of pneumocystis and side effects in patients taking one tablet thrice weekly. The first study[15] found no pneumocystis in 115 patients followed for an average of 20 months (range 3-46); the second[16] found one case of pneumocystis in 64 patients followed for approximately 8 months (primary prophylaxis) or over 9 months (secondary prophylaxis). Twenty-nine percent of the people in the first study experienced side effects (rash, nausea, vomit, rare fever) and 13 percent discontinued therapy; only three of the 64 patients discontinued therapy in the second study.

A third study[17] compared, via retrospective chart review, daily (18 patients) vs. thrice weekly (35 patients) Bactrim. There was one case of pneumocystis. There was a higher incidence of anemia in the thrice weekly treatment group but higher incidences of neutropenia, nausea, and vomiting in the daily treatment group. The incidence of toxicity which required discontinuation of Bactrim was approximately equal in the two groups.

The fourth study, also a chart review,[18] demonstrated a lower incidence of pneumocystis in patients on thrice weekly Bactrim than those on aerosolized pentamidine (7 percent vs. 20 percent with a total of almost 100 patients). All of these studies were relatively small chart reviews, as opposed to large, controlled studies, and thus provide strong suggestive, though not conclusive, data about the effectiveness of one Bactrim tablet three times per week.

## Dapsone With or Without Pyrimethamine

The general consensus in the medical community is that there is not enough data to determine the efficacy of dapsone in preventing pneumocystis, but that it is expected to be approximately as effective as Bactrim. The most serious toxicity associated with dapsone is hemolytic anemia; patients should have their G6PD (glucose-6-phosphate dehydrogenase, an enzyme) levels tested before taking dapsone because the anemia can be severe in patients with a G6PD deficiency.

A study with almost 200 people presented at the June, 1990, Sixth International Conference on AIDS found a statistically non-significant difference in the incidence of pneumocystis and the length of time to infection between a group treated with aerosolized pentamidine (100 mg every two weeks) and dapsone (100 mg twice a week). Although not statistically significant, the dapsone group did have a slightly lower incidence and a slightly longer disease-free interval.[19]

Dapsone was compared with Bactrim in a study presented at the Fifth International Conference on AIDS in Montreal;[20] two out of 173 in the dapsone group vs. none of 48 in the Bactrim group developed pneumocystis. Only 10 percent of the dapsone group experienced adverse reactions requiring termination of therapy, as opposed to 38 percent of the Bactrim group. Treatment was studied for an average of eight to nine months. Importantly, patients who were allergic to one drug generally tolerated the other.

Two short, small studies presented at the Sixth International Conference on AIDS looked at the safety and effectiveness of dapsone plus pyrimethamine.[21] Anemia was the primary toxicity and was usually tolerable. Nausea, vomiting, and rash also occurred in a small number of participants. No pneumocystis developed in 20 patients with a mean follow up of 6.5 months (range 4-16 months).

## Preventing Toxoplasmosis Too?

Dapsone may have the additional advantage of preventing toxoplasmosis, especially when used with pyrimethamine, one of the standard treatments for this disease. When asked by a doctor in the audience at the Sixth International Conference on AIDS if he believed Bactrim could prevent toxoplasmosis, Dr. Henry Masur from the National Institutes of Health replied that Bactrim was not effective against toxoplasmosis in animals or in the test tube, but that he expected that dapsone plus pyrimethamine or the new Burroughs Wellcome drug 566C80 (see below) would have broad anti-parasitic activity against it, as well as against pneumocystis. Another combination he suggested for further study is dapsone plus trimethoprim for those who are allergic to the sulfamethoxazole in Bactrim. (Note that some physicians and researchers do expect that Bactrim may also prevent toxoplasmosis; this question is being addressed in the two government-sponsored trials discussed above.)

## A Note on Fansidar

Fansidar (sulfadoxine-pyrimethamine) continues to be studied in some European countries, but has largely fallen out of favor as a pneumocystis prophylaxis in the U.S. because of its rare but potentially fatal side effects. It has been associated with a severe allergic reaction called Steven's-Johnson syndrome. For more information, consult the *Physicians' Desk Reference.*

## Experimental Prophylaxi: A Promising New Drug: 566C80

566C80 is a member of an anti-parasitic class of drugs called naphthoquinones. Unlike the treatments now in use, it may be able to destroy the cysts in which pneumocystis lives in a latent state in the human body. It may also be useful in the prevention and treatment of other parasitic opportunistic infections in AIDS, such as toxoplasmosis and cryptosporidiosis.

The drug has been demonstrated by researchers at Burroughs Wellcome and St. Jude's Children's Research Hospital in Memphis, Tennessee, to be effective in test-tube and animal studies.[22,23]

An early human study[24] examined the safety of increasing doses of 566C80 in six groups of four people each. The only adverse reaction was a rash in one person at the highest dose; the rash cleared after the drug was discontinued. More studies are currently underway or being designed to examine the safety and efficacy of this drug in the treatment and prophylaxis of pneumocystis. Those who are interested in more information about these studies can call 800/TRIALS-A for eligibility information and referrals to the appropriate study sites.

For a more complete discussion of the research on this compound, see *Treatment Issues*, volume 4, number 7 (published by Gay Men's Health Crisis, Department of Medical Information, 129 West 20th Street, New York, NY 10011).

## Other Experimental Approaches

The *pneumocystis carinii* organism which causes pneumocystis has characteristics of both protozoa and fungi. Several preliminary animal studies presented at the ICAAC conference examined the effectiveness of a group of compounds that are believed to be effective against the fungal properties of the organism. Researchers from Merck Sharp and Dohme and Eli Lilly presented data on beta-1,3-glucan synthase inhibitors. Beta glucan is a structural component of many fungal cell walls.

The most compelling data[25] compared the effects of one of these drugs, L671,329, with Bactrim and pentamidine in treating rats with pneumocystis. More than 98 percent of the cysts were eliminated in those rats treated with L671,329 after 4 days; those rats treated with the other two drugs showed no significant differences in cyst load after 4 days as compared to control rats. A second beta-1,3-glucan synthase inhibitor, L687,781, was shown to be less potent, but effective, in eliminating cysts (greater than 83 percent after five days of treatment).[26] L671,329 was also reported to be an effective prophylaxis in the immunosuppressed rats.

A third study[27] evaluated cilofungin and echinocandin B in rats and found that the cysts in the lungs were swollen and that the nuclei indicated cell death. The authors of this study suggested that these compounds were effective in both treatment and prophylaxis.

We expect continuing improvement in pneumocystis prevention and treatment, as more information becomes available through pre-clinical research (laboratory and animal studies) and clinical trials.

# REFERENCES

1.  U.S. Department of Health and Human Services, Public Health Service. Guidelines for prophylaxis against *Pneumocystis carinii* pneumonia for persons infected with human immunodeficiency virus. *Morbidity and Mortality Weekly Report (MMWR) Recommendations and Reports.* June 16, 1989; volume 38, number S-5.

2.  Pneumocystis prophylaxis survey results reported in *The Synopsis of the Community Consortium.* July 3, 1990; volume 3, number. 7. [The Community Consortium is a group of health-care providers who are involved in community-based clinical research. The majority of these providers practice in the San Francisco Bay Area.]

3.  Kovacs A, Church J, Mascola L, and others. CD4 counts as predictors of *Pneumocystis carinii* pneumonia in infants and children with HIV infection [abstract F.B.24]. Sixth International Conference on AIDS, San Francisco, June 20-24, 1990.

4.  Hughes WT, Kuhn S, Chaudhary S, and others. Successful chemoprophylaxis for *Pneumocystis carinii* pneumonia. *The New England Journal of Medicine.* December 29, 1977; volume 297, pages 1419-1426.

5.  Harris RE, McCallister JA, Allen SA, Barton AS, and Baehner RL. Prevention of pneumocystis pneumonia. Use of continuous sulfamethoxazole-trimethoprim therapy. *American Journal of Diseases of Children.* 1980; volume 134, number 1, pages 35-38.

6.  Fischl M A, Dickinson G M, and La Voie L. Safety and efficacy of sulfamethoxazole and trimethoprim chemoprophylaxis for *Pneumocystis carinii* pneumonia. *Journal of the American Medical Association.* February 26, 1988; volume 259, pages 1185-1189.

7.  Nielsen T L, Jensen B N, Nelsing S and others. Sulfamethoxazole/trimethoprim as secondary prophylaxis against *Pneumocystis carinii* pneumonia [abstract Th.B.412]. Sixth International Conference on AIDS, San Francisco, June 20-24, 1990.

8.  Kelly J, Keyes C, Marte C, Wolbert J, and Chieffe R. Once daily trimethoprim/ sulfamethoxazole as prophylaxis for *Pneumocystis carinii* pneumonia [abstract Th.B.413]. Sixth International Conference on AIDS, San Francisco, June 20-24, 1990.

9.  Leoung GS, Feigal DW, Montgomery AB, and others. Aerosolized pentamidine for prophylaxis against *Pneumocystis carinii* pneumonia. *The New England Journal of Medicine.* September 20, 1990; volume 323, number 12.

10. McCabe R and Edelstein H. Atypical *Pneumocystis carinii* pneumonia in patients receiving inhaled pentamidine prophylaxis [abstract 426]. Also Denis M, Guidet B, and Lebas J. Clinical data of disseminated *Pneumocystis carinii* infection in 6 AIDS patients receiving secondary prophylaxis with aerosolized pentamidine [abstract 427]. Also Noskin G, Murphy R L, Finn W G, and Timins M. Extrapulmonary *Pneumocystis carinii* in patients receiving aerosolized Pentamidine [abstract 428]. Sixth International Conference on AIDS, San Francisco, June 20-24, 1990.

11. Newsome GS, Ward DJ, and Pierce PF. Spontaneous pneumo-thorax in patients with acquired immunodeficiency syndrome treated with prophylactic aerosolized pentamidine. *Archives of Internal Medicine.* October 1990; volume 150, pages 2167-2168.

12. Geaghan S, Fahey J, McGinty E, and others. Impact of prophylactic aerosolized pentamidine on the laboratory diagnosis of *Pneumocystis carinii* pneumonia [abstract 850]. 30th Interscience Conference on Antimicrobial Agents and Chemotherapy, Atlanta, October 21-24, 1990.

13. Hughes, WT and others. Successful intermittent chemoprophylaxis for *Pneumocystis carinii* pneumonia. *New England Journal of Medicine.* 1987; volume 316, pages 1627-1632.

14. Wolbert J, Keyes C, Chieffe R, Marte C, Kelly J, and Holzman R S. Side effects of prophylactic trimethoprim/sulfamethoxazole are diminished with once daily dosing [abstract 2086]. Sixth International Conference on AIDS, San Francisco, June 20-24, 1990.

15. Lariviere M and Ruskin J. Low dose trimethoprim/sulfamethoxazole prevents *Pneumocystis carinii* pneumonia [abstract 8]. 30th Interscience Conference on Antimicrobial Agents and Chemotherapy, Atlanta, October 21-24, 1990.

16. Stein D S, Terry D, Palte S, Lancaster D J, and Weems J J. Thrice weekly dosing of trimethoprim/sulfamethoxazole for primary and secondary prophylaxis of *Pneumocystis carinii* pneumonia [abstract 854]. 30th Interscience Conference on Antimicrobial Agents and Chemotherapy, Atlanta, October 21-24, 1990.

17. Morgan A, Graziani A, and MacGregor R R. Daily versus intermittent trimethoprim/sulfamethoxazole for *Pneumocystis carinii* pneumonia [abstract 856]. 30th Interscience Conference on Antimicrobial Agents and Chemotherapy, Atlanta, October 21-24, 1990.

18. Catena W, De Luca A, and Perez G. Efficacy of low dose trimethoprim/sulfamethoxazole in pneumocystis prophylaxis [abstract 857]. 30th Interscience Conference on Antimicrobial Agents and Chemotherapy, Atlanta, October 21-24, 1990.

19. Torres R, Thorn M, Newlands J, and others. Randomized trial of intermittent dapsone versus aerosolized pentamidine for primary and secondary prophylaxis of *Pneumocystis carinii* pneumonia [abstract Th.B.407]. Sixth International Conference on AIDS, San Francisco, June 20-24, 1990.

20. Metroka C, Jacobus D, and Lewis N. Successful chemoprophylaxis for pneumocystis with dapsone or Bactrim [abstract T.B.0.4]. Fifth International Conference on AIDS, Montreal, June 4-9, 1989.

21. Ogata-Arakaki D, Falloon J, Lavelle J, and others. The safety of weekly dapsone and weekly dapsone and pyrimethamine as pneumocystis prophylaxis [abstract Th.B.411]. Also Clotet B, Sirera G, Romeu J, Velasco P, Gimeno J M, and Tor J. Twice weekly dapsone-pyrimethamine for preventing *Pneumocystis carinii* pneumonia relapses in HIV infected patients [abstract Th.B.414]. Sixth International Conference on AIDS, San Francisco, June 20-24, 1990.

22. Rogers M D and Lafon S W. *In vivo* and *in vitro* anti-*Pneumocystis carinii* activity of the hydroxynaphthoquinone, 566C80 [abstract 588]. 30th Interscience Conference on Antimicrobial Agents and Chemotherapy, Atlanta, October 21-24, 1990.

23. Hughes WT and others. Efficacy of a hydroxynaphthoquinone, 566C80, in experimental *Pneumocystis carinii* pneumonia. *Antimicrobial Agents and Chemotherapy.* 1990; volume 34, pages 225-228.

24. Hughes W, Kennedy W, Shenep J, and others. Safety and pharmacokinetics of 566C80, a hydroxynaphthoquinone with anti-*Pneumocystis carinii* activity [abstract 861]. 30th Interscience Conference on Antimicrobial Agents and Chemotherapy, Atlanta, October 21-24, 1990.

25. Romancheck J A, Pittarelli L A, and Schmatz D M. A comparative study of the anti-pneumocystis activity of L671,329, trimethoprim/sulfamethoxazole and pentamidine isethionate [abstract 586]. 30th Interscience Conference on Antimicrobial Agents and Chemotherapy, Atlanta, October 21-24, 1990.

26. Schmatz D M, Romancheck M A, Pittarelli L A, Nollstadt K, Bartizal K, and Turner M J. The use of ß 1,3 glucan synthesis inhibitors for the treatment and prevention of *Pneumocystis carinii* pneumonia [abstract 585]. 30th Interscience Conference on Antimicrobial Agents and Chemotherapy, Atlanta, October 21-24, 1990.

27. Rogers M D and Lafon S W. *In vivo* and *in vitro* anti-*Pneumocystis carinii* activity of the hydroxynaphthoquinone, 566C80 [abstract 588]. 30th Interscience Conference on Antimicrobial Agents and Chemotherapy, Atlanta, October 21-24, 1990.

# NIAID RECOMMENDS CORTICOSTEROIDS IN PNEUMOCYSTIS TREATMENT

On October 10 the U.S. National Institutes of Allergy and Infectious Diseases published a note to physicians, "Important Information on the Clinical Benefit of Systemic Corticosteroids As Adjunctive Therapy for *Pneumocystis carinii* Pneumonia in AIDS." Several studies have found that early use of these steroids could cut death rates by half or more in cases of moderate or severe pneumocystis. No benefit was shown with mild disease.

To evaluate these studies, NIAID and the University of California, San Diego, convened a consensus panel in May, 1990. The panel's conclusions, together with two of the studies, will be published in November in *The New England Journal of Medicine*. The note to physicians was published earlier to make the information immediately available.

A copy of the note to physicians, including specific recommendations of the consensus panel, can be obtained by calling 800/TRIALS-A.

# IMUTHIOL APPROVED IN NEW ZEALAND

On October 25 the drug Imuthiol (also known as DTC, or diethyldithiocarbamate, or dithiocarb) was officially approved for marketing in New Zealand—the first country to grant marketing approval. The drug is indicated for persons over 18, who either have a T-helper count under 200, or who have symptomatic HIV infection and cannot tolerate AZT, regardless of T-helper count.

## Comment

Imuthiol has been studied as an AIDS/HIV treatment for years. Placebo-controlled studies have repeatedly found sustained T-helper increases and reduced opportunistic infections in persons using the drug. Nevertheless, in the U.S. there has been widespread skepticism about its efficacy. Also, we do not know why it has not been approved in France, where it was developed by Pasteur Merieux.

*AIDS Treatment News* first covered research on Imuthiol in issue #29, when a multicenter controlled study was taking place in San Francisco and five other U.S. sites. At that time we predicted that "If all goes well, DTC could be approved sometime in 1988." All did not go well, of course; unexpected and sometimes inexplicable delays intervened.

Is this a drug which should have been approved long ago—or are the existing data unconvincing—or, given the drug's safety, are both statements true? We do not know. Imuthiol is one of many potential treatments which deserves in-depth followup; we cannot pursue them all. It is urgent that more people become involved in such investigation.

# ORAL INTERFERON: LOS ANGELES STUDY DOES NOT FIND BENEFIT

An observational study of 167 patients using low-dose oral alpha interferon (the active ingredient in the "Kemron" treatment from Kenya) did not find any beneficial or harmful effect from the treatment. This study was conducted between June and October of 1990 by doctors Paul J. Rothman, D.O., and Robert Jenkins, M.D.; it was organized and financed by SEARCH Alliance, a new community-based research organization in Los Angeles. (For background on SEARCH Alliance, see *AIDS Treatment News* issue #105; for background on the low-dose oral interferon treatment, see issue #101).

The average T-helper count of the volunteers beginning the treatment was 141.4. The average after treatment was 131.8; the difference was not statistically significant (meaning that the difference was small enough that it could easily have been due to chance). Statistical analysis also showed no difference in response between those who started with T-helper counts under 200, compared to those starting with higher counts.

While T-helper counts declined in most study participants, 25 percent had rises of greater than 10 percent in their baseline values. (Note: such rises can be caused by laboratory errors, and/or by the variable course of HIV infection. They do not necessarily mean that these patients benefited from the treatment.) P24 antigen was lower at weeks two and four than at baseline, but higher than baseline at weeks six and eight; neither result was statistically significant.

## Comment

While this study cannot conclusively disprove the treatment—to do that would be almost impossible—it provides practical information that people need now. Supporters of Kemron can argue that there are different kinds of alpha interferon, and the medicine used by these study volunteers was not identical to that used in Kenya. Also, the doses could not be tightly controlled. And this was not a randomized trial, so there could be unknown biases due to self-selection by the volunteers who entered the study.

We find little practical weight in these arguments. There is no reason to believe that the small differences between various versions of alpha interferon could make the difference between a valuable treatment and no effect at all. As for dosage, if it was not controlled then it would have varied over a range which presumably would have included the effective dose in some volunteers; therefore, if the treatment worked at any dose, at least some average effect should have been seen. And it makes little sense to discount this study as not being a randomized controlled trial, since having a placebo or other control group would not have made the drug work any better than it did. People need practical answers quickly, not perfect answers in future years.

We commend SEARCH Alliance for its effectiveness in quickly organizing this study. The group announced its existence only five months ago. It has finished a useful study before most research organizations could have made the decision to start one.

For a copy of the data tabulation and analysis of this study, send a self-addressed stamped envelope to: SEARCH Alliance, 7461 Beverly Blvd., Suite 304, Los Angeles, CA 90036.

## CONGRESS GRANTS FLEXIBILITY IN TRAVEL RESTRICTION: 1992 HARVARD CONFERENCE IS ON

On October 27 the U.S. Congress passed and sent to the President an immigration bill including a provision which allows the Department of Health and Human Services to decide whether HIV-positive visitors can enter the United States. President Bush has said that he will sign the bill.

The travel restrictions had caused over 140 organizations to boycott the June, 1990, Sixth International Conference on AIDS in San Francisco, and could have cancelled the May, 1992, Eighth International Conference planned for Boston. Harvard University, which along with the International AIDS Society is sponsoring the 1992 Conference, had announced that it would withdraw its sponsorship if Congress did not act on the travel restrictions this year (see story in *Science*, September 28, 1990, page 1495). Although over a year remains before the Conference, expensive commitments must be made far in advance, and it might not have been possible to move the meeting elsewhere.

The new law will not by itself end the travel ban. But it clearly makes the Bush Administration and its Department of Health and Human Services responsible for the decision. Public-health experts within HHS had called for removing the travel restrictions for all diseases except tuberculosis. But the White House said that it could not change the policy on HIV (although it could on all other diseases), because HIV alone had been added to the list by Congress, in 1987 legislation sponsored by Senator Jesse Helms (Republican, North Carolina).

The travel restrictions remain in effect, and no immediate change is expected. Health and Human Services must analyze what the new law requires it to do, and then formulate its policies. But the new legislation ends the stalemate under which both Congress and the White House were passing the buck to each other.

Major credit for the improvement belongs to Massachusetts legislators Senator Edward Kennedy and Congressman Barney Frank, and to Harvard University.

## INTERNATIONAL COMPUTER CONFERENCE: CALL FOR EXPERTISE

*AIDS Treatment News* is investigating options for international computer communication about AIDS, by medical scientists and others (see "Proposal: Computerized International Publication of AIDS Research Results," issue #102). One motive for this project had been to substitute for the 1992 Eighth International Conference on AIDS in Boston, when it appeared likely that that Conference would be cancelled due to U.S. travel restrictions on persons with HIV (see article above). Now the Boston meeting is proceeding, but there are other reasons for facilitating computer links for researchers and others involved with AIDS.

The large international meetings occur during five days each year; they would be more productive if participants could develop relationships and initiate projects in advance. Computer communication is available every day of the year, 24 hours a day, from any place with adequate telephone service. "Computer conferences" and traditional face-to-face conferences have different strengths; neither can adequately replace the other.

Our role at *AIDS Treatment News* is not to set up a computer system—we do not have the resources to do so—but to find out what is happening already in international computer communication about AIDS, then tell others what resources are available to them, and how they can gain access.

There is no time for re-inventing the wheel. Therefore we think the system should start with the major academic computer networks which already exist and have links throughout most of the world. From there, "gateway" facilities and organizations can make communication available to those without academic affiliations, including public agencies, private-practice physicians, activist groups, and other community organizations.

For many organizations, fax rather than computers is the appropriate means of communication. Again, gateway organizations can provide links between the computer network and those using fax machines. Therefore, groups can participate in the ongoing electronic conference, even if they have no computer equipment, experience, or access.

If you know about any internationally available computer communication system which is already being used effectively to communicate about AIDS—or if you have other expertise to contribute to this project—contact John S. James at *AIDS Treatment News*, attn: computer, P.O. Box 411256, San Francisco, CA 94141, 415/255-0588.

# Issue Number 115
# November 23, 1990

## DDC/AZT COMBINATION: PROMISING EARLY RESULTS

*by John S. James*

Preliminary results from a dose-finding trial of combination treatment with ddC and AZT suggest that the two drugs together, in small or moderate doses, may work better than standard treatment with AZT alone. These results must be interpreted carefully, however, because the study is still incomplete, and final verification and analysis has not been done; also, it is relatively small, with 48 volunteers. This article reports on the information from this study which has already become publicly known.

The Federally sponsored trial, ACTG 106, is being conducted in Miami and San Diego; principal investigators are Margaret A. Fischl, M.D., and Douglas D. Richman, M.D. The 48 volunteers all had AIDS or advanced ARC, with T-helper counts under 200 when they entered the study. Six different treatment regimens are being compared; the 48 volunteers are divided into six groups of eight each. Five of the six treatment arms combine ddC and AZT; the sixth uses a very low dose of AZT alone. The doses (in milligrams, given every eight hours) are:

| AZT | ddC |
|-----|-------|
| 200 | 0.750 |
| 200 | 0.375 |
| 100 | 0.750 |
| 100 | 0.375 |
| 50 | 0.750 |
| 50 | none |

Since these amounts are given three times a day, the total AZT doses are 600, 300, and 150 mg per day. The high ddC dose is the same as that now being used in the major ddC vs. AZT comparison trials, and the low ddC dose is half that amount. Volunteers were first assigned to the four arms with the higher AZT doses (600 or 300 mg per day). Some groups have been on the treatment for over a year, others for less time.

We have not seen the data, which will of course change as the study progresses. The following overview comes from a recent Project Inform fact sheet, and other published sources cited in the references below.

## Results

Large T-helper increases were found. The Project Inform report cited a median peak increase of 164; the exact figure will change as the study progresses. After reaching this peak, T-helper counts began to decline. We have heard conflicting reports about how far the counts declined, but it is clear that they are above the starting value after one year of the treatment. Both the size of the increase, and the time it was sustained, are much better than with AZT treatment alone—especially for this group of patients, whose median starting T-helper count was under 100. Also, 100 percent of patients in the four treatment arms with the higher AZT doses (600 or 300 mg per day) combined with ddC had increases of at least 50, measured on at least two consecutive tests. These results strongly suggest that the combination treatment has a greater antiviral effect than AZT alone.

What about clinical improvement? Few opportunistic infections have occurred in the study, and all of them occurred within the first few weeks of treatment—none within the remaining time, about 50 weeks for many patients. This clustering of infections early in the study strongly suggests that the regimen was helpful, since with no treatment, the rate of infections would, if anything, have increased. The early infections may have been developing before the treatment's benefit had time to begin. Other clinical improvement was also reported, with median weight gain of about 9 pounds.

Tests will soon be run to look for changes in plasma viral levels, and to see if drug resistance develops during the combination treatment. The researchers do not yet have this information.

## What Should Be Done?

The results already known from ACTG 106 suggest that the combination treatment with ddC and AZT may be substantially better than any standard therapy (i.e., AZT alone), for many patients at least. We do not have conclusive proof, however, because of the relatively small number of volunteers in this study, and because the combination was not directly compared to a standard dose of AZT. Also, this study does not answer the question of how best to use ddC for patients now failing AZT.

What will happen now? The usual procedure would be to run more studies, after finishing this one; with luck, conclusive proof might be available in two years. The problem, of course, is that many people do not have that time to wait. Note that this study applies most directly to those whose HIV infection is relatively advanced.

What should be done is to convene a panel of experts, give them access to all the existing data on ddC and ddI, from all completed and ongoing studies, along with the technical support staff necessary so that they can analyze it. They should be asked whether physicians could provide better care for persons with AIDS or HIV if they had these drugs available, than if they continue to have only AZT. If the answer is yes, for ddC or ddI or both, then the drug(s) should quickly be approved for prescription use, with appropriate labeling, including an explanation of the available evidence which led to approval, and the panel's recommendations to physicians concerning use of the drugs. After approval, postmarketing studies should answer the remaining questions, such as how to best use the drugs for particular patient populations. (Is it better, for example, for patients who have used AZT but are now failing it to switch to ddC or ddI alone, to one of those drugs in combination with AZT, or to alternating use of the drug and AZT?)

## Comment

A number of other studies of human use of ddC are either published, in press, or in process. ddC is being tested alone, in comparison with AZT, and in alternation with AZT. In addition, there are similar studies with ddI; however, the ddI-AZT combination study started later than ACTG 106, so little information is now available. (There is more information now about ddI as a single agent, however, than about ddC; for a review of a recent ddI report, see *AIDS Treatment News* #110.)

Currently, the open-access programs for ddI and ddC have made these drugs available to many patients who cannot use AZT. But these programs are limited because their strict entry criteria exclude many patients who could benefit, without taking individual circumstances into account. Also, they do not allow combination use with AZT—which now seems to be emerging as the best way to use these drugs. And the paperwork required of physicians effectively makes these drugs unavailable to many patients.

The largest ddC and ddI studies are usually set up to compare each of these drugs with AZT. These trials were designed this way because it would have been unethical to test ddC or ddI in a placebo trial, when the standard of care is now AZT. But how these drugs compare to AZT is usually the wrong question, since generally the new drugs will be used for patients who cannot benefit from AZT, or in combination with that drug. The right question is whether physicians can give better care if they have these drugs available in addition to AZT.

The references below list many papers which have already been published on human use of ddC in HIV treatment. But the most important studies are now ongoing. It is urgent that the existing information be brought together and evaluated now, leading to drug approval if appropriate. It would be tragic to wait a year, two years, or more for approval of ddC and ddI, when people need treatment options now.

## REFERENCES

*Note:* This list is not complete. Only the more relevant articles on human use of ddC—especially together with AZT—are included.

American Foundation for AIDS Research. *AIDS/HIV Treatment Directory*. September, 1990; pages 18-19, 43. Also see June, 1990; pages 28-29.

Bozzette SA and Richman DD. Salvage therapy for zidovudine-intolerant HIV-infected patients with alternating and intermittent regimens of zidovudine and dideoxycytidine. *American Journal of Medicine*. May 21, 1990; volume 88, supplement 5B, pages 24S-26S.

Bozzette S, Skowron G, Arrezo J, Spector SA, Pettinelli C, and Richman DD. Alternating and intermittent ddC and AZT in the treatment of persons with advanced HIV infection and hematologic intolerance to AZT [abstract S.B.425]. Sixth International Conference on AIDS, San Francisco, June 20-24, 1990.

Broder S. Pharmacodynamics of 2',3'-dideoxycytidine: an inhibitor of human immunodeficiency virus. *American Journal of Medicine*. May 21, 1990; volume 88, supplement 5B, pages 2S-7S.

Broder S, and Yarchoan R. Dideoxycytidine: Current clinical experience and future prospects— A summary. *American Journal of Medicine*. May 21, 1990; volume 88, supplement 5B, pages 31S-33S.

Dubinsky RM, Yarchoan R, Dalakas M, and Broder S. Reversible axonal neuropathy from the treatment of AIDS and related disorders with 2',3'-dideoxycytidine (ddC). *Muscle and Nerve*. October, 1989; volume 12, number 10, pages 856-860.

Kolata, Gina. Interest grows in licensing shortcut for 2 AIDS drugs. *The New York Times*, Medical Science section, September 25, 1990.

Meng TC, Boota A, Fischl MA, Spector SA, McCaan M, and Richman DD. Phase I/II dose finding study of concurrently administered dideoxycytidine and zidovudine [abstract S.B.426]. Sixth International Conference on AIDS, San Francisco, June 20-24, 1990.

Meng TC, Fischl MA, and Richman DD. AIDS Clinical Trials Group: phase I/II study of combination 2',3'-dideoxycytidine and zidovudine in patients with acquired immunodeficiency syndrome (AIDS) and advanced AIDS-related complex. *American Journal of Medicine*. May 21, 1990; volume 88, supplement 5B, pages 27S-30S.

Merrigan TC, Skowron G, Bozzette SA, and others. Circulating p24 antigen levels and responses to dideoxycytidine in human immunodeficiency virus (HIV) infections. *Annals of Internal Medicine*. February 1,1989; volume 110, pages 189-194.

Merrigan TC and Skowron G. Safety and tolerance of dideoxycytidine as a single agent. Results of early-phase studies in patients with acquired immunodeficiency syndrome (AIDS) or advanced AIDS-related complex. *American Journal of Medicine*. May 21, 1990; volume 88, supplement 5B, pages 11S-15S.

Pizzo PA. Treatment of human immunodeficiency virus-infected infants and young children with dideoxynucleosides. *American Journal of Medicine*. May 21, 1990; volume 88, supplement 5B, pages 16S-19S.

Project Inform, San Francisco. News bulletin, "Combination Therapy," November, 1990.

Richman DD. Susceptibility to nucleoside analogues of zidovudine-resistant isolates of human immunodeficiency virus. *American Journal of Medicine*. May 21, 1990; volume 88, supplement 5B, pages 8S-10S.

Shirasaka T, Yarchoan R, Aoki S, and others. In vitro study of drug-sensitivity of HIV strains isolated from patients with AIDS or ARC before and after therapy with AZT and/or 2',3'-dideoxycytidine (ddC) [abstract Th.A.263]. Sixth International Conference on AIDS, San Francisco, June 20-24, 1990.

Skowron G, and Merrigan TC. Phase II trial of alternating and intermittent regimens of zidovudine and 2',3'-dideoxycytidine in ARC and AIDS [abstract Th.B.23]. Sixth International Conference on AIDS, San Francisco, June 20-24, 1990.

Skowron G, and Merrigan TC. Alternating and intermittent regimens of zidovudine and dideoxycytidine in the treatment of patients with acquired immunodeficiency syndrome (AIDS) and AIDS-related complex. *American Journal of Medicine*. May 21, 1990; volume 88, supplement 5B, pages 20S-23S.

Yarchoan R, Pluda JM, Thomas RV, Pemo CF, McAtee N, and Broder S. Long-term (18 month) treatment of severe HIV infection with an alternating regimen of AZT and 2',3'-dideoxycytidine (ddC) [abstract W.B.P.327]. Fifth International Conference on AIDS, Montreal, June 4-9, 1989.

# ACYCLOVIR RESISTANT HERPES: NEW TREATMENT OPTION?

*by Michelle Roland*

Three anecdotal case reports have recently come to our attention about a potentially effective treatment for acyclovir-resistant herpes. The treatment, an ophthalmic (eye) solution called trifluridine (also called Viroptic, or trifluorothymidine), is available by prescription. It is currently used to treat patients with herpes simplex keratitis, an infection of the cornea of the eye.

The only published report on trifluridine treatment of acyclovir-resistant herpes in a person with HIV infection was presented at the Sixth International Conference on AIDS in San Francisco in June, 1990 [Doherty and others, abstract Th.B.446]. This patient first had acyclovir-resistant herpes lesions which responded to foscarnet. However, a subsequent lesion was resistant to both acyclovir and foscarnet. Two other topical treatments (idoxuridine cream; interferon gel alone) were tried but failed in this patient before she responded to the combination of trifluridine and interferon with "considerable but incomplete healing."

Two other cases were discussed by Harold Kessler, M.D., from Rush-Presbyterian St. Luke's Medical Center in Chicago, at the recent meeting of the AIDS Clinical Trials Group (ACTG) in Washington, D.C. (The ACTG is a research program of the National Institute of Allergy and Infectious Diseases of the National Institutes of Health; it is the group which conducts the bulk of the Federally sponsored AIDS clinical research in this country.) Dr. Kessler emphasized that there is no proof that trifluridine is effective in acyclovir-resistant herpes, because there have been no studies of this treatment. In addition, he knows of a total of only four episodes of herpes in three patients who were treated with this drug. However, he agreed that this information should be made available to patients and physicians before the completion of a controlled study since there are few alternative treatments currently available to people with herpes lesions that are resistant to both acyclovir and foscarnet.

Dr. Kessler described applying a thin film of the solution over a well-cleansed lesion. He then covered the lesion with a thin layer of Polysporin ointment to keep the solution in contact with the lesion. Gauze was placed over the lesion. The medication and dressing were changed three times a day. One patient (with a lesion of three by four centimeters) responded in four to five weeks. This patient relapsed with a lesion that was next to the original one. The second lesion healed within two weeks with treatment with trifluridine. A second patient was treated at another medical center and had a complete response in two weeks.

Dr. Kessler emphasized that this treatment is not a cure for herpes simplex infections. New lesions will occur after treatment with any anti-herpes drug. However, new lesions may be susceptible to acyclovir and/or foscarnet.

An open-label prospective study of this drug is being designed for people with chronic cutaneous herpes which is suspected of being acyclovir resistant. In the meantime, Dr. Kessler has requested that physicians trying trifluridine send viral isolates for acyclovir and foscarnet resistance testing to his laboratory in Chicago so that the effectiveness of trifluridine can be assessed before the official study is under way. *Physicians* can reach Dr. Kessler at 312/942-5865 (Division of Infectious Diseases, Rush-Presbyterian St. Luke's Medical Center, Chicago).

## PML: UPDATED REPORT AVAILABLE

A severe opportunistic viral infection of the brain called progressive multifocal leukoencephalopathy (PML) has long been considered by the medical establishment to be untreatable. But over a year ago Los Angeles activists Lisa and Peter Brosnan published a compilation of literature discussing experimental treatments for PML (see *AIDS Treatment News* #79, #88 and #100), and they have recently completed an expanded, updated edition. The new report includes case histories collected by the authors, the results of an informal PML survey which they conducted earlier this year, a discussion of the known potential treatments, and several articles reprinted from recent medical literature.

Requests for the report can be sent to 3031 Angus Street, Los Angeles, CA 90039. Urgent requests can be called in to 213/666-0751. The cost of copying and mailing the report is $25 for first class delivery, or $30 for express mail. Persons with AIDS are offered the report for $15, for either kind of mailing; it will be sent free if necessary.

Although no single drug has been *proven* to treat PML, no one facing this diagnosis should be told that there is nothing at all to try. Acyclovir, cytarabine, dexamethasone, heparin, interferon, NAC, and vidarabine have all been tried against PML with varying degrees of success. Peter and Lisa's first report undoubtedly saved lives over the past year, and the new edition promises to build on that accomplishment.

## PNEUMOCYSTIS STEROID CONTROVERSY

*by John S. James*

On November 14 *The New York Times* published a front-page story alleging that news of a consensus panel's recommendation for using steroids in treating certain cases of pneumocystis had been delayed for five months, in part because researchers feared that announcing the information earlier would jeopardize publication of their results in prestigious medical journals. Much press and television coverage followed; *The New York Times* published a followup story on November 16, and a brief note on November 18 ("The Week In Review" section). *AIDS Treatment News* was credited with bringing this story to public attention; our role, however, was minimal, as everything we reported came from a press release and note to physicians from the U.S. National Institute of Allergy and Infectious Diseases (NIAID). We had refrained from adding any comment of our own, as we were torn between criticizing the delay and praising NIAID for calling the consensus panel in the first place and disseminating the recommendations without waiting for journal publication. In AIDS and in other diseases as well, there is a great need for a respected body to determine when a health emergency exists, call experts together to recommend appropriate changes in the standard of care, and then get the recommendations promptly to the physicians who need them.

There is legitimate concern that some researchers or officials may be blamed unjustly for delaying news of the steroid decision. The consensus panel met in May, and NIAID released the results in October. However, there were serious medical issues concerning the recommendations, issues which could not be resolved in a day. Meanwhile, much of the steroid information was publicly available, having been reported at medical meetings and in some journal articles; in San Francisco, a survey by the Community Consortium found that 67 percent of their physicians who responded had already used steroids in this situation. We are not close enough to this issue to know what, if anything, should have been done differently to disseminate the information more rapidly.

Yet the issues raised by these events are clearly real ones. There are glaring deficiencies in how new medical information is communicated to physicians. Some problems do stem from news embargos imposed by some medical journals; many researchers do not believe the public assurances that these embargos do not apply to AIDS or other emergencies. Other problems occur after publication; for example, there are thousands of journals, and physicians have little time for reading. European journals, for instance, often never come to the attention of the U.S. medical community. The development of professional bodies to cut through the noise and focus on what is most important seems to be hindered by the tendency of such groups to be too conservative (the safest position for guarding against future lawsuits or criticism). All too often the final result is a medical mainstream ignorant of relevant research— surrounded by mavericks often working on the fringes of respectability. This system poorly serves the public interest.

The recent controversy over steroid use in pneumocystis succeeded where other efforts failed in alerting all physicians to this treatment development. It also made clear that the public will not stand for unnecessary withholding of lifesaving information. And hopefully it will focus professional attention on the larger problems in medical communication, and on how the dissemination of urgent treatment information can be improved.

## GLYCYRRHIZIN CORRECTION AND UPDATE

*by Denny Smith*

Last May 18, in issue #103 of *AIDS Treatment News*, we published an article on the experimental treatment glycyrrhizin. Since then, we received a communication from Paul Bergner, the editor of *Medical Herbalism*, correcting two points made in that report. The first error in our article regards the exact chemistry of glycyrrhizin. While we believed that it was one of the sulfated polysaccharides, it is actually considered a glucoside, resulting in a significantly different pharmacological profile.

The other inaccuracy involves our inference that glycyrrhizin is used in Europe as a treatment for stomach ulcers. At least some of the European preparations derived from the root of *Glycyrrhiza* have actually been "de-glycyrrhizinated" for use in treating ulcers, since they rely on other components of the plant for their therapeutic effect. We appreciate these corrections, and any others from concerned readers.

Mr. Bergner also mentioned the possible use of the Koenigsburg urine test, which might alert doctors and their patients to possible adverse reactions to glycyrrhizin, before symptoms appear. Persons interested in *Medical Herbalism* can write to P.O.Box 33080, Portland, OR 97233.

**November 23, 1990**

Incidentally, we have found that the Japanese product called Glycyron 2 is available at San Francisco's Healing Alternatives Foundation, a buyers' club which is able to handle mail orders. The number for Healing Alternatives is 415/626-2316.

## WOMEN AND HIV CONFERENCE, DEC. 13–14, WASHINGTON, DC

*by Laura Thomas*

There will be a conference on women and HIV in Washington, DC, on December 13-14, 1990. The conference is free, and is targeted at women with HIV, health care providers, and AIDS service providers. The goals of the conference are to: identify research needs, provide up-to-date treatment information on women with HIV and improve the quality of care they receive, identify the social and economic barriers facing women with HIV and how they affect research, and identify community resources and educate participants on the special needs of women at risk. The conference will be organized in four basic tracks: epidemiology, psychosocial and social issues, education and prevention, and treatments and clinical issues.

The conference was called by the National Institutes of Health after pressure to do so from AIDS activists, especially the women of ACT UP/New York and ACT UP/DC. While this conference will not be as comprehensive or accessible as we would like, it is at least a recognition on the part of the Government that there **is** a problem, and it is a step forward for the NIH in dealing with the issues of women and HIV.

To register or request more information, call Carol Gordon or Debra Steward at 301/770-0610, or 301/770-3153 after 5 pm Eastern time. Interested people should call immediately to get the registration form and send it in, because registration forms should be in by November 30, and space is filling up fast. Attendance is limited to the first 1,000 people, with 100 spaces reserved for women with HIV. Women with HIV infection should note that on their form.

A committee is working to raise money for transportation for women who would not otherwise be able to get to the conference. Individuals who would like to donate money or frequent flyer miles towards travel scholarships can send their donation to: Women and HIV Conference Travel Fund, c/o Denise Rouse, DC Women's Council on AIDS, 725 8th Street, SE, Washington, DC 20003.

People interested in possible scholarships should contact Denise Rouse of the DC Women's Council on AIDS at 202/544-8255.

The conference is also trying to find free community housing in Washington for women with limited funds. Anyone who lives in the Washington area and is able to house a conference participant for a few days can contact Kate Perkins at 301/496-0545.

Many AIDS activists want to get together Saturday, December 15, after the conference, to share information, compare notes, and plan their next steps. Conference participants who are interested in meeting with other activists, women with HIV, and service providers should plan to stay through Saturday. Information will be posted at the conference as to where this meeting will be.

# WORLD AIDS DAY: WOMEN AND AIDS

*by Laura Thomas*

December 1 is World AIDS Day, and the World Health Organization has chosen "Women and AIDS" as this year's theme. There will be actions and events all over the world to mark the day, many of them focusing on women and HIV.

The World Health Organization's very conservative estimate is that there are over three million women with HIV in the world, most of them in Africa. In fact, one in 50 women in sub-Saharan Africa is infected with HIV, and one in 700 in North America. AIDS is the leading cause of death for women ages 20-40 in major cities in the Americas, Western Europe, and Africa. By 1992 over four million infants will have been born to mothers with HIV, and about a million of the babies will themselves be infected.

In the United States women are the fastest growing group of people with HIV, yet remain invisible in the epidemic. AIDS is the leading cause of death for women ages 25-34 in New York City, and women with AIDS die four to six times faster than men with AIDS. However, the Centers for Disease Control still refuse to include the opportunistic infections specific to women in their list of AIDS-defining infections. This means that many women with HIV are misdiagnosed or even undiagnosed, and do not receive the treatment or services they need. It also makes it very difficult for women with HIV to get the immediate disability benefits they need once they become sick, and women have died while waiting for their benefits.

ACT UP/Network, the national network of direct action AIDS activist groups, has declared November 26-December 3, 1990 a "Week of Outrage." During the week, ACT UP groups across the country will hold demonstrations to draw attention to the issues of women and HIV infection. Chicago, San Francisco, Seattle, Los Angeles, and Austin, are among the cities demonstrating. For more information, contact your local ACT UP, or call Saundra Johnson at 312/829-6797. The Week of Outrage will culminate on Monday, December 3, with a large demonstration at the Centers for Disease Control in Atlanta, to demand that the CDC expand their definition of AIDS to include the infections and symptoms common to HIV-infected women. For more information about the action in Atlanta, contact ACT UP/Atlanta at 404/286-6247.

# *AIDS TREATMENT NEWS* OUTREACH ASSISTANCE REQUESTED

*by Tim Wilson*

Since early this year we have been aware and concerned that many people who could benefit from the information in *AIDS Treatment News* do not have access to it. In June we began developing an outreach campaign in order to reach a larger audience of HIV-impacted populations with our treatment message, and now we request *your* assistance with this project. As one of our subscribers, you can be part of our support structure and help us succeed in our overall mission of getting the word out about important treatment options and public policy issues.

The staff of *AIDS Treatment News* is requesting the assistance of our subscribers in the following outreach areas:

•  **New 800 subscription number.** Help us spread the word that interested parties can now call **1-800-TREAT-1-2** (1-800-873-2812) for *AIDS Treatment News* subscription information (*Note*: this is *not* a treatment information hotline). Ask your local community AIDS service organizations, HIV testing and counseling centers, buyers' clubs, publications, bulletin boards, universities, etc., to update their AIDS resource lists to include this new number.

Our 800 number is currently valid in the 48 contiguous United States and in Canada. The correct number for local San Francisco calls, for other geographic areas, and for all non-subscription business is 415/255-0588. Help us make sure that our current numbers are listed in appropriate places in your community, and listed accurately.

•  **Medical professionals, libraries, friends.** Does your doctor or other health professional, your HMO or medical center, subscribe to *AIDS Treatment News*? What about your local public library, or college or university library, or the human resources department where you work? Do you have friends or loved ones who would benefit from the information in *AIDS Treatment News*? Please encourage others to subscribe. Remember that we support our work almost exclusively through subscriptions; in order to maintain complete editorial independence, we accept no advertising.

•  **Special Assistance Fund.** Although we offer a substantial 60 percent discount on subscriptions "for persons with AIDS/HIV with financial difficulties" (and as many as 70 percent of our subscribers use that rate at one time or another), the reality is that many subscribers reach a point at which they can no longer afford even the discounted price. Our policy has always been to extend such subscriptions without charge in order to continue the dissemination of valuable treatment information to persons living with AIDS, struggling community-based organizations, prisoners without resources, health departments in a budget crunch, etc., and we do not want to change that policy. However, the need continues to grow faster than we have been able to generate full-rate subscriptions which subsidize these free extensions.

We have established a Special Assistance Fund for those who want to support our "free extension" program. We are asking for donations of $20 (equivalent to one six-month extension) and $40 (equivalent to one 12-month extension or two six-month extensions), or multiples thereof. We will track this income separately, and make the information about revenue generated for this fund available to any of our subscribers who request it. *AIDS Treatment News* is not a 501(c)(3) non-profit organization for which donations are tax-deductible; editor/publisher John S. James operates as a sole proprietor. However, we bring a strong not-for-profit consciousness to our work—we are working to save lives, not in business to make money—and we hope that you will support this worthwhile program so we are not forced to change our policy.

We would like to take this opportunity to thank all of our subscribers who have sent unsolicited contributions to us in the past. These donations have helped tremendously in allowing *AIDS Treatment News* to continue our "free extension" program to this point.

# Issue Number 116
# December 7, 1990

## DDI AND DDC APPROVAL EFFORT—INTERVIEW WITH MARTIN DELANEY

*by John S. James*

Martin Delaney, co-founder of Project Inform, has been actively involved since August in the effort to obtain rapid evaluation and, hopefully, approval of ddI and ddC. We asked him to outline what is happening in this effort.

Before working full time in AIDS, Mr. Delaney taught negotiation and other business skills to corporate teams. Recently he has communicated extensively with the researchers studying ddI and ddC, and with other experts from the sponsoring pharmaceutical companies, the FDA, the National Institutes of Health, and activist organizations.

**JJ:** You are optimistic on early approval. What are the reasons for optimism?

**MD:** I have had extensive meetings with the parties—the FDA, the researchers, the companies, and other activists. There are some uncertainties about how the data will be evaluated, but there is a clear commitment on the FDA's part in making this process happen. The discussions are about how they can make it happen, not whether. The question is, how can we evaluate the data in this circumstance, and make a scientific case that what we are seeing is predictive of the usefulness of the drug?

The issues are not unique to ddI or ddC. These are broader issues for all AIDS drugs in the near future. We will not have placebo studies, so we must find ways to make comparisons to existing AZT data, and to a better picture of the recent natural history of AIDS since the beginning of pneumocystis prophylaxis. If these issues did not come up now for these drugs, they would come up for whatever drugs are next. There are scientific hurdles, but there is also a strong commitment to clear these hurdles, to find a scientifically valid way to do it.

There are no simple answers here. The simple answers have already been rejected by FDA. For example, they do not feel that T-helper increases—even for a longer period than produced by AZT—is, by itself, adequate proof of the drug, unless it is corroborated by other data. But others hotly dispute this view, arguing that T-helper increases alone should be enough.

The FDA does not want to be the obstacle; it recognizes the critical urgency of making the two drugs available. So they are saying that they want a joint decision, a collective decision-making process to explore all these issues, with scientists in other research and development agencies—for example, the National Cancer Institute, and the AIDS Clinical Trials Group of the National Institute of Allergy and Infectious Diseases, as well as activist experts—on how the NDA (New Drug Application, with the detailed data on the drug) should be submitted. The FDA has agreed that it is safer politically to seek expert consensus in this way; if it made the decision alone without consultation, it would be highly vulnerable if something went wrong. In the FDA's view, this decision is a watershed event. We do not want them to make it alone.

**JJ:** The biggest questions seem to revolve around what constitutes proof of efficacy.

**MD:** Absolutely. The debate will hinge partly around the meaning of drug-induced T-helper increases. Statisticians are finding that T-helper counts definitely associate with survival outcome—especially that the risk is greater when the count falls below 50.

The tougher question is, if the T-helper counts are so predictive, does increasing the counts by use of a drug predict increased survival, as a higher count does in the natural history (without treatment)? Most researchers instinctively believe it does [that an antiviral which increases T-helper count probably does improve survival]. But the FDA argues that no one has yet proven this point.

Recent statistical analysis suggested that the benefits of AZT are greater than what would be predicted simply by the T-helper increase. Why that is so is unclear. The T-helper count may not tell us all we need to know about the immune system; the benefit of AZT may be greater than this count alone would suggest. None the less, others argue that increased T-helper counts are one useful predictor of a drug's efficacy.

The National Cancer Institute, for example, says that in all its studies, any antiviral drug which has kept the T-helper count above 50 seems to keep people alive. In the NCI studies, only one patient who remained above 50 has died in the last four years. Samuel Broder, M.D., director of the NCI, strongly believes that this data alone validates the usefulness of drug-induced T-helper increases [as an indicator of clinical or survival benefit from the drug].

The long-term clinical picture, as measured by the number of opportunistic infections or by survival, is harder to evaluate than people would like, because the easiest point of comparison is the old AZT studies. And most of those were done without pneumocystis prophylaxis. So the FDA is reluctant to use them for comparison, arguing that more recent data includes other variables besides the drug. So now Bristol-Myers is collecting data from several major clinical centers in the country—not just ddI data, but also case-history data from patients not given ddI, to get a better picture of the natural history of AIDS with pneumocystis prophylaxis. Perhaps this data can be used as a valid comparison; but of course much work is required.

Another outcome which FDA will consider will be overall clinical improvement, such as weight gain, or Karnofsky scores (a rating of overall health). If you put each of these pieces together, and if they are coherent, I think there is no question that FDA will grant the approval. But they do not want to approve the drugs on T-helper counts alone, without this other data.

There should also be some input from virology markers. Plasma viremia data (measuring the amount of virus in the blood) should be available by January.

If you keep your eye on all of these pieces of the picture, you don't get nervous with every new rumor that sweeps part of the country.

**JJ:** What else is at stake here, beyond the short-term availability of ddI and ddC?

**MD:** A great deal is at stake. If the FDA cannot find a way to accept this kind of data as proof of drug effectiveness, it will have no choice but to demand the re-use of survival as the sole endpoint in future studies. In other words, we test the drug until some of the patients die. And this would require a return to the routine use of placebo controls. We cannot allow this to happen.

**JJ:** If a drug is known to be an antiviral, known to be effective against HIV at concentrations reached in the body—and if there is no reason to suspect that the drug raises T-helper counts directly—then if T-helper counts consistently go up when the drug is given to persons with HIV, it seems hard to explain that effect other than by an antiviral action of the drug. Average T-helper cell counts do not rise spontaneously, without treatment, in any known group of persons with AIDS or HIV. It is hard for us to understand waiting months or years for conclusive proof of benefit, after it is already clear that a drug does show a substantial antiviral efficacy in patients.

Usually the FDA's Antiviral Advisory Committee meets for only a day or two, with little or no staff support. How can it possibly give the ddI and ddC decisions the attention they deserve, in view of the extensive data about these drugs, and the major issues regarding interpretation of the data?

**MD:** The committee probably could not do this by itself. Therefore, it will be assisted by other leading researchers brought in as consultants, who have expertise on these particular drugs. A special meeting of the nation's top experts, probably in early February, will seek a consensus on whether these drugs should be approved. In practice, this process must go through the existing structure of the FDA advisory committees.

**JJ:** There has been concern that neither company (Bristol-Myers for ddI, or Hoffmann-La Roche for ddC) has yet submitted its NDA (New Drug Approval application) to the FDA.

**MD:** The companies do seem to be on schedule for submission of that data. It would be a mistake to submit it too early, before they knew what the FDA wanted of them.

I have reassurances that Bristol-Myers will be submitting its NDA shortly after the advisory committee meeting, probably in February. Hoffmann-La Roche has not yet looked as closely at its data, but they have said that they intend to submit their NDA early in 1991.

**JJ:** What timetable do you see for a decision on approval of these drugs?

**MD:** The advisory meeting date has not yet been set, but should be in early February. I see at least one of the NDA applications coming in about a week after that time. Then it would take at least 30 days for the FDA to analyze the data; they may have to ask more questions of the company. All things considered, I think it's a do-able target to get both drugs out by March of 1991. Anything much beyond that, and we should raise the temperature politically.

The consensus building is most important, because it will set a standard of how we look at these urgent approvals in the future. We do not ask the FDA to decide all by itself in an ivory tower. Instead, we want a collective decision with input from all the people who are working in this field.

**Note:** On December 19, a multi-city press conference will explain the movement for early ddI and ddC evaluation. Project Inform and other organizations involved in this issue will take part.

As of this week, 35 organizations have signed a consensus statement circulated by Project Inform (with much help from ACT UP/Golden Gate and Mobilization Against AIDS), calling for urgent review of ddI and ddC. Also, the Community Consortium, a medical group representing almost all of the physicians who have an HIV practice in San Francisco, issued a separate statement urging expedited review of the data on these drugs, with a decision on licensing as soon as possible. In addition, at least 25 members of Congress have signed a letter to the FDA by Congresswoman Barbara Boxer (D-Greenbrae, CA) urging immediate review of ddI and ddC.


# OPPORTUNISTIC INFECTION PROJECT LAUNCHED BY ACT UP/NEW YORK: "COUNTDOWN 18 MONTHS"

*by Denny Smith*

Most of the opportunistic infections identified with AIDS are considered treatable to some degree. But in nearly every instance, the treatments are limited by their side effects or their unreliability for obtaining a consistent response, especially against recurrent infections. Research into better drugs for opportunistic infections has never approached the intensity of attention or funding afforded to research in primary HIV infection.

A campaign to find safer and truly definitive treatments, within a year and a half, for five of the most lethal AIDS-related infections has been inaugurated by ACT UP/New York. This project, dubbed "Countdown 18 Months," was formally launched November 12 during the latest session of the AIDS Clinical Trials Group (ACTG).

The idea was first proposed by Garance Franke-Ruta, and developed by her with fellow members of ACT UP/New York's Treatment and Data Committee. Motivating the campaign are two well-founded assertions:

• A dramatic advance in controlling HIV progression is inevitable, but it may develop too far in the future to prevent many currently asymptomatic seropositives from progressing to symptoms. And it is not of immediate use to thousands of people already battling secondary opportunistic infections.

- The resources now exist with which to replace the haphazard "aim and wince" handling of opportunistic infections, and 18 months is not an unrealistic span in which to mobilize these resources.

A crucial condition for the success of this project will be the development of effective working relationships with persons in pharmaceutical companies and government agencies.

The five infections targeted by Countdown 18 Months are pneumocystis pneumonia, CMV retinitis and colitis, toxoplasmosis, MAI, and the fungal infections— cryptococcosis, histoplasmosis and candidiasis. A 44-page planning document distributed by ACT UP/New York describes the rationale and goals of the plan; it also includes an in-depth look at existing treatments for these infections, experimental treatments now being tried, ways to obtain experimental treatments, reference for more information, and a select contact list of persons involved in AIDS research.

Requests for copies of *The Countdown 18 Months Plan* can be sent, with a small donation if possible, to ACT UP/New York, c/o Countdown, 135 W. 29th St., 10th floor, New York, NY 10001. Information regarding how to work on the Countdown project can be obtained from Garance Franke-Ruta, 212/532-0280 or 212/675-5170, or from Derek Link, 212/529-2368 or fax, 212/529-5997.

## COMPUTERIZED CLINICAL TRIALS LOCATER OPENS IN SAN FRANCISCO

A new service at Davies Hospital in San Francisco will search a database of local clinical trials and prepare a printout with description and contact information for all trials for which a patient may qualify. Anyone with AIDS or HIV may use this service. At present, only trials in the San Francisco Bay Area are listed; however, the system could be customized by medical or research institutions elsewhere.

This service, called Trials Search, differs from other clinical-trial information systems now in use. For example, the government-sponsored AIDS Clinical Trials Information Service provides a free telephone number (800/TRIALS-A) which anyone can call to ask questions about clinical trials in their area. However, the 800/TRIALS-A system is not set up to accept a patient's medical profile and automatically match the trials against it. Another computerized trials system, running at San Francisco General Hospital, keeps a database of potential volunteers and searches that database when one of its trials needs subjects. But in this system, volunteers sign up and do not know when (or if) they will be contacted; the Trials Search system, by contrast, operates at the potential volunteer's initiative, and provides a list of possible trials immediately. We do not know of any other service which does this.

To use Trials Search, the patient fills out a one-page form, indicating past and present opportunistic infections (from a list of 20), past and present treatments (from a list of 18) and present laboratory-test values (nine are requested: T-helper count, white blood count, hematocrit, etc.; patients can obtain the values from their physician's office). This simplified medical history includes the most important information used in the inclusion and exclusion criteria for most clinical trials. Trials Search cannot, of course, tell for sure whether a patient will qualify for entry into a particular study; only the researchers running each trial can make that decision. But Trials Search can rule out the great majority of trials for which the person could not possibly qualify. (In the San Francisco area, about 80 clinical trials are currently running; Trials Search typically locates about ten to 15 of these, on the average, for each client.)

The patient's medical form, which can be anonymous, is mailed or taken in person to Trials Search. It takes only about a minute for a trained operator to enter the patient's information, and the computer then prints a list of likely trials. There is a small fee for this service: no more than $7 per search, with reduced rates for persons with low income. This fee pays approximately a third of the cost of running Trials Search, which has also received small grants from the Bay Area Physicians for Human Rights, from AT&T, and from an anonymous individual. The project's organizers hope to acquire more substantial funding, after usage of the system proves that it is meeting a need.

If medical centers in other areas want to install this system, it would be technically easy because the only equipment needed is a Macintosh computer with a laser printer. There is no telephone or network connection to any other system. Little computer expertise would be required. However, no decision has yet been made about whether to distribute the software; and documentation would need to be written to instruct personnel at other medical centers on how to install and operate the system.

Trials Search is now open for persons with AIDS or HIV (in San Francisco or elsewhere) who want to find out about San Francisco area trials for which they may qualify. For more information, call Jay Seward, at the Institute for HIV Research and Treatment of Davies Medical Center, 415/565-6368, 10 a.m. to 4:30 p.m. weekdays except Wednesdays.

# NEW DNCB STUDY OPENS

A pilot study of the potentially immune-enhancing substance dinitrochlorobenzene (DNCB) is being co-sponsored by Project Inform and Children's Hospital in San Francisco. DNCB was once in wide use by the HIV "treatment underground," but the lack of a standard dose and application at the time produced mixed results. Because DNCB was unpatentable, the mainstream AIDS research establishment seldom pursued it seriously as an HIV treatment.

DNCB is in common use, however, as a diagnostic lab test applied topically to the skin, to assess delayed hypersensitivity in immune function; it has also been tried experimentally to treat alopecia, warts, and melanoma. Available as an industrial solvent, particularly in photographic development, DNCB has been reported to elicit an immunomodulatory activity from CD8 cells, and from Langerhans cells, which are considered a pivotal connection between the body's dermatological and immunological systems. When brushed onto a small area of the skin, DNCB gradually provokes a systemic immune reaction like that caused by poison oak or poison ivy, apparently inducing Langerhans cells to step up their capacity for signaling the proliferation of T-cells.

This study of DNCB is innovative for its plans to observe any correlation between skin and blood markers; it is designed only to monitor people who have already chosen to use DNCB (with or without AZT). It will be supervised by an HIV-knowledgeable physician on staff at Children's Hospital, Rafael Stricker, M.D. The protocol for the study was written by Dr. Stricker and Joseph Brewer of Project Inform. For information about participating, interested persons can call 415/552-7464.

## IN MEMORIAM: TEMPLE MINNER, DAVID SMYTH

Philadelphia AIDS activist Temple Minner died November 19. A vocal force in the local treatment and services scene, Temple helped to build the Philadelphia organization "We the People," and with Kiyoshi Kuromiya he co-founded the respected *Critical Path AIDS Project* newsletter. We spoke to Temple frequently on the phone and we will miss his help and his strong convictions.

San Francisco writer David Smyth died October 24. David was fervently involved in treatment issues, and had contributed valuable research and writing in the past to *AIDS Treatment News.*

## SAN FRANCISCO: CARE BILL HEARING, DECEMBER 11

The San Francisco HIV Health Service Planning Council is holding a public hearing for community input on the needs and priorities for HIV services in San Francisco. The Council has been appointed by Mayor Agnos to set the priorities for allocating the Ryan White CARE bill disaster relief money. The legislation directs the money to be used for direct health care, both inpatient and outpatient, and for support services for people with HIV; the money cannot be spent on education or prevention. San Francisco will be receiving approximately $6.4 million with an additional $6.4 million available through competitive grants. The Council is required to come up with a plan for spending the money by February 1991, so they are working on a very short timeline.

The public hearing is being held to listen to the needs and priorities that the people of San Francisco feel are the most urgent and important. The Council has asked that speakers present their top priorities and identify what type of services they would suggest to meet those needs. Individuals who cannot attend the hearing are encouraged to send in written comments and suggestions.

The hearing will be December 11, 1990 from 3-6 pm, at the Department of Public Health, 101 Grove Street, room 300. Written comments should be sent as soon as possible to HHSP Council, c/c DPH AIDS Office, 25 Van Ness, 5th Floor, San Francisco, CA 94102.

## Comment

The Council wants to hear from individuals about the most important needs and priorities for HIV services, and about existing service gaps. You can help by letting it know about any problem areas where you have first-hand knowledge or experience.

One area that we believe especially needs more funding is benefits counseling—helping persons with AIDS or HIV obtain public benefits or private insurance to which they are legally entitled. Unfortunately, institutions have an incentive to complicate their forms and procedures to keep from paying money due. There are cases of applications being stalled in the hope that persons with AIDS will die before benefits have to be paid. It can be difficult for persons who are ill to protect themselves, without assistance.

Two organizations, AIDS Benefits Counselors and the San Francisco AIDS Foundation, provide different kinds of benefit assistance. The AIDS Foundation teaches people how to apply; AIDS Benefits Counselors provides one-on-one assistance with applications, and organizes volunteer attorneys when needed for appeals.

Anyone with first-hand knowledge about problems in obtaining benefits should contact the Council at the address above. Which organizations have been most effective in providing assistance? Where could additional funding do most good?

## ACT UP AFFILIATES, BUYERS' CLUBS, AND PWA COALITIONS, DECEMBER 1990

For ACT UP affiliates not included below, call ACT UP Network in San Francisco, 415/861-7505. For PWA Coalitions, call NAPWA (National Association of People With AIDS) in Washington, D.C., 202/429-2856. This list only includes organizations with a publishable phone number. We will publish an international list later.

If you know of any organization which should be listed here but was omitted, please call Denny or Laura at *AIDS Treatment News, 415/255-0836.*

The identification codes below are "A" for ACT UP or similar activist group, "B" for Buyers' club, and "C" for PWA Coalition.

ALASKA
> Anchorage, Alaskans Living With HIV  907/272-6210  "C"

ARIZONA
> Tucson, PACT Buyer's Club  602/322-9808  "B"
> Tucson, PWA Coalition  602/322-9808  "C"

CALIFORNIA
> Long Beach, ACT UP  213/435-4346  "A"
> Los Angeles, ACT UP  213/669-7301  "A"
> Los Angeles Buyer's Club  213/748-1295  "B"
> Mendocino, ACT UP/Redwood Region  707/485-5867 "A"
> Oakland, ACT UP/East Bay  415/420-8864  "A"
> Orange County, ACT UP  714/744-6878 "A"
> Sacramento, ACT UP  916/552-1996 "A"
> San Diego, Being Alive  619/291-1400 "C"
> San Diego, Alliance 7  619/281-5360 "B"
> San Francisco, ACT UP/Golden Gate  415/252-9200 "A"
> San Francisco, ACT UP/San Francisco  415/563-0724 "A"
> San Francisco, Healing Alternatives  415/626-2316 "B"
> San Francisco, PWA Coalition  415/553-2560 "C"
> Santa Barbara, ACT UP  805/569-3299 "A"
> West Hollywood, Being Alive  213/667-3262 "C"

COLORADO
- Denver, ACT UP 303/830-0730 "A"
- Denver, Health Action Project 303/894-8650 "B"
- Denver, PWA Coalition 303/837-8214 "C"

CONNECTICUT
- New Haven, ACT UP 203/562-2622 "A"
- New Milford, PWA Coalition 203/624-0947 "C"

DISTRICT OF COLUMBIA
- Carl Vogel Foundation 202/293-5153 "B"
- DC, ACT UP 202/728-7530 "A"
- Lifelink 202/546-3166 "C"
- Oppression Under Target (OUT!) 202/234-3614 "A"
- The Positive Woman 202/745-1078 "C"

FLORIDA
- Broward County, PWA Coalition 305/784-0314 "C"
- Coconut Grove, Cure AIDS Now 305/856-8378 "C"
- Dade County, PWA Coalition 305/576-1111 "C"
- Ft. Lauderdale, PWA Health Alliance 305/763-7723 "B"
- Jacksonville, PWA Coalition 904/387-9350 "C"
- Miami, ACT UP 305/576-1111 "A"
- Miami, Body Positive Resource Center 305/576-1111 "C"
- Orlando, Action Now 407/351-6930 "A"&"B"
- Palm Beach, PWA Coalition 407/845-0800 "C"
- Sarasota, AIDS Manasota 813/954-6011 "B"
- Tallahassee, ACT UP 904/847-7445 "A"

GEORGIA
- Atlanta, ACT UP 404/286-6247 "A"
- Atlanta, PWA Coalition 404/874-7926 "C"

ILLINOIS
- Central Illinois, ACT UP 309/827-6841 "A"
- Chicago, ACT UP 312/509-6802 "A"

INDIANA
- Indianapolis, PWA Coalition 317/637-2720 "C"

KANSAS
- Kansas City, ACT UP 816/753-5930 "A"
- Wichita, ACT UP 316/269-1183 "A"

LOUISIANA
- New Orleans, ACT UP 504/944-4546 or 522-5105 "A"
- New Orleans, PWA Coalition 504/945-4000 "C"
- Shreveport, ACT UP 800/OUTCRYS "A"

MAINE
- Portland, ACT UP Maine 207/774-7224 "A"
- Portland, PWA Coalition 207/773-8500 "C"

MARYLAND
- Baltimore, ACT UP 301/837-5203 "A"
- Baltimore, PWA Coalition 301/625-1677 "C"
- Hyattsville, PWA Coalition 301/464-6964 "C"

MASSACHUSETTS
> Boston, ACT UP  617/492-2887  "A"
> Boston, PWA Coalition  617/859-8333  "C"
> Provincetown, ACT UP  508/487-2063  "A"
> Springfield, PWA Coalition  413/734-8844  "C"

MICHIGAN
> Detroit, Friends PWA Alliance  313/836-2800  "C"
> Grand Rapids, PWA Coalition  616/235-1372  "C"

MINNESOTA
> Minneapolis, ACT UP/MN  612/870-4214  "A"
> Minneapolis, The Aliveness Project  612/822-7946  "B"&"C"

MISSISSIPPI
> Jackson, PWA Coalition  601/353-7611  "C"

NEW HAMPSHIRE
> Newmarket, Positive Action  603/659-8442  "C"

NEW JERSEY
> Bergenfield, PWA Coalition  201/944-6670  "C"
> Central Jersey, ACT UP  201/247-9404 "A"
> Newark, Community Project for PWAs  201/824-5900X228  "C"
> New Jersey Caucus, 201/757-3306 "A"

NEW MEXICO
> Albuquerque, NMAPLA  505/266-0342  "C"

NEW YORK
> Buffalo, Niagara Frontier AIDS Alliance 716/852-6778"C"
> Long Island, ACT UP  516/338-4662  "A"
> Long Island, PWA Coalition  516/756-2354  "C"
> New York City, ACT UP  212/564-AIDS  "A"
> New York City, PWA Coalition  212/532-0568  "C"
> New York City, PWA Health Group  212/532-0280  "B"
> Syracuse, ACT UP  315/475-1544  "A"

OHIO
> Columbus, ACT UP  614/444-8137  "A"

OREGON
> Portland, ACT UP  503/284-0262  "A"

PENNSYLVANIA
> Allentown, PWA Coalition  215/433-5444  "C"
> Philadelphia, ACT UP 215/222-8815 "A"
> Philadelphia, We The People  215/545-6868  "B"&"C"
> Pittsburg, Cry Out!  412/683-9741 "A"

PUERTO RICO
> ACT UP 809/721-4353 after 5 p.m. "A"

RHODE ISLAND
> Providence, ACT UP/Rhode Island  401/461-4191  "A"
> Providence, Lifeline PWA Coalition  401/421-5344  "C"

TENNESSEE
> Nashville, People Living With AIDS  615/385-1510 "C"

TEXAS

        Austin, ACT UP  512/477-AIDS  "A"
        Austin, PWA Coalition  512/472-3784  "C"
        Dallas, Buyers' Club  214/826-7455  "B"
        Dallas, GUTS 214/621-6817 "A"
        Dallas, PWA Coaltion  214/941-0523  "C"
        Houston, ACT UP  713/433-9818  "A"
        Houston, PWA Coalition  713/522-5428  "C"

UTAH

        Salt Lake City, PWA Coalition of Utah  801/359-9619  "C"

WASHINGTON

        Seattle, ACT UP  206/726-1678  "A"
        Seattle Treatment & Education Project  206/329-4857

# Issue Number 117
# December 21, 1990

## 1991: TREATMENTS TO WATCH

*by John S. James*

Two years ago we published a list of treatments we believed would be most important in 1989 (see "Footnote," below). Here is our list for next year. We based our selection primarily on the chance that a treatment could have a practical impact or show major progress in 1991.

Despite the pessimism of most of 1990, we find more grounds for hope now than for a long time. First, there might now be changes in the FDA approval process to enable vitally important AIDS drugs to be developed rapidly, which has not been possible before. (AZT was developed rapidly, but in several ways it was a special case which could not be copied by others.) Also, good candidate drugs are coming out of laboratories faster today than ever before. And some potential treatments which have been in process (or in limbo) for years may now be ready to advance toward usefulness in the foreseeable future.

There is more depth of interest today than ever before in changing the policies and procedures which made the sacrifice of part of a generation inevitable. But major problems remain. Some of the worst delays in treatment development—especially in the often-secret preclinical phase, and sometimes in the U.S. Patent Office—have barely been touched by policy change or advocacy. Research funding is becoming more critical, as money is taken away from research to pay for AZT or other patient care. Congressional advocacy for treatment access has barely begun. To avoid major unnecessary delays and obstacles, community intelligence, communication, coalition, and pressure must continue.

Here are the treatments we are following most closely for 1991:

**(1) ddC and ddI approvals.**

Although there is no conclusive proof yet, there are strong reasons to believe that either or both of these drugs would be important in medical practice—that physicians

**460**

could save many more lives with these drugs in addition to AZT, than with AZT alone. For both drugs, the toxicities and the precautions required are well known. ddI, for example, has already been given to 15,000 people for HIV treatment, through the expanded access program. ddC has not been given to as many people, but it has been in human trials longer than ddI, and it is probably the safer of the two, as it does not cause pancreatitis, the most serious toxicity of ddI.

Both drugs are now available to some patients under expanded-access programs. But it is essential that they become available as prescription drugs, for several reasons: (1) The expanded-access programs do not allow combination with AZT—probably the best way to use ddC, and perhaps ddI also. (2) Many patients who should have access do not meet the criteria for these programs, criteria which could not possibly have been designed to take the full facts of each individual case into account. (3) While the drugs are now "free," the laboratory tests required—and the physician time required to fill out forms—are not. These costs, seldom covered by insurance, create greater economic barriers and inequality than paying for the drugs would cause.

ddC (although not ddI) is well suited to underground use; in fact a ddC underground has existed sporadically for about two years. But regular prescription access would be far better, offering more reliable quality control, regulatory oversight, private and public insurance coverage, and better opportunities for data collection to improve future therapy.

ddC may also be ideal for Third World use, as it costs only pennies a day to manufacture; it has been sold for years, for laboratory use, by chemical-supply companies. Also, management of ddC toxicity requires training of the health-care provider and of the patient, but (unlike with AZT or ddI) it does not require blood tests or other Western medical technology, which is economically inaccessible to much of the world's population. ddC could become the first scientifically tested treatment available to much of the world, forcing a re-examination of the almost universal policy of writing off those already infected and leaving them to die. While U.S. approval would not be legally required for use of the drug elsewhere, it would provide essential credibility and avoid the suspicion that would be aroused by any U.S.-based effort to provide to others a drug not approved for domestic use.

Why is there any issue about whether these drugs will be approved? The problem is that despite the weight of information suggesting that the drugs do work, there is no single stack of paper which makes a flawless academic case for efficacy. Each study is either small, and/or unfinished, and/or has no control group for exact comparisons, and/or looked at T-helper counts or other markers, instead of death or major disease progression. And the many patients—probably many thousands—who have improved on the expanded-access programs are dismissed because they are not part of a controlled trial. To get perfect data to prove these drugs could take another two years. That is why there is the growing demand that the existing data be analyzed now, and that the drugs be approved if they show "substantial evidence" of efficacy. (See definition of "substantial evidence" from the Senate Report on the Drug Amendments of 1962, quoted in *AIDS Treatment News* issue #112.)

**(2) New antibiotics for opportunistic infections: azithromycin, clarithromycin, liposomal drugs, and others.**

Important new treatments for opportunistic infections should be approved in the U.S. or otherwise become more available in 1991. Azithromycin, for example, might be an important advance for toxoplasmosis, MAC (also called MAI), and possibly cryptosporidiosis. Azithromycin has been an approved drug in Yugoslavia for about two years; it is also approved in some other countries in Eastern Europe. In the U.S. the NDA (New Drug Application, or permission to market the product as a prescription drug) was applied for in 1990; with luck azithromycin could be available by prescription in the U.S. in 1991. The labeling will probably recommend it for other purposes than the infections usually associated with AIDS—simply because those trials were conducted first—so insurance reimbursement may be difficult.

Recently the U.S. sponsor of azithromycin, Pfizer Inc., began a compassionate-use program for persons with toxoplasmic brain infections who have failed conventional therapies or are known to be intolerant to the drugs. Physicians can call Michael DeBruin, M.D., at 203/441-5701, or fax 203/441-5702, for information about enrolling their patients. Unfortunately, azithromycin has not been available in the U.S. through buyers' clubs or otherwise from abroad; at least one physician, however, was able to obtain some for a patient through contacts in Eastern Europe.

Clarithromycin, a drug closely related to azithromycin, is approved in Ireland and some other European countries; its U.S. NDA was applied for in 1990, again for conditions not usually related to AIDS. This drug shows considerable promise for MAC (see *AIDS Treatment News* #113 for more information about both clarithromycin and azithromycin).

As we reported in issue #113, it is possible to obtain clarithromycin in the U.S. We have heard two reports so far summarizing the resulting early experience with MAC. One was that clarithromycin was highly successful; the other account also reported success, but was cautious because of the small number of patients so far. In New York the PWA Health Group has circulated a survey to physicians asking for results of using clarithromycin for MAC, after four months of treatment. But clarithromycin has only been available there for about two months so far, so none of the forms have yet been returned.

Both azithromycin and clarithromycin are used orally. Both are chemically related to erythromycin.

Liposomal gentamicin (TLC G-65), another antibiotic, is now in trials for treating MAC. Liposomes are microscopic structures of fats; they are used to improve the delivery of certain drugs to where they are needed in the body, increasing effectiveness and reducing toxicity. TLC G-65 delivers gentamicin inside of macrophages, where MAC organisms would otherwise be protected against the antibiotic. Besides gentamicin, other liposomal drugs now being developed for AIDS-related conditions are amphotericin (a powerful antifungal, now in trials for treating cryptococcal meningitis), and daunorubicin (a chemotherapy agent being developed as a potential treatment for KS).

Besides new treatments—our focus in this article—more is being learned about how best to use the conventional treatments already available. These studies are also important, since it is too early to know whether the new drugs (for toxoplasmosis, for example) will work better than existing ones. If the new drugs are successful, the ones already in use will probably still be best for some situations.

**(3) Hypericin.**

Hypericin is an antiviral found in low concentrations in St. John's wort, a plant which has long been used in herbal medicine. *AIDS Treatment News* covered hypericin extensively from late 1988 through early 1990; see issues #63, #91, and #96 for major reports. We are overdue for an update—in part because we have waited for clinical trials, which have been about to start since last summer. Only the trials will tell for sure whether hypericin is useful for treating HIV. But what we know today suggests that this antiviral is likely to be valuable and deserves high-priority attention:

• In laboratory tests hypericin worked well against HIV. And in animals it worked much better than AZT in preventing death from other retroviruses. (It has been very difficult to infect animals with HIV, so animal retroviruses were used instead of HIV for this test.) For background on antiviral effects of hypericin, see two articles in *Proceedings of the National Academy of Sciences, USA*: Meruelo D and others, "Therapeutic agents with dramatic antiretroviral activity and little toxicity at effective doses: Aromatic polycyclic diones hypericin and pseudohypericin," July 1988, pages 5230-5234; and Lavie G and others, "Studies of the mechanisms of action of the antiretroviral agents hypericin and pseudohypericin," August 1989, pages 5963-5967.

• There is much human experience with oral use of hypericin, especially since St. John's wort extracts with standardized hypericin concentration are sold over the counter in Europe as an antidepressant. The concentration of hypericin in these extracts is very low, probably too low for effective anti-HIV use. But far larger doses of the pure chemical have been given to animals without harm.

• A small community-based trial in San Francisco did find a modest rise in T-helper counts in some patients after use of the herbal extracts—an average 12 percent rise, sustained during the four months of the trial, for those patients who started with high T-helper cell counts. However, this preliminary study did not seek or obtain statistical significance. Another trial with St. John's wort extract is now ongoing at the Community Research Initiative in New York.

In short, all the elements are in place to suggest that hypericin should prove to be useful. It works well in laboratory and animal tests. It has been used in humans, although in low doses (but animal studies suggest that, with the pure chemical instead of crude herbal extracts, the doses can be greatly increased). In addition, there are two other reasons why this potential treatment may be important:

• The mechanism of action is completely different from that of AZT. If hypericin does work, it will provide physicians with a new class of anti-AIDS drug—not just another nucleoside analog like ddC or ddI. New possibilities for combination and other therapy will be opened up.

• Hypericin also has activity against some other viruses, including CMV and herpes simplex. A recent test found anti-CMV activity at a concentration of one microgram/ml—about the concentration at which a typical antibiotic is active against bacteria. (Barnard DL and others. Characterization of the anti-human cytomegalovirus activity of three anthraquinone compounds. Interscience Conference on Antimicrobial Agents and Chemotherapy, Atlanta, October 21-24, 1990, abstract #1093.) Unfortunately, it would be difficult to achieve this blood level with the readily available St. John's wort preparations.

However, tests reported in a European patent application for use of hypericin as an antiviral (European patent application number 87111467.4, Yeda Research and Development Ltd., Rehovot, Israel, filed August 7, 1987) found much greater activity against herpes simplex; these laboratory tests reported inhibition at 2.5 nanograms (0.0025 micrograms)/ml. Although acyclovir, a safe and effective standard treatment for herpes, is already available, new treatments are needed for acyclovir-resistant strains. The herbal extracts already available at buyers' clubs should be tested for this purpose.

Underground research with higher doses of hypericin (as a potential HIV or CMV treatment) would be possible, since chemical extraction of hypericin from the St. John's wort plant is relatively easy. We hope that the ACTG (AIDS Clinical Trials Group, of the U.S. National Institute of Allergy and Infectious Diseases) trial planned to start soon at New York University will make underground research unnecessary.

The AIDS Clinical Drug Development Committee of the ACTG put hypericin in its highest priority category in May 1990. It is hoped that the first trial with pure hypericin (not the very-low-dose herbal extracts) can start early next year.

What is needed now is a first look at efficacy of hypericin, to test whether or not this drug may be a "home run" in the treatment of HIV. If so, far more resources would be made available than are now being applied to its development. If not, then we could afford to wait for the larger, and probably slower, trials which would be needed to determine whether it could make a more modest contribution.

**(4) Compound Q.**

We have not followed compound Q (trichosanthin) closely, as we have left this treatment to Project Inform, which is directly involved in the research. Reports we have received, not only from Project Inform but also from individuals who have used the drug, are usually good. It is well known that there are serious risks in using this treatment; expert supervision is essential, because occasionally there are severe side effects which could be fatal if not treated immediately.

At this time, the physicians and researchers testing compound Q are still learning how to use it best. Large-scale "pivotal" trials—those designed to lead to drug approval—may need to wait until more of this preliminary research is finished.

**(5) Protease inhibitors.**

This class of drugs has attracted intense interest among major pharmaceutical companies. Much of the work is secret, however; therefore it has been difficult to cover this area well.

Protease is an enzyme which is necessary for HIV to reproduce. When a new copy of the virus is being created by an infected cell, a single long string of amino acids (the components of protein) is produced. This single string must be cut in the right places to form the pieces which need to be assembled in a new virus. The protease, which is on one end of the original string, does this cutting. If the protease does not work, defective copies of the virus are formed, and they cannot reproduce.

HIV protease is only created by infected cells; it has no normal function in the body. Protease inhibitors are drugs to temporarily or permanently disable this enzyme, without harming normal cells.

Different protease inhibitors are being developed by different companies. At least one is expected to enter Federally funded human trials (within the ACTG system) within the next few weeks.

**(6) Tat gene inhibitors.**

"Tat" is a gene of HIV which regulates viral activity. Human trial of drugs to inhibit the tat gene may begin in early 1991.

### (7) Non-nucleoside-analog RT inhibitors.

Reverse transcriptase (RT) is an enzyme necessary for reproduction of HIV; it is not used by human cells. Therefore, RT is a natural target for anti-HIV drugs.

AZT, ddC, and ddI are RT inhibitors. But they are also nucleoside analogs—meaning false building blocks of DNA. Because they can sometimes interfere with human DNA, drugs in this class tend to be toxic and cause side effects.

But other drugs, which are not nucleoside analogs, can also inhibit RT. Some of these may have effective anti-HIV activity without the toxicity of nucleoside analogs. A number of companies are developing such drugs (see "Drug Concerns Make Big Strides in AIDS Work," *The Wall Street Journal*, December 7, 1990); until recently, however, this work received little public attention.

One group of non-nucleoside RT inhibitors which has been well known is the TIBO derivatives (see *AIDS Treatment News* issue #97). An early human test in Europe of one of these drugs may have been disappointing; according to AmFAR's *AIDS/HIV Treatment Directory*, "no significant immunologic or virologic improvement was noted" in the 10-patient dose-escalating trial. Other TIBO derivatives may be tested.

Another kind of non-nucleoside RT inhibitor is BI-RG-587, described below in this issue.

### (8) Kaposi's sarcoma: anti-angiogenesis treatments.

The much-rumored new KS treatment in Japan, mentioned by Dr. Robert Gallo of the U.S. National Cancer Institute (see *AIDS Treatment News* issue #99) is believed to be a drug which prevents abnormal angiogenesis (growth of blood vessels). Apparently this drug is difficult to produce, and U.S. researchers have not been able to obtain enough for human tests. Therefore they are looking for substitutes; one possible substitute, pentosan polysulfate, is now being tested at the National Institutes of Health. We have heard mixed reports about pentosan.

Angiogenesis treatments are also likely to be important for cancer, as solid tumors must cause blood-vessel growth in order to obtain nourishment and grow beyond a small size. (In KS, the abnormal blood-vessel growth itself is the main problem.) Since new blood vessels do not normally grow in adults, except in wound healing, drugs to stop this growth may be feasible for treatment use.

A important report on a new anti-angiogenesis compound appeared in *Nature*, December 6, 1990 (Ingber and others, "Synthetic analogues of fumagillin that suppress angiogenesis and suppress tumour growth," pages 555-557). In mice the compound inhibited solid-tumor growth with few side effects. This report does not mention KS or AIDS, however, so it may not receive the attention in the AIDS community which it deserves.

# Footnote: January 1989 Predictions

Almost two years ago (issue #72) we listed the following as likely to be important in 1989: ddI; passive immunotherapy; hypericin; compound Q; Chinese anti-infection herbs; FLT (fluorodeoxythymidine); AzdU; d4T; and soluble CD4. Looking back after two years, it is striking how little has been accomplished for most of them, in view of the seriousness of the AIDS emergency. Most remain today as they were then: still promising, still untested. Several remain on our current list for next year.

## BI-RG-587: NEW ANTIVIRAL READY FOR TRIALS?

A December 7 report in *Science*[1] on laboratory and animal tests of a new AIDS antiviral has generated more than usual interest. Many AIDS laboratory findings appear in technical journals and are then picked up by the press, but most are not heard from again. The reason for the greater interest in this drug seems to be that the major practical bases have been covered well. With luck, U.S. human trials could begin by early or mid 1991.

The antiviral, named BI-RG-587, was found by a systematic strategy for synthesizing and screening chemicals likely to be active against HIV-1 reverse transcriptase (RT), but without the toxicity of the nucleoside analog RT inhibitors such as AZT, ddC, and ddI. BI-RG-587 inhibited several strains of HIV-1 at low concentrations (under 50 nM) in cell cultures. Over 8,000 times the concentration was needed to be toxic to human cells. The chemical was so specific to HIV-1 that it had no effect on HIV-2, or on any other virus tested; this great specificity may help to reduce side effects. BI-RG-587 was also effective against HIV-1 strains obtained from four patients using AZT; we do not know the concentration used in these tests.

In animals, BI-RG-587 could be given orally. In monkeys, a single dose produced plasma levels 35 to 140 times the concentration needed to inhibit HIV-1 in the cell-culture tests, and these levels were maintained during an eight-hour period. In chimpanzees, 600 times the required concentration was achieved. The drug did cross the blood-brain barrier very well in the animal tests.

BI-RG-587 is a simple molecule which appears not difficult to synthesize—important so that if it proves effective, there will not be delays due to manufacturing problems.

The developer of BI-RG-587—Boehringer Ingelheim Pharmaceuticals, Inc., Ridgefield, Connecticut—was not previously known to be working on AIDS. However, rumors were furiously circulating shortly before the December 7 announcement, suggesting that the German parent company was starting tests of an AIDS drug.

*AIDS Treatment News* has learned that the U.S. company has plans to file an IND (Investigational New Drug application) in January 1991, and has hopes of starting a U.S. trial by March.

Despite encouraging laboratory results, only human trials can tell if the drug will work. Another non-nucleoside RT inhibitor—a TIBO derivative, the first one tested in humans—showed similar promise in laboratory and animal tests, but seems not to be effective in patients. Other companies also are developing their own lines of non-nucleoside RT inhibitors. No one knows in advance which ones will be successful. But what can be done is to make sure that there are no unnecessary obstacles or delays in finding out.

## REFERENCES

1.  Merluzzi VJ, Hargrave KD, Labadia M, and others. Inhibition of HIV-1 Replication by a Nonnucleoside Reverse Transcriptase Inhibitor. *Science*. December 7, 1990; volume 250, pages 1411-1413.

# Issue Number 118
# January 4, 1991

## NEW MERCK ANTIVIRALS IN HUMAN TESTS

Merck & Co. is conducting human trials on two new antivirals, known as L-697,639 and L-697,661. The trials began in Europe about a month ago, and are about to begin at the U.S. National Institutes of Health in Bethesda, Maryland. According to a Merck spokesman quoted in the *Los Angeles Times* (December 22, business section), company scientists screened 23,000 compounds to find these two, then moved them from the laboratory to human tests in the remarkably short time of six months. An NIH spokeswoman quoted in the same article said that 40 asymptomatic HIV positive volunteers were enrolled in the study at NIH.

These drugs are non-nucleoside RT inhibitors—that is, they block the enzyme reverse transcriptase (RT) without also being nucleoside analogs—false building blocks of DNA. AZT, ddC, and ddI are RT inhibitors which are nucleoside analogs. It is hoped that non-nucleoside drugs can be found with very little toxicity—since the enzyme reverse transcriptase is found only in retroviruses and has no use in the human body, while nucleoside analogs can in some cases affect human DNA. Other non-nucleoside RT inhibitors are the new Boehringer Ingelheim drug BI-RG-587 discussed in *AIDS Treatment News* #117, and the class of drugs called TIBO derivatives being developed in Europe by Janssen.

We have heard that other companies have one or more non-nucleoside RT inhibitors in pre-clinical development, but have not announced them. Reverse transcriptase appears to be a practical target for anti-HIV drug development, since the enzyme is well known and chemicals to block it can presumably be screened by laboratory assays, without the special laboratory facilities needed for handling live virus. It is important that more of these potential treatments be tested, since only one drug in five which enters human trials ever reaches marketing approval.

# DDC/DDI APPROVAL UPDATE

*by John S. James*

Much AIDS news today concerns the campaign for a rapid FDA evaluation of the experimental AIDS antivirals ddC and ddI—the issue we listed as the most important treatment development to watch in 1991 (*AIDS Treatment News* #117.) The decisions now being made will affect not only these drugs, but *all* critically important AIDS antivirals in the future; they will determine whether any future AIDS treatment, no matter how well it may work, could possibly travel the development and regulatory pipeline without many months or years of medically unnecessary delay. We are now seeing the beginnings of major changes; but at the same time there is widespread confusion, and sometimes chaotic miscommunication.

The meaning of the current controversies cannot be understood without background on the situation which now exists, and how it developed.

## Background: The Problem

Neither ddC nor ddI are new; both could have been developed and approved at about the same time as AZT. ddC was delayed because of early toxicity; it was not known until later that the right dose was about 200 times less than the dose of AZT or ddI. As for ddI, it was well into human trials two years ago—and the subject of a loud and sometimes bitter public dispute between Ellen Cooper, M.D., chief of the FDA's Division of Antiviral Drug Products, and Samuel Broder, M.D., director of the U.S. National Cancer Institute; the occasion was the first hearing of the Lasagna Committee, which issued its report on approval of new drugs for cancer and AIDS on August 15, 1990 (for background on this report, see *AIDS Treatment News* #110). The dispute, an advance echo of what is happening today, concerned the FDA's refusal to approve the NCI's plan to begin testing ddI as a treatment for children with AIDS under two years old; the U.S. National Cancer Institute was ready to start this ddI trial two years ago, but apparently the FDA wanted tests on adults to be finished before the tests with children began. (For detailed newspaper coverage of the ddI dispute of two years ago, see "Cancer Institute: AIDS Drugs Unduly Delayed," by Michael L. Millenson, *Chicago Tribune*, January 5, 1989, and "The Battle over FDA Drug Policy; The Pressure Is On to Speed New AIDS and Cancer Drugs through the Agency's Slow Approval Process," by Laurie Garrett, *Newsday*, February 14, 1989.)

Two years later, one activists spoke of the spreading "ripple of terror that the trials [running now for ddI and ddC] are not what should have been designed." It seems that nobody thought through how the information to be generated by these trials—scheduled to run for about 18 months more—would be used to support drug approval. One effect of this lack of planning is that AZT, the first AIDS antiviral to reach FDA approval, shut the door behind it, keeping all rivals out. This happened despite the clear need for new therapies—shown most compellingly by epidemiological data suggesting that AZT has extended average survival after AIDS diagnosis by no more than several months. (This survival data includes patients not receiving AZT because of drug intolerance or other reasons; the benefit of AZT for those who do use it might be greater.)

Much of the reason for the current complexity, confusion, and miscommunication stirred up by the push for early evaluation of ddC and ddI is the need to retrofit to cover for mistakes of the past. These mistakes occurred because of lack of higher-level oversight and planning in the AIDS research process. Key positions have long been vacant, or filled with people unwilling to deal effectively with AIDS.

One of the problems in the current development of ddC and ddI is the lack of definition of what the trials are trying to prove. Normally, the goal would be to prove efficacy (i.e., that the drug works better than no treatment) for some group of patients. It should not be necessary to prove that the new drug is better than standard therapy—or even equal to it, because many patients cannot use the standard therapy, and because combination treatment using both the new and standard treatment is highly promising.

But since it would be unethical to run a placebo trial, ddC and ddI are being compared to AZT instead. Statistical efforts were made to use the old AZT-vs.-placebo trial of four years ago to allow ddC and ddI to be mathematically compared with a placebo, even though no real placebo is being used in the current trial. This desperate attempt to forge a case for approval out of ill-designed trials seems to have led to some of the recent controversy.

If the new drugs must be compared to AZT, then the next question is whether they must be proved superior, or only equivalent, to merit FDA approval. Equivalence, of course, would be the standard preferred. But there are statistical complications in proving equivalence. For example, in a trial to test whether one drug is better than another, the incentives are for researchers to run a tight, clean study, so that if there is a difference, it will be found. But in a test for equivalence, the incentives are for researchers to run a sloppy trial, because failure to find a difference means success. For this and other reasons, there is confusion now over whether proof of equivalence will be enough for approval of ddC or ddI, or whether proof of superiority will be required.

There are other problems with the current ddC and ddI trials, and with the regulatory process. One concern is that companies do not usually submit their data to the FDA until their NDA (New Drug Application) is finished; the FDA prefers to get the data all together, in order to save staff time. But an NDA is a large document, typically consisting of many volumes of paperwork. Anyone familiar with the influence of corporate and organizational cultures would expect that any time one organization generates such a document and passes it to another for evaluation, many points of disagreement or friction will almost certainly be found. Without inside knowledge of the operations at the FDA, we cannot know whether this potential problem does or does not in fact cause serious, avoidable delays. (If it does, procedures could be changed to encourage earlier collaboration for NDA review of critically important drugs.)

Two years ago, NCI's Dr. Samuel Broder saw that no new AIDS antivirals would be approved unless procedures were changed. "If we have to compare every drug to AZT, with death as the endpoint of a trial, we're going to be in a situation where it will be very difficult to get any other antiretroviral approved for AIDS. It took us two years to get AZT out—how long do you think the next one will take? Five years, ten years? That's unacceptable!" (Quoted in *Newsday* article cited above; the comments were addressed to Dr. Ellen Cooper of the FDA. The context of the discussion was ddI. Dr. Cooper replied with the question, "Why don't you want to see a year's research in clinical trials on an antiretroviral before approval?")

Two years later, the trials of ddC and ddI still have months or years to run—and as we pointed out above, they are not well focused on the important questions. This is the context of the growing movement to ask the FDA to call in the existing data now, look at all that is known about these drugs, and approve them if there is "substantial evidence" that they work.

## San Francisco Physicians Seek Early ddl, ddC Review

On December 26, 1990, two San Francisco physicians' organizations, representing almost all physicians with large AIDS/HIV practices in the San Francisco area, filed a formal petition with the FDA urging that Agency to use its existing statutory authority to expedite submission of existing data on ddI and ddC, and then make a decision on marketing approval by March 1, 1991. The petitioning organizations are:

(1) The Community Consortium, which consists of over 180 physicians, nurses, physician's assistants, and other licensed health care providers. The Community Consortium has been conducting community-based trials of AIDS treatments since 1986; one of its trials made major contributions to FDA approval of aerosol pentamidine for pneumocystis prophylaxis.

(2) The Bay Area Physicians for Human Rights, an organization with over 200 members dedicated to quality health care for lesbians and gay men. BAPHR has long been involved in AIDS policy issues; for example, it was the first organization to issue safer sex guidelines.

This petition is especially important for several reasons:

• It shows that the call for rapid evaluation of ddI and ddC (and of other drugs which may be equally promising in the future) has the clear support of the leading AIDS physicians in the San Francisco area, who are among the most experienced in the world. As far as we know, there was no opposition to the petition within either medical organization.

• It cites specific sections in the Code of Federal Regulations which show that the FDA has the clear legal authority and also the mandate to expedite the approval of critically important drugs for life-threatening illnesses.

• It also calls on the FDA to use its authority to establish and publish criteria by which antiretroviral drugs will be judged for approval, which would provide guidance for pharmaceutical companies and reduce the confusion which now prevails.

• The 11-page petition document itself (including 55 technical references) is the best single statement of the case for early approval of these drugs.

• The petition will become part of the Congressional Record, available for easy reference by members of Congress.

The initiative and the legwork for this petition were provided by San Francisco activists Jim Driscoll and Barry Freehill, with medical guidance and leadership by Donald Abrams, M.D., Chairman of the Community Consortium. The idea of using a petition was suggested by Sidney Wolfe, director of the Public Citizen Health Research Group.

The petition is open for endorsements by other organizations. Persons interested in receiving a copy should send a large self-addressed stamped envelope to: Jim Driscoll or Barry Freehill, c/o Community Consortium, 3180 - 18th Street, Suite 201, San Francisco, CA 94110.

## Congressional Letters Support Expedited ddI and ddC Review

On November 27 Congresswoman Barbara Boxer (Democrat, California) released a letter from 25 members of Congress to the new Commissioner of the FDA, David A. Kessler, M.D., asking for early review and possibly early release of ddI and ddC. Congresswoman Boxer stated, "It is imperative that incoming FDA Commissioner Kessler make this a top priority. His background, as an AIDS pediatric physician from a Bronx public hospital, well qualifies him to take a fresh look at medical evidence supporting these drugs."

Congressman Jerry Lewis (Republican, California), Chairman of the House Republican Conference, wrote a separate letter supporting early review of these drugs.

Congressional involvement is important because in the past, the FDA has often faced criticism from Congress for approving a drug too soon, but almost never for delaying approval. These letters provide cover for the FDA, and greatly reduce the concern that fear of Congress might prevent it from moving as rapidly as it otherwise could.

Mobilization Against AIDS first asked Congresswoman Boxer to draft the letter and circulate it in Congress; she immediately agreed to do so. To obtain a copy of that letter, write or call Mobilization Against AIDS, 1540 Market St., #160, San Francisco, CA 94102, 415/863-4676.

Paul Boneberg of Mobilization Against AIDS pointed out that obtaining such assistance from members of Congress is not difficult, if local organizations choose to develop an appropriate relationship with their representatives.

## Project Inform Consensus Statement on ddI, ddC Approval

The first consensus statement in support of early licensing of ddI and ddC has been circulated by Project Inform. Over 25 organizations and a number of physicians have signed.

On August 16 Martin Delaney of Project Inform first wrote to Doctors Ellen Cooper and Paul Beninger of the Division of Antiviral Drug Products of the FDA, warning them that early approval of ddI and ddC was about to become a major public issue, and exploring possibilities for expediting evaluation and approval of these drugs.

The first draft of the Project Inform statement called for early approval of the drugs, not just early review. Some physicians objected to this draft, saying that they had not seen the data, and therefore could not know whether or not the drugs were ready for approval. Later drafts of the Project Inform statement—as well as the physicians' petition, and the Congressional letter, both described above—took these reservations into account, and called on the FDA to rapidly review the existing data, and approve the drugs if justified.

## Ellen Cooper Resigns As Antiviral Chief

Late last month Dr. Ellen Cooper asked to be reassigned within the FDA and leave her job as chief of the Division of Antiviral Drug Products. Most activists who worked with Dr. Cooper consider this development bad news, since no one else at the FDA has her experience with AIDS drugs. It is widely agreed that her job generated intolerable pressures.

In an interview published in *The Wall Street Journal*, December 24, 1990, Dr. Cooper cited the conflict between four groups—people with AIDS, pharmaceutical companies, scientists running trials, and regulators (at the FDA). (It is notable that this list did not include a fifth group—the frontline physicians with large AIDS/HIV practices.) She commented that "Politics has become paramount, but science should have a role." She said that she was open to using T-helper counts (or other measurements short of death or disease progression) to prove drug efficacy, "but there's got to be an analysis of the data by statisticians, researchers, and clinicians. That's just starting now."

One incident which must have contributed to job pressure concerns recent letters from Dr. Cooper to Bristol-Myers and to Hoffmann-La Roche concerning standards for approval for ddI and ddC. We have not seen these letters nor talked to anyone who has. Apparently they address the problems with using the old AZT-vs.-placebo trial as a basis for interpreting the data from the current ddI-vs.-AZT and ddC-vs.-AZT trials.

These letters have barely been mentioned in the press, but behind the scenes they generated a storm of controversy, because they were widely interpreted as taking back decisions already made and requiring data that everybody knew would not be available—in effect, therefore, saying that the FDA will not approve either drug at this time. There may have been a misunderstanding, however, because others believe that the purpose of these letters was not to rule out approval, but rather to ask the companies to put forward their best case for the drugs. Without seeing the letters, we cannot know what message was intended, and whether a different message may have been received.

## Comment

We are too far from Washington to cover what is happening inside the Government in AIDS treatment research and development, or in other AIDS policy; we wish there were a Washington-based newsletter to do so. We do have impressions on why Dr. Cooper's job has been such a difficult one, and on how that position could be made more workable in the future.

Over a year ago this writer was at the FDA for a class which the Agency had very commendably organized for community-based research groups; we were there as a member of San Francisco's Community Research Alliance (now the Project Inform Community Research Alliance). One lecture concerning a highly technical aspect of clinical trials was given by Dr. Cooper. We commented to an FDA staff member present that we were surprised that the head of the division would be prepared to speak on such a specialized area. He answered, with obvious respect for Dr. Cooper, that she could speak equally well on any aspect of clinical trials and the FDA's role in regulating them.

We see Dr. Cooper as a top expert on clinical trials, but one who in fact had two jobs—not only the scientific job she wanted and could do well, but also a political job in addition. Due to lack of national leadership on AIDS from higher levels of government, Dr. Cooper had become not only the leader of the antiviral division at FDA, but also, in effect, the sole umpire to judge the standards of approval for all AIDS antiviral drugs—and in consequence, *the* designer of national policy on how to respond to the epidemic, in so far as development of antiviral drugs is concerned—development on which the life of everyone with HIV depends. There is no way that such a role could not be political.

The best outcome now might be for the FDA to separate the two jobs. Then Dr. Cooper could return to being head of the antiviral division, without also having to singlehandedly set national policy on AIDS drug development and take up the slack created by leadership default from the President on down. The head of the antiviral division is three levels below the Commissioner of the FDA; the political decisions (such as whether to insist on new technical standards now if the practical consequence is that nothing will be approved) are ultimately the responsibility of higher levels. There now is a Commissioner of the FDA—David A. Kessler, M.D., who was installed on December 3, after the office had long been vacant—so this best outcome might now be possible.

## ASPIRIN UPDATE: WARNING, PROMISE, AND CALL FOR INFORMATION

*by John S. James*

Last August 17, *AIDS Treatment News* published an in-depth look at the possibility that ordinary aspirin might have a role in AIDS treatment—as an immune modulator, not just for minor symptom relief. One of the physicians we interviewed, Joseph Sonnabend, M.D., in New York, called recently to warn us of the importance of medical monitoring with aspirin use—especially the need to follow platelet count. He has seen one case of serious hemorrhage in a patient with a rapidly falling platelet count, who was taking two 325-mg aspirin tablets four times a day. Fortunately, this person recovered.

Dr. Sonnabend suggests that anyone with a platelet count of under 100,000, or who has ever had thrombocytopenia (low platelet count), should have frequent medical supervision if they use aspirin, or other drugs which can interfere with blood clotting. Anyone with HIV should be monitored by their physician if they use aspirin.

Background note: platelets assist in blood clotting. Platelet counts often decline in persons with HIV infection. For unknown reasons, this decline is usually less serious than if the same numbers occurred in persons without HIV—and platelet counts often become normal again as HIV infection progresses. Bleeding problems due to low platelets have been rare with HIV infection; but the case mentioned above shows that risk does exist, and appropriate precautions are necessary.

## A Report of T-Helper Improvement

We have heard of one case of an unexpected major improvement in T-helper count after low-dose aspirin use. We are reluctant to mention a single case until there is confirmation; but here, the patient was in an NIH epidemiological study and has very good data available—quarterly T-helper and other blood counts from a quality-controlled lab for the last six years. We also chose to mention this case because it suggests that an easy-to-organize community-based trial could tell quickly if the effect is real, or just a chance result in one case.

This patient's T-helper count had declined for four years, then stabilized at an average of about 500 with AZT; he has taken 500 mg of AZT per day for two years. He started taking a single 325-mg buffered aspirin tablet per day near the end of August, 1990. His last T-helper count before starting aspirin was 553. By mid September the count was unchanged at 556, although the helper/suppressor ratio had changed from .56 to .78. By mid November the count was 895, and by mid December it was 968 (the November test was to apply for a different NIH study). The T-helper percent and helper/suppressor ratio showed substantial increases. There was no other change in therapy or other known factor which would explain these improvements.

The patient had selected the low dose (one aspirin a day) because of a report[1] that an even lower dose (one aspirin every other day) had the greatest effect in increasing both interleukin-2 (IL-2) and interferon gamma in healthy volunteers. In this study, IL-2, which stimulates the growth of T-cells, was increased to two to three times baseline levels by low-dose aspirin.

## Questions for a Clinical Trial

• The first question for a trial to answer is whether aspirin can have any consistent effect in raising T-helper counts, or if the effect reported above was just happenstance or only applied to one patient. Clearly it would be easy to run a trial with low-dose aspirin, and follow T-helper counts for at least three months.

Some other questions:

• Is antiviral therapy (in this case, AZT) necessary? Stimulating the growth of T-helper cells without antiviral therapy might increase the growth of the virus. We have heard good results from studies which combined IL-2 and AZT; one early report found a T-helper increase of over 300 during IL-2 therapy, although the increase disappeared after treatment was stopped[2]. (As we went to press, we learned that results of an important trial at Stanford University of combination HIV treatment with IL-2 and AZT have recently been published; we could not obtain this paper by press time.) If low-dose aspirin does indeed stimulate the body to produce more of its own IL-2[1], then aspirin might be an alternative easier to obtain, safer, and of course less expensive than the experimental pharmaceutical IL-2.

• Could this treatment approach also work for persons with lower starting T-helper counts? A community-based trial could accept volunteers with a range of T-helper values. Then—if any significant effect is seen—the researchers could look for a dose-response relationship.

## Call for Information

Any information about long-term use of aspirin, and its effect (or lack of effect) on T-helper counts, could be helpful for designing such a trial. If you have information we should know about, contact John S. James at *AIDS Treatment News*.

## REFERENCES

1.    Hsia J., Simon GL, Higgins N, Goldstein AL, and Hayden FG. Immune modulation by aspirin during experimental rhinovirus colds. *Bulletin of the New York Academy of*

*Medicine.* January 1989; volume 65, number 1, pages 45-56. (Note: the data cited above was from volunteers who did not have colds.)

2. Bartlett JA, Blankenship K, Waskin H, Sebastian M, Shipp K, and Weinhold K. Zidovudine and interleukin-2 in WR2 HIV infected patients: Evidence for stimulated immunologic reactivity against HIV [abstract S.B.421]. Sixth International Conference on AIDS, San Francisco, June 20-24, 1990.

**Note:** For background on aspirin, and what is known or not known about its different mechanisms of action, see the latest *Scientific American*, January 1991, pages 84-90.

# WOMEN AND AIDS CONFERENCE REPORT
*by Laura Thomas*

The first National Conference on Women and HIV Infection was held December 13-14, 1990, in Washington, DC. It marked the first time that so many women with HIV, care providers, and activists had met specifically to talk about women and AIDS. The main issues discussed at the conference were the need for adequate health care for women with HIV infection, the lack of knowledge about the progression of disease in women, the problems of women and clinical trials, and the difficulties of doing education and prevention for women. This is a preliminary report of some of the information from the conference.

Some of the most interesting statistics presented proved conclusively what we already knew: health care makes a difference. Pat Kloser, M.D., from the Newark Women's AIDS Clinic, showed that the women who were cared for in her clinic averaged 70.4 weeks between AIDS diagnosis and death, as compared to the women who went through the emergency room and hospital system there, who averaged only 27.5 weeks.

The clearest recommendation for care was that women with symptomatic HIV disease should get cervical and anal Pap smears every six months, followed up by colposcopies if necessary. Pap smears are recommended for all women once a year, and men with HIV may be interested in having anal Pap smears done, as well. A Pap smear is a test for unusual, possibly pre-cancerous cells. Women with suppressed immune systems are especially vulnerable to infection with HPV (human papilloma virus) which causes cervical and other anogenital cancers. While there are not yet any truly effective treatments for cervical cancer or HPV infection in people with HIV, early detection and treatment offers the best hope of keeping it under control. Pap smears should become part of every woman's health care regimen, and we have heard that they are now going to be included in the standard of care for participants in AIDS Clinical Trials Group clinical trials.

There seems to be some evidence that the antimicrobial action of the PCP prophylaxis TMP-SMX (Bactrim or Septra) is causing vaginal candidiasis, or yeast infections, in women. It is well known that antibiotics such as penicillin can cause such infections, which many women have self-treated with acidophilus or yogurt, although we have not heard of any women on Septra taking acidophilus to counter the candidiasis. Vaginal candidiasis is also very common in women with HIV, so it may be hard to tell whether it is caused by Septra or not. TMP-SMX may also be preventing some of the HIV-related bacterial pneumonias that many women and injection drug users are getting.

Conflicting data was presented on the interaction of methadone and AZT. One clinician stated that methadone lowered levels of AZT in the blood, and another said that it nearly doubled AZT levels. Many recovering injection drug users are on methadone, so this will be an important drug interaction to study. As a group, injection drug users in clinical trials showed the same compliance rates as gay men did, debunking the myth of IDUs as irresponsible people. In fact, the most important predictor of compliance in a Boston trial of AZT was the belief in the efficacy of AZT, not the participant's drug-using status or transmission route.

One woman with AIDS described her frustration at being unable to find a doctor who was willing to operate on her cervical cancer. Doctors discussed their difficulties in getting and keeping good nurses. Many women talked about the need for substance abuse treatment, and made it clear that they could not take care of their HIV infection without taking care of their substance use, and vice versa. We were encouraged to hear of community-based clinics for women with HIV; but speakers noted that women enter the health care system everywhere, and there are few obstretics and gynecology physicians, or emergency room personnel, who are trained to care for women with HIV.

# Issue Number 119
# January 18, 1991

## TREATMENT STRATEGIES:
## INTERVIEW WITH PAULA SPARTI, M.D.

*by Denny Smith*

For a practical look at AIDS treatment advances, we interviewed Paula Sparti, M.D., who maintains a large HIV and family practice in Miami, Florida. Dr. Sparti also participates in the recently reconvened immune-based therapies group at the National Institutes of Health (NIH).

Traditionally, most AIDS/HIV treatments have been divided into antivirals, treatment or prophylaxis for opportunistic infections, and immunomodulators. New developments in these areas include combinations of antivirals (for example AZT with ddC, or with interferon, or with compound Q), and multiple opportunistic infection prophylaxis (using drug combinations to prevent most or all of the common OIs, not only pneumocystis).

Immunomodulators (agents which might fight HIV by affecting the body's various natural immune mechanisms rather than by acting on the virus directly) may account for the most numerous and least understood approaches. Since immune responses involve elaborate "cascades" of precise, sequential events in the body, attempts to alter a certain immune activity can prove even more complicated than the prospect of developing treatments which act against HIV directly. We hope to cover specific immunomodulators in upcoming issues of *AIDS Treatment News*.

---

**DS:** I want to pose some questions to you which we at *AIDS Treatment News* are often asked to answer, such as when to start anti-HIV drugs; what combinations of drugs look feasible; when to start prophylactic measures; is there such a thing as planning for infections, or planning access to various drugs?

**478**

The notion of immunomodulation is gaining momentum now, but the spectrum of potential agents and rationales is overwhelming. Also, and perhaps most urgently, many people are facing the prospect of AZT resistance, with unanswered questions about the prospective antivirals—ddI, ddC, and compound Q.

**PS:** In deciding when to begin antiretrovirals, I monitor bloodwork every three months, because I have seen a number of people who have had precipitous T-helper cell drops in a six month period of time. I have also been following some patients for nine or ten years who have had very stable counts. So I look for a sustained decline in helper cells and the T-cell ratio, more than just an absolute count that drops below 500 once or twice. I have two or three people who have had absolute T-helper cell counts below 500 since 1981, and who have been completely stable without an antiretroviral; without a doubt they would have been damaged a long time ago had I started them on nucleoside analogs.

I try much more to follow how stable people are, their percentage of T-helper cells, and their helper/suppressor ratio, rather than an absolute cell count. If you follow the absolute count over a long period of time, you can see that it goes up and down, and it is very dependant on an individual's total white count and lymphocyte count on a given day.

I haven't found that beta 2 microglobulin is very helpful. Sometimes I will see an increase in the beta 2 and the neopterin before a decline in immune competence. I'm finding that the p24 antibody [not to be confused with p24 antigen] is probably much more sensitive; I am just now getting fairly consistent results on quantitative p24 antibodies. You can follow them, and if they begin to fall, it may herald a fall in T-helper cells as well.

When I do start people on antiretrovirals, I start them on AZT alone. For years I have been starting people on 400 to 600 mg daily, for a typical 150 lb. person. There is community access to other drugs, and I know a number of my patients who are choosing to add ddC to their AZT.

I think there is a lot more myopathy [muscle disorder] associated with AZT than other people seem to be reporting. I have had some patients on AZT for up to four years, and they may not have obvious myositis [muscle discomfort]; they don't necessarily show significant increases in their CPKs, but they experience progressive wasting and muscle loss. There were a number of sessions at the last ACTG meeting elaborating the effect of AZT on mitochondria of muscle, and of ddI and ddC on nerve mitochondria. So although early intervention is very, very important, I think we still have to remember how toxic nucleoside analogs are.

**DS:** Would such myopathy be distinct from anything HIV alone might cause?

**PS:** It is distinct. HIV myopathy is inflammatory, for the most part. We can do a muscle biopsy here at the University of Miami and distinguish inflammatory myositis from a necrotic kind of cell death caused by AZT. And the difference is important to know, too, because if it *is* inflammatory and not due to AZT, you can treat it with non-steroidal anti-inflammatories, and if it's really bad you can treat it with short term steroids. You could stop the AZT to see if the myopathy or weight loss stops. But the problem is that it takes a long time to develop the myopathy and a long time to reverse it. It's not wise to have people off of an antiretroviral for the time it would take to decipher the problem, unless you have an effective substitute. A biopsy can help you know what you're dealing with.

**DS:** Is there any immediate way to mitigate the AZT-related myopathy?

**PS:** One of the things that comes to mind, considering the mitochondrial defect related to myopathy, is coenzyme Q-10 [not to be confused with compound Q], which supposedly helps the function of the mitochondria. This isn't strictly scientific, but I know that in Japan, coenzyme Q-10 is given to decrease the cardiac damage resulting as a side effect of adriamycin. It's available here by prescription.

**DS:** You know it's also available without a prescription at local buyers' clubs.

**PS:** Yes, and at health food stores, but I was thinking that for people who have insurance, a prescription may help to pay for it. Another solution to myopathy, and side effects generally, will be combinations of low-dose AZT with low-dose ddI or ddC, which are less likely to cause myopathy, or the neuropathy seen with higher doses of the single drugs.

**DS:** Regarding nucleoside combinations, do you think it's better to use them together in low doses, or to alternate them?

**PS:** I think that using them together is better; the likelihood of postponing resistance could be better in a simultaneous combination than in an alternating regimen. But that's the kind of thing we don't know for sure yet. I'll be happier when we have more to combine than two nucleoside analogs!

**DS:** Are there non-nucleoside candidates you feel strongly about?

**PS:** Well, I'm interested again in Ampligen, as an adjunct, as something used in combination with other drugs. It's now planned for phase I and phase II studies combining it with AZT. Ampligen may make AZT more active.

**DS:** Ampligen seems to have been hard to categorize as either an antiviral or an immunomodulator.

**PS:** Right, it may have activity of both. It's mismatched double-stranded RNA.

**DS:** Are you optimistic about compound Q?

**PS:** Well, I know Martin Delaney and Drs. Alan Levin and Larry Waites are very much behind it. I'm not negative about Q, I just haven't seen the same results they've reported. I also haven't had as much experience as they've had. I have followed maybe 30 or 40 people who have used Q, while they have seen hundreds. I would probably need more exposure to see the results they're seeing. I *have* noticed that a few people who were on AZT or ddI with slowly declining bloodwork seem to have been stabilized with the addition of compound Q. So, although I don't have a lot of experience, I think with some people I'm seeing a stabilization benefit from Q, and perhaps a modest increase in T-helper cells.

**DS:** Have you seen any serious toxicities from Q?

**PS:** Nothing life-threatening, but quite a few allergic reactions; fortunately the Q doesn't stay in the body very long, so we just stop the infusion and give IV Benadryl, and epinephrine if we need it. In subsequent treatments we premedicate those people with Hismanal, and Decadron too, if warranted, for several days before their infusion and also the day after. This way we've been able to reinfuse people who have had reactions.

**DS:** Other antivirals or experimental agents you're interested in?

**PS:** I am anxious to see what happens with the non-nucleoside RT inhibitors. Merck and Upjohn have several possibilities. The sooner we get results the sooner we get expanded options. I have also been eager to see trials of hyperimmune HIV globulin, or passive immunotherapy, get started. Medicorp has not had the funding to sponsor a major protocol, but Abbott Laboratories, which is much larger, may be able to back one.

**DS:** What about some popular community treatments, like oral interferon, NAC, and hypericin?

**PS:** NAC is more popular than hypericin, in which interest seems to have faded for lack of controlled clinical trial results. With NAC, a number of people report increased energy and appetite. I think there is a good rationale behind NAC, since it purportedly increases glutathione levels, which are deficient in virally infected cells. But the real benefits and dosage are uncertain, so again, we need clinical trials for quantitative results.

I have seen absolutely nothing with oral alpha interferon. I have heard of people who claimed increases in T-helper cell counts, but I have not been able to find anyone in my practice or our local community who has been able to show a sustained increase from oral interferon.

**DS:** That's pretty much what I have heard from other physicians. However, another antiviral I wanted to ask you about was the injectable alpha interferon, approved by the FDA to treat Kaposi's sarcoma. Anthony Fauci seems to talk a lot about it in terms of a potential HIV agent.

**PS:** I think the limitation there is that you have to use it early in HIV disease. If you use it later, you risk further compromise of the immune system. People with higher T-helper cells can tolerate interferon, and if you combine it with low-dose AZT you can obtain significant increases in T-helper cells as well as diminish their KS lesions. One of the factors is that late in HIV disease, endogenous [naturally occurring] levels of interferon are high, anyway. Simply adding more is not going to be helpful in that case.

I think interleukin [IL] is more interesting. The interleukins 2, 4, and 7 have a lot to do with T-cell proliferation and maturation. Of course IL-2 can be very toxic, but apparently you can use less of it if you combine it with IL-4. I think this is the beginning of being innovative with immunomodulation. When you have been treating HIV for several years, you have a lot of patients with less than fifty T-helper cells, but who are not ill yet. We're desperately trying to find ways to increase the T-helper cells.

**DS:** I have spoken to a couple of people who have tried lithium as a way to boost their helper count, but I understand that it only produces a broad, non-specific increase in white cells.

**PS:** A few of my patients wanted to take lithium, but you're right—if you're not increasing the number of mature T-helper cells, then it's not going to be really helpful. You may get a sort of artificial sense that T-cells have increased, because you've elevated the total white count, but not necessarily the percent of functioning, mature T-helper cells.

**DS:** Any thoughts on isoprinosine or Imuthiol (DTC)?

**PS:** Those two, and levamisole as well, have been receiving a lot of interest out here. Several recent reports show that levamisole increases cell-mediated immunity. Imuthiol has been studied much more in Europe than in the U.S., and it now is available in New Zealand. People here have tried an industrial grade DTC, or antabuse as a DTC substitute. We just need more results of controlled clinical trials to know for sure. Isoprinosine is something which more of my patients used back in 1984 and '85, not so much lately.

People should give more consideration to transfer factor. It may be a crude lymphocyte extract, with an indeterminate mixture of lymphokines, but I have definitely seen people whose energy and well-being improved on transfer factor. Perhaps it suppresses some of the herpesviruses. I had two patients in the past couple of years with CMV retinitis who chose not to go on ganciclovir, yet both of their infections were stabilized while on transfer factor. The people at the NIH are not prone to pursue transfer factor—their position would be that this is just a concoction of various biological products, and it would be difficult to attribute a response to any one of its constituents. So verifying its worth may be a job for a community-based research group.

I have been trying quite a bit of intravenous immune globulin (IVIG) in some of my patients with very low T-helper cells. It's clear to me that their ability to produce antibodies to specific antigens is severely damaged. [IVIG supplies antibodies.] The results are anecdotal, but I have seen benefits in people with chronic sinusitis and chronic bronchitis after several months on IVIG.

**DS:** If you had a proven immunomodulator right now, when would you give it to patients? Would it be helpful to asymptomatics, including those with healthy blood markers?

**PS:** Well, we know so little about immunomodulation, it's difficult to say for sure. But agents that cause T-cell proliferation, the interleukins, for example, would probably work better when the T-cells are higher, when stem cells are in better shape. If your bone marrow is wiped out, there's not much for the interleukin to work with. If we had something that would help cell-mediated immunity, then using it early might avoid some of the down-spiraling which results from immune-complex disease and inflammation.

**DS:** It sounds like you're saying that immunomodulation should have specific targets.

**PS:** The more I learn, the more I realize how incredibly intricate the immune cascade is. You can't just throw an interleukin into somebody's body and obtain a known effect. You have to know how to use it and when to use it, in what dose and in what frequency. I'm excited that the immune-based therapy group is back together at the NIH.

**DS:** Regarding opportunistic infections, and prophylactic measures to thwart them, I spoke to Dr. Larry Bruni, who practices in Washington, DC, who suggests that not only does HIV infection allow other pathogens to cause infections, but those secondary infections might transactivate HIV, or enhance HIV progression, as well. So both things may be happening in tandem. What do you think about that, and the role of prophylaxis for the various AIDS-associated infections?

**PS:** I definitely believe that when people get sick, whatever that "sick" is, it affects viral replication and it affects their T-helper cell count. I have been using more and more multiple opportunistic infection prophylaxis. A lot depends on the toxicity of the drugs in question. Some of the studies being designed to address prophylaxis, other than for pneumocystis, are a little disturbing in that they use an inflexible, uniform T-helper cell cut-off of 200, even though infections do not appear uniformly at 200 helper cells. Most infections other than pneumocystis don't appear above 100, or even 50, T-helper cells.

Given that, I tell those patients that, although there is no proof that a certain drug will prevent an infection, my recommendation is for a prophylaxis. I offer fluconazole, 100 mg a day, to prevent cryptococcal meningitis in people who already need an antifungal for candidiasis. I see who can tolerate pyrimethamine, 25 mg a day, to try to prevent toxoplasmosis. In people with symptoms of herpesvirus infections, including leukoplakia, I use acyclovir liberally. And I think multiple prophylaxing works. I now have many more people who are three or four years past their first OI. That is different from what was happening a while ago, when people would die within the first year or two of an initial opportunistic infection.

**DS:** Is it useful first to check people for past exposure to a certain infections?

**PS:** Oh yes, we always do that. We always test for toxoplasmosis, which is common in Florida, as well as CMV, Epstein-Barr, herpes simplex. If people are negative, you can avoid the drugs and their possible side effects.

**DS:** Do you see many identifiable mycoplasma infections?

**PS:** I keep mycoplasma in mind, and if I see someone with interstitial pneumonitis, or pulmonary problems that I can't really explain, or they're just not getting better, I liberally use doxycycline. You can give it intravenously if necessary, or orally if they are not that ill.

**DS:** Have you seen results from doxycycline?

**PS:** You cannot always know what you're treating, and you see some strange things. I have seen thrombocytopenia resolve temporarily on doxycycline, for no apparent reason. Recently there was a relevant article in the *Tropic*, which is the Sunday magazine of the *Miami Herald*. It asked if the people at the NIH are missing the boat by having just one paradigm, the antiviral paradigm, and not looking at the importance of cofactors, and the autoimmune part of this disease.

But if you ask me whether *Mycoplasma incognitus* is more important than syphilis, or CMV, or HIV, I really doubt it. Of all the possible cofactors, so many are present, including some we may have not even identified yet. Mycoplasma is only the newest kid on the block.

**DS:** Do you see patients who use recreational drugs, and are some of those drugs a risk for aggravating HIV progression?

**PS:** Well, opiates are known to cause immune suppression. Interestingly, some of my patients are still using naltrexone, which is an opiate antagonist. One of them, anecdotally, has been using it for five years now, and he has had totally stable T-helper cells.

I think that the use of opiates is immunosuppressive, as are cocaine and alcohol. Narcotics are compromising also because they chip away some of the will to live, the will to fight. Some of my drug abusers want to feel better, but they don't want to do the work required to feel better. For them it's "too much trouble to eat, too much trouble to take a deep breath," or to get to appointments. The will to live is part of being a long-term survivor.

I think antidepressants are probably helpful. Depression itself can deplete T-helper cells. There is a fair amount of evidence that antidepressants used to treat chronic fatigue syndrome can achieve some beneficial immunomodulation—increased natural killer cell activity, sometimes increased T-helper cells.

**DS:** Do you think there are particular AIDS diagnoses that frequently get overlooked?

**PS:** Nothing stands out, although I think sometimes people do not get treated at all because their complaints are simply chalked up to AIDS. I hope that's unusual.

I push to make a diagnosis if at all possible. If someone has got a fever, I don't wait for something horrible to happen; I begin a comprehensive workup. It is important to treat something before it gets out of hand. If someone has a fever, part of a fever workup should be sending them to an ophthalmologist to have them checked for CMV retinitis that may not yet be causing visual disturbance. You may have to check for cryptococcal antigen even though they might not have a headache. It requires a sixth sense. Some practitioners who do not have a daily familiarity with AIDS don't know to diagnose and treat aggressively, and when their patients are finally seen by AIDS experts, they are really sick, and more difficult to treat.

**DS:** What would you like to see added to the current treatment picture?

**PS:** I'm anxious to see a lot more things evaluated. I would like to see more results on photopheresis. There are some interesting discussions of low-dose total body irradiation as a method of decreasing suppressor cells, with a consequent increase in helper cells. There are so many potential therapies out there to be evaluated, and I'm frustrated because I want them all to be evaluated as soon as possible. Now that I am working within the NIH, I see that there's a handful of people who make most of the decisions.

Maybe we will be able to get them to really look at more substances, and new procedural ways of doing things, and not to be so immediately negative. You would think that under the circumstances they would give anything and everything the benefit of the doubt. It will be interesting to see what happens in the next year or so.

## MAJOR FDA MEETING ON DRUG APPROVAL STANDARDS, FEBRUARY 13 AND 14

*by John S. James*

Crucial issues on how to prove efficacy for new-drug approval will be considered at a meeting of the FDA's Antiviral Drug Products Advisory Committee on February 13 and 14, near Washington, DC. The meeting is open to the public.

The Wednesday, February 13, session concerns endpoints in AIDS trials, and the role of CD4 and other laboratory markers as indicators of clinical benefit. While this meeting is not scheduled to consider ddC and ddI, those drugs clearly provide its immediate context and rationale.

On Thursday, February 14, the Committee plans to focus on AZT, especially followup on the trials which supported expanded indications for treatment (T-helper counts to 500).

While there has been little public attention to this meeting, there has been much activity behind the scenes, especially preparations by scientists. Since AIDS treatment activists from around the country will be in Washington on those days, there may also be activist meetings before and after the antiviral committee meets.

The Antiviral Drug Products Advisory Committee is scheduled to meet at the Holiday Inn Crown Plaza, Rockville, MD, at 8:30 a.m. on both days.

## Comment

Here is a scenario which we find useful for organizing our thoughts for this meeting. Suppose that in the near future an AIDS or HIV treatment is found which works very well—either a single drug, or more likely, a combination. Suppose that almost everyone who uses the treatment becomes healthy again (except for any irreparable damage which might have been caused by severe illness): weight and energy return, all blood work becomes normal, and there are no opportunistic infections or new malig-nancies, as long as patients keep taking the treatment. Assume that the toxicities are small or manageable.

The question is, "What would happen then"—and what should happen?

## The present system

Under the current system it does seem clear what *would* happen. First, if the treatment were a combination of new drugs, it would not be tested at all, because the FDA almost never allows a trial of more than one unapproved drug at the same time. All but one of the drugs would have to go through the entire approval process separately, proving itself alone compared to AZT. Then, years later, the combination could be tried.

Suppose the new treatment were a single drug, so that the above problem was not an issue. The first bottleneck—organizing corporate commitment and funding—would already have occurred. Waiting for the patent office could have delayed the project for a year or more. Then, if luck were bad, additional years could have been spent in litigation.

We have not investigated the detailed requirements for animal testing. But we have heard from persons familiar with this area that they are often grossly excessive and irrational.

Next comes the process of getting approval for phase I (dosage and toxicity) human trials. Here the biggest problem is juggling busy peoples' schedules to get the required people and papers into the same room at the same time. Perhaps the IRB or other required body does not finish its other business in time, so the drug is postponed for weeks or months until the next meeting. Then some of the people cannot attend, and the trial is postponed again.

Finally the phase I trials actually start. They often take more than a year, because one group must take the drug for an extended time at a very low dose, before the next group starts at the next dose, etc. for a number of different doses. Traditionally, these phase I trials were planned to run until toxicity was found, even if it became clear that the drug showed efficacy at a non-toxic dose. The higher doses that would never be used still had to be tested. (ddI was substantially delayed for this reason.)

Next comes the design of phase II comparative efficacy trials. Traditionally this is done by research physicians, with no input from the "front line" physicians experi-enced in treating patients. Therefore the resulting trials can be difficult to administer, and often have trouble recruiting patients.

The early steps in drug development, before phase II, are outside the scope of the Antiviral Drug Products Advisory Committee. Now we come to the later steps in development, where the public pays attention, creating pressure for reform, and therefore meetings like the one in February. (The earlier steps do not generate such pressure, because they are usually secret until human trials begin. The public does not see the inefficiency, and until recently, was simply told that good science takes time, and that the only issue was whether or not to weaken the scientific process.)

Today there is much confusion about what standards to use to judge efficacy of AIDS drugs. The traditional ones, which still prevail, are illustrated by the large ongoing trials of ddI and ddC. The original idea was that each new drug would be compared with a placebo—and the trial would have to prove superiority of the drug, by accumulating a statistically significant number of deaths or major opportunistic infections in the placebo group. When it became unethical to use a placebo in a trial designed to end in death or major illness, AZT was simply substituted for placebo, and the goal of drug equivalence was more or less substituted for superiority. No one thought through the effects of these changes on the trial design.

With or without these complications, it was necessary to wait for deaths or OIs in the volunteers not receiving the treatment being tested. Therefore, even if the new treatment cured everybody instantly, it would still take many months or years to meet the efficacy standards set for these trials.

Because deaths in the AZT group occur slowly, these studies need to be very large and/or run for a long time (for example, 18 or 24 months) to expect to attain statistical significance. Hundreds of volunteers are required. Each trial needs to run identically at a number of major medical centers in order to find enough qualifying volunteers, creating major delays for administration as well as for recruitment. (For example, the IRB for each site must meet to approve the study—and each IRB meets on its own schedule. Each IRB must either accept or reject the study exactly as given—it cannot change any of the science, or the data will not be compatible. Since IRBs do not like to serve as rubber stamps, they exercise themselves by making insignificant changes in the informed consent form which the volunteers will sign—the only changes they are allowed to make. The study then has a separate consent form for each site—a minor, almost humorous problem, compared to the others.)

When the trial finally begins, a group of experts called a Data Safety Monitoring Board meets periodically during the trial and secretly unblinds the data, to stop the study for ethical reasons if extreme differences between the groups are found. But in practice, the standards for stopping the trial early are extremely severe. Therefore the Data Safety Monitoring Board serves more as a public-relations cover than as a real protection for patients; but because its deliberations are secret, the public does not realize this fact.

An additional problem now is the lack of clarity about what will be considered evidence of drug efficacy. Proof that a new drug is *superior* to AZT, in *preventing death and major disease progression*, is the most conservative possible standard. The problem with this standard is that for reasons cited above it will take a very long time to meet this level of proof, even if the drug is in fact better. In addition, a drug which is only equally effective as AZT—or even less effective—could save many lives, if it has different toxicities, is effective in different patients, or has unique value in combination with AZT or other drugs. What is happening today, however, is that companies are confused about what standards the FDA will use; therefore they are reluctant to submit their data, and the FDA does not see it.

These operational problems explain why, years after AZT approval, no new AIDS antiviral has been properly tested and approved, although attractive candidate drugs have long been available. The problems continue because no one is in charge of the national response to the epidemic, so no one has the authority to correct them.

## What Should Be Done?

The hope is that the February 13 meeting will reduce the confusion by recommending a viable efficacy standard. What might such a standard be?

There is considerable movement toward a consensus of accepting improvement in T-helper cell count (or percent), together with at least some measurement of clinical improvement, such as regained lost body weight, as proof of efficacy for an antiviral (unless, of course, there is some good reason to reject the evidence; we are not suggesting that approval would be automatic). Part of the rationale is that there seems to be no group of persons with HIV whose average T-helper counts will increase over time without treatment; the direction is always down. If a drug increases T-helper count by means of its antiviral effect—a result which can be seen within eight to 12 weeks, about a tenth the time required by a trial which looks for death or major disease progression—and there is no reason to believe that the drug would increase T-helper cells by any mechanism other than inhibiting the virus which causes AIDS—then it is hard to believe that the drug is not having an effect on the disease. Requiring some measure of direct patient benefit is an additional precaution; it should cause little objection, as few physicians or patients would want to use a drug if there was no direct evidence that patients using it got better.

If a drug (or combination of drugs) can pass this test, then it should be considered to have met the efficacy standard for approval—at least in the current emergency. Otherwise, the practical consequence of maintaining the current system is that *all* new AIDS antivirals will be delayed for years, the new generation of drugs such as protease inhibitors will not be developed expeditiously, and tens of thousands of deaths will be guaranteed.

We have heard little opposition to changing the efficacy standard for AIDS antivirals along the lines of the developing consensus described above. The issue is not whether there should be a change, or even what the change should be—although academic arguments will likely be raised concerning any particular proposal. The real issue is whether anything will get done, given the lack of coordination and high-level leadership on Federal AIDS policy.

## PEPTIDE T: NEW ACCESS OBSTACLES

*by John S. James*

For several months there have been increasing reports of difficulty in obtaining peptide T, an experimental treatment which is generally agreed to be safe and is in clinical trials. (*AIDS Treatment News* last covered peptide T in issue #84.) Recently the situation came to a head when two buyers' groups had their supplies cut off, due to Federal action against two different suppliers; in one of these cases, Ron Woodruff of the Dallas Buyers' Club sued the FDA, and lost in Federal court in San Francisco. We started investigating, but soon learned that *Treatment Issues*, the treatment newsletter published by Gay Men's Health Crisis in New York, was already working on this problem. "Peptide T Access Blocked," by Wayne Kawadler, was published last week in *Treatment Issues*, volume 5, number 1, January 10, 1990.

[Note: To obtain a copy, send a note asking for the peptide T issue to: GMHC, attn: Medical Information, 129 West 20th St., New York, NY 10011, or call Wayne Kawadler at 212/337-1950. Also note: *Treatment Issues* is published ten times a year by Gay Men's Health Crisis. There is no charge for a subscription, but a $20 per year contribution ($40 international) is suggested if possible. A $10 contribution is suggested for all back issues, for the last three years. To request a subscription, write or call to the number above. Note that that number is only for *Treatment Issues*; for other AIDS information, call the GMHC hotline at 212/807-6655.]

We will not restate Mr. Kawadler's article, but it included the following points:

• FDA agents recently visited Peninsula Laboratories, in Belmont, California, and told them that some of their peptide T, sold for animal research, "was actually being used by people and that the commerce must stop." [Note: Peptide T, like most experimental drugs, can be sold as a chemical for research or industrial purposes without advance approval; but if intended for human use, it can only be sold to someone with an IND (Investigational New Drug approval), i.e., permission from the FDA to conduct human trials.] This FDA action against Peninsula Laboratories led to the unsuccessful lawsuit by Ron Woodruff. Peninsula Laboratories had previously provided peptide T used in clinical trials.

• Carlbiotech, a pharmaceutical company in Denmark, recently received a contract to provide peptide T for a clinical trial at the University of Southern California. At about the same time, the FDA wrote to Carlbiotech and told them not to sell peptide T to anyone without an IND.

• The FDA has a well-known policy of allowing importation for personal use of limited amounts of drugs approved elsewhere but not in the U.S., under certain conditions. Apparently peptide T does not meet the guidelines for this policy, however, since it is not approved as a drug in any country.

• One clinical trial of peptide T now recruiting—a five-year study at Yale for intravenous drug users—will enroll 24 volunteers per year. The protocol for the study at the University of Southern California is not yet final; current plans are for a six-month placebo study to enroll 150 volunteers. [We called the U.S. AIDS Clinical Trials Information Service, 800/TRIALS-A, and it had no information on peptide T trials now recruiting.]

## Comment

Peptide T has been a hidden but appalling scandal for years. *AIDS Treatment News* first covered this drug four years ago, on January 16, 1987 (issue #22). At that time we reported that the drug had been given to four terminally ill patients in Sweden, and their condition had improved. We concluded that January 1987 article with an unfortunately prophetic paragraph:

"The public, through its AIDS, medical, and other public-service organizations, must continue to watch the development of peptide T, as well as other treatment research. In the past, too many promising AIDS treatment leads have been strangled in red tape or left on the shelf to collect dust instead of being tested promptly. Only continuing public vigilance can make sure it doesn't happen again."

Later, we heard a credible (but not confirmed) report that the Swedish research had been stopped by U.S. pressure.

It would take a book to trace the convoluted history of peptide T and investigate the many allegations of wrongdoing in its history. What happened to this drug is a grotesque microcosm of problems with drug development in this country. We do recommend such a study for a serious researcher; many hundreds, if not thousands, of pages of documentation are available. (For starters, see "Peptide T" in *Treatment Issues*, volume 3, number 1, February 6, 1989, published by Gay Men's Health Crisis, New York; also see "Peptide T and the AIDS Establishment," *Boston* magazine, June 1990.)

Does the drug work? Our understanding is that it was originally intended to be an antiviral, and did show such activity in laboratory tests; the mechanism of action was believed to be similar to that of soluble CD4, i.e., preventing the virus from binding to and entering uninfected cells. But human tests which looked for antiviral activity were disappointing, and as a result, some researchers lost interest. Clinical trials have, however, repeatedly found neurological or other symptom improvements. [See, for example, reports on human trials at the Sixth International Conference on AIDS, San Francisco, June 20-24, 1990—abstracts number S.B.459, S.B.501, S.B.505, and 2183.]

And personal reports we have received do suggest that the drug is helping—even if the mechanism is not known. For example, one of the people whose supply was recently cut off told us that he had been trying AIDS treatments for years, and had been through the "placebo effect" many times, enough to tell that his improvement with peptide T was not just a psychological effect from trying a new treatment.

We do not know how difficult it will be to get peptide T in the future. Unfortunately, the drug is rather expensive. It is usually administered by injection; it can also be prepared for nasal use, although that route is less efficient.

One big unanswered question is why would the FDA move against peptide T now? Everyone agrees the drug is safe. Furthermore, as far as we know, it is not being and has not been promoted. Instead, a few people learned that the drug was especially helpful for them—sometimes by volunteering for FDA-approved trials and then having their drug cut off when the trial ended— and quietly found ways to obtain a supply, either from U.S. or international sources. This system has continued for many months, if not for years, and as far as we know there have been no problems, no complaints. When there are many real problems to worry about, why would the FDA move now on a non-problem, when doing so will not do anyone any good, and may cause some people serious harm?

Until now the AIDS community has had only a sporadic interest in peptide T, because other issues are more important—for example, the early evaluation of ddC and ddI—and beyond that, the development of workable efficacy standards for an epidemic emergency. The new generations of drugs now beginning human trials—from Merck, Boehringer Ingelheim, Hoffmann-La Roche, and a number of other major pharmaceutical companies—must have a rational development path, so that they do not waste the two years or more that the current system requires. Our main focus must naturally be on the most critical issues.

But access issues will not go away. For no matter what happens in FDA and drug-development reform, for years to come there will be many people who face death or irreparable injury because of lack of approval of treatment they need, when they are in fact right about their need for the drug, and the FDA and its experts are in fact wrong (or, more commonly, have not yet evaluated the drug, or even seen or tried to see the data). The FDA-suggested alternative of an individual compassionate IND is seldom available for AIDS. No community can abandon its people when they are sacrificed for bureaucratic convenience.

One of the problems we will face is bad court decisions left over from the decade-old battle against laetrile, a dubious cancer remedy. Under decisions of the U.S. Supreme Court (and also of the California Supreme Court), patients and their physicians have no right to treatment access; instead, the FDA makes that decision (but only when pharmaceutical companies, for their own reasons, ask it to). If the system is corrupt or ineffectual, or if the experts are incompetent, mistaken, or (most commonly) just too busy, then the patient has no recourse except to die or obtain treatment underground.

It is important to realize that this monstrous outcome occurred because the courts were asked to decide the wrong question. Laetrile advocates proposed that persons terminally ill should have the right to try anything, since the alternative was death. This position hardly seems unreasonable. But the problem is that the courts saw that they were being asked to put the terminally ill outside of the regulatory process entirely, in effect declaring open season for any hustler ready to take advantage of their desperation. This the courts were unwilling to do.

What the courts should have been asked instead was to give the ultimate access decision, in extreme cases, to the patient and physician—but to clearly distinguish this right of access from the marketing or promotion of unproven drugs. Currently, the laws control both drug access, and drug marketing (forbidding unsupported claims); but the mainstay of unapproved-drug regulation is in fact the control of claims (at least in California, which has some of the strictest health-fraud regulation in the nation). In one case, for example, a California physician was arrested after treating a patient with a drug the physician had invented. We heard later that State authorities said they did not object if the patient continued to receive the treatment, by getting a pharmacist to formulate the drug; their objection was to statements made by the physician to patients, apparently heard by an undercover agent. We do not propose this case as a model; it does, however, illustrate the difference between control of access and control of claims. We suspect that if the courts had been asked to respect the autonomy of the terminally ill, but without at the same time removing them from regulatory protection, the decisions might have been different.

Unfortunately, it takes a long time for court rulings to change. One resource we should mention for those who have to fight the access issue now is the book *Catastrophic Rights* (subtitled *Experimental Drugs and AIDS*), by John Dixon, president of the British Columbia Civil Liberties Association (published by New Star Books, Vancouver, 1990). The phrase "catastrophic rights" refers to expanded rights of treatment access by persons who are catastrophically ill; the book develops this concept through discussion and analysis of relevant legal, medical, and scientific issues.

Above all, we believe that the best single strategy for the AIDS or other patient communities in fighting for treatment access is the development of medical consensus. When mainstream, respected experts who are familiar with a treatment have a well-supported belief that the treatment is valuable, then courts are reluctant to stand in their way. But we must also remember that while medical consensus will defeat most *philosophical* obstacles to treatment access, it will often not defeat the commercial and practical ones—as illustrated by drugs like fluconazole and EPO, which were not readily available until long after physicians realized they needed them. Nothing will replace continued hard work by activist and medical organizations to discover the real source of the obstacles, and ways to eliminate or circumvent them.

# FLT: (FLUOROTHYMIDINE) UPDATE

On December 21, 1990, *AIDS Treatment News* mentioned FLT, an antiviral that we had listed two years ago as an important potential AIDS/HIV treatment. FLT is being developed by Lederle Laboratories (a division of American Cyanamid Company), and has already begun human trials.

Stanley A. Lang, Ph.D., project director at Lederle Laboratories, provided correct information. He explained that a very early phase I trial, a single dose human study, has been finished; such studies are used to test pharmacokinetics, meaning how well the drug is absorbed, how long it stays in the body, etc. The drug was found to be very well absorbed orally, and it remains in the blood long enough that it would be used only twice daily. Now Lederle is about to start a phase I/II trial with 50 volunteers at three sites: Sloan Kettering in New York, Johns Hopkins in Baltimore, and the University of North Carolina in Chapel Hill. This trial will use five different doses, with each tested for four months.

In laboratory tests the drug has worked well against strains of HIV taken from patients. (Many earlier drug-development efforts went astray when they used the more convenient laboratory cultures of HIV in such tests; these viruses, which have been cultured for years in laboratories, are different from those found in patients.) FLT also (like most new antivirals being tested) is effective against virus strains which are resistant to AZT—despite the fact that FLT is chemically similar to AZT.

Unfortunately, FLT also shows toxicity in animal tests, especially bone-marrow toxicity like AZT. AIDS drug expert Raymond F. Schinazi, Ph.D., was quoted in the December 13, 1990, *Medical Tribune* as saying that FLT "is one of the most potent compounds around. A promising drug, but it has to be used with a lot of caution."

# FAACTS: ALTERNATIVE TREATMENT INFORMATION AVAILABLE

*by John S. James*

A new volunteer group, assisted by specialists in computerized searching of medical and scientific literature, is providing information from journal articles and abstracts to AIDS libraries, activist organizations, clinics, and others interested in treatment alternatives.

FAACTS (Facts on Alternate AIDS Compounds & Treatments) has currently assembled a total of 750 pages of information, on 16 topics. The treatments currently covered are: astragalus, Carrisyn, DHEA, DNCB, glycyrrhizin, DTC (Imuthiol), IL-2, isoprinosine, levamisole, NAC, passive immunotherapy, peptide T, AL 721 and blue-green algae (both treatments covered in one packet together), THA, and transfer factor.

Each of the 15 packets contains 25 to 45 pages of information, including five or more selected journal articles, plus additional abstracts.

For information on how to obtain the individual packets, or the complete set (in two binders) plus updates as available, call FAACTS, 415/548-9654, or write to 5337 College Avenue, Suite 517, Oakland, CA 94618.

## Comment

We joined the advisory board of FAACTS because we consider the organization a much needed effort to help provide in-depth treatment information. While the same material is available in medical libraries, most people do not have access to a medical library; even if they did have access and knew how to use the library, there would still be the problem of selecting relevant information. The frustration was well expressed recently by one AIDS treatment activist, who went to a buyers' club for information about DHEA, and found "one page of nothing."

This project began when two information specialists offered to do computer literature searches for a friend with AIDS. They wanted to make the service available to more people, and FAACTS was formed to do so. FAACTS is being coordinated by Peter Moreland, who can be reached through the phone number or address above.

# Issue Number 120
# February 1, 1991

## THE EPIDEMIC AND THE WAR

*By Denny Smith*

When San Francisco was struck by the Loma Prieta Earthquake in October 1989, the American public, the governments of California and the United States, and the international media devoted weeks of attention to the rescue stories and recovery efforts. Congress arranged for speedy economic help to the Bay Area, and insurance companies took out full page ads for many days running to facilitate any claims their customers needed to file. The Vice-President came to survey the tragedy, to express his deep concern and that of the President as well.

For those San Franciscans who had already endured eight years of lives lost to the AIDS epidemic, the intensity of the response to the earthquake evoked mixed emotions. No Vice-President ever visited the injured in San Francisco General's AIDS ward. Rather, the White House seldom mentioned AIDS in the ten years of the epidemic.

No insurance company ever placed eloquent ads in city dailies offering to assist with the payment for HIV treatments. In contrast, many insurers have gone to some trouble to back out of coverage for legitimate treatments. In the first issue published after the earthquake, *AIDS Treatment News* commented that "in two days, national institutions mobilized as they have never done in eight years of AIDS," and that outside of communities immediately affected by the epidemic, there had not been "even a pale shadow of the mobilization that the far less deadly earthquake has called forth."

Now, much of the world is traumatized by a new disaster: the war in the Middle East, which is commanding the attention and the assets of many nations, their citizens and their news media. Every day, headlines convey the war's urgency, economic futures are reassessed, and the greatest political gravity is assigned to the crisis.

**494**

And once more, people who have been struggling with chronic disasters in their lives and their communities are faced with discrepancies in their government's priorities. One week after the resort to warfare, the death toll from AIDS in the U.S. passed 100,000. AIDS has killed more San Franciscans in a decade than have died in the past century of wars and earthquakes combined. The day after bombings against Iraq began, San Francisco Mayor Art Agnos wrote in the *San Francisco Examiner*, "The war we wanted was a war against AIDS, homelessness and poverty." In the United States today, AIDS is the second leading cause of death of men ages 25 to 44. Who will decide when the vast human resources now poured into technology for ending life can be used instead to build technology for preserving life?

Besides diverting attention from the AIDS crisis, the war has impeded research and care due to staff shortages, as medical professionals are sent to the Gulf. Long-term financial impacts on medical research are not yet known, but almost certainly they will be severe. Clearly the war will do no good for AIDS or any other medical research and care; the question is what damage will be done and how much. We plan to report as necessary on these consequences of the Gulf War, but not to let it divert our attention from the war against AIDS.

## IMMUNE GLOBULIN PROVES VALUABLE FOR TREATING CHILDREN, POSSIBLY ADULTS
*by Denny Smith*

Immune globulin is a concentrated and purified solution rich in antibodies from pooled human blood. It has been tested for some time in children with HIV, and some adults, as a method of bolstering their immunity to various bacterial infections. The antibody protection obtained from immune globulin is considered a short-term, passive immunity. The drug is a licensed treatment, often used as a way of conferring some measure of immunity against hepatitis and measles immediately following a perceived exposure to those viruses; it has also been used for reversing low platelet counts related to immunodeficiency.

On January 17 the National Institute of Child Health and Human Development announced results of a study of intravenous immune globulin (IVIG) involving 372 children (from two months to 12 years of age) which found significant benefits in the group receiving monthly IVIG, compared to those given a placebo. The data was gathered at 28 trial sites beginning March 1, 1988, and the recommendation to end the study was made January 10 of this year, after a Data Safety Monitoring Board discerned the study's trend.

IVIG was shown to decrease the number of bacterial infections and hospitalizations, and to increase the time between infections. These benefits were more dramatic in the children with higher T-helper cell counts. Although the children with less than 200 helper cells gained some protection compared to their counterparts in the placebo group, the improvement was not considered significant.

Other than mild brief rashes, few side effects were observed from the IVIG. The particular product used in the study was supplied by the Berkeley firm of Cutter Biological, which agreed to continue supplying free IVIG to any study participant.

Many children in both the placebo and treatment arms were at some point of the study also treated with AZT or aerosol pentamidine; neither of these appeared to influence the effect of IVIG. Physicians can obtain more details of the study, known as protocol ACTG 045, by calling 800/TRIALS-A. The press release announcing the study's results also noted that by the end of November of last year, the Centers for Disease Control had recorded 2,734 cases of AIDS in children under age 13, and that two to ten times that many more children in the U.S. may be HIV-infected; of these a disproportionate number are children of color.

For a thorough discussion of IVIG in clinical pediatric AIDS care, we refer readers to an article by E. Richard Stiehm, M.D., of the Division of Immunology at the University of California in Los Angeles, published in the December 1989 issue of *AIDS Medical Report*. In addition to controlling chronic bouts with bacterial infections, Dr. Stiehm suggests that IVIG might effectively be included in the treatment regimens for some serious opportunistic infections in children, such as CMV pneumonia and respiratory syncytial virus. Oral formulations of immune globulin have been used against cryptosporidial diarrhea.

## Adults May Also Benefit

IVIG is receiving more notice recently for treating adults with AIDS, and not just to treat ITP, or low platelets. Paula Sparti, M.D., an experienced HIV clinician in Miami, told us that some of her adult patients who are troubled with chronic infections like sinusitis and bronchitis have improved noticeably after several months of IVIG infusions (see interview with Dr. Sparti in the last issue of *AIDS Treatment News*, #119). These patients have low T-helper counts, in contrast to the lesser response associated with low T-helper counts in the children's study.

There are a number of reasons why results with adults and children may not be comparable. For example, the value of immune globulin for children comes from the contribution of antibodies to help children's inexperienced immune systems resist unfamiliar infections. In healthy adults, the immune system has already collected a larger "repertoire" of protective antibodies through years of exposure to the environment's microbes. But various kinds of immunodeficiency in adults, including AIDS, can deplete their acquired immunity, increasing susceptibility to common infectious agents.

Alan Levin, M.D., an immunologist working with adult HIV patients in San Francisco, presented related information at a recent community forum. Dr. Levin explained that a substantial value of immune globulin in treating HIV symptoms, aside from the simple transfer of antibodies, is a regulatory effect on inflammatory processes which characterize HIV infection, and on the immune dysfunction set in motion with the inflammation. He cautioned that IVIG can cause headaches, and rarely, anaphylactic reactions, and is very expensive. However, the cost in many instances has been reimbursed by health insurance, especially if the therapy is prescribed for treatment of repeated infections.

# CALIFORNIA: HEALTH INSURANCE NOW AVAILABLE FOR PERSONS WITH AIDS

*by John S. James*

California residents can now buy health insurance regardless of health status—meaning that no one is too sick to qualify—under a new state program beginning February 1. This program, the State of California Major Risk Medical Insurance Program, subsidizes insurance companies to provide health coverage to persons otherwise uninsurable due to chronic illness.

Major Risk policies are comparable to standard commercial health insurance; they do cover prescription drugs, including off-label use of approved drugs, as well as experimental drugs provided under an FDA-approved "treatment IND." The cost to the individual is set by law to be about 25 percent more than what a healthy person of the same age would pay for the same coverage—meaning that the policy can be highly beneficial for persons with costly medical problems.

This program is funded by money from the tobacco tax approved by a voter initiative. Medical high-risk programs are also being developed in some other states.

The Major Risk program in California has some important limitations:

• Currently there is only enough money for 10,000 people. According to one estimate, 25 times that many Californians are now uninsured due to health status. Therefore enrollment may close in a few weeks or months; the best time to get coverage is now.

• Like other health insurance, these policies are expensive, especially for older persons, since rates are based on age. (Besides age, rates are also based on location, on which plan is chosen, and, for families, on number of dependents.)

• To be able to serve more people with limited funds, the Major Risk policies have a payment cap of $50,000 per year, and $500,000 for the life of the program. In most cases this cap will not be a problem for persons with AIDS, since treatment usually does not cost that much.

• As with many commercial policies, there is a deductible, which is $500 per year. After the patient has paid that amount, the insurance covers 80 percent. For an individual, the maximum out of pocket for a year is $2000 for an individual ($3000 for a family); after that, the insurance pays 100 percent, up to the cap mentioned above. The plan covers physicians, hospitals, prescription drugs, and a number of other services including outpatient, emergency care, rehabilitation, and some psychiatric care; it does not cover some services, such as glasses or dental.

• So far three companies have joined the Major Risk program. All of them are "preferred provider" plans, meaning that patients need to use physicians on the list of the company they select, or pay a larger part of the cost out of pocket. Therefore, before joining the Major Risk program, a person should contact local offices of each of the three companies (see below) for a list of physicians in their area. Such checking may be particularly important for persons who live in rural areas, where fewer physicians are located.

• There will be a short delay, probably one to two months, between applying for the policy and receiving coverage, which starts on the first of the month after the application is processed. Therefore persons should not wait until they are hospitalized or otherwise need major care, but should obtain the insurance in advance.

• Another reason for not waiting is that starting July 1, there will be an additional 90-day waiting period for coverage of pre-existing conditions. At this time, however, no such waiting period applies.

• Under current regulations, persons who enroll and then drop out of the plan, such as for nonpayment of premiums, will need to wait a year to get back in. The intent of this requirement is to make the program operate as insurance, with people paying into it when they are healthy, instead of being a subsidy for which people enroll only when they have major medical costs.

• The Major Risk program is only available for persons who live in California. If one moves out of the state, the insurance ceases. Besides non-residents, two other groups are not eligible for Major Risk: those who are eligible for COBRA coverage, and those who are eligible for Medicare *both* part A and part B.

• This program will continue from year to year without additional legislation. The California legislature may expand the program in the future; it could, of course, possibly decide to discontinue it.

## For More Information

Applications for Major Risk Medical Insurance will be accepted starting February 1; coverage should begin on some policies as of March 1. Interested persons can send an application request to MRMIP, 744 P St., Room 1077, Sacramento, CA 95814, or phone 916/324-4695.

The three companies which have now signed up are Blue Cross, Blue Shield, and Pacific Mutual. Persons will need to select one of these when they apply for the program. Theoretically, the coverage is the same from any of the companies, because a state-appointed board decided what expenses would and would not be covered; however, different physicians have enrolled with the different companies as preferred providers. To find out which local physicians are on the preferred provider list for each company, contact each company and ask for a PPO directory for the Major Risk Medical Insurance Program. Phone numbers for the three companies now participating in the program are: Blue Cross, 800/333-0912; Blue Shield, 800/351-2465; and Pacific Mutual, 800/854-3027.

Some persons may also want to check with the state government to see how well the companies have performed in the past. Under the newly elected Commissioner of Insurance, John Garamendi, the California Department of Insurance will now release the number of complaints received about each company. Another way to check is to ask one's physician's office which companies are best at paying on time, etc.

A one-day seminar on California's Major Risk program, for patients, physicians, and medical organizations, will be held Friday, February 22, in Oakland. For more information, call Strategic Health Systems, 714/777-8824.

## History and Acknowledgement

Legislation authorizing the Major Risk program was passed over a year ago (Title 10, California Code of Regulations, Chapter 5.5), but at first little happened. Later, when thousands of people had their health insurance suddenly cancelled as companies withdrew coverage, legislators received many complaints from constituents, and the legislation was implemented. A board was appointed to set up the program; it had the authority to sell insurance directly, but chose instead to work with insurance companies who chose to participate, in order to provide coverage more quickly.

A few private citizens worked closely with the board while it was designing the program; their influence led to important improvements, such as coverage for off-label and treatment-IND drugs. One of these citizen-experts, Stan Long of Los Angeles, provided us with much of the background on the program.

The Lobby for Individual Freedom and Equality (LIFE), a gay and AIDS lobby in Sacramento, also helped in drafting the regulations.

# AIDS TREATMENT NEWS 1991: FOCUS AND PLANS

*by John S. James*

The new year provided an occasion to examine our mission and direction, and ask how we would like to change. What issues affect our decisions on what to cover, or not cover, in *AIDS Treatment News*? In this article we step back for a more philosophical overview of how we try to operate.

There have long been public concerns about the lack of AIDS information, and also about being overwhelmed by the glut of it. How can there be both too little information and too much at the same time? We suspect that this paradox is possible because most published information is not useful. Again and again we hear complaints that press stories of the latest treatment advances have no followup, and no way for readers to do anything with the information. These stories have little value except to say that something happened.

We suspect that this problem arises because the press no longer provides the information needed for people to fulfill their ostensible roles as sovereign citizens. The press gets many stories essentially free by opening itself to manipulation by those with something to put over. Some publications do resist this system; the *Wall Street Journal*, for example, must provide useful reports, because its readers are deemed important, and they use the information in making financial decisions. And many individuals throughout the media bring as much integrity to their jobs as they can get away with. But we think that this analysis—that a hidden role of the media is to strip the public of its sovereignty, to package the audience for sale to powerful interests—best explains the irrelevance of most news reports to readers' lives. This problem is hardly unique to AIDS, but it is less noticed in most other areas, where people seldom use public information in making real decisions. The life and death urgency of AIDS treatment decisions exposes the inadequacy of most of what comes through the usual media channels.

The corrective, then, is to respect the reader as a person making his or her own assessments and decisions. The goal should be to provide quality intelligence which might be useful to that person—not to predetermine what the decisions should be and then try to bring that outcome about. These goals may seem obvious—yet most people in the health-information business (or in any business, for that matter) are not allowed to operate this way. A drug company, for example, has an institutional commitment to its own products; its employees are not likely to put forth an analysis which favors the competition.

We believe that our effort to avoid such institutional bias helps to explain the success of *AIDS Treatment News*. Avoiding this bias does not, of course, mean not having a point of view. On the contrary, a point of view is usually essential for making complex information intelligible. How, then, do we distinguish what beliefs are or are not legitimate for guiding our coverage in this newsletter? One distinction is between having a belief but remaining willing to change when new evidence becomes available vs. not being willing to change because of what one has published in the past. Another standard we use is to try to assure that our writing would be useful even to readers with a different or opposite point of view.

Two less obvious, more philosophical dynamics help our efforts to keep the material in *AIDS Treatment News* relevant and useful:

• In business management, there is a saying that results are obtained by applying resources to opportunities, not to problems. We can benefit from this principle because we can select, from the entire range of AIDS treatments, what we want to work on. If a drug is found to be less than promising, or if our research bogs down for any reason, we can move quickly to something else. If, for example, researchers are secretive, we can choose another treatment to write about. (Secrecy and intrigue are often used to enhance the value of something which would not succeed on its own. Most new drugs do begin their life in secret; but at that stage they are not available as treatment options, and therefore not of immediate interest to our readers.)

Almost nobody else involved in AIDS treatments has the journalist's freedom to move at will to where opportunities are best. Scientists at pharmaceutical companies, for example, are constrained to work on their companies' products—even if it becomes apparent that other treatments are better. University scientists, theoretically free to study anything, may need years to change research direction, because of the need to find new sources of funding, or to obtain specialized facilities or training.

• How do we select which treatments to cover from among hundreds of possibilities? Of course there is no formula. But one mental tool has proved helpful for this kind of unstructured decision. Like the gardener who provides a fertile bed, plants many seeds, and then selects the plants which grow best, one can provide a fertile ground for many different hypotheses, ideas, or treatment options, and see which ones continue to do well over time. Whenever we learn about a new viewpoint, a new way of judging, evaluating, or prioritizing the available theories or treatment options, we apply it to the various potential treatments as a test. Those treatments which continue to look strong under all or almost all points of view remain leading candidates; those which fail any of the evaluation viewpoints are weakened. The strongest candidates for the purpose at hand (for us, to write articles about) emerge from this process organically.

This approach gives answers in weights or probabilities, not as a definite yes or no. It moves directly to the practicality of each treatment in a single integral process, without making a special stop at the question of efficacy. This is different from the philosophy now prevailing in drug development and regulation, which makes proof of efficacy the most critical part of the process. Obviously efficacy is essential; but in practice, we often have no exact knowledge of it, and cannot put all decisions on hold until we do.

Other criteria we use in deciding what treatments to investigate and write about are more immediate and straightforward:

• We have long believed that one of the best AIDS survival strategies at this time is to try a number of safe and well-supported treatment possibilities, keeping the ones which seem to help and discarding the others, to find treatment combinations which work best for oneself. This process is an individual one; the same treatments may not work for someone else. At *AIDS Treatment News* our most important function is to provide accessible treatment information, to help increase and improve the options available.

• We also cover public policy issues which affect treatment research and development, to help the AIDS community work together toward better drugs in the future. This work is essential, because individual decisions alone are not yet enough for most people's survival. We need better treatments, and therefore we need high quality, well planned, practical research; community involvement is critically important for assuring it.

• We seldom rush to be the first with the news. Instead, we talk with people who are well informed about treatments, and we prefer to report a new development after it has already acquired some knowledgeable following, rather than before. It is hard to judge a treatment early in its history, when little data is available; also, most potential drugs in early development will ultimately fail. So instead of competing for scoops, we let the community of experts judge first; then we contribute by bringing together the most important information and making it easy to understand.

In evaluating expert or other opinions, we consider the credibility and also the motives of the source. More trustworthy information comes from reputable physicians and scientists who are putting their reputations on the line, or from people in the AIDS community who have no financial or other personal conflict of interest and are motivated only to find good treatments. Less trustworthy information comes from promoters with products to sell.

• Occasionally we learn about a treatment which clearly needs more attention than it is getting, and then we may publish one or more major articles, without waiting for expert consensus. Sometimes we have been right, sometimes not; often no one yet knows. Examples include our reports on AL 721 (April 1986), aerosol pentamidine (January 1987), dextran sulfate (May 1987), fluconazole (September 1987), DHEA (January 1988), hypericin (August 1988), ddI (January 1989), roxithromycin and azithromycin (March 1989), NAC (October 1989), aspirin (August 1990), and clarithromycin (October 1990). We consider these articles among the most important work we have done.

• We are less impressed than some others by theories, unless they have at least some preliminary practical results which support them. Even leading scientists sometimes make the mistake of going directly from a theory to a complex, costly, and time-consuming trial or other project, without finding ways to do quick checks first to see if their theory seems to be working in practice. As a result, their projects may never get off the ground, or may tie up substantial resources for no good purpose. Today's understanding of AIDS is far more primitive than the public realizes, than the experts' clean charts and pictures suggest. For now, therefore, theories serve mainly as guides or suggestions for what might be tried; they are not descriptions of what is actually happening with the disease.

• When *AIDS Treatment News* began, we planned to cover "experimental and alternative" treatments. (Later we changed the wording of our statement of purpose to "experimental and complementary," to emphasize that non-standard treatments should not replace good conventional medical care, but rather add to it.) Our original plan was not to cover conventional treatments, since physicians and patients would have better sources for this information. But recently some of our most valuable articles, as judged by what our readers tell us, were closer to conventional medicine—for example, the overview of pneumocystis prophylaxis (November 1990). Interviews with leading HIV physicians have also been important; we hope to have more of them in the future.

• Some readers feel that we have become too conservative; they want more coverage of "alternative," non-mainstream treatments. We agree that more coverage is needed, but we have mixed feelings on this issue. When we began over four years ago, useful mainstream research was almost nonexistent; the leading edge of AIDS treatment was in the underground. But today the leading edge is often in major pharmaceutical companies or medical centers. We must cover the most important news from wherever it occurs.

Most of the treatments which are outside of the medical mainstream but still in widespread use (for example, garlic, exercise, or acupuncture) have not been rejected on the basis of evidence, but rather not studied because they lack commercial potential. Some may well be of value; and it is important in any case to provide unbiased information on treatments which people are using. Perhaps we underemphasized complementary treatments in 1990. But it is hard to evaluate treatments when little has been published in mainstream medical and scientific literature.

• One dilemma is that the advances which ultimately may be most important, such as the rational design of new chemical entities, may have no near-term relevance to our readers, as the substances are not available, or not suitable for use because of unknown risks. Still we need to cover this news so that our readers will be oriented to what is happening. Perhaps the most important issue now facing the community is how to reform the regulatory process so that important potential advances (for example, the new Merck or Boehringer Ingelheim non-nucleoside drugs, or the protease inhibitors now being developed by many pharmaceutical companies) will have a rational development path, without the senseless delays which have so far been imposed. People need to realize that there are potentially major advances now entering human trials, in order to understand how critical this issue is.

## Geographical Issues

When we write about treatments, it does not matter where the news comes from, as long as we can substantiate it. But when we cover treatment activism, are we a national publication, or are we partial to San Francisco and the West Coast, where we are located?

We want to provide national coverage, and therefore we make efforts to avoid a San Francisco bias. But we also believe it would be a mistake to aim to be entirely geography-free. Obviously we can attend more meetings locally than in other areas such as New York or Washington; we can know the local people, projects, and issues better. Part of our mission is to report to a national audience from San Francisco. If, for example, we were located in Washington, DC, we would publish the same news about new treatments, but otherwise we would focus on Federal activities affecting treatment development—which we cannot cover in depth from San Francisco.

## Covering the News

Should *AIDS Treatment News* focus more effort on in-depth reports on stories which appear in the general news media, providing the background which the news stories do not? At this time we have decided not to. The main reason is that we have found that most treatment news reported in the general media is not valuable. To say so in print would require research time to verify each case, directing our time, attention, and space in the newsletter to what is *not* important. Another reason is that, as explained above, we prefer to wait and hear what the community of experts has to say before deciding which treatments to cover. The media, however, is most interested in a story when it is new, and at that time the expert evaluation we seek may not be available.

## Medical and AIDS Publications

Should we specialize in abstracting AIDS news from medical journals? Again we have decided not to. One reason is that at least two newsletters already perform this function: *ATIN: AIDS Targeted Information Newsletter* (for subscription information, call 800/638-6423, or 800/638-4007 in Maryland); and *Acquired Immune Deficiency Syndrome Newsletter*, 1680 N. Vine St., Suite 1006, Los Angeles, CA 90028.

## Let Us Know

Much of our information comes from readers; we pay careful attention to all correspondence and comments we receive. Please let us know if you have any ideas about how we could make *AIDS Treatment News* more useful to you or to others.

# NEWS NOTES

## British Study: People with AIDS Living Twice As Long

A study of medical records, published January 25 in the *British Medical Journal*, found that AIDS survival doubled between 1984 and 1987, from a median of 10 months to 20 months, among patients treated at St. Mary's Hospital in London. According to a Reuters report on the study (we have not yet obtained the original article), deaths from pneumocystis dropped from 46 percent in 1986 to 3 percent in 1989.

KS and lymphoma were increasing as causes of death, apparently because people were living longer due to improved prevention and treatment of other AIDS complications.

## Hospital Deaths Higher for Uninsured

A study of over half a million discharge records of patients hospitalized in the United States in 1987 found that the in-hospital death rate was 1.2 to 3.2 times higher among uninsured patients, in 11 of 16 groups which were analyzed. The study also found that although uninsured patients were in worse condition than privately insured patients when they entered the hospital, they were discharged sooner.

The study was published January 16 in the *Journal of the American Medical Association*.

## BRM (Biological Response Modifiers) Conference, March 22–24 in Québec City

The First International Congress on Biological Response Modifiers will be held March 22-24, 1991 at the Hilton International Québec, Québec City, Canada. The conference is organized by the Inter-American Society for Chemotherapy.

The following description is from the conference brochure:

"The exciting and challenging field of BRM represents a revolutionary approach to the treatment of several pathological processes. BRM offers the potential for the development of breakthrough therapies against cancer and a wide range of infectious conditions, including AIDS.

"As the First International Conference on Biological Response Modifiers, this meeting is of immediate importance to physicians involved in both clinical practice and investigative research, as well as research scientists from academia, the pharmaceutical industry, and biotechnology organizations."

A list of scientific topics includes: BRM in AIDS, BRM in cancer, BRM in bacterial, parasitic, fungal and viral diseases, BRM as antiviral agents, BRM and the immune system, BRM and hematopoiesis, BRM and anti-HIV drugs, colony stimulating factors, other growth factors, interferons, interleukins, tumor necrosis factor, leukotrienes, and platelet activating factor.

[Note: the term "biological response modifiers" is not new, but the area is now receiving intense scientific interest. The phrase has sometimes been used interchangeably with "immune modulators," but "biological response modifiers" is more general, in that the same mechanisms which control the immune system also control growth and other functions of many cells.]

The conference will be held in English.

For more information, call Michel G. Bergeron, M.D., 418/654-2705, or 418/654-2715 (fax).

# HIV Entry Ban Will Be Removed

On January 23 the U.S. Department of Health and Human Services formally published a proposal to end the restrictions against travelers and immigrants with HIV entering the United States. Leprosy and several sexually transmitted diseases were also removed from the list, leaving tuberculosis as the only disease for which persons will be excluded. The new rule will not take effect until June 1.

The HIV visitor ban caused major problems for the International Conference on AIDS in San Francisco last June. Over 100 organizations, including the International League of Red Cross and Red Crescent Societies, the British Medical Association, and the European Parliament, boycotted the conference because the travel restrictions had no medical rationale and made it difficult for delegates to attend. Later, Harvard University said that it would withdraw its sponsorship of the 1992 Conference unless the restrictions were changed.

The Department's intent to remove the ban was widely reported in early January 1991.

# Issue Number 121
# February 15, 1991

## AZT: DIFFERENT FOR PEOPLE OF COLOR?

*by John S. James*

Data released this week from a U.S. Veterans Administration (VA) study suggested that early treatment with AZT (for persons with T-helper counts of 200 to 500) might not be helpful to Blacks and Latinos, and might even be harmful. (The study did not question later treatment, for anyone with T-helper count under 200.) But three other studies found no racial difference in the effect of AZT. And scientists reviewing the VA study found the data "fragile," and suggested that it may well have resulted just by unlucky chance. There is widespread concern that results which could well be due to errors or statistical happenstance may discourage people from seeking medical care.

The study, called VA Cooperative Study 298, was conducted at veterans' hospitals in Houston, Los Angeles, Miami, New York, San Francisco, and Washington, D.C., and at the Walter Reed Army Medical Center. Volunteers entering the trial had to have T-helper counts of 200 to 500, and symptoms of HIV infection but not AIDS, to be eligible. They were randomly assigned to either an early treatment group, which received AZT immediately, or a later treatment group, which received a placebo at first. Later, when T-helper counts dropped below 200 on two successive visits, the placebo was stopped and all participants in the study received AZT. All AZT doses were 1500 mg per day—about three times what most physicians use today. The goal of the study was to learn whether starting AZT early would increase survival and delay progression to AIDS. The trial was **not** designed to look for racial differences.

For ethical reasons, study participants were offered pneumocystis prophylaxis when it was officially recommended. Also, when AZT was officially approved for early use, study volunteers were notified, and some switched from blinded treatment (either AZT or placebo) to AZT, at their request.

### Overall Results

A total of 338 volunteers were enrolled in this study; 170 were assigned to receive early treatment (AZT immediately), and 168 assigned to receive placebo at first. The average age of the volunteers was about 40; about two thirds of them were white, one third Black or Latino.

The trial was stopped as planned in January 1991. When the data was analyzed for all volunteers together—not broken down by race—it was found that early treatment did clearly delay progression to AIDS; 44 patients in the delayed-treatment group, but only 25 in the early-treatment group, developed AIDS. But early treatment showed no benefit in preventing death; 23 in the early-treatment group died vs. 19 assigned to delayed treatment. (This difference is too small to be statistically significant, meaning that it could easily have occurred by chance.)

Two notable results of the study were that of six cases of dementia, all were in the late-treatment group, suggesting that AZT may have helped in preventing that condition. Also, of six cases of lymphoma, five were in the late-treatment group, suggesting that AZT may also have reduced the risk of lymphoma.

## Racial Differences

The researchers were surprized at these inconsistent results, so they looked more closely at the data to see what was happening. They checked to see if results were different for IV drug users compared to other patients, but no difference was found.

When they checked for racial differences, they combined the data for Blacks and Latinos, in order to have enough data in each group to run statistical tests. For the minority groups, they found no statistically significant benefit of AZT in delaying progression to AIDS. But the statistics on death were especially disturbing; nine Black or Latino volunteers in the early treatment group died, but only one who received later treatment. Also, early AZT treatment did not show the same benefit in T-helper count for the people of color as it did for whites.

No one knows why this entirely unexpected result occurred. Researchers who reviewed the study have suggested a number of reasons to be skeptical about the results until more is known:

• No other study has found a racial difference in response to AZT. Three major AZT studies were analyzed to look for such a result, but none was found. How could three studies find no racial difference in response to AZT, while a fourth finds a **nine to one** difference among minorities with early AZT treatment, vs. a survival advantage among whites? One obvious possibility is that this difference in deaths happened by unlucky chance, and did not reflect any real differences in how races respond to AZT.

• Another concern is that the VA study was analyzed by "intent-to-treat" rules, meaning that volunteers were counted in the treatment groups to which they were randomly assigned—regardless of anything that might happen later. There are advantages to this kind of analysis, but there are also disadvantages; in the VA study, for example, deaths were counted the same whether they were AIDS related, or due to other causes including murder, suicide, traffic accident, or diseases not believed to be related to HIV. We have not seen any analysis of the study with these unrelated deaths excluded.

A particular problem with intent-to-treat rules in this case is that when AZT was approved for persons with 200 to 500 T-helper cells, study participants had to be given a choice to switch to AZT if they wanted; it would not have been ethical to give a placebo to persons in that T-helper range without their consent. Many of the volunteers assigned to the later-treatment arm did choose to switch; but under the intent-to-treat rules, they had to be counted as late treatment, even if their AZT actually began early. This change did not affect persons assigned to early treatment, who were receiving AZT already.

• This study was not designed to look for racial differences. It is easy to get misleading results when a study is analyzed later in ways not originally planned or intended.

• Because the study was finished in January and presented to other researchers in February, there was no time to complete the analysis, or to thoroughly check the results.

• One theory being considered is that some races might absorb AZT less well than others, when the drug is taken orally. This possibility seems unlikely to account for the VA results, however, since the dose used in that study was three times too high. Unless the differences were enormous, poor absorption would have been a benefit (in reducing side effects), not a detriment.

On February 14 a number of physicians reviewed the VA data. Almost all of them said that it would not affect their practice of medicine, except that it might become one more item to be discussed with the patient when the decision was made as to whether or not to start AZT. No one wanted to change the official FDA "labeling" which suggests that AZT be considered for HIV-positive persons with T-helper counts under 500.

## Concerns

The executive director of the National Minority AIDS Council, Paul Kawata, urged caution in interpreting these preliminary findings. "We must not send people of color with HIV infection underground. This study has the potential to take away hope for HIV infected minorities. It is much too early to draw any definitive conclusions."

And Reggie Williams, executive director of the National Task Force on AIDS Prevention, said that "We can not afford to give Black people...any more excuses not to get tested, into early intervention modes and yes, into clinical trials. Nor can we afford to give those in government research and policymaking positions a reason to further marginalize us from our fair share of whatever is out there that may prolong life with HIV."

## NAC: MAJOR LABORATORY STUDY SUPPORTS AIDS TREATMENT THEORY

*by John S. James*

A laboratory study by Anthony Fauci, M.D., and other scientists at the U.S. National Institute of Allergy and Infectious Diseases, and at the Cornell University Medical College in New York City, has confirmed and extended earlier work by Dr. Leonard A. Herzenberg and colleagues at Stanford University suggesting that n-acetylcysteine (NAC) can inhibit growth of HIV. NAC is used in many European countries to treat bronchitis; it is not approved for this use in the United States, but has been available for over a year through buyers' clubs.

For background on this drug, see "NAC: Bronchitis Drug May Slow AIDS Virus," *AIDS Treatment News* #88; also see issues #92 and 93. Despite widespread public interest and some scientific interest in the drug, no U.S. controlled trial has yet begun; there are rumors of a trial in Europe, but no results have been published. One monitoring study, in which persons using NAC kept diaries, was organized by the Fight for Life Committee, an AIDS activist group in North Lauderdale, Florida, in 1989. Preliminary results, which were positive, were summarized in *AIDS Treatment News* #92.

No laboratory study can prove that a drug is helpful for people; only clinical trials can do that. But laboratory studies can suggest which drugs should have priority for trials, and what effects to look for (and therefore how the trials should be designed). The recently published laboratory results will certainly increase interest in NAC—not as a potential cure or means to control HIV or AIDS entirely, but as a safe and available treatment which may be considerably helpful for some patients.

## The New Study

The recent NAC study, by a group headed by Fauci and by Alton Meister, M.D., of Cornell, was published February 1 in *Proceedings of the National Academy of Sciences, USA* (volume 88, pages 986-990). Here is an overview of how this research was conducted, and what it found.

The experimenters used a line of cells created in the laboratory which have HIV as an inherited part of their DNA. These cells have been used for studies of why HIV is usually latent for many years, and only later becomes active and causes serious disease. The researchers used three chemicals which are known to greatly stimulate HIV activity in these cells: PMA, tumor necrosis factor, and interleukin 6 (IL-6); two of these, tumor necrosis factor and IL-6, are normally found in the body and are known to be markedly increased in persons with AIDS. The researchers tested NAC (and also two related substances) to see if they could prevent this stimulation of viral activity caused by each of the three chemicals. In all three cases, NAC did prevent most of the stimulation of the virus.

NAC is believed to work primarily by increasing the level of glutathione in cells. Glutathione is necessary for life; it helps cells produce energy, and it also helps protect them against oxidation; in addition, it may be an immune modulator, necessary for T-cell activation. A German scientist, Dr. Wulf Droge, at the German Cancer Research Center in Heidelberg, had found that glutathione levels were deficient in cells of persons with AIDS, and that the deficiency worsened as the disease progressed; he was the first to suggest NAC as a potential AIDS treatment, since it is known to raise glutathione levels.

Dr. Droge's work came to the attention of Doctors Leonard Herzenberg and Leonore Herzenberg, who are husband and wife and both members of the Genetics Department at Stanford University. The Herzenbergs brought NAC as a possible AIDS treatment to the attention of the U.S. scientific community. In June 1990 their team published results, in the *Proceedings of the National Academy of Sciences*, showing that NAC inhibited HIV replication in a variety of laboratory tests.

The new study by Fauci, Meister, and others confirmed the Herzenbergs' results. Also, to make sure that NAC was indeed working by raising glutathione levels, the researchers ran similar experiments, using glutathione itself, and also a glutathione derivative, instead of NAC. All three substances did inhibit HIV infection—probably by more than one mechanism. NAC was found to have an additional antiviral effect which the other two did not have. These effects, especially the latter, are not well understood. The research with NAC, as well as its immediate importance in supporting the need for clinical trials of this drug, is leading to further insights on how HIV becomes activated in cells—understanding which could lead to treatments designed to keep the virus permanently inactive.

## Comment: Practical Consequences

Anecdotal reports suggest that a minority of people who try NAC feel much better, with benefits such as increased energy and appetite, but that most do not notice any change. We checked with buyers' clubs and found that a number of people have continued to use NAC during the last year, but that the demand has been limited when no new scientific information and resulting media coverage has come out.

The following suggestions have come from our conversations with several people familiar with NAC:

• Persons who try the treatment and feel markedly better during the first two weeks should definitely continue. In these cases, NAC may be correcting an abnormally low level of glutathione within cells.

• If no change is noticed, then it is hard to tell whether or not the treatment is doing any good. In some people, T-helper counts have increased, but it may take months to get this effect. There are suggestions that NAC may help stabilize people with HIV infection, or may speed recovery from opportunistic infections, but it is too early to know if there is any real benefit.

• The best formulations of NAC are generally believed to be those made in Europe for treating bronchitis. Three different kinds are available from the PWA Health Group, 212/532-0280; this buyers' club will fill mail orders. Doses used generally range from 600 to 1800 mg per day, with those who are more seriously ill using the higher doses. While glutathione itself is sold in some health-food stores, one expert we talked to said that it would **not** be effective.

U.S. researchers have been trying to start a clinical trial of NAC for the last two years, but commercial and bureaucratic obstacles have prevented any such study from starting. Researchers at the U.S. National Institutes of Health are now seeking FDA permission to begin a trial.

## NEUROPATHY: ANSWERS EMERGING?

*by Denny Smith*

Neuropathy has become a problem for many people with HIV infection, and can develop for a variety of reasons. Fortunately, it might be controllable with a number of promising treatments, many already available for other purposes.

The progression of HIV alone can apparently lead to two different disorders of the peripheral nervous system. One kind is a painful sensory dysfunction resulting from the degeneration of the axon, the component of nerve cells responsible for conducting impulses. The other, less frequent, neuropathy results in a motor weakness caused by an inflammatory process which damages the myelin covering the nerve fibers. This kind may resemble "myopathy," a discomfort or fatigue of muscle fibers, which is also identified with HIV or with long-term use of AZT.

Other possible causes of neuropathy include some opportunistic infections and tumors, as well as some of the drugs used in HIV/AIDS therapies (such as ddI, ddC, interferon, and certain chemotherapies). Distinguishing the cause or type of neuropathy is important for deciding which treatment approach to take. Discontinuing a medication from which neuropathy has been known to result may resolve the symptoms completely, especially if done in a timely manner. But if an infection or medication is determined not to be the cause, nerve conduction tests may help with a diagnosis.

Much of the previous medical literature discussing neuropathy came from experimental approaches for the often painful neuropathy experienced by people with diabetes. Research into diabetic neuropathy has suggested a number of possibilities, and achieved some limited successes.

Among these are a number of treatments already licensed for other indications: piroxicam, plasmapheresis, calcitonin (nasal spray), capsaicin, antiarrhythmia drugs like mexiletine and lidocaine (intravenous), antidepressants such as nimodipine, imipramine, desipramine or fluoxetine, anticonvulsants like phenytoin, and narcotics for very painful neuropathy.

Some others, regarded generally as investigational agents, are coenzyme Q-10, gamma-linolenic acid, prostaglandin E1, and tolrestat.

We interviewed two physicians familiar with aspects of HIV-related neuropathy: Ari Ganer, M.D., of the Santa Clara Valley Medical Center, and Harry Hollander, M.D., at the University of California San Francisco.

Dr. Hollander told us that, although the rationales for trying some of these drugs theoretically would apply to HIV as well as to diabetic neuropathy, their side effects are **not** dependably uniform: a treatment reported to be safe in one situation might not be so in the other. He told us that antidepressants are usually tried first for symptomatic relief; if they fail, he follows with an anticonvulsant, noting that the course of neuropathy and the sequence of drug choices are variable for every patient.

Dr. Ganer and Dr. Stanley Deresinski are studying mexiletine to treat HIV-related neuropathy in a controlled clinical trial sponsored by a community-based research organization, the AIDS Community Research Consortium (ACRC). This trial is funded by the American Foundation for AIDS Research (AmFAR), and has two sites south of San Francisco, both of which are open to more participants. This study employs the "crossover" design, so that for the first half of the study, some patients will be given mexiletine, the others a placebo. After a short "washout" period, the placebo and active drugs are switched. Neither the investigators nor participants know when active drug was given until the study is finished.

Nevertheless, patterns are often apparent in crossover trials if the treatment is making a difference. Dr. Ganer said that he is encouraged by preliminary impressions of the study: some people have obviously experienced significant relief from the symptoms of neuropathy during part of the trial. The only measures of response in the study are the patients' reports of pain or pain relief.

Brian Camp, R.N., the clinical coordinator of the Redwood City site, shared similar impressions, and hopes to see neuropathy studies expanded in scope and number.

Of the other agents discussed as potential treatments for HIV-associated neuropathy, Dr. Ganer thinks capsaicin is a good candidate for clinical trials, alone or in combination with mexiletine. Two pharmaceutical preparations containing capsaicin are already marketed for treating the discomfort of herpes zoster (shingles) lesions. Both are supplied as creams; one of them, Axsain, contains a 0.075% concentration of capsaicin, and the other, Zostrix, contains 0.025%. [Note: capsaicin is the component of hot peppers which makes them hot.]

If the mexiletine trial proves useful, Dr. Ganer hopes to expand HIV neuropathy trials to test capsaicin, or other agents. He remarked that surprisingly little attention has been paid to this common problem. The current trial is recruiting people with neuropathy resulting from HIV, but future studies will probably accept people with drug-induced symptoms as well. Persons interested in this study can contact the Santa Clara Valley Medical Center site at 408/299-5588, or the Redwood City site at 415/364-6563.

AmFAR has granted the ACRC funding for expanded trials. Of course, since mexiletine, capsaicin and some of the other possibilities mentioned above are already available by prescription, physicians and patients have access to those drugs now, without enrolling in a trial. Meanwhile, *AIDS Treatment News* welcomes anecdotal reports of experience with treating neuropathy from our readers.

# REFERENCES

Parry, GJ, Kozu H. Piroxicam may reduce the rate of progression of experimental diabetic neuropathy. *Neurology*, volume 40, number 9, pages 1446-1449, September 1990.

Zieleniewski W. Calcitonin nasal spray for painful diabetic neuropathy. (letter) *The Lancet*, volume 336, number 8712, page 449, August 18, 1990.

Boulton AJ, Levin S, Comstock J. A multicentre trial of the aldose-reductase inhibitor, tolrestat, in patients with symptomatic diabetic neuropathy. *Diabetologia*, volume 33, number 7, pages 431-437, July 1990.

Nakamura Y, Takahashi M. Clinical application of prostaglandin on peripheral neuropathy. *Nippon Rinsho*, volume 48, number 6, pages 1224-1228, June 1990.

Jamal GA, Carmichael H. The effect of gamma-linolenic acid on human diabetic peripheral neuropathy: a double-blind placebo-controlled trial. *Diabetic Medicine*, volume 7, number 4, pages 319-323, May 1990.

Kastrup J, Petersen P, Dejgard A. Intravenous lidocaine and cerebral blood flow: impaired microvascular reactivity in diabetic patients. *Journal of Clinical Pharmacology*, volume 30, number 4, pages 318-323, April, 1990.

Egbunike IG, Chaffee BJ. Antidepressants in the management of chronic pain syndromes. *Pharmacotherapy*, volume 10, number 4, pages 262-270, 1990.

Masson EA, Boulton AJ. Aldose reductase inhibitors in the treatment of diabetic neuropathy. A review of the rational and clinical evidence. *Drugs*, volume 39, number 2, pages 190-202, February, 1990.

Hollander, H. Peripheral neuropathy and HIV infection. *AIDSFILE*, volume 3, number 2, page 1, June 1988.

# TREATMENT LIBRARY: BOOKS AND NEWSLETTERS

*by John S. James*

An organization or an individual can set up a basic AIDS library for relatively little cost. A few reference books, newsletters, and referral phone numbers are most important as the core reference materials. After that, there are many directions in which a library can evolve, and specialization is appropriate, as few could afford to be comprehensive. This article provides an annotated list of basic materials, a starting point which will make an AIDS treatment library immediately useful.

The section on reference books, below, is central; an AIDS treatment library can provide a core of current information and make itself useful for under $200. The other lists, of AIDS newsletters and of "alternative" information sources, include more optional items, which some libraries will choose not to carry. We have not included academic medical and scientific journals in this article.

The standard medical books can best be found at a bookstore with a good medical department (in San Francisco, for example, we usually check the bookstore at the University of California San Francisco Medical Center, 500 Parnassus Avenue—or the medical section of Stacey's Books, 581 Market Street). If no store is convenient, the books can usually be ordered from the publisher. For newsletters, we include contact or ordering information.

## Reference Books

• **Introductory handbook for patients.** *Early Care for HIV Disease*, by Ronald A. Baker, Ph.D., Jeffrey M. Moulton, Ph.D., and John Charles Tighe, 1991, published by the San Francisco AIDS Foundation, 415/863-2437, or 800/367-2437 (from Northern California), $9.95. This 108-page book, released last week, is a first introduction for persons who have learned that they are HIV positive. It includes topics such as finding a doctor, understanding blood tests, nutrition and food safety, drugs (including AZT, ddI, and ddC, interferon, GM-CSF, and combination therapies), clinical trials, expanded access, paying for medical care and obtaining public assistance when necessary, and finding psychosocial support. An excellent resource list includes phone numbers for local and national hotlines throughout the United States, six different Spanish hotlines, a Filipino hotline, addresses and phone numbers for over two dozen minority AIDS organizations, and an annotated list of 20 AIDS newsletters and other publications; an organization with an AIDS library might want to photocopy this hotline and resource list for easy reference by library users. The book includes a glossary to define the medical terms it uses.

• **Medical dictionary.** *Webster's Medical Desk Dictionary*, Merriam-Webster Inc., Springfield, Massachusetts, 1986, $21.95, is clearly written and accessible to a general audience. If you want a more technical dictionary, consider *Dorland's Illustrated Medical Dictionary*, W.B.Saunders Company, Philadelphia, 1988; Dorland's is written primarily for physicians.

• **Drug book(s).** We usually use *Nursing91 Drug Handbook*, Springhouse Corporation, Springhouse, Pennsylvania, 1991, $21.95. It is updated every year, and the information it presents on each drug is practical and well written. This handbook is organized by classes of drugs, rather than one alphabetical list, so patients can learn about other potential treatment options, which might be necessary if a drug prescribed for them causes side effects.

Many people use the *Physicians' Desk Reference* (the "*PDR*") as their basic book on approved drugs. The 1991 edition is available now in bookstores for $49.95. It is thorough and authoritative, as it contains the official "labeling," what the FDA allows drug manufacturers to say about each drug. The PDR is not as convenient to use as the nursing handbook; for example, it is organized by drug manufacturer, not by type of drug. But the PDR is more thorough, especially on side effects. A good library should consider both.

Another option is *Handbook of Drugs for Nursing Practice*, by Virginia Karb and others, the C.V. Mosby Company, St. Louis, 1989, $28.95. We would choose this book over the other two except for the fact that the latest edition now available is two years old, and AIDS drug information changes rapidly.

• **AIDS textbook.** We recommend *The Medical Management of AIDS*, Second Edition, by Merle A Sande, M.D., and Paul A Volberding, M.D., W.B. Saunders Company, Philadelphia, 1990, $45. This book, edited by two professors at the Department of Medicine of the University of California San Francisco, was written by dozens of leading AIDS experts. Chapters include early HIV infection, dermatologic care, oral manifestations of AIDS, gastrointestinal disease, neurologic complications, hematologic manifestations, and cardiac, endocrine, and renal complications. There are also chapters on pneumocystis, toxoplasmosis, cryptococcal meningitis, fungal infections, mycobacterial diseases, salmonella and other encapsulated bacteria, herpes virus infections, and malignancies. Other sections examine epidemiology, prevention of transmission, pathogenesis, children with AIDS, and legal issues. Most chapters have dozens of references. This book is written for physicians; the general reader will need a medical dictionary to follow parts of it. Be sure to get the second edition, since the first was published in 1988 and is now out of date.

• **Directory of AIDS treatments.** The *AIDS/HIV Treatment Directory* is published by the American Foundation for AIDS Research, 1515 Broadway, Suite 3601, New York, NY 10036-8901, 212/719-0033, updated quarterly, $30 per year. This directory focuses primarily on experimental treatments now in clinical trials for HIV, opportunistic infections, malignancies, and other AIDS-related complications. The entries are continually updated; sometimes drug information appears in the *Directory* before it is published anywhere else. Besides the listings of treatments and clinical trial sites, editions include other useful information; for example, the December 1990 issue includes an article on combination therapies, a list of compassionate use and treatment IND programs, a list of community-based trial organizations, a list of U.S. AIDS Clinical Trials Group centers, an index of drug manufacturers, a glossary, and an extensive list of AIDS newsletters and other information sources.

• **How to get medical benefits.** *The AIDS Benefits Handbook*, by Thomas P. McCormack, Yale University Press, 1990, is "a brief encyclopedia of income, health, and housing programs for the disabled," including information on state-by-state variations. It explains SSDI, SSI, AZT assistance, Medicaid, General Assistance, Emergency Assistance, Food Stamps, and others, including "several programs of real potential for aiding PWAs, but which are far less well known to the AIDS advocacy community and therefore not used nearly to their potential: the Hill-Burton, state or local indigent medical assistance and private charity programs available in many hospitals; State Supplementary Payment (SSP) programs to finance PWA group housing in 'board and care homes'; and state-run drug (and even health insurance) subsidy programs." [Note: a brief announcement of this book appeared in *AIDS Treatment News* #105.]

## Treatment Newsletters

At last count, there were well over 100 periodical publications devoted solely to AIDS. We cannot evaluate them all; if we have missed some which you believe should be listed, please let us know. Note that this list does not include many specialized newsletters, such as local clinical-trials directories, or newsletters not primarily about treatment.

The first three listed below often cover some of the same material as *AIDS Treatment News*, with articles on treatments and interviews with physicians. Of the four, *BETA* is probably the most conservative; *AIDS Treatment News* is usually regarded as most willing to venture outside of the medical mainstream.

• *Treatment Issues*, published ten times a year by the Gay Men's Health Crisis, 129 West 20th St., New York, NY, 10011, $20 suggested donation for a one-year subscription.

• *PI Perspectives*, published several times a year by Project Inform, 347 Dolores, Suite 301, San Francisco, CA, 94110. 415/558-9051 from San Francisco and other countries, 800/334-7422 from rest of California, 800/822-7422 from U.S. locations besides California; $25 suggested donation for information packet and subscription.

• *Bulletin of Experimental Treatments for AIDS* (*BETA*), published four times a year by the San Francisco AIDS Foundation, $35 per year. For subscription information call 415/863-AIDS from San Francisco and other countries, 800/327-9893 from elsewhere in the United States, 415/861-3397 for information about bulk orders.

*Positive News* is another newsletter also published quarterly by the San Francisco AIDS Foundation. It is free and appears in four languages: English, Spanish, Tagalog, and Chinese. Described by the Foundation as "a low-literacy newsletter on issues affecting people with HIV infection," *Positive News* contains little treatment information; it is important because it provides AIDS information in several languages.

• *Notes from the Underground*, published six times a year by the PWA Health Group, 31 West 26th St., 4th Floor, New York, NY, 10010, 212/532-0280, $35 individual, $75 institutions/physicians; send a self-addressed stamped envelope for a free sample copy. The January 1991 issue includes articles on azithromycin, a guide on where to get non-approved drugs, an article on pricing at the PWA Health Group (which is a non-profit buyers' club), and important testimony by executive director Derek Hodel to the Congressionally-mandated AIDS Research Advisory Committee.

• *Treatment & Research Forum,* published monthly by the Community Research Initiative, 31 West 26th Street, 3rd floor, New York, NY 10010, 212/481-1050, donation requested. Includes information on drugs being studied by the Community

Research Initiative, one of the oldest and largest community-based AIDS research organizations, and other treatments of interest.

• *AIDS Medical Report*, published monthly by American Health Consultants, 67 Peachtree Park Drive, NE, Atlanta, GA, 30309, 800/688-2421, $149 for subscription ($199 with CME credit). Written for physicians, this newsletter usually has one in-depth, practical report per issue on standard-of-care treatments.

• *Critical Path AIDS Project*, published monthly by the AIDS Library of Philadelphia, 32 N. 3rd St., Philadelphia, PA, 19106. 215/545-2212, $15 or contribution of choice for subscription, free to people with HIV. Publishes in-depth articles, often reprinted from elsewhere, on treatments, as well as prevention and services, including listings of support groups in the Philadelphia area.

• *AIDS Medicines in Development*, quarterly survey of most investigational agents currently in AIDS research, published by the Pharmaceutical Manufacturers Association, 1100-15th St., NW, Washington, DC, 20005. No cost; send written request for subscription.

• *Treatment Update*, and *Traitement Sida*, published by AIDS Action Now!, 517 College Street, Suite 324, Toronto, Ontario, Canada M6G 1A8. 416/944-1916. Varied subscription prices. Notes on research and treatment ideas.

• *STEP Perspective*, published by the Seattle Treatment Education Project, 1535-11th Ave, Suite 203, Seattle, WA, 98122. 206/329-4857. $15 or more suggested contribution for subscription. Well researched articles on treatment studies.

• *Washington HIV News*, Box 3933, Merrifield, VA 22116-3933, 202/797-3590. Published in cooperation with the Whitman-Walker Clinic, *Washington HIV News* includes medical news and education, and information about new treatments, especially those in clinical trials. Subscriptions (four issues) are free for persons with AIDS, otherwise $8 individual rate, $80 institutional rate. Phone or write for free sample issue.

• *ATIN: AIDS Targeted Information Newsletter*, sponsored by the American Foundation for AIDS Research, published monthly by Williams and Wilkins, P.O. Box 23291, Baltimore, MD 21203-9990, 800/638-6423 (in Maryland call 800/638-4007), $125 per year individual, $275 institution. This review of the medical and scientific literature on AIDS has several hundred citations in each issue, with brief reviews, sometimes quite technical, of the most important articles.

• The treatment committees of at least three ACT UPs now publish newsletters. Some articles report on treatments, others discuss business, such as meetings with pharmaceutical companies or government agencies. Because these groups are in the forefront of treatment activism, the newsletters include information not otherwise available. For more information, call the numbers below:

• ACT UP/New York Treatment and Data Committee: *The Treatment and Data Digest*. Call Mike Barr at 212/982-8206, or Chris DeBlasio at 212/420-8432.

• ACT UP/Los Angeles Treatment and Data Committee: *Treatment Issues Report*. Call Wade at 213/841-2631, or the ACT UP office at 213/669-7301.

• ACT UP/Golden Gate Treatment Issues Committee: *Treatment Issues Report*. Call the ACT UP office at 415/252-9200, or Michael Wright at 415/864-6305.

# Alternative (Complementary) Treatment Information

It is hard to judge information about potential treatments which are in some way outside of the medical mainstream. Some guidelines can be given, however:

• Even for non-mainstream treatments, there is almost always some background information published in credible medical or scientific journals; if there were not, the proposed treatment would clearly not be ready for use except by qualified research institutions. (Persons should be aware, however, that unscrupulous promoters sometimes provide impressive-looking but irrelevant references, knowing that most people will not follow up and discover that the cited articles do not support the claims the promoter is making.)

• Besides the medical literature, the background and motives of those interested in the treatment can be considered. Is the information about it coming from a nonprofit or community-based AIDS organization, or from a promoter with a scheme to make money?

• Particular danger signs are secret remedies, or any attempt to keep patients from obtaining standard medical care, or from discussing all treatments they plan to use with their physicians. Quacks often try to cut their victims off from other information sources, to increase their own control.

Patients should tell their physicians about all treatments they are considering; both parties should seek to build relationships where this is possible. Physicians are busy; few have time to follow the latest research on everything their patients may be interested in, and some are threatened when patients ask questions they cannot answer. Still, complementary treatments should be discussed, in case there is important information, especially precautions or other safety concerns, which may apply particularly to the individual patient because of his or her health status, or because of drugs the physician has prescribed. [Note: We prefer the term "complementary" to "alternative," to emphasize that any unproven treatment possibilities should be used in addition to good-quality standard medical care, not instead of it. Also note: for more information on the physician-patient relationship, see "Managing Your Doctor," by Michelle Roland, *AIDS Treatment News* #111.]

**Disclaimer**: We have listed the following information sources as a starting point for a complementary-treatment section of an AIDS library. But we cannot be as confident about non-standard treatment information as we can be about standard medical information, such as that found in medical dictionaries or in drug handbooks. While we believe that the following sources are usually correct in summarizing information from the medical and scientific literature, we could not check everything; in addition, some of the writers have strong viewpoints or preconceptions which need to be taken into account. We urge readers not to rely on any single source as authoritative, but to follow up by seeking additional information about any treatment options which interest them.

This list is not complete; there are many useful publications not included here. Some entire areas are omitted—Chinese medicine, for example—not because we dismiss them, but because we are not prepared to cover them well.

The items listed below are extremely diverse. We cannot vouch for all of the information they contain. We have listed each item because we believe that some of our readers will want to know about it.

The books may be available in AIDS sections of gay or medical bookstores. For newsletters, and sometimes also for books, we include mailing addresses and telephone numbers.

• *Surviving AIDS*, by Michael Callen, Harper Collins Publishers, 1990. This is not primarily a book about treatments, but rather is based on interviews with long-term survivors. The author, one of the founders of both the People with AIDS Coalition and the Community Research Initiative in New York, was diagnosed with AIDS in 1982 (before the term "AIDS" existed), and given a short time to live; he is still alive and active today, over eight years later. Aside from the interviews, other chapters include "Why Some Survive," "The Propaganda of Hopelessness," "Making Sense of Survival" (summarizing what he learned from his continuing study of survivors), "What I Would Do If I Were You," and "The Case Against AZT."

• *Living with the AIDS Virus*, by Parris M. Kidd, Ph.D., and Wolfgang Huber, Ph.D., 1990, HK Biomedical, Inc—Educational Division, P.O. Box 8207, Berkeley, CA 94707, phone 415/527-6871. This 182-page book provides an easy-to-read overview of most of the better-known complementary and experimental treatments. While there are chapters on AZT and the biology of HIV, the main emphasis is on nutritional approaches, especially egg lecithin lipids (i.e., AL-721) and "natural" antioxidants, reflecting Dr. Kidd's background as a consultant on nutritional supplements.

• HEAL (Health Education AIDS Liaison) is preparing an updated version of its *AIDS Information Packet on Alternative & Holistic Therapies for AIDS*. We have not seen this packet, which should be available in about three weeks; the previous version was 150 pages. HEAL requests a donation of $12.50 or more for the packet, but will send it without charge to anyone who cannot afford to donate. HEAL, a nonprofit organization, holds treatment meetings in New York; it also plans to publish a quarterly newsletter. For more information, send a self-addressed stamped envelope to: HEAL, P.O. Box 1103, Old Chelsea Station, New York, NY 10113, or call 212/ 674-HOPE.

• *Nutritional Influences on Illness*, Melvyn R. Werbach, M.D., 1988, 1990, Keats Publishing, Inc., New Canaan, Connecticut, 203/966-8721, $17.95 (paperback). This 504-page book by an assistant professor at the University of California Los Angeles School of Medicine is **not** about AIDS—which does not even appear in the index. Instead, the book has chapters on 92 different diseases, each one reviewing the medical and scientific literature suggesting that certain foods or nutrients may be helpful (or in some cases harmful) in its treatment. While few of the conditions covered are AIDS related, persons with AIDS or HIV might find ideas worth trying.

• *Smart Drugs and Nutrients*, by Ward Dean, M.D., and John Morgenthaler, 1990, B&J Publications, Santa Cruz, CA 800/669-2030. This book, released in January 1991, is subtitled "How to Improve Your Memory and Increase Your Intelligence Using the Latest Discoveries in Neuroscience." It is not about AIDS; instead it reviews scientific studies of several dozen drugs which some researchers believe may improve mental functioning. Drugs are regularly prescribed for this purpose in some countries, but in the U.S. the concept has so far not been accepted. We mention the book here for research interest, because of the possibility that some of the drugs might be helpful in treating AIDS-related neurological problems. As far as we know, however, no studies to test this possibility have ever been done.

A two-part article on cognition-enhancement drugs is also being published by *Megabrain Report: The Psychotechnology Newsletter*, P.O. Box 2744, Sausalito, CA 94965.

• *Forefront Health Investigations,* published six times a year by MegaHealth Society, P.O. Box 60637, Palo Alto, CA 94306, 408/733-2010. Originally called *Journal of the MegaHealth Society* and focusing on "health information on life extension and biological technology," *Forefront* recently changed its name and has begun to include more information on AIDS and HIV; for example, the December 1990 issue includes an article on anabolic steroids as a proposed treatment for wasting syndrome, and an article on yeast infections (not AIDS-related, but possibly useful with AIDS). The previous issue discussed combining AZT with ddC or with ddI.

# Issue Number 122
# March 1, 1991

## KAPOSI'S SARCOMA TREATMENT OVERVIEW
*by Michelle Roland*

With the increasing use of pneumocystis prophylaxis, anti-retroviral treatment, and subtle improvements in the management of opportunistic infections, people with AIDS are living longer today than several years ago. Unfortunately, as people live longer, increasing numbers are having to cope with complications of Kaposi's sarcoma (KS) and lymphoma, and more people are dying from these conditions. For this reason, we are presenting a comprehensive article covering standard and experimental treatments for KS. We hope this article will provide a clear picture of both current and future potential treatment options.

We will briefly discuss standard approaches for treating isolated cutaneous (skin) lesions, including intralesional chemotherapy, radiation, and liquid nitrogen. In addition, experimental approaches for cutaneous lesions will be reviewed. Some of these, like intralesional interferon and topical tretinoin (retin-A), are available by prescription for other uses. Others, like 5-FU collagen matrix, are still in clinical trials or earlier stages of development.

For disseminated KS (involving either internal organs and/or many skin lesions), we will discuss the use of interferon, standard chemotherapy, and chemotherapy drugs which are available for other indications, such as oral and intravenous etoposide (also called VP-16). Some newer chemotherapy agents, including liposomal daunorubicin, liposomal doxorubicin, and piritrexim, are still in clinical trials or earlier stages of development. Growth factors (also called colony stimulating factors) like GM-CSF and G-CSF appear to be effective in limiting the bone marrow damage associated with chemotherapy and interferon; we will describe their FDA (U.S. Food and Drug Administration) approval status and informal expanded access programs.

A discussion of an exciting new class of compounds called anti-angiogenesis agents will follow. These drugs work by an entirely different mechanism than do the chemotherapy drugs. They include experimental compounds like the Japanese drug brought to widespread attention by Robert Gallo, M.D., from the National Cancer Institute, fumagillin analogues, and PF4. Pentosan is an anti-angiogenesis compound currently in clinical trials sponsored by the National Institutes of Health. Finally, we will discuss the experimental use of agents such as Vitamin D derivatives and synthetic heparin/steroid combinations as anti-angiogenesis compounds.

A discussion of the broad area of biological response modifiers, a growing area of interest in the treatment of HIV infection and cancer, will include descriptions of the experimental compound IL-2 and the prescription drug levamisole. We will also describe the immunomodulatory and anti-angiogenic properties of cimetidine, an ulcer medication, and its potential utility in KS. In addition, we will outline the current status of the Prosorba column, an approach we first discussed in 1989 (issue #75) and briefly mention the application of hyperthermia in KS.

## Standard Treatment Options

The choice of standard treatment approaches for KS today depends on the location and extent of the lesions, the individual's overall immune status (usually determined by T-helper cell counts and other laboratory markers), and the bone marrow production capacity, especially the neutrophil count. (Neutrophils are a type of white blood cell important in fighting bacterial infections.)

## Limited Skin Lesions

A small number of skin lesions causing cosmetic problems can be treated with injections of small doses of a cancer chemotherapy drug called Velban (vinblastine) and/or with radiation therapy. Some clinicians freeze the lesions with liquid nitrogen, causing the cells to die and the lesions to fade.

## Disseminated (Widespread) KS

Alpha interferon (INF-alpha, INTRON A, Roferon) is an FDA-approved treatment for people with KS and a T-helper cell count greater than 200. It has been shown to have an anti-HIV effect as well as an anti-KS effect and is being studied, alone and in combination with AZT, for both indications. Preliminary results suggest that lower doses of each drug used together (3-5 million units interferon plus 600 mg AZT per day) may be more useful than either drug alone with respect to both antitumor and antiviral effects; a larger proportion of people are responding to the combination than would be expected to respond to interferon alone[1]. Alpha interferon is usually used in people who have disseminated internal or skin lesions but may also be used if there are only a few lesions.

Interferon has been shown to be much more effective in people with higher T-helper cell counts (over 400) who have not had a previous opportunistic infection. It is also more effective in people who do not have fever, night sweats, or weight loss.[2] Studies combining chemotherapy agents (either vinblastine or VP-16/etoposide) with interferon have been disappointing, showing increased toxicity and a lower response rate than expected with either agent used alone. A recent study looked at the ability of patients to tolerate increasing doses of interferon after completing chemotherapy (adriamycin, bleomycin, and vincristine). It was hoped that the interferon would maintain the regression of the lesions, reducing the need for ongoing chemotherapy. Again, the results were disappointing overall, although two patients with higher T-helper counts (350-400) were able to tolerate the interferon and responded well to the therapy during this short study.

While there has been a great deal of interest in interferon in both KS and HIV, the side effects are significant. Although rarely life-threatening, the flu-like symptoms, including chills, headaches, fatigue, muscle aches, and low grade fevers, can be debilitating and affect quality of life.

New types of interferon are also being studied. These include beta interferon and variations of alpha interferon. One such variation, consensus interferon, is a single molecule made of the seventeen different alpha interferon molecules which have been identified. As far as we can tell, no distinct advantages of any specific product have yet been demonstrated.

The other standard approach to the treatment of widespread KS is cancer chemotherapy. The specific choice of which drugs to use depends on the individual's blood counts and medical history, including a history of peripheral neuropathy since some of the drugs might aggravate this condition. The most commonly used regimens today are a combination of bleomycin and vincristine, with or without adriamycin (doxorubicin), or alternating vincristine and vinblastine. Some clinicians include etoposide (VP-16) or use variations of the combinations described above. A complete review of a series of single agent and combination chemotherapy clinical trials by Donald Northfelt, M.D., can be found in the September 1990 issue of *AIDS Medical Report,*[3] published by American Health Consultants. A copy of volume 3, number 9 can be purchased for $13.25 by calling 800/688-2421. (Also see *AIDS Treatment News* issue #73 for a discussion of the specific toxicities of the different chemotherapeutic drugs.)

It is unfortunate but important to note that although significant lesion improvement has been seen with several chemotherapeutic regimens, survival time has often not been prolonged. There appears to be a high rate of bacterial and other infections occurring in patients receiving chemotherapy for KS. Two obvious but important suggestions were made in a recent paper reporting on a trial of chemotherapy plus aerosolized pentamidine for pneumocystis prophylaxis: 1) it is essential to use pneumocystis prophylaxis drugs, and to consider prophylaxis for toxoplasmosis and other opportunistic infections, and 2) use of growth factors which stimulate the bone marrow to produce specific types of blood cells, like G-CSF (granulocyte colony stimulating factor) or GM-CSF (granulocyte-macrophage colony stimulating factor), should be considered in an attempt to reduce the bone marrow suppressive effects of chemotherapy.

## How to Obtain G-CSF and GM-CSF

The difference between G-CSF and GM-CSF is that G-CSF only stimulates the production of cells called granulocytes (especially neutrophils, a type of granulocyte), whereas GM-CSF also stimulates the production of cells called macrophages. Some clinicians, researchers, and activists believe that G-CSF would be a better choice for use in people with HIV infection because macrophages serve as a reservoir of HIV and some other infectious agents.

G-CSF, manufactured by Amgen Inc., (trade name: Neupogen) was approved by the FDA for marketing on February 21, 1991. This product was approved for patients with cancer who are using chemotherapy which suppresses white blood cell production. The approval does not include HIV- or KS-specific indications. Although any doctor can prescribe a drug for any use once it has been FDA-approved, securing reimbursement from insurance companies and Medicaid/Medicare may prove to be difficult for off-label use of the drug.

Amgen has established a "Safety Net" program for uninsured and medically needy patients. This program requires that both the patient and physician qualify. Physicians must complete an application form and purchase the G-CSF directly from Amgen. Patients will be eligible if they are uninsured and earn a combined family income of less than $25,000 per year or if they are insured, earn a combined family income of less than $25,000 per year, and have significant out-of-pocket expense for the product. *Physicians only* can call 800/272-9376 for more information on this program.

Preliminary studies suggest that GM-CSF is helpful in reducing neutropenia (low neutrophil counts) and the incidence of infections in people being treated for KS. See *AIDS Treatment News* #110 for background on GM-CSF in lymphoma treatment and *AIDS Treatment News* #108 for information on its use with ganciclovir for CMV infections). Clinical trials are testing GM-CSF's ability to reduce bone marrow damage caused by the chemotherapy, interferon/AZT combinations, and a variety of other treatments in people with HIV infection. For information on ACTG-sponsored trials which include GM-CSF, call 800/TRIALS-A.

Two variations of GM-CSF are being developed by four different pharmaceutical companies. We spoke with Carol Colvin, Pharm. D., the professional services manager at Immunex Corporation in Seattle. She explained that Immunex, in collaboration with Hoechst-Roussel Pharmaceuticals, is developing one product while Schering-Plough and Sandoz are jointly developing a slightly different product. According to Dr. Colvin, Immunex's product has been recommended for approval by the FDA Biological Response Modifiers Advisory Committee and the company is awaiting general FDA approval. She said that such approval has historically come a couple of months after Advisory Panel recommendation. An application for approval has also been filed with the FDA for the Schering/Sandoz product. This application has not yet been recommended by the Advisory Committee.

Immunex's initial application seeks approval only for patients with cancer receiving bone marrow transplants followed by high-dose chemotherapy. Again, reimbursement for off-label use of this product may be difficult. Immunex has established a reimbursement hotline to assist physicians in getting insurance companies to pay for the product and a patient assistance program for those patients who have exhausted all other avenues of paying for the drug. According to Dr. Colvin, both of these lines will be open, and the price of the drug will be announced, on the day FDA approval is received. How well these programs actually function remains to be seen.

Until GM-CSF is approved, physicians may try to get the drug through expanded access for patients with low neutrophil counts. A representative of Schering-Plough said that the drug may be supplied to individuals on a case-by-case basis, but would give no further details. Physicians can call the company at 800/526-4099 for information about enrolling specific patients

Immunex *does not* have an expanded access program for HIV-positive patients, purportedly because of limited experience with the use of GM-CSF in people with AIDS. In spite of a growing sense of the utility of GM-CSF in a wide variety of HIV-associated conditions, and an increasing collection of data in these situations, Immunex has no plans to include HIV-positive patients in its compassionate-use program.

## Experimental Approaches to Treat Individual Lesions

•  Intralesional interferon. Terrance Chew, M.D., a hematologist-oncologist studying this approach at St. Francis Hospital in San Francisco, explained that the interferon might have an immune-stimulating and anti-HIV effect in the lesion itself and that injecting it locally would reduce the toxic side effects experienced with systemic injections. He told us that he is able to get high concentrations of the interferon in the lesions and that the approach is "worth pursuing." He recommended its use for people with high T-helper cell counts.

A small study (seven patients) published in the abstract book of the Sixth International Conference on AIDS in San Francisco suggested that all lesions treated with intralesional interferon responded in thickness, size, and color, but that patients with higher T-helper cell counts and without any prior opportunistic infection experienced a larger response. Dr. Chew's study calls for three injections per week; the study from the Conference used daily injections for four weeks, followed by three injections per week. Intralesional Velban, liquid nitrogen, and radiation therapy usually require significantly fewer treatments.

•  Topical tretinoin gel (Retin-A). Another abstract from the Sixth International Conference on AIDS described the use of topically applied 1% All Trans Retinoic Acid (tretinoin) gel for cutaneous KS. Although only eight people were studied, all treated lesions showed a reduction in color and size of the nodules as compared to lesions which were untreated or treated only with the oil used in the gel. One patient had a complete response after two weeks; five experienced a 50% reduction in size and firmness of their lesion(s) after three months. Retin-A is used in the United States for the treatment of severe cases of acne.

A note on retinoids: Tretinoin is a vitamin A derivative known as a retinoid. Other retinoids available in the United States include isotretinoin (Accutane) and etretinate. [The use of accutane and etretinate has been limited in women because they both cause severe birth defects. Etretinate should not be used for an undetermined period of time *even before becoming pregnant* because it takes an unknown amount of time to be eliminated from the body.] Topical and systemic retinoids have been found to be useful, by themselves and in combination with alpha interferon, in various benign (non-cancerous) and cancerous growths of the skin and mucous membranes. Each of the retinoids tested has different efficacies in different conditions, including hairy leukoplakia (accutane) and molluscum contagiosum (retin-A). Unfortunately, it has not been possible to achieve therapeutic doses of natural Vitamin A to treat the human cancers which have been studied.

Given the growing interest in retinoids for the prevention and treatment of a wide range of cancers and non-cancerous growths, we believe that research in the possible application of retinoids for the management of KS, by themselves or in combination with other treatments, should be designed and conducted promptly. In the meantime, it is important to remember that there are serious toxicities associated with some of the retinoids; any use of these drugs should be undertaken with medical advice and careful monitoring by a physician. It is also important to realize that the only data available on the use of a retinoid in KS is the small study mentioned above. In addition, the conditions for which the retinoids have been shown to be useful may involve different mechanisms than those which cause KS.

• 5-FU Collagen Matrix. This experimental treatment is currently being tested for use in HIV-negative people with anal or genital warts. We mention it here because an intralesional implant trial for the treatment of KS had been listed in the Community Consortium's *Directory of HIV Clinical Research in the (San Francisco) Bay Area* since the Summer 1990 issue. The KS trial was supposed to take place in the offices of a doctor in San Francisco with a large HIV practice. When we contacted his office we were told that the company had pulled out of the study for unknown reasons. A worker at the HIV-negative anogenital wart study site in San Francisco told us that the FDA had put a hold on testing the drug in HIV-positive people. When we contacted the drug company, Matrix, to discuss the status of their product, all we were told was that the trials were on hold and would not be starting soon. Further messages have not been returned.

5-FU is a cancer chemotherapy drug. Collagen is a structural component of the skin and connective tissue. The collagen matrix was developed to help keep the chemotherapy agent in the lesion longer. We do not know if this treatment would have any advantages over currently existing KS therapies. All we do know is that there is a bit of a mystery around why the planned trial has been discontinued before it even started.

## Experimental Chemotherapy Treatments

Non-standard cancer chemotherapy drugs which have been studied in KS include oral and IV formulations of etoposide (VP-16), liposomal daunorubicin, doxorubicin (also being developed in a liposomal form), piritrexim, epirubicin, idarubicin, and mitoxantrone. As far as we can tell, the most useful drugs from this list at this time are etoposide, liposomal daunorubicin, and piritrexim.

• Etoposide (VP-16). An oral formulation of etoposide is currently being evaluated for safety and dosage at five hospitals associated with the government-sponsored AIDS Clinical Trials Group (ACTG). The drug is being administered weekly for 52 weeks. The advantage of an effective low-dose oral chemotherapy drug would be in its ease of administration and milder side effects. We spoke with Susan Krown, M.D., Chair of the ACTG Oncology Committee, who told us that the study is accruing rapidly and proceeding without any problems. The oral formulation of VP-16 is approved for the treatment of a specific type of lung cancer.

Dr. Krown told us that until now other drugs, such as bleomycin and vincristine, with or without adriamycin, have often been used as first line treatment in KS. However, she said that VP-16 might be used earlier more routinely if the results from the ACTG study are positive. Some clinicians currently use either IV or oral VP-16 (weekly or monthly) in combination with other chemotherapy drugs. Others are trying the oral form daily in very low doses for several weeks.

• Liposomal daunorubicin. Liposomes are small spheres of fat into which drugs can be placed. The hope with liposomal technology is that toxic drugs can be targeted more specifically, and at higher concentration, to the areas where they are needed. It is thought that the liposomal drugs will leak in those areas in which there are abnormal blood vessels and will target the abnormal cells that comprise the KS lesions. Daunorubicin is a cancer chemotherapy drug.

We spoke to Dr. Chew about his plans for two studies with this drug. No patients have been enrolled in his studies yet due to problems with drug supply. At this stage, the drug company has promised him only a small supply and he plans to enroll patients on a first-come-first-served basis when the drug is available. He will consider patients with widespread KS which has not responded to treatment or has never been treated. He will try to include patients with the greatest need first, when the drug supply is limited. For more information about this trial, please call Drew Catapano at (415) 775-4321, extension 2512.

The original trial has been written to include 16 patients. Dr. Chew agreed that if this initial trial is promising, future trials should be designed to look at the efficacy of the liposomal daunorubicin in combination with other chemotherapy agents and/or biological response modifiers (immunomodulators) like interferon. An abstract presented at a recent scientific meeting claims that daunorubicin has an anti-HIV effect in test-tube studies. Dr. Chew said he felt that there is not yet sufficient data to support that conclusion.

Dr. Chew told us that liposomal daunorubicin has been under study for 2 years at the University of Southern California in Los Angeles and that it has shown promise. We spoke with Sue Cabriales, R.N., the research nurse who administers the drug to patients in that trial. There are currently 15 people enrolled in the trial, and the drug company is just beginning to analyze the data. The drug is administered every two weeks over a 40-minute period. Ms. Cabriales told us that it is a very easy drug to deliver because it does not cause local tissue damage, unlike many cancer chemotherapy drugs.

Although the data have not yet been analyzed, Ms. Cabriales gave us her unofficial impression of the drug. Toxicities appear to be minimal, with some fatigue, mild nausea, and increased cholesterol and triglyceride levels. Depressed blood counts have been observed, but it is unclear whether they are due to the liposomal daunorubicin, AZT, or some other factor. The drug appears to arrest the further development of KS in many patients and, in some cases, reduces lesion size. However, the disease does progress if the treatment is stopped. The longest a patient has been on the trial is over one year.

• Liposomal doxorubicin (adriamycin) is being developed by another drug company using a different technology. Dr. Chew expects it to be available for clinical trials within six months.

• Piritrexim is an experimental compound similar to the chemotherapy drug methotrexate. It is not yet approved by the FDA for any indication. Two studies have been conducted in people with KS at the University of Miami. The first used two courses of piritrexim alone, followed by a combination of piritrexim with interferon. This study has been completed. A second study using only piritrexim was initiated to look at the safety and efficacy of using the drug in low doses on a daily schedule. This study will be completed within weeks.

We spoke with the principal investigator of these two studies, Margaret Fischl, M.D., from the University of Miami School of Medicine. She explained that piritrexim had been shown to have some success in solid tumors, suggesting that it may be useful for KS. So far, the drug has been relatively well tolerated, with skin rashes and depressed white blood cell counts among the common side effects. The two most important findings so far, according to Dr. Fischl, are: 1) as with alpha interferon, piritrexim appears to be most useful in early KS, where tumor regressions have been seen, and 2) there is both test-tube and human evidence to suggest that piritrexim may also be useful in preventing pneumocystis pneumonia. Dr. Fischl explained that daily dosing with a low dose seems to be superior to the cyclic schedule used in the first study.

Dr. Fischl plans to present the data from these two studies to the ACTG for consideration of future studies. She told us that the main question that needs to be considered in deciding where to go next with this drug is whether or not piritrexim will have any significant advantage over alpha interferon. She pointed out that interferon does show activity against HIV in addition to early KS, whereas piritrexim does not have any anti-HIV activity.

• A number of small studies have also been conducted with the chemotherapy drugs doxorubicin (adriamycin), epirubicin, idarubicin, and mitoxantrone. In general, results have been inconsistent or not dramatic. Test-tube studies have suggested that mitoxantrone should be pursued, whereas previous clinical studies have been disappointing. Dr. Chew told us that data which is awaiting publication suggests that idarubicin, recently approved for acute leukemia, acts more quickly than daunorubicin in leukemia and thus might be more effective in KS. We will continue to follow developments in new chemotherapy drugs for KS.

## Anti-Angiogenesis Compounds

With the exception of a single trial (of pentosan, described below), the U.S. government-sponsored clinical trials in KS have focused on the use of chemotherapy and interferon by themselves and in combination with anti-retrovirals and the white blood cell growth factors (GM-CSF and G-CSF) discussed earlier in this article. However, a growing number of scientists working in the areas of cancer and basic research are focusing their attention on an entirely different class of compounds, those which interfere with angiogenesis (the growth of new or abnormal blood vessels).

Most solid tumors rely on an abundant blood supply, provided by an extensive network of blood vessels, for their growth. Anti-angiogenesis research has generated an intense level of scientific interest because of the theoretical possibility of being able to "starve" solid tumors by preventing further blood vessel development. These compounds may be useful in KS because KS appears to be a proliferation of abnormal blood vessels. It is believed that many of the growth factors involved in the development of blood vessels in solid tumors are the same as those involved in the development of KS lesions.

Over the past several months we have published reports on the much-publicized Japanese compound first brought to public attention by Robert Gallo, M.D., of the U.S. National Cancer Institute (see *AIDS Treatment News* issues #99 and #100) and fumagillin analogues (see *AIDS Treatment News* issue #117). These are both believed to interfere in angiogenesis. None of the compounds we have reported on in these articles are currently available by prescription or for purchase from other sources; they are still in the very early stages of development by pharmaceutical companies and/or university laboratories. However, they have immediate importance for research, and potential long-range importance for treatment.

These compounds and/or others in the same class may prove to be more specific and thus less toxic than the cancer chemotherapy drugs which are currently in widespread use for KS. Although many of the most promising compounds are still in very early preclinical development, some drugs in this class are currently being used for other conditions. This means that they are available for scientists to study both in laboratory experiments and in clinical trials with humans now. Some physicians and researchers in the AIDS community, including Joseph Sonnabend, M.D., from New York, have been discussing, writing about, and urging further research in this area for several years.

Hundreds of compounds are being studied in laboratories around the world for their anti-angiogenic properties. A computer search revealed over 1,000 articles in the scientific literature in this area. The retinoids mentioned earlier in this article are believed to have anti-angiogenic properties. We will describe briefly only a few additional compounds, including pentosan, PF4 (platelet factor 4), fumagillin analogues, vitamin D3 analogues, and a synthetic heparin/steroid combination. These are not necessarily the most promising compounds, nor the most available; they are simply the ones which have received the most attention so far in the AIDS research, treatment, and activist communities.

It is our strong belief that the experts in the field of angiogenesis and cell differentiation, whether or not they are involved in HIV, should be actively recruited by the government-sponsored research agencies to share their knowledge, theories, data and expertise in the effort to find safe and effective treatments for KS.

• Pentosan is a sulfated polysaccharide being studied for safety and dosage at the National Cancer Institute (NCI). Pentosan is an anti-coagulant which is believed to have both anti-HIV and anti-KS properties. We spoke with James Pluda, M.D., who is directing this study. So far, three doses have been studied in groups of three to six patients. Patients in the lowest dose group have been receiving the drug for several months. Some patients using the second dose showed some anti-coagulant effects; therefore, it was decided to test an intermediate dose rather than trying to increase the dose any further. Other side effects seen so far have included reversible liver function test abnormalities, and thrombocytopenia (decreased platelet count).

Dr. Pluda explained that this drug does not kill the KS cells; it just stops their growth, so it takes some time to see an effect. He emphasized that he does not know how to use this drug safely yet, and that people who have obtained it should only use it with the careful monitoring of a physician experienced with the drug. All slots for the NCI study have been filled.

• rPF4 is a recombinant (genetically engineered) version of a protein which is found in platelets, a type of blood cell. It has been found by researchers at Repligen Corporation to inhibit angiogenesis in test tube studies and in animals with a variety of different tumors. It does not cure the tumors, but prevents further growth.

According to Theodore Maione, Ph.D., principle investigator of the animal studies, the activity of the compound has been specifically targeted to the cell type found in blood vessels (endothelial cells). KS lesions include a large number of fast growing endothelial cells. Therefore, it is hoped that PF4 will specifically target the cells which comprise the KS lesions. While no formal toxicity tests have been conducted yet, no toxicities have been observed in animals.

rPF4 is not yet ready to enter human trials. After animal testing is completed, Dr. Maione told us that Repligen will file an application with the FDA to do testing in people with KS. The initial studies will use intralesional injections to determine if there is a local tumor response. The FDA application will not be filed until the end of 1991. In the meantime, Repligen is scaling up production of the compound.

• Fumagillin analogues are synthetic variations of a naturally occurring antibiotic. We asked Donald Ingber, M.D., Ph.D., the author of a recent article in *Nature*, about these compounds. He told us that fumagillin itself is too toxic to be used in humans but that the synthetic analogues have shown tumor response in every solid tumor tested in animals to far. As with PF4, the tumors generally do not regress, but their growth stops. Dr. Ingber described these compounds as very specific to growing tumors and non-toxic. He anticipates that therapy with this type of compound would be life-long, as with diabetes.

No tests have yet been conducted in humans. The drug company, Takeda Chemical Industries, Ltd., is attempting to increase production of the compounds in order to begin clinical trials, hopefully, within the next two years. These trials may not, however, be in people with KS. The company is also involved in an active search for other anti-angiogenesis compounds.

• "Gallo's Japanese KS Drug." For background on the scientific and political issues involved in this area, refer to Project Inform's *PI Perspectives*, issue number 9, October, 1990 (National 800/822-7422; California 800/334-7422) and *AIDS Treatment News* issue #99.

• Vitamin D3 analogues also appear to have anti-angiogenesis properties in test-tube studies. Vitamin D3 itself was not found to be effective in these studies. The authors suggest that these vitamin D3 analogues may work by a similar mechanism as the retinoids discussed earlier in this article.

• Synthetic heparin substitutes in combination with specific steroids have been found to inhibit angiogenesis in two experimental models. Heparin is a potent anti-coagulant; however, fragments of the compound which have lost their anti-coagulant properties retain anti-angiogenic activity when combined with certain steroids. The most potent heparin substitute reported on in this paper was beta-cyclodextrin tetradecasulfate. This compound actually stimulated angiogenesis when used alone, but was inhibitory in combination with a steroid.

The heparin substitutes were combined with the steroid hydrocortisone or with a hydrocortisone derivative which has lost most of its steroid properties. We have spoken with many physicians and researchers about this particular combination. Without exception, two concerns were raised. The first was the need to use heparin substitutes rather than heparin in order to avoid the anti-coagulant effects. The second was that steroids have been shown to stimulate the growth of KS when they have been given to patients for other purposes. Therefore, while heparin substitutes and steroid derivatives which lack the usual steroid properties appear to be a potentially useful anti-angiogenic combination, a standard heparin/steroid combination could be more harmful than helpful.


## Biological Response Modifiers in KS

Another area of intense scientific interest is in the use of immune modulators, or biological response modifiers, in the treatment of a wide variety of illnesses, including cancer and HIV infection. Many of the biological response modifiers being studied now are compounds which the body's cells produce naturally as a part of the immune response or in normal blood cell production (IL-2, the interferons, G-CSF, GM-CSF). Some others are drugs which have been used for completely different indications, but are suspected to have biological response modifier properties as well (cimetidine, levamisole), and some technologies have been developed specifically for this purpose (Prosorba column).

Many people believe that one of the keys to managing HIV infection will be combining one or more biological response modifier(s) with various antivirals and prophylactic agents. It is hoped that the biological response modifiers will, in a sense, give the immune system a "boost" in fighting the various infections, cancers, and KS associated with HIV infection.

• Interleukin-2 (IL-2) is a naturally occurring compound which is being studied in people with KS at the U.S. National Institutes of Health. A small study of IL-2 and AZT has recently completed enrollment. A second study is using IL-2 plus alpha interferon in people with HIV infection, including people with KS. We were unable to reach anyone at the NIH or at Cetus Corporation about these studies, and thus we are not sure of the safety or efficacy of IL-2 in people with KS.

A study published in 1989 showed exacerbation of KS in three of four patients using a combination of IL-2 and beta interferon. It was suggested by the authors of that study that investigators who use IL-2 should avoid intermediate to high dose bolus (injection over a very short period of time) therapy. In addition, it was suggested that levels of an undesirable type of interferon, gamma-interferon, be monitored in these patients and that therapy be adjusted if these levels increase significantly.

It will be important to know whether these changes were made in the NIH studies and, if so, how such changes have affected the outcome of people with KS who are using IL-2.

• Cimetidine (Tagamet) is an ulcer medication which has been found to have both anti-angiogenic and immunomodulatory effects. We first reported on the use of cimetidine in patients with KS in 1989 (see *AIDS Treatment News* #80). Interest in studying this drug for use in HIV and cancer has been nearly nonexistent since that time. We have heard speculation that there might be little interest in further studies because the patent is running out in the next year, significantly decreasing the drug's profitability.

A small study performed by Thomas Smith, M.D., from the Massey Cancer Center in Richmond, Virginia, was recently published as a letter in the *Journal of the National Cancer Institute*. Of the eight patients treated for skin, oral, and/or gastrointestinal KS lesions, one experienced a complete response, one a partial response, and one a mixed response. There were no subjective or objective toxicities reported.

We spoke with Dr. Smith who told us that his impression is that cimetidine is most effective in people with relatively high T-helper cell counts. He explained that it seems to be useful in skin and oral lesions, not just in gastrointestinal lesions. Cimetidine appears to enable Natural Killer (NK) cells, the immune system's main defense against cancer, to fight the KS.

Dr. Smith believes that cimetidine will ultimately be most useful in combination with cancer chemotherapy and/or other biological response modifiers. He also told us that patients who cannot tolerate low doses of alpha interferon, his first choice treatment in combination with AZT, may benefit from cimetidine.

Dr. Smith did not know of anyone else studying cimetidine. Because of the small patient population where he practices, he is not planning future studies of this drug in people with KS. If he gets funding, he will be studying the drug in patients with cancer.

• Levamisole is also a prescription drug which may have some immunomodulatory function. Originally approved for the treatment of worms, its approval was recently expanded to include the treatment of advanced colon cancer (stage C) when it is used in combination with fluorouricil, a cancer chemotherapy agent. Although it is ineffective alone in colon cancer, it appears to enhance the effect of the chemotherapy in this particular case.

This is another drug about which we have spoken to many researchers and clinicians. Although none of them seemed greatly enthusiastic about it, we believe that a small pilot study should be conducted to determine if levamisole might have any efficacy in KS, given its limited toxicity, immunostimulatory properties, and utility in enhancing chemotherapy in colon cancer.

• We first discussed the Prosorba™* Column (Protein A) in 1989 (see *AIDS Treatment News* issue #75) when we described the four year experience of Dobri Kiprov, M.D., at Children's Hospital in San Francisco. Dr. Kiprov and others conducted a Phase I study of the Prosorba column in people with KS and reported a response rate of 42%. Because of the relative safety and efficacy demonstrated in this early clinical trial, Dr. Kiprov told us that he feels that further studies should be pursued rapidly. (*Prosorba is a registered trademark of IMRE Corporation.)

The Prosorba column is used to remove circulating immune complexes from the blood. These complexes, comprised of antibodies and antigen, are believed to play a role in suppressing the immune system. Therefore, it is believed that the Prosorba column may be effective against both KS and HIV.

Frank Jones, Ph.D., CEO of IMRE Corporation, the manufacturer of the Prosorba column, told us that financial difficulties have delayed additional studies in people with KS. However, a Phase II protocol is written, and Dr. Jones hopes to implement it at up to five institutions some time this year. This clinical trial will involve about 100 patients and run for one and a half to two years.

Dr. Kiprov suggested that the Prosorba column should be tested in combination with other biological response modifiers, such as interferon. According to Dr. Kiprov, these combinations are being used to treat people with breast cancer in Europe. He also believes that such combinations may be effective in treating the primary HIV infection.

The Prosorba column is currently approved for use in idiopathic thrombocytopenia purpura (platelet count below 100,000/mm³). Dr. Jones told us that some U.S. physicians are currently using it in KS even though it is not yet approved for that indication.

## A Note on Hyperthermia

Whole body hyperthermia made dramatic press headlines and was quickly dismissed as an HIV "cure" by most researchers, clinicians, and activists last year. However, the local or regional use of heat to enhance chemotherapy treatment or radiation has been and continues to be evaluated in a wide number of cancers by researchers throughout the world. Hyperthermia may well prove to be a useful adjunctive therapy in the treatment of cancer and KS.

## Conclusion and Comment

There are two general approaches to take in dealing with KS. The first is to take the existing therapies available today, combine them or refine them, and try to make them as effective as possible, with the minimum amount of toxicity. This is being done by the ACTG, the US government-sponsored group which has the biggest responsibility for testing AIDS-related drugs. The latest plans for ACTG trials include combining chemotherapy drugs with the newer anti-retrovirals ddC and ddI, in the hopes that these combinations will be less toxic than AZT with chemotherapy. The importance of the use of GM-CSF and, by assumption, G-CSF in KS has also been demonstrated by ACTG studies; as these drugs become available, they will probably have a small but significant impact on the lives of people with KS.

The second approach which must be taken is to recruit the basic research experts to work on understanding the mechanisms involved in KS and to develop novel approaches to dealing with this condition. When advances in understanding are made, as they are being made in the area of angiogenesis, these advances need to be applied to people as quickly as is safely possible. Preclinical screening tests need to be conducted to compare a large number of compounds to find the most effective and safest. Then some agency needs to be ready to go with human trials. We believe instituting this approach should be a very high priority among those who set research policy in KS.

## REFERENCES

1.    Fischl, MA, Krown, SE, Lane, HC, and others. Alpha interferon: the questions and answers. *PAACNOTES*. May/June, 1990; volume 2, number 3, pages 115-121.

2. Krown, SE. The role of interferon in the therapy of epidemic Kaposi's Sarcoma. *Seminars in Oncology.* June 1987; volume 14, number 2, supplement 3, pages 27-33.

3. Northfelt, DW. Clinical presentation and treatment of AIDS-related Kaposi's sarcoma. *AIDS Medical Report.* September 1990; volume 3, number 9, pages 99-114.

4. Gill, GS, Rarick, MU, Bernstein-Singer, M, and others. Interferon-alpha maintenance therapy after cytotoxic chemotherapy for treatment of acquired immunodeficiency syndrome-related Kaposi's sarcoma. *Journal of Biological Response Modifiers.* 1990; volume 9, pages 512-516.

5. Shields, PG, Dawkins, F, Holmlund, J, and others. Low-dose multidrug chemotherapy plus *Pneumocystis carinii* pneumonia prophylaxis for HIV-related Kaposi's sarcoma. *Journal of Acquired Immune Deficiency Syndromes.* 1990; volume 3, number 7, pages 695-700.

6. Krown, SE, Paredes, J, Bundow, D, and others. Combination therapy with interferon-alpha (INF-alpha), zidovudine (AZT), and recombinant granulocyte-macrophage colony-stimulating factor (GM-CSF): a phase I trial in patients with AIDS-related Kaposi's sarcoma. Sixth International Conference on AIDS, San Francisco, June 20-24, 1990 (abstract #S.B.513).

7. Tschechne, B, von Wussow, P, Schedel, I, and others. High dose intralesional recombinant interferon-alpha-IIb-treatment in HIV-1-infected patients with Kaposi's sarcoma. Sixth International Conference on AIDS, San Francisco, June 20-24, 1990 (abstract #2100).

8. Bonhomme, L, Fredj, G, Averous, S, and others. Topically applied all trans-retinoic acid for the treatment of Kaposi's sarcoma. Sixth International Conference on AIDS, San Francisco, June 20-24, 1990 (abstract #2090).

9. Lippman, SM, Shimm, DS and Meyskens, FL. Non-surgical treatments for cancer: retinoids and alpha interferon. *Journal of Dematol Surgical Oncology.* August 1988; volume 14, number 8, pages 862-869.

10. Lippman, SM and Meyskens, FL. Vitamin A derivatives in the prevention and treatment of human cancer. *Journal of the American College of Nutrition.* August 1988; volume 7, number 4, pages 269-84.

11. Editorial. A carrot a day keeps cancer at bay? *The Lancet.* January 12, 1991; volume 337, page 81-82.

12. Filio, LG and Gaudreault, R. Effect of daunorubicin on HIV-1 infected U937 and HUT 78 cells. 30th Interscience Conference on Antimicrobial Agents and Chemotherapy, October 21-24, 1990, Atlanta (abstract #534).

13. Qu, BX and Steiner, R. AIDS-associated Kaposi's sarcoma: identification of new drug candidates for treatment. *Proceedings of the Annual Meeting of the American Society of Clinical Oncology,* 1990.

14. Maione, TE, Gray, GS, Petro, J, and others. Inhibition of angiogenesis by recombinant human platelet factor-4 and related peptides. *Science.* January 5, 1990; volume 247, pages 77-79.

15. Maione, TE and Sharpe, RJ. Development of angiogenesis inhibitors for clinical applications. *Trends in Pharmacological Sciences.* November 1990; volume 11, number 11, pages 457-461.

16. Ingber, D, Fujita, T, Kishimoto, S, and others. Synthetic analogues of fumagillin that inhibit angiogenesis and suppress tumor growth. *Nature.* December 6, 1990; volume 348, pages 555-557.

17. Oikawa, T, Hirotani, K, Ogasawara, H, and others, Inhibition of angiogenesis by vitamin D3 analogues. *European Journal of Pharmacology.* 1990; volume 178, pages 247-250.

18. Folkman, J, Weisz, PB, Joullie, MM, and others. Control of angiogenesis with synthetic heparin substitutes. *Science.* March 17, 1989; volume 243, pages 1490-1493.

19. Gill, P.S., Loureiro, C., Bernstein-Singer, M. and others. Clinical effects of glucocorticoids on Kaposi sarcoma related to the acquired immunodeficiency syndrome (AIDS). *Annals of Internal Medicine.* June 1, 1989; volume 110, pages 937-940.

20. Krigel, R.L., Padavic-Shaller, K.A., Rudolph, A.R., and others. Exacerbation of epidemic Kaposi's sarcoma with a combination of interleukin-2 and beta-interferon: results of a phase II study. *Journal of Biological Response Modifiers*. 1989; volume 8, number 4, pages 359-365.

21. Tsuchida, T., Tsukamoto, Y., Segawa, K. and others. Effects of cimetidine and omeprazole on angiogenesis in granulation tissue of acetic acid-induced gastric ulcers in rats. *Digestion*. 1990; volume 47, pages 8-14.

22. Smith, T.J. and Kaplowitz, L.G. Pilot study of cimetidine in the treatment of Kaposi's sarcoma in patients with acquired immunodeficiency syndrome. *Journal of the National Cancer Institute*. January 16, 1991; volume 83, number 2, pages 139-141.

23. Moertel, C.G., Fleming, T.R., Macdonald, J.S. and others. Levamisole and fluorouricil for adjuvant therapy of resected colon carcinoma. *The New England Journal of Medicine*. February 8, 1990; volume 322, pages 352-358.

# Issue Number 123
# March 15, 1991

## TOXOPLASMOSIS: 566C80 STUDY
## OPENS IN SEVEN CITIES

*by Michelle Roland*

A pilot study of the experimental compound 566C80 in patients with toxoplasmosis who have failed or who are intolerant to standard therapy has recently opened at eight sites in seven U.S. cities (see list below). 566C80 has wide spectrum anti-protozoal activity, and is being tested against pneumocystis as well as against toxoplasmosis. (For more information about the drug, see "Pneumocystis Prophylaxis Overview," *AIDS Treatment News* #114.) This article is based on our interview with the study coordinator at San Francisco General Hospital; we have not called the other sites.

According to SFGH research coordinator Rebecca Coleman, Pharm. D., this trial is essentially a mechanism for compassionate access for people who have failed standard treatment with pyrimethamine and sulfadiazine. Dr. Coleman stated that each patient will be considered individually under the inclusion and exclusion criteria, especially concerning presence of other active infections requiring medication.

566C80 is an oral drug; it will be administered for a total of 42 days. The study requires all patients to be hospitalized for at least four days; then they will be followed as outpatients weekly for two weeks, every two weeks for a month, and then monthly for a total of six months. Patients who respond to treatment *may* be eligible to receive maintenance doses of 566C80 indefinitely. According to Dr. Coleman, the company is committed to ongoing access but has not yet received FDA approval for such a program. She explained that the FDA is expected to grant incremental approvals— perhaps for several months at a time—to supply the drug when necessary, after the conclusion of the study.

To be eligible for the trial, patients must have a positive diagnosis of toxoplasmosis and no evidence of any other infection or cancer of brain tissue. Patients who appear to have *failed* standard treatment will be required to have a brain biopsy. Symptoms of toxoplasmosis must not have improved after at least 21 days of standard therapy, or must have progressed after at least 14 days of treatment. Patients *intolerant* to standard therapy may also qualify for this trial. They will not be required to have a brain biopsy if other diagnostic tests suggest toxoplasmosis.

Patients must be at least 13 years old, and women must have a negative pregnancy test. During the first three weeks of treatment, neither AZT, ddI, ddC, Bactrim, dapsone, clindamycin, nor any experimental treatment will be allowed.

The drug will be provided by Burroughs Wellcome, but all other costs will be the responsibility of the patient. To facilitate reimbursement by third party payers, the diagnostic tests and frequency of clinic visits have been established to reflect standard care practices. The staff at SFGH will work with each patient and referring physician to receive prior authorization of coverage from third party payers.

## Trial Sites and Physicians

Physicians with a patient to enroll should contact one of the following physicians. According to a representative of Burroughs Wellcome, these sites are open; however, we were unable to call by press time to confirm that each is ready. Additional sites are expected to open in the future. This trial is not yet listed with the AIDS Clinical Trials Information Service (800/TRIALS-A).

San Francisco (2 sites): San Francisco General Hospital, John Stansell, M.D., 415/821-8313; Ralph K. Davies Hospital, Gifford Leong, M.D.

Oakland: Merritt-Peralta Medical Center, Patrick Joseph, M.D.

Los Angeles: Los Angeles County/USC Medical Center, Fred Sattler, M.D.

Portland: Oregon AIDS Task Force/Research and Education Group, Jim Sampson, M.D.

New York: Harlem Hospital, Wafaa El Sadr, M.D.

Baltimore: Johns Hopkins Hospital, Judith Feinberg, M.D.

Durham: Duke University Medical Center, Hetty Waskin, M.D.

# DDC: DEVELOPER SPEEDS FDA APPLICATION

Hoffmann-La Roche, the developer of the anti-HIV drug ddC, has arranged with the U.S. Food and Drug Administration to submit its New Drug Application (NDA) for that drug in sections as they are ready, for stepwise review by the FDA, instead of the usual procedure of waiting until the whole NDA is finished. The company estimates that the submission process should be completed by midyear. In addition, Hoffmann-La Roche will seek marketing approval for ddC in combination with AZT, as well as approval for use of ddC alone as an alternative to AZT. These efforts to speed the approval are important for several reasons:

• Each NDA is a large document, with many volumes of paperwork; it is submitted by one large organization (a pharmaceutical company) for evaluation by another (the FDA). In any such procedure, the differences in corporate culture between the organizations, as well as the effects of staff turnover, will invariably lead to points of friction, requiring sometimes lengthy negotiations to resolve. This organizational dynamic alone can lead to major delays in drug approval, quite aside from any substantive scientific, medical, or policy questions. Submitting the NDA in sections allows early issues to be addressed immediately, and later frictions to be reduced as the individuals involved develop working relationships.

• The FDA has traditionally leaned strongly toward first evaluating a drug by itself, and considering combinations only after efficacy has been shown for the drug alone. ddC, however, is showing unexpectedly good results in combination with AZT, in a small study. (See *AIDS Treatment News* #115 for early news about this combination. The study results have not yet been formally published.) If Hoffmann-La Roche had not applied for combination approval at this time, then the combination data would have been irrelevant to the FDA's evaluation of the NDA, and the drug would have been judged without this strong support.

• AIDS treatment activists had also feared that ddC approval would be delayed by the serious staff shortages at the FDA—that the Agency could not afford to assign people to evaluate the NDA for ddC until the NDA for ddI was finished. The staff shortages are very much a problem; but at least the wait behind ddI seems unlikely to happen with ddC.

There are still concerns about how much if any of the data from the major controlled trials now ongoing can be used in the current evaluation of ddC (and also ddI). Some experts fear that using the data being generated by these trials, before the trials have ended, might bias the studies or even lead to their discontinuation. The existing studies are automatically reviewed anyway, by a Data Safety Monitoring Board (DSMB); however, the DSMB operates secretly, even from the FDA, and it only looks for extreme differences between the study drugs, differences which would make it unethical to continue the study. For drug approval, the question is not whether the new drug is very different from an already-approved therapy, or even whether the two are equivalent; instead, the key question is whether the new drug has efficacy and value as a treatment. We are concerned that ddC (and ddI) may be evaluated without considering all of the important existing data. We do not know how this complex issue will be resolved.

# PNEUMOCYSTIS PROPHYLAXIS: STUDY SUGGESTS LOWER BACTRIM DOSE

A study of hospital records, published February 23, 1991, in *The Lancet*, has suggested that low-dose co-trimoxazole (also called Bactrim, Septra, sulfamethoxazole-trimethoprim, etc.—there are many different names for this drug) was more effective than aerosol pentamidine for preventing pneumocystis, may also help prevent toxoplasmosis, and had fewer side effects than the larger Bactrim doses used in other studies to prevent pneumocystis. And the cost of this form of pneumocystis prophylaxis, when generic versions of the drug are used, is about a hundred times less than the cost of aerosol pentamidine; the drug can cost about $10 per year, making this therapy potentially available to everyone.

The patients studied were members of Kaiser Permanente Medical Care Program in Los Angeles. Since Kaiser patients usually get all their care from Kaiser clinics and hospitals, and obtain their prescriptions from Kaiser pharmacies, uniform records of visits and prescriptions were available. 116 patients met all the criteria for this study: consecutive prescriptions for co-trimoxazole between December 1986 and June 1988, symptoms of immune deficiency, a diagnosis of AIDS or ARC, and either previous pneumocystis and/or T-helper count under 200. All records were reviewed until June 1990, or until the patients died; no one was lost to followup. The co-trimoxazole dose used by these 116 patients was one DS (double strength) tablet every Monday, Wednesday, and Friday.

No patient had pneumocystis while on this treatment. Of the 116 patients in the study, 71 had previously had pneumocystis, and they were followed on the prophylaxis for an average of 18.5 months. Those who had not had pneumocystis previously were followed for an average of 24.2 months. By contrast, without prophylaxis, half of the patients who have had pneumocystis would be expected to relapse within eight months, according to published data from other studies; and more than half of symptomatic patients with T-helper counts less than 200, but who have never had pneumocystis, would probably develop the disease within 24 months.

These results were better than those with aerosol pentamidine. The same Kaiser center found that 10 percent of patients who had previously had pneumocystis relapsed within one year, despite 300 mg of aerosolized pentamidine once per month.

Also, there were no cases of toxoplasmosis among the 116 patients treated with the low-dose co-trimoxazole. There were cases of the disease among those treated with aerosol pentamidine (which could have no effect on toxoplasmosis, because very little of the drug leaves the lungs). However, there were not enough cases to show for sure that co-trimoxazole was preventing the disease; the fact that no one developed toxoplasmosis might have been a result of the therapy, or it might have been coincidence.

Side effects believed due to co-trimoxazole—especially rash, fever, and nausea—occurred in 28 percent of the 116 patients. But only in nine percent (of the 116) were they severe enough to require permanently stopping the drug. (In some other cases, the co-trimoxazole was stopped for seven to ten days, and then could be restarted.) Side effects almost always began within the first month if they occurred at all. In no case were they life-threatening or otherwise very severe.

# PNEUMOCYSTIS PROPHYLAXIS IN CHILDREN: NEW GUIDELINES

*by Michelle Roland*

Because the immune systems of children and infants are very different from those of adults, HIV infection often manifests itself uniquely in these populations. Therefore, standard treatment and prophylaxis guidelines in adults often have little relevance for infants and children. Clinicians and parents of HIV-infected children know that these children develop pneumocystis long before their T-helper counts have declined to the usual adult threshold of 200 to 300. However, almost no data exist on T-helper counts in healthy, non-HIV-infected infants and children, let alone in those with HIV infection.

A working group convened at the National Pediatric HIV Research Center at Children's Hospital in New Jersey has reviewed a series of studies of the natural history, treatment, and prevention of pneumocystis in infants and children. Their recommendations for pneumocystis prophylaxis are being published by the U.S. Centers for Disease Control in the March 15 *Morbidity and Mortality Weekly Report (MMWR)*. The full text will be reprinted in the *Journal of the American Medical Association (JAMA)* on April 3. Copies can be obtained from the National AIDS Information Clearinghouse by calling 800/458-5231 after about mid-April.

Pneumocystis is a common opportunistic infection in infants with HIV. Ninety percent of young children with pneumocystis have had T-helper counts below 1500. Infants without HIV infection may have normal T-helper counts around 3,000 and as high as 5,000—far higher than adult values; as they grow older, the counts decline to adult values. In contrast, the T-helper percentage values are comparable between children and adults. The new recommendations take these differences into account.

Although these recommendations are a vital step toward improving the standards of health care available to infants and children, advocates for children with HIV have noted that the AIDS Clinical Trials Group (ACTG), the government-sponsored clinical trials system, is conducting little research on preventing and treating opportunistic infections in children. Understanding these illnesses, and testing agents to prevent and treat them, must become higher priorities in the immediate future.

# AIDS AGENCY RAIDED IN ORLANDO; AZT SEIZED

On March 7 the Florida Department of Law Enforcement (FDLE) raided the Orlando, Florida, office of Trans-Aid and the home of its founder and director, Alfredo Martinez-Garcia. AZT and other medications were seized. No criminal charges have been filed. In the week after the raid, the Florida AIDS Legal Defense and Education Fund received 75 calls, mostly from AIDS service organizations and PWA groups afraid that they, too, might be raided.

## Background

Alfredo Martinez-Garcia started Trans-Aid Support Services, Inc. in March 1988 after his lover died of AIDS. Alfredo, as he is commonly known, is well known in the Orlando area and elsewhere for his AIDS service work.

The target of the raid appears to be the widespread practice of giving away unused expensive medications left by someone who has died, or by someone who has decided to discontinue use of medicines they have purchased, to other patients who have prescriptions for the drugs but are unable to afford them. It is usually illegal for anyone except certain medical professionals to distribute prescription drugs, even by giving them away without charge. Until now, however, law enforcement authorities have not sought out such cases. The Orlando raid has raised fears that this policy might be changing—possibly under pressure of an AIDS hysteria in Florida which started after it was learned that a dentist there may have transmitted HIV to patients.

According to an affidavit by the FDLE on which the search warrant was based, the Florida investigation of Trans-Aid goes back at least to July 1989; it was apparently begun by the Inspector General's office of Florida's Health and Rehabilitative Services. By January 1991 the FDLE had become involved. Agents with electronic monitoring visited Trans-Aid, and an informant posing as a person with AIDS, and using a fictitious file of blood-test results, began calling Alfredo and asking for drugs. According to law-enforcement officials quoted in the *Orlando Sentinel*, the informant received AZT twice and another drug once during the three-month investigation by FDLE.

## Comment

The Florida Legal Defense and Education Fund has scheduled a March 19 meeting in Tallahassee between State officials and AIDS service organizations. Almost all AIDS organizations have clients who obtain AZT through friends or through patients' networks because they could not afford the drug otherwise. There are widespread fears that trying to police this activity would damage the bonds between State agencies, non-government agencies, and patients—as well as raising class and access issues, and wasting resources needed elsewhere. Many feel that with the health-care system desperately needing reform, self-help efforts like Trans-Aid should be encouraged, not squelched.

In the current case, there is some question among lawyers and others involved as to whether it would be best to organize a high-profile public defense of Alfredo and Trans-Aid, or to focus on a low-key effort to develop a compromise—for example, an arrangement for a physician to visit Trans-Aid periodically to distribute free drugs to patients with prescriptions for them. One physician has already volunteered to do so.

Certainly Alfredo and Trans-Aid deserve community support. For at least three years Alfredo has dedicated his life to serving the AIDS community, so he should have our support when he needs it. Also, it is important to establish that a legitimate AIDS organization will receive an effective legal defense, and public defense if appropriate. To avoid the development of politically motivated prosecutions, officials must know that forays against such groups will be difficult, expensive, unpopular, and unprofitable. We hope this case will be settled quickly, however, without the need for a national cause celebre, which would consume community resources which could better be focused elsewhere.

Trans-Aid does need money for legal defense; how much is needed depends on whether criminal charges are filed. Alfredo cannot personally afford the legal assistance needed even to seek return of his personal prescriptions, which were seized with the other medications.

Persons who want to contribute can send a check to Trans-Aid, 4618 Canna Drive, Orlando, FL 32809; Trans-Aid is a non-profit organization. Because future needs are uncertain, persons may want to call Alfredo first, to be better informed about the current situation. He can be reached at Trans-Aid, 407/839-0945 (day), or 407/352-2352 (evenings).

# LABOR UNIONS CHAMPION INSURANCE, CARE FOR HIV

*by Denny Smith*

Two San Francisco labor unions have implemented HIV care programs which could serve as models for other organizations. The programs concern insurance coverage for HIV treatments, and a long-term union effort to improve HIV care at a major medical center.

## Restaurant Workers Win HIV Coverage

Local 2 of the San Francisco Hotel Employees and Restaurant Employees Union has become the first trade union in the U.S. to acquire and fulfill a health benefits contract which includes substantial and explicit coverage for members with AIDS/HIV-related expenses.

The contract language specifying the coverage was won over a year ago by the 12,000 unionized workers in the City's pivotal hotel and restaurant industry. However, the benefits became available only recently, after the first employer contribution was made in November of 1990.

The Local 2 fund will reimburse for experimental as well as prescription drugs, co-insurance payments and deductibles, lab work, homecare, non-disposable medical equipment, and even non-medical expenses such as food, rent, utilities, and transportation. Coverage is provided by a special fund created from monthly, progressive contributions from employers, and will compensate for any legitimate health care refused reimbursement by the employee's regular insurer.

We spoke to Jack Gribbon, who works for the Local and who designed the care package. He is familiar with the specific difficulties in negotiating health benefits for his members, and for union contracts in general. Antagonisms over health coverage were integral to four of every five labor disputes in this country in 1989.

Mr. Gribbon said that in spite of the model language of his union's contract, many people with HIV continue to be marginalized or ignored in health care benefits negotiations. He shared with us an anecdote typifying inadequate HIV coverage in union contracts, from last year's conference of the International Foundation of Employee Benefits. These annual conferences are attended by trustees representing business, labor, and community service agencies. When the dilemma of how to cover HIV infection as a pre-existing condition came up for discussion, someone suggested that HIV simply become a basis for complete exclusion from insurance coverage. Mr. Gribbon, together with allies at the conference, strongly protested and proposed the exact opposite: that people with HIV or AIDS be able to expect the same comprehensive coverage afforded their co-workers. Mr. Gribbon would like to see other employers and unions use the Local 2 fund to negotiate the language of their own health care contracts.

## Hospital Workers Take Stand For Patient Care

Local 250, Hospital and Institutional Workers Union of the Service Employees International Union (SEIU), has fought for over five years for the needs of members with HIV, for workplace safety, and for the patients served by the Local. This fight has been waged through the Local's "AIDS Education Committee," which is open to participation from any union member and has enjoyed strong backing from both local and national SEIU leadership. The committee's "Train the Trainer" programs have helped Local members distinguish between real risks for exposure to HIV and irrational fears, and to respect the rights of patients while assuring the safety of caregivers.

The first achievement of Local 250's AIDS Education Committee was the creation of an inpatient AIDS ward at Kaiser Hospital in San Francisco, a development which greatly improved the medical care for patients there. Previously, Kaiser patients hospitalized with AIDS-related complications often experienced inconsistent care, marred by inexperience with treating HIV on the part of some attending physicians and by fears of "catching" AIDS on the part of some hospital staff.

Kaiser-Permanente is a health maintenance organization (HMO) with clinics and medical centers throughout California and, to a lesser degree, several other states. HMOs operate as a combined health insurer and health-care provider; they are expanding in the United States. This writer was employed at the San Francisco Kaiser facility in 1986, a year before joining the staff of *AIDS Treatment News*. When dissatisfaction with the care of persons with AIDS became a serious issue, we met with several co-workers to enlist the support of our union, of the San Francisco Human Rights Commission, and of sympathetic Kaiser doctors, nurses, and technicians, to effect a change in Kaiser's AIDS care.

A series of negotiations with the hospital administration led to an acknowledgement that the problems were unacceptable. Plans were developed for a ten-bed ward devoted exclusively to caring for patients with AIDS, and the ward was to be staffed by caregivers fluent in the latest standards of AIDS treatments.

Kaiser implemented the plan in good faith, with input from the union and from employee representatives. A comprehensive AIDS-care orientation was provided to everyone who volunteered to work on the ward. We have since heard generally good reports of the ward from the San Francisco PWA community. Kaiser's *out*patient care has not always shared this response. In fact, repeated negotiations between Kaiser and a community activist group called KPAU (Kaiser Patient Advocacy Union) produced less progress and more friction on both sides than did the earlier situation. We plan to report on the status and goals of Kaiser, and of KPAU, in a future article.

# THYMOPENTIN: PROMISING IMMUNOMODULATOR

*by Denny Smith*

Thymopentin, also known as TP-5, is a synthesized derivative of thymopoietin, a naturally-occurring hormone responsible for inducing T-cell precursors to differentiate and mature. A study at the Istituto di Patologia Medica in Bari, Italy, reported thymopentin-related increases in T4 cells and some improvement in symptoms for 21 people. Two studies of thymopentin published at the Sixth International Conference on AIDS pointed to stabilization of T-helper counts and p24 antigenemia in asymptomatic and mildly symptomatic patients during treatment with thymopentin. One of the studies was too small to see differences in disease progression. In the larger study, none of the treated patients progressed to symptoms, compared to four of the placebo patients who did progress. No side effects were attributed to thymopentin (Abstracts #S.B.484 and S.B.485).

We spoke to Kathy Labriola, L.V.N., who managed a third thymopentin trial for Marcus Conant, M.D., a well-known San Francisco physician and researcher. Ms. Labriola shared the preliminary results of this trial, which was concluded last July but has not yet finished a statistical analysis. The study enrolled 100 asymptomatic participants and lasted one year. No other HIV drugs were used, except that for six months of the study, ten people were taking AZT. Participants receiving active drug were given 50 mg once a week. (In the previous studies of thymopentin, the same dose was given three times a week.)

When the trends of symptom development were identified, thymopentin clearly showed some protective benefits. Of those participants getting a placebo, 21 developed some observable symptoms, compared to only 13 receiving thymopentin. Nobody who received the drug in the study progressed to AIDS, but two who were in the placebo group did. In addition, four in the placebo group developed serious cases of herpes zoster, or shingles, two experienced outbreaks of genital warts, and eight were troubled by fungal skin infections. In the treatment group, four people noticed skin infections, but none experienced shingles or warts.

Serologic markers were not as descriptive. The placebo group experienced a slightly sharper decline in average T4-helper cell counts, and the ratio of T4 to T8 cells, than did the treatment group. However, two participants receiving thymopentin became mildly positive for p24 antigenemia, while everyone on placebo remained antigen-negative.

Dr. Conant is now recruiting for a trial of thymopentin combined with AZT. The number for more information is 415/923-0555.

Several other thymus preparations have been under study in AIDS research as possible immunomodulators. These include thymosin, thymostimulin, thymomodulin, thymic humoral factor, calf thymus lysate, and thymus implants. We will report any significant news of these agents as they develop.

## REFERENCES

Thompson, S E and others. Effects of thymopentin on disease progression and surrogate markers in HIV infection-A one year study. Abstract #S.B.484, Sixth International Conference on AIDS, San Francisco, June 20-24, 1990.

Conant, M and others. Twenty-four week double blind evaluation of thymopentin treatment on disease progression in HIV infected patients. Abstract # 485, Sixth International Conference on AIDS, San Francisco, June 20, 1990.

# NEW FDA COMMISSIONER TESTIFIES ON AIDS DRUGS

On March 6 the new FDA Commissioner David Kessler, M.D., told Senator Edward Kennedy's Labor and Human Resources Committee that the FDA would not obstruct drugs for AIDS or other life-threatening diseases. According to reporter Nick Bartolomeo of the gay newspaper *The Washington Blade*, Dr. Kessler told the Committee that the FDA had more than 350 applications for testing new AIDS drugs and other treatments—which Dr. Kessler described as "the pipeline of things to come." Dr. Kessler also said that "if the mission [of the FDA] is to protect public health, the Agency has an obligation to reach for the data. We can't sit back passively." A short article on the hearing appeared in the *Blade* on March 15.

Dr. Kessler also discussed conditional approval, a proposal to allow earlier drug approval on condition that the developer continue scientific testing. (Note: such agreements have been made in the past, but often broken by the developer. New legislation might be needed for conditional approval, since at present it is not clear that the FDA has the authority to enforce such agreements.)

An article on the hearing in the March 17 *San Francisco Examiner* mentioned the testimony on avoiding delays in approval of important new drugs. The *Examiner* article focused primarily on Kessler's call for stronger enforcement to prevent abuses such as fraudulent data submitted for generic drugs, or misleading drug claims in advertisements directed to the public.

# Issue Number 124
# April 5, 1991

## TREATMENT STRATEGIES:
## INTERVIEW WITH LARRY BRUNI, M.D.

*by Denny Smith*

To help promote strategic, individualized programs for controlling HIV disease, we interviewed Larry Bruni, M.D., a Washington, D.C., physician who has maintained a large HIV practice for several years. Dr. Bruni is known as an innovator in the care of his patients; a Cable News Network (CNN) interview with him should air later this month.

**DS:** For people who are still above 500 T-helper cells, what do you look for to make decisions about intervention in the progression of HIV?

**LB:** The various blood markers aren't very useful at that point, so I look carefully at the clinical picture. I've come to regard anything except a broken bone as possibly related to HIV. That may be a fallacious assumption, but better to be too vigilant, rather than trivialize something like a rash or headaches that could be tied into disease progression. I don't dismiss anything. When people worry that they are being hypochondriacal, I tell them that they're not. By just recording patients' complaints in their charts, I can sometimes discern a pattern of symptoms. Small things that would ordinarily go unnoticed may be significant. For example, when I examine the ears, I look for small bubbles behind the eardrums. These can be caused by infections of mycoplasma, which sometimes colonize the middle ear. I'm more willing to try doxycycline than to tell the patient "don't worry about it."

**DS:** When do blood markers become noteworthy?

**LB:** Well, the T-4 helper cell counts and percentages are important because, of course, progressive depletion of helper cells is the hallmark of HIV infection. But you can't rely on this alone, partly because the methods of counting the cells are not absolutely precise; there are many calculations involved in deriving the final "count."

**DS:** That's a good point, because I think a lot of people, including myself, don't understand all the calculations involved in lab results. We often assume that the total blood cell population is ordinarily stable, so any variation in one component is alarming.

**LB:** No one should be alarmed by small variations. Also, the percentage of T-helper cells is more revealing than the absolute count.

**DS:** When someone who is on AZT experiences a drop in T-helper cells, is that ever attributable to a drop in the overall white count, which can in turn be attributed to AZT?

**LB:** Yes. So I don't routinely put people on nucleoside analogs [AZT, ddI, ddC] for T-helper cell counts above 500. But there are circumstances that may warrant the use of AZT in that range, particularly clinical symptoms that indicate disease activity. For example, if someone is having repeated bouts of genital warts.

**DS:** In other words, a relatively minor problem which is resistant to normally success-ful treatment may be a signal of HIV activity.

**LB:** Not only that, but I think HIV would be a rather indolent [slow to change] infection if it weren't for all the other infections our bodies have to process at the same time. I don't really make a distinction between opportunistic infections and the idea of cofactors. I teach my patients that HIV disease is a slow process if not for other things that push it, such as other infections, exposure to sunlight, etc. And infections can transactivate each other. While the warts are allowed to recur by HIV, HIV is stimulated by the wart virus. So for both practical and theoretical reasons, we need to control this cycle by controlling any problem that is potentially chronic, like bronchitis or adenovirus colitis.

**DS:** In light of that, what are some of the things you look for in patients who would ordinarily think of themselves as asymptomatic?

**LB:** Sinus infections, skin rashes, fungal infections of the toenails, athlete's foot that is persistent, prostate infections, and of course, headaches and fatigue. Headaches, especially, are too often chalked up to "tension," but since stress can contribute to immune dysfunction, and to emotional dysphoria, I think even a tension headache may deserve intervention.

**DS:** You mentioned sunlight as a cofactor.

**LB:** Yes, even before studies were published about its effect on HIV, sunlight was known to provoke herpes outbreaks. Strong sunlight, probably the ultraviolet rays, can impair immune response. You don't have to worry about the regular exposure during daily activities. I'm talking about laying out in the sun, or playing volleyball in your swimsuit for hours at a time. T-helper cell counts drop almost invariably after someone spends a long weekend at the beach.

**DS:** I understand that you favor the empirical use of antibiotics, when a set of symptoms is eluding any particular diagnosis or treatment. Is there a concern that antibiotic drugs could suppress the immune system further?

**LB:** I haven't really seen any systemic damage from antibiotics. Indeed, my own experience is that a course of antibiotics frequently perks up the immune picture. The first antibiotic I tried on an empirical basis was doxycycline, in 1988, based on Stephen Caiazza's ideas.

**DS:** Since HIV isn't affected directly by antibiotics, this must be a way of dealing with cofactors in hiding.

**LB:** It often seems that something else is driving the infection. The notion that latent syphilis may be treated this way is interesting. I can't think of any topic in medical school that professors were more smug about than syphilis treatment. "We know everything there is to know about this disease," they'd say. Reminds me of the character in Voltaire's *Candide*.

**DS:** Dr. Pangloss!

**LB:** Yes, as though we live in the best of all possible worlds, and we know everything we need to know. But meanwhile, one treatment they were using to treat syphilis failed to cross the blood/brain barrier, and those people may be chronically infected with syphilis, including many people with HIV.

**DS:** So the cerebrospinal fluid could be "reseeding" the body, and doxycycline may be dealing with it?

**LB:** I've had some excellent results with doxycycline; tetracycline, as well, will cross the blood/brain barrier. I try it in people who have a residual indicator of syphilis in their blood. And now we know that we could be treating mycoplasma infections empirically, too. I have actually seen rises in T-helper cells in some patients during treatment with doxycycline.

**DS:** How do patients and physicians make judgment decisions together?

**LB:** Physicians need to be willing to make some intuitive judgments, because we won't find advice in the medical journals, whose reports invariably end with something like "not statistically conclusive, more investigations needed." Patients can be limited by their preconceptions. I still get patients who say to me, "I'll try anything except AZT." "Why won't you try AZT?" "Because it's poison." Yet studies clearly show that when we use AZT correctly, we can improve the quality and the length of life.

**DS:** So you're trapped between patients who do not like the primary option available, and a medical establishment which cannot seem to improve the options.

**LB:** Well, I'm really happy now that we have ddC, even if people have to use the "gray market" version. I think ddC works, without horrible side effects. Now routinely, when I start people on AZT, after three months I tell them it's time to switch to ddC. Another three months, we return to AZT, and I continue alternating like that.

**DS:** What's the rationale for rotating instead of using them together?

**LB:** Well, it takes about three months for AZT side effects to appear, at the current low doses. This dosing may avoid indefinitely those predictable drops in white cells and hemoglobin. By using them separately, you can also see how each drug affects each patient.

**DS:** You've mentioned AZT and ddC, but not ddI.

**LB:** For a year and a half, our office has been overwhelmed by the paperwork associated with ddI. And the manufacturer's criteria for ddC eligibility are ridiculous. I'm ready to forego all that if patients can reliably obtain ddC through the buyers' clubs.

**DS:** Are there other important treatments that patients can get through the buyers' clubs?

**LB:** In addition to ddC, I'm glad to see the clubs carrying levamisole [a potential immunomodulator] and clarithromycin [a new antibiotic]. I started recommending levamisole to patients last November, before it was approved by FDA for use in colon cancer. When it became available by prescription, I started slowly, not being familiar with its use and wishing to avoid toxicities. Now I give it to people who do not improve on more standard therapies. I think it holds great promise as an immunomodulator.

**DS:** Is clarithromycin still looking promising for treating MAI, cryptosporidiosis, or toxoplasmosis?

**LB:** I've replaced all the old MAI drugs with clarithromycin and ciprofloxacin. The dose we're trying is eight pills [250 mg each] of clarithromycin daily, which unfortunately is expensive. I'm seeing some weight gain, and reduced fevers. These patients feel it's working. I'm trying the related drug azithromycin to treat toxoplasmosis in several patients who were obviously failing the pyrimethamine/sulfa combination. It's too early in follow-up to say for sure, but I think it will work. I'm also advocating some prophylaxis in people who have been exposed to *Toxoplasma*, and who have dropped below 200 T-helper cells. I believe azithromycin and clarithromycin probably will become the best drugs with which to treat toxo or prevent active infections. Anecdotally, two of my patients with cryptosporidiosis found complete relief from the diarrhea within five days on azithromycin, and after ten days of treatment they maintained normal bowel function and regained all their lost weight for months.

**DS:** Something we have been hearing a lot about lately is gall bladder inflammation and bile duct obstructions. Is this becoming a common HIV-associated trouble?

**LB:** Very common. This is usually a condition called acalculous cholecystitis, meaning an inflammation which is not caused by gallstones. The cause could be any of a number of pathogens, like CMV, cryptosporidiosis, or other parasites. But the drugs we give to treat those infections do not penetrate the gall bladder very well, making it sort of a reservoir of infection. The signs are abdominal pain, often connected with diarrhea. Since this tends to persist and not respond to antibiotics, the best treatment seems to be removal of the gall bladder. You can get along nicely without a gall bladder, and the surgery should improve both appetite and nutrient absorption.

**DS:** Getting back to the empirical use of treatments, you have found IVIG [intravenous immune globulin] useful, haven't you?

**LB:** It can be very helpful, also very expensive. It's valuable for treating the kind of recurring bacterial infections that a healthy immune system ordinarily handles, especially sinus infections. It is also a good complement to use with ganciclovir when treating CMV pneumonia or colitis. Adding it to therapy for retinitis does not help much, according to studies which have been completed.

**DS:** Can you make immune globulin specific, engineer it to be concentrated in certain antibodies?

**LB:** It's not engineered so much as graded for counts of particular antibodies. I use Gammagard, made by Baxter, because it has the highest concentration of anti-CMV antibodies.

**DS:** Do you have any advice about nutritional supplements?

**LB:** I have recommended a short list of supplements for several years, and have recently added NAC and coenzyme Q-10 to that list.

**DS:** Why has interest in coenzyme Q been revived recently? [Note: do not confuse coenzyme Q with compound Q.]

**LB:** It might be helpful for countering some of the heart muscle degeneration being reported now in connection with HIV infection.

**DS:** I saw one such report that alerted physicians to the possibility of HIV cardiac abnormalities, and that some symptoms casually attributed to lung involvement, like fatigue and shortness of breath, instead could be implicating the heart.

## Research Politics

**DS:** What are some of the politics affecting the clinical care picture today?

**LB:** I see the Food and Drug Administration and the National Institutes of Health as having a symbiotic relationship with the pharmaceutical industry. They are in a codependent relationship. People on both sides have their complaints, but they do not seriously analyze themselves. Congress plays along with the game, too, funding and regulating the relationship. And as in codependency, something like a disaster has to happen for a real change to occur. No one is presently in charge of an overall plan for AIDS. But you watch—five years from now, when straight teenagers are dropping like flies, then AIDS will become a national priority. Of course, we will probably have a new administration by then, too. Meanwhile, we need clinicians and researchers to talk to each other, to try to build solutions to the problems of HIV disease. Instead of obsessing on basic research, we must constructively analyze what the problems are, and start acting on priorities toward the solution. Plan the work and work the plan. No organization in the world is doing that now.

**DS:** Perhaps we should aim for solutions that fit the problem, instead of problems that fit someone's solution.

**LB:** Exactly right. And we need innovators. More AZT studies are not innovative. The non-innovative answers are not solutions. They are solutions in search of problems, as you said. And all the while researchers around the world traipse around their own little garden path, doing their own personal research. By contrast, we could harness that creative thinking, and integrate this research chaos into a bigger picture. One model I've worked with is the National Community Research Initiative, in Washington, D.C. We began by developing computer software, called CRIS, to let physicians keep up with each other's experiences, to correlate all the raw data of our practices. We've developed a database that can work as a total clinical management system. We can directly download results of bloodwork from the laboratory by modem into the database. This technology could help to share statistics, to generate statistically valid correlations. In my office we will soon have a computer work station in each patient examination room, so we can have the patient's history and treatment experiences and all lab work at our fingertips.

**DS:** It would seem that physicians in different countries, using different therapies, could use the database to learn from each other.

**LB:** Yes, this information is eminently exportable. Communication technology is an innovative, useful approach.

# CLARITHROMYCIN: ABBOTT SEEKS COMPASSIONATE ACCESS FOR MAC

Abbott Laboratories has contacted the U.S. Food and Drug Administration (FDA) and proposed a draft protocol for compassionate use of clarithromycin for persons with AIDS who have mycobacterium avium complex (MAC, also called MAI).

Clarithromycin, a new broad-spectrum antibiotic approved in 20 countries but not yet in the United States, has quickly become a major concern of treatment activists. MAC is one of the most widespread opportunistic infections, and conventional treatment (usually a "cocktail" of four or five antibiotics) is often unsatisfactory. Early research results and practical experience both suggest that clarithromycin is much more promising than any of the standard treatments. Persons with MAC have imported the drug, but it is expensive, and often financially burdensome or unavailable, since unapproved drugs are seldom covered by insurance. It is hoped that some form of compassionate treatment access can fill the gap until the drug can be financed in the same way as other medical care. We do not know how long it will take for Abbott's preliminary proposal for compassionate use to be completed and implemented.

Clarithromycin was first developed for uses not related to AIDS. For these purposes the drug is less critical, because other satisfactory treatments are available. Clarithromycin has the advantage of broad-spectrum activity; according to Abbott's April 1 news release, it "has been shown to be active against all significant respiratory pathogens as well as against the full range of community-acquired skin and gastrointestinal infections."

For more information on clarithromycin, see *AIDS Treatment News* #109 and #113. Also see the interview with Larry Bruni, M.D., in this issue. For information about obtaining the drug now, call the PWA Health Group, 212/532-0280, or LABC/Staying Alive, 213/748-1295.

# ELEVEN PERCENT ENTIRELY HEALTHY TEN OR MORE YEARS AFTER HIV SEROCONVERSION

A major San Francisco study of AIDS progression is finding that about 11 percent of persons infected with HIV are completely healthy ten or more years later; they not only have no HIV-related symptoms, but also have normal T-helper counts. A formal report on intensive studies of some of these patients is being prepared for publication. Meanwhile, a March 25 article in the *San Francisco Examiner* brought current findings to wider public attention. Researchers are trying to find out why the disease progresses very slowly (if at all) in some people; such knowledge might be useful in developing treatments.

The data is emerging from the Clinic Study, conducted by the San Francisco Department of Public Health (DPH) and the U.S. Centers for Disease Control. The Clinic Study began as research on sexually-transmitted hepatitis B, before AIDS was known; 6,705 gay or bisexual men who visited San Francisco's sexually-transmitted disease clinic from 1978 to 1980 were recruited, and frozen blood samples were saved. Later it was found that 489 of them were either HIV positive when they entered the study, or became positive at a known time between 1978 and the present. Because the approximate time of seroconversion is known, this cohort is providing some of the best information anywhere on how AIDS develops.

Of the 489 whose time of seroconversion is known, 341 were found to be HIV positive more than ten years ago, between 1977 and 1980. As reported last November[1], 49 percent of these men had died of AIDS, ten percent currently had AIDS, 19 percent had ARC, 3 percent had lymphadenopathy but no other symptoms, and 19 percent had no clinical symptoms of AIDS or HIV. [Note: Survival is almost certainly better today; these percentages are for persons infected by 1980, years before antiretrovirals, pneumocystis prophylaxis, and other treatment improvements were in use.] Today more than half of that 19 percent—11 percent of the 341—not only have no symptoms, but also have normal T-helper counts.

We asked Susan Buchbinder, M.D., of the AIDS Office of DPH, whether the statistics on disease progression suggest that some of the 11 percent would never become ill, or if they were only the extreme end of the statistical distribution of slow disease progression. She said that no one knows at this time—but that in either case, information about why HIV infection behaves differently in these people might help in developing treatments.

One of the major theories being studied now in conjunction with the San Francisco City Clinic is that certain blood cells, perhaps CD8 lymphocytes, secrete an unknown substance which helps to keep the virus in check. The group at the University of California San Francisco Medical Center, headed by virologist Jay Levy, M.D., has been investigating this possibility for several years. Other researchers, including Dr. Buchbinder and Alison Mawle, Ph.D., of the U.S. Centers for Disease Control, are investigating another kind of white blood cell, the cytotoxic lymphocyte.

Dr. Buchbinder asked us to let our readers know that any gay or bisexual men who visited San Francisco's STD clinic from 1978 to 1980, and have not already been in contact with the research team, could call to see if they have frozen blood stored. They must give permission for their blood to be used for research. Persons who participate in research can learn about their own health history and status, and also they will be contributing to knowledge which could help to improve HIV treatments. Those who may have blood stored can call Paul O'Malley at the Clinic Study, 415/554-9030.

## REFERENCES

1. Rutherford GW, Lifson AR, Hessol NA and others. Course of HIV-I infection in a cohort of homosexual and bisexual men: an 11 year follow up study. *British Medical Journal* November 24, 1990; volume 301, pages 1183-1188.

# CMV: ORAL GANCICLOVIR STUDIES OPEN

*by Michelle Roland*

Two clinical trials testing oral ganciclovir in people with CMV infection have recently opened at seven centers around the United States. The larger study is for people with *newly diagnosed* CMV retinitis. The second trial is designed to evaluate the effects of food on the absorption of oral ganciclovir. It will last eight days and is open to people with a past or present CMV *infection* (documented by a positive CMV culture or the presence of antibodies against CMV) without any evidence of CMV-related *disease*.

Note that most people have been exposed to and infected with CMV at some time in their lives, but only some will develop symptoms related to that infection.

## Background on CMV Treatments

Intravenous (IV) ganciclovir (also called DHPG, or Cytovene) is currently the only FDA-approved treatment for CMV retinitis, a sight-threatening infection of the eye. People who have been diagnosed with CMV retinitis are generally given ganciclovir twice a day for two to three weeks (induction phase) followed by daily infusions five to seven days a week for the rest of their lives (maintenance phase). If a person experiences a progression of their disease during the maintenance phase, they are generally re-induced with twice a day ganciclovir for another two to three weeks.

If the treatment fails to prevent progression of the retinitis after repeated inductions, or if the side effects of the ganciclovir are too serious to continue treatment, people may choose to try the experimental drug foscarnet. Although this compound is not yet FDA-approved, it is usually available to people in these situations through an expanded access program. Foscarnet is also an IV drug.

Several oral and other experimental anti-CMV drugs are currently in various stages of development. The oral compound which has been studied most is ganciclovir. In early studies it was found that the drug was not well absorbed; therefore, quantities much larger than the IV dosage must be taken to achieve concentrations high enough to be effective.

## CMV Retinitis Study

The new study in people with CMV retinitis will compare oral and IV ganciclovir as maintenance treatment, after all participants have received a three week induction course with IV ganciclovir. This is an extremely important study because it will answer questions about the relative safety and efficacy of the oral and IV formulations. If the oral compound is found to be about as safe and effective as the IV drug, data from this study may lead to FDA licensing of oral ganciclovir.

To be eligible for this study, the CMV retinitis must have been diagnosed, and no anti-CMV drugs may have been used, within one month of enrollment. Participants cannot have *persistent* diarrhea or other gastrointestinal symptoms, because these are some of the potential side effects of oral ganciclovir. Participants must be at least 13 years old. Because this drug causes birth defects in animals, both males and females will be required to use birth control, and women will be required to have a negative pregnancy test.

Initiation or resumption of AZT will be allowed after the first five weeks of the study. ddI may be initiated or continued at any time during the study. ddC is not yet allowed, but an amendment may be written to include ddC and/or combination antiretroviral therapy at some point during the study as more data becomes available about the efficacy of these treatment approaches.

After the first three weeks of twice daily IV infusions of ganciclovir, participants will be randomized to receive either oral ganciclovir (two capsules six times a day while awake) or IV ganciclovir (once a day, seven days a week). Some patients treated outside of this study would only receive IV ganciclovir five days a week after the first two to three weeks, depending on blood counts and the preference of the patient and the physician. Randomization to the IV arm of this study may therefore require more infusions than is common in some physicians' clinical practices.

The study lasts for a total of 23 weeks. The ganciclovir and all clinic visits and lab work required by the study will be provided free of charge. If the drug still appears to be safe at the end of the study, all participants will be eligible for oral ganciclovir through another Syntex protocol, as long as they are willing to be followed on the protocol.

At press time the study drugs have been shipped to the seven sites listed below. We have confirmed that the study is open in Boston, Miami, and San Francisco/Davies. The Washington, D.C., site will not be enrolling patients until early May for the retinitis study, but is currently accepting participants for the food absorption study described below. We were not able to contact the San Francisco (Children's Hospital) or Galveston sites before going to press, but have been told by the clinical research associate at Syntex that they are all ready to enroll patients.

**Chicago:** Rush-Presbyterian-St. Luke's Medical Center. Contact person: Pam Urvanski, 312/942-5865.

**Boston:** Beth Israel Hospital. Contact person: Jocelyn Loftus or Mary Ann Lee, 617/735-4103.

**Miami:** Miami Veteran's Administration Medical Center. Contact person: Tommy Stapleton, 305/324-3267, or Debra Fertel, M.D., 305/324-4455. Please note that because this is a Veteran's Administration hospital, all veterans are eligible for the study, and individual non-veterans will be considered.

**San Francisco:** Davies Medical Center. Contact person: Ed Freeman, 415/565-6617.

**San Francisco:** Children's Hospital. Contact person: Jaime Geaga or Toby Dyner, M.D., 415/750-6529, or David Busch, M.D., 415/923-3883.

**Galveston:** University of Texas Medical Branch. Contact person: Karen Waterman, 409/761-4979.

**Washington, D.C.:** Georgetown University Hospital. Contact person: Cari O'Leary, 202/687-6845, or Anne Byrne, 202/687-8087, or James P. Lavelle, Jr., M.D., 202/687-8826.

Additional sites in San Francisco, New York , Detroit, and San Diego are expected to receive the study drug and start enrolling patients within the next few weeks. For more information on the current status of the trial in these areas, call 800-TRIALS-A. Syntex will be updating information available through that number on at least a monthly basis.

## Study of the Effect of Food on Absorption

This study is open to people who have been infected with CMV at some time in the past but do not have any signs of CMV disease. Participants must have a T-helper count above 200. The study lasts only eight days. It requires multiple blood samples on two days, single blood samples on several other days, regular telephone contact, and strict timing of medication and meals. Participants must be willing to stop taking most drugs, including all antiretrovirals, for 12 days. Because this study is not expected to provide any benefit to the participants, and does entail a significant amount of travel and inconvenience, participants will be paid $300 at the completion of the trial.

This is also an important study; it is crucial to learn how to maximize the absorption of oral ganciclovir, while minimizing its side effects. The trial is being conducted at the San Francisco (Davies Medical Center only) and Washington, D.C., sites listed above, both of which are currently enrolling participants.

# FIRST NATIONAL CHILDREN WITH HIV/AIDS AWARENESS DAY

*by Michelle Roland*

The First National Children with HIV/AIDS Awareness Day will be held on the Mall near the Capitol Building in Washington, D.C., on Tuesday, June 11, 1991. This event is being spearheaded by the Sunburst National AIDS Project, an organization which sponsors a summer camp for HIV-positive children and their families. Supporting organizations include the Names Project, the U.S. Department of Maternal and Child Health, the National Education Association, the Children with AIDS Project of America, the Parents' Pediatric AIDS Coalition of California, the Children with AIDS Foundation in Boston, the AIDS Resource Foundation for Children in New Jersey, and the Minnesota AIDS Project. Newman's Own is the first corporate sponsor to offer its support.

To continue building national awareness of pediatric AIDS issues, a joint resolution is being submitted to both Houses of Congress to designate June 10-16 as Pediatric AIDS Awareness Week.

The organizers of the National Children with HIV/AIDS Awareness Day plan to educate the public about the various modes of pediatric AIDS transmission, the all-inclusive range of ethnic and social groups affected, and the ever-increasing number of babies, children, and teenagers with AIDS. They hope that this attention will influence Congress to allocate more funding for AIDS research and direct services. Finally, the Day's events will provide support to families affected by AIDS, and remembrance of children who have died from AIDS-related conditions.

The organizers are looking for professional athletes and celebrity speakers, fundraising assistance, and additional corporate sponsors. Volunteers to help in Washington on June 11 are also needed. The Sunburst AIDS Project is requesting participation of school systems throughout the country to increase awareness about children with HIV/AIDS and to support the Awareness Day; four states (California, Minnesota, Mississippi, and Tennessee) have already endorsed this program, called the Butterfly Project. Local Congressional representatives may be contacted by phone or mail to support the Pediatric AIDS Awareness Week (H.J. Resolution 91). If you would like to help in any area, or would like more information, call Sunburst National AIDS Project in Brooklyn at 718/763-8095, or in Petaluma, California, at 707/769-0169, or write to 148 Wilson Hill Road, Petaluma, CA 94952.

# LAWSUIT CHALLENGES PATENT ON AZT

A lawsuit prepared by Public Citizen, a nonprofit public interest group founded by Ralph Nader, has challenged Burroughs Wellcome's 1988 patent on AZT (brand name Retrovir). The lawsuit claims that the patent is invalid because "the company did not conceive, develop or demonstrate the utility of the drug, nor did it name all of the inventors in its patent application," according to a March 19 press release from Public Citizen. "This lawsuit will establish the public's right to a fair price, and it gives the government a vehicle to challenge Burroughs Wellcome's monopoly." Plaintiffs include the PWA Health Group in New York, and two individuals in Washington, D.C., who are using AZT.

Burroughs Wellcome's press release of the same date claimed that its scientists "were the first to conceive the use of the chemical AZT for the treatment of HIV infection in humans"—the basis of the company's use patent, and that challenging the patent now, "more than five years after its filing...could have a chilling effect on innovation in the United States and could discourage future AIDS research." The press release also states that the company has supported "in whole or in part, more than 90 Retrovir-related clinical trials involving some 10,000 patients worldwide," and that the current price of approximately $2,200 per year for the dose of 500 mg per day "represents a 70 percent reduction in cost of therapy as a result of price decreases and reduced dosage since the drug was first marketed in 1987."

# Issue Number 125
# April 19, 1991

## AIDS ANTIVIRALS: A NEW GENERATION

*by John S. James*

Advances in understanding the life cycle of HIV have quietly led to the development of many potential "designer drugs" for treating HIV disease. Several of the new drugs are now beginning human trials. Because of the advances they represent, we believe there is more hope now than ever before for improvements in AIDS treatment. But optimism should remain cautious, because there have been many disappointments in the past.

At least five of the new drugs have already been given to humans in early tests:

• L-697,661 and L-697,639 (sometimes called the "L-drugs"), developed by Merck & Co. These drugs are of a class called non-nucleoside-analog reverse-transcriptase inhibitors. (This means that they block the viral enzyme reverse transcriptase, but—unlike AZT, ddC, and ddI—they are not nucleoside analogs; hopefully they can avoid the toxicity which may be inherent in that class of drugs.) L-697,661 is now recruiting for phase II trials at the National Institutes of Health, near Washington, DC, and also at the University of Alabama in Birmingham (see announcement below).

• A Hoffmann-La Roche tat inhibitor (drug which blocks the protein produced by the tat gene of HIV). Without the tat protein, HIV becomes inactive. This drug is now beginning human trials at Johns Hopkins in Baltimore; we do not have details at this time. Later, the drug may also be tested for specific activity against KS (Kaposi's sarcoma).

• BI-RG-587, being developed by Boehringer Ingelheim Pharmaceuticals, Inc. There has been much interest in this drug since publication of laboratory results in *Science*, December 7, 1990 (see *AIDS Treatment News* #21). Unfortunately, it has recently been learned that there is less human experience to date than had been widely assumed (see BI-RG-587 article, below).

- At least one and probably two companies have conducted early human tests of protease inhibitors (which block another enzyme which is necessary for HIV). Little information is available at this time.

Many other new antivirals have been created by pharmaceutical companies. Some have not reached human testing yet; others are not being actively developed, sometimes because they seem to have no advantage over other drugs ahead of them in the development and regulatory pipeline.

What is notable about these antivirals is that the researchers familiar with them are convinced that they probably will work. Laboratory and animal testing has shown that they do stop the virus, they do get absorbed and into cells where they are needed, and they are nontoxic in animals. The main questions to be answered are whether there is any unexpected toxicity or other problem with human use; and of course doctors need to learn the best ways to use each drug in practice—dose, schedule, combinations with other antivirals, possible problems with viral resistance, etc.

None of the new drugs is expected to cure AIDS; as with AZT, treatment will have to be continued indefinitely. And no matter how good a drug looks in theory, no one can be sure that it will work until it has proven effective in human use.

One reason for caution is that the last time the research community expressed similar optimism about a new drug—soluble CD4—that drug turned out to be worthless as a treatment. The current situation, however, is different in several ways. The case for soluble CD4 was based largely on theory; for it to work in the body, many things had to happen, and some of them could not readily be tested in advance. By contrast, the mechanism of action of the new drugs is better understood, and more suitable to laboratory and animal tests.

In addition, many new antivirals are now being created, and most of them are very different from each other. Any problem found with one is unlikely to also affect the others. If even one drug works as expected, the result will be a major improvement in treatment for HIV, compared with the current therapy with AZT alone.

Which of the new drugs looks best at this time? It is impossible to tell, because most of the data is secret; even if it were available, only rough and uncertain comparisons could be made from the laboratory and animal results. For the AIDS community, the most important ones now are those which are moving fastest into human trials and (if warranted) FDA approval. By this measure, Merck's L-697,661 is now ahead.

The current system for approval of new drugs by the FDA (which controls how drugs are developed by pharmaceutical companies) is grossly unsuited to the needs of the current situation—a fact which will increasingly become a public issue. Some of the main problems:

- The current focus is on proving efficacy—which is not the central issue with the new antivirals. Unless endpoints other than death or disease progression are accepted as good enough for drug approval, years will be wasted arranging for enough people in trials to sicken or die on AZT to provide statistical proof that a new drug works better.

- Combination therapies will almost certainly be better than single drugs for HIV treatment. But combinations are not tested until late in the development process, because the FDA wants proof of single-drug efficacy first, and also because pharmaceutical companies are reluctant to cooperate in testing their rivals' products.

• Major problems can also arise in getting the large organizations involved—pharmaceutical company, FDA, and often NIH as well—to work together effectively. There has been little national planning and coordination to see that such problems are worked out.

• Notorious shortages of staff, facilities, and money at the FDA prevent that agency from doing its work efficiently. For example, NDA (New Drug Application) documents are delivered to the FDA in boxes, by truck, because the FDA does not have appropriate computers—making data analysis very costly in staff time. Pharmaceutical companies would gladly help provide the tools needed, but that would raise issues of control. Apparently the FDA wants to develop the needed systems itself—a commendable intention, but without resources, little will happen and the current deadlocks will remain.

These are some of the practical problems that will determine how soon the new drugs are tested and made available to those who need them.

*AIDS Treatment News* will focus increasingly on the new generation of antivirals, including those listed above, as more news becomes available. Meanwhile, we will continue to cover what we believe are the most promising of the older treatments—such as the AZT/ddC (or ddI) combination, or hypericin—as well as other treatment news of interest to the community.

# L-697,661 PHASE II TRIALS AT NIH, AND IN BIRMINGHAM

*by John S. James*

A phase II trial of L-697,661 (also called L-661), an important new antiviral developed by Merck & Co., will begin soon at the U.S. National Institute of Allergy and Infectious Diseases (NIAID) near Washington, D.C.; about 75 volunteers will be enrolled. A similar but not identical trial will be conducted at the University of Alabama in Birmingham.

## NIAID Trial (Near Washington, DC)

To be eligible for the NIAID trial, volunteers must be HIV-positive, have a T-helper count of over 200, and have a positive titer for plasma viremia. (The Birmingham trial may later accept persons with lower T-helper counts.) Volunteers must be between 18 and 60 years old, and either never have taken AZT or have taken it for no more than a total of six months; they must not have a history of serious intolerance to AZT. They cannot take any investigational drug, AZT, or other HIV treatment within four weeks of beginning the study. They cannot currently have any OI, dementia, wasting syndrome, or malignancy (other than muco-cutaneous KS). They cannot have significant kidney or liver disease.

The reason this particular trial excludes persons who have taken AZT for more than six months is that viral resistance to AZT may have developed after long-term use. Because anyone entering this trial might be assigned to the AZT arm, such resistance could falsely bias the results against AZT.

Once in the study, volunteers will be randomized to five groups: 25 mg of L-661 twice a day, 100 mg three times a day, 500 mg twice a day, AZT 100 mg five times a day, or placebo. After 12 weeks, those receiving either the placebo or AZT will be re-randomized to one of the three L-661 groups. The study will be evaluated every six weeks, and continued for another six-week period as long as results warrant. It will look for changes in "surrogate markers" (such as T-helper count, plasma viremia, etc.).

All drugs are taken orally. No hospitalization is required, but weekly visits are necessary during the first part of the trial. To obtain the best possible data, volunteers will keep diaries and work closely with a case manager.

L-661 has been given in single-dose or short-term studies to several dozen people so far, with no significant adverse effects.

For more information, or to volunteer for this study, call Donna O'Neill, R.N., at 800/772-5464 ext. 312 or 301/402-0980 ext. 312, or Susan Haneiwich at the same phone numbers, ext. 403.

## Birmingham, Alabama Trial

The trial at the University of Alabama is similar; however, there will be no placebo. Three doses of L-661 will be compared against the usual dose of AZT. This trial has just begun; it is seeking 60 volunteers with T-helper counts between 200 and 500. Later, a similar trial in Birmingham will need 60 additional volunteers with T-helper counts under 200.

The trial for persons with lower T-helper counts is planned to start in about a month. The reason for starting first with T-helper counts from 200 to 500 is to get good information quickly about any toxicity of the drug. Such side effects could be masked by AIDS symptoms in persons who are more seriously ill.

Weekly visits are required during the first six weeks of these trials. Because of the safety precautions needed during early experience with a new drug, it is strongly preferred that volunteers stay in Birmingham during the first six weeks they are on the study.

For more information, or to volunteer for the Birmingham trial, call 800/822-8816, or 205/934-9999, and ask for information about the new L-661 study.

## L-Drug Support Group

An "L-drug" support group for persons in any trial of L-661 (or of the related drug, L-697,639), or who are considering volunteering, has been organized by AIDS activist Bill Bahlman. He can be reached at 212/929-4952, or by mail at 496-A Hudson St., Suite J-11, New York, NY 10014.

## Comment

L-661 is one of the most important AIDS treatments now being tested. The NIAID and Birmingham trials are very well designed to obtain information quickly without undue risks to participants:

• A placebo is often necessary to obtain definitive data quickly—which is especially important with this drug. The NIAID placebo arm will last for only 12 weeks (a limited risk) and then those in that arm will be given the active drug. Since there are five arms to the study, there is only one chance in five of getting the placebo. By contrast, previous studies often asked persons with serious HIV disease to take placebos for much longer, sometimes for two years.

• These studies are designed to look for improvement in bloodwork or in clinical condition of patients, instead of looking for disease progression or death, as phase II studies have often done. With "surrogate markers" instead of death or serious disease, statistically reliable results can be obtained much faster, and with fewer volunteers (which avoids additional delays in organizing and conducting the trials).

• These studies will produce drug-drug and (in the NIAID study) drug-placebo comparisons, as well as dose-response information. The doses, based on earlier laboratory, animal, and human studies, vary over a wide range, which is appropriate with this drug, since the range between effective and toxic doses may be very large. Dosage information will be obtained quickly, early in the clinical-trials process; then it will be available to guide all later trials or other uses of the drug.

• This trial will produce data continuously, because of the six-week evaluations; it will not be necessary to wait for a year, two years, or more to know whether the drug is working. And there is no arbitrary endpoint; the study will continue as long as warranted. The same trial which produces short-term results rapidly will go on to produce long-term results as well, instead of wasting this opportunity, as most studies in the past have done. This design also provides the drug to volunteers, instead of cutting them off at the "end" of the study.

## BI-RG-587: ACT UP URGES FASTER EFFICACY TRIAL, LEARNS DOSES NOT TESTED YET

On April 11, ACT UP/Golden Gate in San Francisco wrote to the Primary Infection Committee of the ACTG (AIDS Clinical Trials Group, funded by the U.S. National Institute of Allergy and Infectious Diseases) urging an immediate trial to test BI-RG-587 in comparison with AZT, and with the combination of those two drugs. Jesse Dobson of ACT UP had heard that such a study might be delayed until BI-RG-587 could be tested with ddI, so that a number of combinations could then be tested together—the cleanest way scientifically to run a study. The point of the letter, and of separate demands by ACT UP/Golden Gate, was to urge that the testing of BI-RG-587 with AZT go forward now, and not wait for dosage data on combining the drug with ddI.

After the letter was sent, activists learned from sources within Boehringer-Ingelheim, the drug's developer, that no more than twelve people have yet received BI-RG-587— and none of them has received more than a single dose. The comparison with AZT could not be started yet, because, under the current drug-development system, a dosage safety trial of BI-RG-587 needs to be done first. Activists are surprised and disappointed that a dosage trial has not been conducted yet.

**April 19, 1991**

Laboratory and animal data on BI-RG-587 was published last December 7 in *Science*. However, the drug to be tested in clinical trials is apparently not the same as the one published there, but a chemical variant of it. The delay in trials might have been caused by changing the drug to a new one presumably believed to work better. On the other hand, it is common for pharmaceutical companies to present or publish data on their second-best drugs, keeping the best ones secret. If that happened here, the delay would be unlikely to be due to a late change in drugs.

Activists suspect that the delay in trials may be caused by coordination difficulties within one or more of the government agencies involved with this drug. This example suggests that even for the most promising treatments, the system cannot be trusted to work by itself, without consistent oversight.

# HYPERICIN UPDATE

*by John S. James*

Hypericin is an antiviral found in a common plant, St. John's wort, a medicinal herb. Unfortunately, there is very little of the chemical in the plant, and laboratory and animal studies suggest that the dose available in common herbal preparations is too small to be effective. People with AIDS or HIV have used these herbal preparations for about two years, with mixed reports but no clear evidence of benefit. [For more background on hypericin, see coverage in *AIDS Treatment News*, especially issues #63, #91, #96, and #117].

A clinical trial using chemically synthesized hypericin could start as early as May at New York University Medical Center/Bellevue Hospital, the University of Minnesota at Minneapolis, and Boston Beth Israel Hospital. This trial was scheduled to start in the summer or fall of 1990, but was delayed by difficulties in preparing sufficient drug. Enough hypericin is now available.

We received the following summary from Fred Valentine, M.D., the principal investigator:

"The study is designed for HIV-infected individuals with less than 300 CD4 cells (i.e., T-helper count under 300), with or without symptoms, who have not taken any antiretroviral drug for one month prior to starting hypericin. Increasing doses of hypericin will be administered intravenously twice a week to successive groups of individuals to determine the maximum tolerated dose. Plasma viremia, p24, cellular viremia, and change in CD4 T-cells will be measured to determine what doses may be effective. It is important that individuals entering this trial of hypericin do not take AZT, ddI, ddC, or other antiretroviral agents, because these agents might have increased toxicity when taken with hypericin, and because the effects of the drugs would interfere with the ability of the trial to measure the effect of hypericin on viremia, p24, and CD4 cells."

It is important to study this potential treatment because:

• In one animal study, hypericin worked much better than AZT against a mouse retrovirus which is used to screen possible anti-retroviral compounds. (HIV itself could not be used in these tests, because ordinary mice cannot be infected with the human virus.)

- Animals can tolerate large amounts of hypericin with little toxicity. The levels which are expected to be antiviral can easily be reached.

- Hypericin's mode of action against HIV in the laboratory is entirely different than that of AZT, suggesting that hypericin might provide an important therapeutic alternative, either alone or in combination with AZT.

- In laboratory tests, hypericin also reduced viral activity in whole human blood freshly drawn from HIV-positive patients. Data suggests that it can work in both lymphocytes (e.g., T-helper cells) and monocytes (e.g., macrophages). The test with whole blood is important because it shows activity against the "wild" virus strains found in patients, not only against the strains which have been bred for years in laboratories.

- Laboratory tests have also shown activity against certain other viruses, including herpes and possibly CMV.

- In small doses, hypericin has already been in widespread human use for years, both as an "alternative" HIV treatment, and as an antidepressant in Europe.

- Hypericin should be convenient to take. Animal studies suggest that it can be given orally—and may only need to be taken twice a week to maintain effective blood levels.

There are also disadvantages. Human toxicity of large doses is not known. Possible problems to watch for are elevated liver-function tests (sometimes seen with the herbal extract, although not necessarily caused by hypericin), and phototoxicity (extreme sensitivity to sunlight or other ultraviolet light, a problem seen in farm animals when they eat large amounts of the plant).

## Comments

The trial described above plans to test hypericin doses up to 2 mg per kg of body weight (about 150 mg for an average adult), providing that no serious toxicities are seen before that level. By contrast, the herbal tablets most commonly sold in buyers' clubs contain 250 mg of 0.14 percent hypericin, or 0.35 mg of the drug—hundreds of times smaller than the highest dose planned for the trial. The tablets and other herbal preparations contain many chemicals, and taking very large doses would involve serious risks.

We have heard that it is not very difficult to chemically extract relatively pure hypericin from the St. John's wort plant; the plant is common in most of the world. At this time, however, we do not know of any source where the chemical is available. (We have not looked for it, because of the risks of trying a new drug; it seemed better to wait for the clinical trial, which will test hypericin with very close monitoring for possible toxicity.)

One factor delaying this drug was the need to develop an improved synthesis procedure which will be suitable for large-scale commercial use. If researchers had used the plant material first, they would have had to repeat animal and human testing after the synthetic version became available. FDA-required animal toxicity testing, done in specialized labs, can cost hundreds of thousands of dollars, creating major barriers to drug development by all but large or well-financed companies.

One problem which no one anticipated is that the synthetic material has not proven as effective as the plant material in antiviral tests in animals (although it is still effective). It is not known why this is so.

Another finding which anyone researching hypericin should know is that animal tests have found that some preparations of the chemical are less orally available than others, for reasons now unknown. If one hypericin extract fails to work, then blood tests could be used to make sure the chemical is being absorbed. A different extraction procedure might work better.

The chemical mode of action of hypericin may involve a singlet oxygen; if so, certain antioxidants might reduce its effectiveness.

What should have been done two years ago, and still should be done now, is to chemically extract enough hypericin from the plant to treat a few people and see whether or not there is a clear, dramatic benefit. If there is, then the resources would be found to make the treatment available quickly, by whatever means is best. On the other hand, if the results of this early efficacy test are negative or unclear, then the development of the drug can proceed on its present course.

This approach, of an early, rapid test for a possible "home run" drug, may be impossible in the current regulatory system. It may happen instead underground.

## Hypericin Technical Articles

These articles and abstracts are relevant to the development of hypericin as a possible antiviral. Also see the previous issues of *AIDS Treatment News* cited above.

Barnard DL, Huffman JH, and Wood, SG. Characterization of the anti human cytomegalovirus (HCMV) activity of three anthraquinone compounds [abstract #1093]. 30th Interscience Conference on Antimicrobial Agents and Chemotherapy, Atlanta, October 21-24, 1990.

Chu CK, Schinazi RF, and Nasr M. Anti-HIV-1 activities of anthraquinone derivatives in vitro [abstract #M.C.P.115]. V International Conference on AIDS, Montreal, June 4-9, 1989.

Cooper WC and James JS. An observational study of the safety and efficacy of hypericin in HIV+ subjects [abstract #2063]. VI International Conference on AIDS, San Francisco, June 21-24, 1990.

Degar S, Lavie G, Levin B, and others. Inhibition of HIV infectivity by hypericin: Evidence for a block in capsid uncoating [abstract #I-16]. HIV Disease: Pathogenesis and Therapy, University of Miami, March 1991.

Kraus GA, Pratt D, Tossberg J, and Carpenter S. Antiretroviral activity of synthetic hypericin and related analogs. *Biochemical and Biophysical Research Communications.* 1990; volume 172, pages 149-153.

Lavie G, and Meruelo D. Inhibition of retrovirus-induced diseases by two naturally occurring polycyclic aromatic diones hypericin and pseudohypericin [abstract #C.501]. V International Conference on AIDS, Montreal, June 4-9, 1989.

Lavie G, Valentine F, Levin B, and others. Studies of the mechanisms of action of the antiretroviral agents hypericin and pseudohypericin. *Proceedings of the National Academy of Sciences, USA.* August 1989; volume 86, pages 5963-5967.

Lavie G, Mazur Y, Lavie D, Levin B, Ittah Y, and Meruelo D. Hypericin as an antiretroviral agent; mode of action and related analogues. *Annals of the New York Academy of Sciences.* 1990; volume 616, pages 556-562.

Lavie G, Meruelo D, Daub M, and others. Retroviral particle inactivation by organic polycyclic quinones: A novel mechanism of virucidal activity characterized by diminution of virus particle derived reverse transcriptase enzymatic activity [abstract I-27]. HIV Disease: Pathogenesis and Therapy conference, University of Miami, March 1991.

Meruelo D, Lavie G, and Lavie D. Therapeutic agents with dramatic antiretroviral activity and little toxicity at effective doses: Aromatic polycyclic diones hypericin and pseudohypericin. *Proceedings of the National Academy of Sciences, USA.* July 1988; volume 85, pages 5230-5234.

Meruelo D, Degar S, Levin B, Lavie D, Mazur Y, and Lavie G. Inactivation of retroviral particles by hypericin: Possible role of oxidative reactions in the antiretroviral activity [abstract I-29]. HIV Disease: Pathogenesis and Therapy, University of Miami, March 1991.

Schinazi RF, Chu CK, Babu JR, and others. Anthraquinones as a new class of antiviral agents against human immunodeficiency virus. *Antiviral Research.* 1990; volume 13, pages 265-272.

Takahashi I, Nakanishi S, Kobayashi E, Nakano H, Suzuki K, and Tamaoki T. Hypericin and pseudohypericin specifically inhibit protein kinase C: possible relation to their antiretroviral activity. *Biochemical and Biophysical Research Communications.* December 29, 1989; volume 165, number 3, pages 1207-1212.

Tang J, Colacino JM, Larsen SH, and Spitzer W. Virucidal activity of hypericin against enveloped and non-enveloped DNA and RNA viruses. *Antiviral Research.* 1990; volume 13, pages 313-326.

Valentine F, Meruelo D, Itri V, and Lavie G. Hypericin: efficacy of a new agent against HIV in vitro [abstract #M.C.P.18]. V International Conference on AIDS, Montreal, June 4-9, 1989.

Valentine FT. Hypericin: A hexahydroxyl, dimethyl-naphthodianthrone with activity against HIV in vitro and against murine retroviruses in vivo [oral presentation, published abstract]. HIV Disease: Pathogenesis and Therapy, University of Miami, March 1991.

Weiner DB, Lavie G, Williams WV, Lavie D, Greene MI, and Meruelo D. Hypericin mediates anti-HIV effects in vitro [abstract #C.608]. V International Conference on AIDS, Montreal, June 4-9.

Wood S, Huffman J, Weber N, and others. Antiviral activity of naturally occurring anthraquinones and anthraquinone derivatives. *Planta Medica; Journal of Medicinal Plant Research.* 1990; volume 56, number 6, pages 651-652.

# DDI WARNING: DON'T TAKE DAPSONE AT SAME TIME

The U.S. Division of AIDS has issued a warning to physicians that patients using ddI and also using dapsone, a drug for pneumocystis prophylaxis, should not take the drugs within two hours of each other. The problem is that dapsone requires an acid environment in order to be dissolved; but ddI cannot tolerate an acid environment, so it is taken with a buffer to neutralize stomach acidity. The lack of acidity causes the dapsone not to be absorbed.

Jacobus Pharmaceutical Company, the manufacturer of dapsone, brought the problem to the attention of the Division of AIDS after several cases of pneumocystis were found in patients who were taking both drugs. At least 11 cases of pneumocystis have occurred within 10 to 130 days after starting therapy with the two drugs together.

This problem could also affect other drugs which require an acid stomach—for example, ketoconazole.

The following recommendation is included in Safety Memo 013 of the Division of AIDS:

"Recommendation: The Division of AIDS and Jacobus Pharmaceutical Company recommend that clinicians contact all patients who are receiving both ddI and dapsone by telephone and advise them to take dapsone two hours prior to ddI."

The memo also says that if patients cannot take dapsone at least two hours before ddI, they should wait until two hours after. The two drugs should not be taken within two hours of each other.

## ADVOCACY PROGRAM FOR HEALTH PROVIDERS WITH HIV

*by Denny Smith*

The American Association of Physicians for Human Rights (AAPHR), a national organization of gay and lesbian physicians, is sponsoring an effort to protect the rights and livelihoods of doctors and other health workers from proposals requiring disclosure of their HIV status. The "Medical Expertise Retention Program, The National Program for Physicians With HIV Disease" is directed by attorney Ben Schatz, who will assist and advocate on behalf of seropositive health workers.

Recently, alarm bells have been clanging in the media and professional organizations over allegations that patients are at risk for contracting "the AIDS virus" when they are under the care of a dentist or physician with HIV. Ironically, many physicians with HIV have had to compensate for years of their colleagues' AIDS phobia by providing more than their share of the care required by thousands of Americans with HIV.

For information about AAPHR's program, or to make a tax-deductible contribution, interested persons can call 415/864-0408.

### Comment

This is a crucial civil rights issue for anyone involved in the AIDS epidemic. The concern voiced for the "safety of the patient" echoes the older "safety of the physician" campaigns waged against seropositive patients. In both situations the issue of safety has been finessed to serve other agendas.

Health workers should be observing "universal" blood and body fluid precautions with all of their patients, for their own safety and that of their patient as well. If universal precautions are observed, there remains no compelling reason to compromise the privacy of health workers, or their patients, with HIV. Hepatitis and other serious infections have amounted to a far greater risk than HIV in the healthcare setting. But HIV has garnered far more hysteria—a dangerous mismatch between perception and reality.

If alarmists achieve their goals, then physicians, dentists, and nurses will be discriminated against openly, and no other sector of the workforce or general population would be exempt from similar bias. Many competent care-givers could be removed from their positions unfairly and needlessly, and the loss of those experienced in caring for HIV would impoverish the quality of medicine generally for everyone needing HIV care.

# HIV IMMIGRATION: NEW THREAT, AIDS ORGANIZATIONS NEEDED

As reported previously in *AIDS Treatment News*, the U.S. Department of Health and Human Services (HHS) recommended that HIV—along with all other diseases except active tuberculosis—be dropped as grounds for excluding visitors and immigrants from the United States. But conservative Republicans are now pressuring President Bush to overrule the HHS recommendation and keep HIV as grounds for exclusion, at least for permanent immigrants.

Apparently the argument this time is avoiding medical-care costs to the government, rather than fear of contagion. Our understanding is that existing law already allows immigrants to be excluded if they are likely to require government expense. The real issue, then, is whether HIV should be singled out from all other diseases for automatic exclusion not based on public-health requirements.

At least one-hundred organizations have already signed an April 16 consensus letter supporting the recommendation of HHS that HIV not be used to bar U.S. entry by visitors or immigrants. Signers include the American Public Health Association, United States Conference of Mayors, American Red Cross, National Hemophilia Foundation, American Foundation for AIDS Research, San Francisco Department of Public Health, American Jewish Committee, AIDS Action Council, San Francisco AIDS Foundation, and the Eighth International Conference on AIDS.

The letter has already been submitted to HHS Secretary Louis Sullivan, but an addendum with other signers is being prepared. If your AIDS, medical, or other organization could sign this letter, contact Dana Van Gorder, Harvard AIDS Institute/ Eighth International Conference on AIDS, 617/495-2318, or 617/495-2863 (fax).

# Author Index

## A

Adams, Brock, 395–396
Adiel, Ellie, 131
Agnos, Art, 495
Alonso, Kenneth, 300, 329
Armstrong, Donald, 120
Auer, Lisa, 408

## B

Bachrach, Sara, 268
Bahlman, Bill, 560
Baird, Barbara, 371
Baker, R. A., 513
Barr, David, 185
Bartolomeo, Nick, 543–544
Barton, Keith, 47
Baseman, Joel B., 210
Basso, Will, 132
Baucom, Irene, 421
Beilenson, Anthony, 251
Bergeron, Michel G., 504
Bergeson, Marian, 348
Bergner, Paul, 445
Berman, Phil, 334
Bersani, Leo, 57
Berzofsky, Jay, 334
Bihari, Bernard, 111, 113, 119, 265, 348
Blecman, Marty, 15–23
Boneberg, Paul, 111, 472
Boxer, Barbara, 452, 472
Bozette, Sam, 427–428
Bramhall, S. Jeanne, 55–56
Brenneman, Douglas, 102
Brewer, Joseph, 455
Bridge, Peter, 103
Broder, Samuel, 97, 110, 317, 450, 469–470
Broderick, Bonnie, 388
Brosnan, Peter L., 43, 151, 262
Bruni, Larry, 415, 483, 545–551
Buchbinder, Susan, 552
Burzynski, Stanislaw, 264
Busby, Steven, 266
Busch, David, 554

Bush, George, 379, 395, 437, 567
Byers, Vera, 243, 308
Byrne, Anne, 554

## C

Cabriales, Sue, 526
Caiazza, Stephen, 547
Callen, Michael, 119, 518
Camp, Brian, 512
Campbell, Duncan, 164
Campbell, James, 365
Canessa, A., 352
Capaldini, Lisa, 255–262
Cardona, Lysette, 243
Castle, Chris, 321
Chew, Terrance, 524
Colvin, Carol, 523
Conant, Marcus, 128, 185–186, 232, 245, 334, 430, 543
Coonan, Kathy, 148
Cooper, David, 128, 329
Cooper, Ellen, 99, 111, 374, 377, 469–470, 472
Cooper, William C., 220
Corey, Lawrence, 417
Cranston, Alan, 238
Crimp, Douglas, 57
Crystal, Ronald G., 181
Cummins, Joseph M., 271, 273

## D

Dean, Ward, 518
DeBlasio, Chris, 516
DeBruin, Michael, 414, 462
Delaney, Martin, 4, 24, 28, 72, 98, 111, 148, 347, 472, 480
Deresinski, Stanley, 511
Dharmananda, Subhuti, 194
Dieterich, Douglas, 214
Dixon, John, 491
Dobson, Jesse, 561
Dodd, Caroline L., 422

# Subject Index

## A

Foscarnet
  availability, 207
  for CMV infections, 206, 222, 356–357
  dose limiting neurotoxicity, 356
  expanded access, 383–384
    costs of, 385
    800 number for, 384
    eligibility criteria, 384–385
    physicians' responsibility, 385
  and ganciclovir
    concurrent/alternate use of, 357
    trials for, 26–27
  information, 800 number for, 88
  *in vitro* anti-HIV/herpesvirus activity,
    207
  salvage trials (San Francisco), 16, 88
  toxicity, 206, 356
Foscavir. *See* Foscarnet
5-FU collagen matrix. *See* 5-Fluorouracil
    collagen matrix
Fukushima Medical College (Japan),
    glycyrrhizin studies, 293
Fumagillin analogs
  availability, 528
  effects on tumor growth, 465
  for Kaposi's sarcoma treatment, 529
Funding of research
  AIDS lobby and, 249–252
  attacks on, 225–228
  demographic obstacle to consensus/
    coalitions, 228
Fungal infections
  fluconazole for, 218
  and HIV, 546
Fungal properties, *pneumocystis carinii*, 432
Fusidic acid, anti-HIV activity, 46
Fusidin. *See* Fusidic acid

# G

G6PD deficiency, 431
GALAPAC. *See* Gay and Lesbian Political
    Action Committee
Gall bladder
  inflammation of, 549
  removal of, 549
Gallo's Japanese KS Drug, 528–529
Gammagard (Baxter), 549
Gamma-linolenic acid, for neuropathy, 511
Ganciclovir
  for CMV colitis, 355–356
  for CMV infections, 81, 190, 206
    administration schedule, 355
    concurrent/alternate use with
      foscarnet, 357

  dosage, 355
  oral, 358
  CMV resistance to, 343
  and ddI for CMV infections, 222
  effectiveness, time-limited, 354
  FDA recommendation against approval
    of, 85
  and foscarnet, trials for, 26–27
  with immune globulin, 549
  intraocular administration, 206, 222
  intravenous, for CMV retinitis, 552–554
  intravenous administration, 206
  mail-order, 131
  maintenance therapy, 355–356
  neutropenia, GM-CSF effects, 206
  new drug approval, 26, 81
  oral
    absorption, food effects, 554–555
    bioavailability, 333
    for CMV colitis, 333
    for CMV retinitis, 552–554
    formulations, 206
  resistance to, 354
  side effects, 354
  status review by FDA, 4
  synergism with eflornithine, 206
  Syntex and, 79
  toxicity, 206, 222
Gantrisin (sulfisoxazole), anti-HIV report,
    46
Garlic, for cryptosporidiosis, 214
Gastrointestinal tract, toxoplasmosis
    infection, 351
Gay and Lesbian Advocates and Defenders,
    268
Gay and Lesbian Political Action Committee
    (GALAPAC), lobbying programs,
    250–251
Gay Men of Color Consortium, award by
    San Francisco Dept. of Public Health,
    248
Gay Men's Health Crisis (New York), 57
  endorsement of consensus statement, 305
  indomethacin study, 362
  parallel track consensus statement, 114
  *Treatment Issues. See Treatment Issues*
  World AIDS Day (12/1/89), 170
G-CSF. *See* Granulocyte-colony stimulating
    factor
Ge-132. *See* Germanium sesquioxide
Genelabs (Redwood City, Calif.)
  compound Q contribution, 243
  compound Q IND, 76
  compound Q phase II trials, 123
  compound Q supply to PICRA, 123
Genentech

# N

NAC. *See* N-Acetyl-L-cysteine

NAIC. *See* National AIDS Information Clearinghouse

Naltrexone, 484

Names Project (San Francisco)
International AIDS conference boycott list, 321
support of Children with HIV/AIDS Awareness Day (6/91), 555

NAN. *See* National AIDS Network

Naphthoquinones, for pneumocystis prophylaxis, 432

NAPWA. *See* National Association of People with AIDS

Narcotic drugs, for neuropathy, 511

NAS. *See* National Academy of Sciences

National Academy of Sciences, ACTG committee, 192

National AIDS Information Clearinghouse, food videotape release, 161

National AIDS Network (NAN)
endorsement of consensus statement, 305
*Multi-Cultural NOTES on AIDS Education and Service*, 249

National Assembly of State Arts Agencies, 305

National Association of Black and White Men Together, National Task Force on AIDS Prevention, 247

National Association of Community Health Centers, Inc., 305

National Association of People with AIDS (NAPWA)
ddI parallel track negotiations, 111
endorsement of consensus statement, 305
parallel track consensus statement, 114
World AIDS Day (12/1/89), 170

National Association of Social Workers, 305

National Association of State Alcohol and Drug Abuse Directors, 305

National Black Gay and Lesbian Leadership Conference and Health Institute (2/90: Atlanta, Ga.), 247–249

National Cancer Institute
antiviral in blue-green algae, 134–136
commercial production of algal sulfolipids contract, 253
ddI long-term study results, 372–373
ddI study, 25
dipyridamole research, 36–37
Kaposi's sarcoma
potential treatment, 269
treatment in Japan, 244–245

National Committee to Review Current Procedures for Approval of Drugs for Cancer and AIDS (Lasagna Committee), 379–380, 400–402
"FDA Standard for Effectiveness of New Drugs," 400–402

National Community Research Initiative (D.C.), CRIS software, 550

National Education Association, support of Children with HIV/AIDS Awareness Day (6/91), 555

National Gay and Lesbian Task Force
consensus statement endorsement, 305
lobbying programs, 252
parallel track consensus statement, 114
World AIDS Day (12/1/89), 170

National Gay Rights Advocates
parallel track consensus statement, 114
waiver for HIV-positive U.S. visitors, 157

National Heart, Lung, and Blood Institute, glutathione research, 181

National Hemophilia Foundation, 305

National Institute of Allergy and Infectious Diseases (NIAID)
AZT
approval for early use, 233
clinical trials, 37
low- vs. high-dose trial, 126
Community Programs for Clinical Research on AIDS, 89
corticosteroids recommendation for pneumocystis, 435
ddI
access negotiations, 83–85
phase I trial, 25
dipyridamole clinical trials, 37
Emprise grant
application, 263
withdrawal of, 266
fluconazole recommendation for cyptococcal meningitis, 298–299
and foscarnet "salvage" protocols, 16
HIV transmission to infants during pregnancy, 128
interferon alpha/AZT *in vitro* research, 136
L-697,661 trials, 559–560
MAI treatments, 47
mycoplasma meetings, 210
NAC inhibition of HIV growth, 508–510
parallel track proposal, 77–79
participation in HIV Awareness Week (6/89), 40
politics of early treatment and, 87

with sulfadiazine
    pulse-dosing, 352
    for toxoplasmosis, 44, 306, 351
    synergism with interferon gamma, 352
    for toxoplasmosis, 483
    with trimethorprim, for PML, 43

## Q

Quan Yin Healing Arts Center (San
    Francisco), 194–195

## R

R82150
    antiviral effectiveness, 318
    clinical trials, 318
    development, 224
    dosage, 318
    human experience with, 224
    inhibition of HIV, 224
    selectivity of, 224
    TIBO derivatives, 318, 320
Racial differences, in response to AZT, 506–
    508
Radiation-resistant HIV expression *in vivo*.
    *See* R-HEV test
Radiation therapy
    intralesional, 524
    for Kaposi's sarcoma, 138
    for lymphoma, 196–197, 261
Ralph K. Davies Hospital, 566C80 trial, 536
Randomization, in rapid screening trials, 375
Randomized controlled trials
    characterization, 121–122
    ethical concerns, 243
Rapid screening trials. *See* Clinical trials,
    rapid screening
Rashes
    Bactrim-related, 428, 430
    and HIV diagnoses, 257
    hypericin effects, 8
    immune globulin-related, 495
    piritrexim-related, 527
    Stevens-Johnson syndrome and, 10
    trimethoprim-sulfamethoxazole-related,
        330
Raw foods, MAI infections and, 47
Raw meat, cautions for *Toxoplasma*-infected
    persons, 306
Raw vegetables, cautions for *Toxoplasma*-
    infected persons, 306
Raymond-Poincaré Hospital/University
    René-Descartes, 107

Receptor binding
    glycyrrhizin sulfate effects, 293
    Iscador effects, 186
Red blood cells. *See also* Blood cells
    AZT/interferon alpha effects, 340
Red Crescent Society, 202
Reference materials. *See also* Information
        services
    AIDS textbooks, 514
    complementary/alternative treatment
        information, 517–519
    directory of AIDS treatments, 514
    drug books, 513–514
    FAACTS (Facts on Alternate AIDS
        Compounds & Treatments), 492–
        493
    handbook for patients, 513
    hypericin articles (technical), 564–565
    medical benefits, 514–515
    medical dictionaries, 513
    treatment newsletters, 515–516
Renal failure, germanium-related, 164–165
Replication, viral. *see* Viral replication
Repligen Corporation, 529
Research
    alternative program for, 193–194
    computerized publication proposal, 285–
        286
    conflicts of interest in, 309–313, 422–
        424
    funding
        attacks on, 225–228
        by Congress, 249–252
        demographic obstacle to consensus/
            coalitions, 228
    HIV treatments in 1990, 190
    improvements needed in, 304
    incentives for pharmaceutical companies,
        236–237
    lack of leadership, 276, 278, 313–314,
        473, 487
    mainstream view of, 29–30
    price incentives for drug development,
        236
    priorities
        consensus statement, 304–305
        organizations concerned with, 314–
            315
    publications embargos, 311–312
    response-surface methodology, 342
    toxoplasmosis situation, 353
    traditional power structure, 424
Research designs
    *AIDS Treatment Research Agenda* (ACT
        UP/New York), 79–80
    clinical trials, 63–70

# W

# AIDS: Books that can help

☐ *AIDS Treatment News:* Volume 1  (Issues 1 through 75)
by John S. James

The first 75 issues of the widely respected newsletter which described all manner of standard and experimental treatments for AIDS and related conditions. Completely indexed, this is the only easy-to-use reference suitable for the layperson as well as professionals.
$12.95 paper, 560 pages

☐ *Living in Hope:* A 12-Step Approach
by Cindy Mikluscak-Cooper, R.N. and Emmett E. Miller, M.D.

The first and only 12-step program for people who are HIV-positive, or at risk for infection. Using daily affirmations and guided imagery, this book provides powerful tools for coping, change, and healing.
$12.95 paper, 300 pages

☐ *Serenity* Second Edition by Paul Reed

Emotional support and guidance for people with HIV, and their families, friends, and caregivers. Leads readers from despair to action to hope.
$6.95 paper, 128 pages

☐ *The Q Journal:* A Treatment Diary by Paul Reed

An intimate journal, detailing one author's experimental treatment with the new drug, Compound Q. Probes many issues surrounding AIDS—loss, hope, research, treatment, anger, coping, and the courage to go on living.
$8.95 paper, 176 pages

☐ *Psychoimmunity and the Healing Process*
Third Revised Edition by Jason Serinus, C.H.T.

A compendium of alternative therapies for AIDS and immune dysfunction that can be used in addition to conventional medical care.
$12.95 paper, 400 pages

☐ *Extended Health Care At Home* by Evelyn M. Baulch

Step-by-step advice on coping with the problems that arise during any extended home health care: finding a home nurse, dealing with physical and emotional issues, obtaining supplies and equipment. Includes a section on the special needs of people with AIDS.
$9.95 paper, 272 pages.

☐ *Face to Face:* A Guide to AIDS Counseling

by James W. Dilley, Cheri Pies, & Michael Helquist

A guide to dealing with emotional and psycho-neurological problems encountered with AIDS—suitable for patients or counseling professionals. Addresses the special needs of various affected populations—minorities, IV drug users, women, and gay men.
$14.95 paper, 350 pages

☐ *AIDS Law for Mental Health Professionals*

by Gary James Wood, J.D., et al

The legal and ethical issues confronting therapists when they treat people infected with or concerned about HIV infection, with an emphasis on California law.
$19.95 paper, 272 pages

# Gay fiction and literature

☐ *Loving Someone Gay* revised edition

by Don Clark

A classic guide for family members, friends, or others learning to accept a loved one who is gay. This revised edition has new material on gay politics and activism, and on coping with AIDS.
$8.95 paper, 290 pages

☐ *...So Little Time* by Mike Hippler

Over 50 essays on gay life, from an award-winning columnist, on topics ranging from politics, family, sports, and travel, to religion, sex, AIDS, and role models. Includes some of Hippler's most popular pieces, including *Dear Abby, Am I Too Gay?, How to Meet Lesbians*, and the wrenching *Visit to an AIDS Ward*.
$11.95 paper, 288 pages

☐ *Kvetch* by T.R. Witomski

A humorous collection of scalding, controversial essays from a master of searing wit, including *101 Things to Do with a Straight Man, How to Cruise the Met*, and *Zeitgeist or Poltergeist: Why Gay Books Are So Bad*.
$7.95 paper, 132 pages

☐ *Longing* by Paul Reed

Hailed by the *New York Times* for its style, this haunting novel of gay life in the San Francisco of the early 1980's also made the *Christopher Street* bestseller list.
$7.95 paper or $14.95 cloth, 192 pages

Available from your local bookstore, or order direct from the publisher. Please include $1.25 shipping & handling for the first book, and 50 cents for each additional book. California residents include local sales tax. Write for our free complete catalog of over 400 books and tapes.

Ship to:

Name _____

Address _____

City _____ State ____ Zip _____

Phone _____

Celestial Arts

P.O. Box 7327

Berkeley, CA 94707

For VISA or Mastercard orders

call (510) 845-8414